Handbook of Security and Privacy of AI-Enabled Healthcare Systems and Internet of Medical Things

The fast-growing number of patients suffering from various ailments has overstretched the carrying capacity of traditional healthcare systems. This handbook addresses the increased need to tackle security issues and preserve patients' privacy concerns in Artificial Intelligence of Medical Things (AIoMT) devices and systems.

Handbook of Security and Privacy of AI-Enabled Healthcare Systems and the Internet of Medical Things provides new insights into the deployment, application, management, and benefits of AIoMT by examining real-world scenarios. The handbook takes a critical look at existing security designs and offers solutions to revamp traditional security architecture, including the new design of efficient intrusion detection algorithms, attack prevention techniques, and both cryptographic and noncryptographic solutions. The handbook goes on to discuss the critical security and privacy issues that affect all parties in the healthcare ecosystem and provides practical AI-based solutions.

This handbook offers new and valuable information that will be highly beneficial to educators, researchers, and others.

Agbotiname Lucky Imoize, Department of Electrical and Electronics Engineering, Faculty of Engineering, University of Lagos, Akoka, Lagos, Nigeria.

Valentina Emilia Balas, Department of Automatics and Applied Software, Faculty of Engineering, Aurel Vlaicu University of Arad, Arad, Romania.

Vijender Kumar Solanki, Department of Computer Science and Engineering, CMR Institute of Technology (Autonomous), Hyderabad, TS, India.

Cheng-Chi Lee, Research and Development Center for Physical Education, Health, and Information Technology, Department of Library and Information Science, Fu Jen Catholic University, New Taipei City 24205, Taiwan; Department of Computer Science and Information Engineering, Asia University, Taichung City 41354, Taiwan.

Mohammad S. Obaidat, Life Fellow of IEEE, Fellow of AAIA, and Fellow of SCS, Distinguished Professor, University of Jordan, Amman, Jordan.

Artificial Intelligence (AI): Elementary to Advanced Practices

Series Editors: Vijender Kumar Solanki, Zhongyu (Joan) Lu, and Valentina E Balas

In the emerging smart city technology and industries, the role of artificial intelligence is getting more prominent. This AI book series aims to cover the latest AI work, which will help the naïve user to get support to solve existing problems and for the experienced AI practitioners, it will assist to shedding light for new avenues in the AI domains. The series will cover the recent work carried out in AI and its associated domains, it will cover Logics, Pattern Recognition, Natural Language Processing (NLP), Expert Systems, Machine Learning, Block-Chain, and Big Data. The work domain of AI is quite deep, so it will be covering the latest trends which are evolving with the concepts of AI and it will be helping those new to the field, practitioners, students, as well as researchers to gain some new insights.

Artificial Intelligence (AI)
Recent Trends and Applications
Edited by S. Kanimozhi Suguna, M. Dhivya, and Sara Paiva

Deep Learning for Biomedical Applications
Edited by Utku Kose, Omer Deperlioglu, and D. Jude Hemanth

Cybersecurity
Ambient Technologies, IoT, and Industry 4.0 Implications
Gautam Kumar, Om Prakash Singh, &Hemraj Saini

Industrial Internet of Things
Technologies, Design, and Applications
Edited by Sudan Jha, Usman Tariq, Gyanendra Prasad Joshi, and Vijender Kumar Solanki

Machine Learning And Deep Learning Techniques For Medical Science
Edited by K. Gayathri Devi, Kishore Balasubramanian and Le Anh Ngoc

Handbook of Security and Privacy of AI-Enabled Healthcare Systems and Internet of Medical Things
Edited by Agbotiname Lucky Imoize, Valentina Emilia Balas, Vijender Kumar Solanki, Cheng-Chi Lee, and Mohammad S. Obaidat

For more information on this series, please visit: www.routledge.com/Artificial-Intelligence-AI-Elementary-to-Advanced-Practices/book-series/CRCAIEAP

Handbook of Security and Privacy of AI-Enabled Healthcare Systems and Internet of Medical Things

Edited by Agbotiname Lucky Imoize,
Valentina Emilia Balas, Vijender Kumar Solanki,
Cheng-Chi Lee, and Mohammad S. Obaidat

CRC Press
Taylor & Francis Group
Boca Raton London New York

CRC Press is an imprint of the
Taylor & Francis Group, an **informa** business

Designed cover image: Shutterstock

First edition published 2024
by CRC Press
2385 Executive Center Drive, Suite 320, Boca Raton, FL 33431

and by CRC Press
4 Park Square, Milton Park, Abingdon, Oxon, OX14 4RN

CRC Press is an imprint of Taylor & Francis Group, LLC

© 2024 selection and editorial matter, Agbotiname Lucky Imoize, Valentina Emilia Balas, Vijender Kumar Solanki, Cheng-Chi Lee, Mohammad S. Obaidat; individual chapters, the contributors

Library of Congress Cataloging-in-Publication Data
Names: Imoize, Agbotiname Lucky, editor. | Balas, Valentina Emilia, editor. | Solanki, Vijender Kumar, 1980– editor. | Lee, Cheng-Chi, editor. | Obaidat, Mohammad S. (Mohammad Salameh), 1952– editor.
Title: Handbook of security and privacy of AI-enabled healthcare systems and internet of medical things / edited by Agbotiname Lucky Imoize, Valentina Emilia Balas, Vijender Kumar Solanki, Cheng-Chi Lee, Mohammad S. Obaidat.
Description: First edition. | Boca Raton : CRC Press, 2024. | Includes bibliographical references and index.
Identifiers: LCCN 2023015691 (print) | LCCN 2023015692 (ebook) | ISBN 9781032438795 (hardback) | ISBN 9781032440798 (paperback) | ISBN 9781003370321 (ebook)
Subjects: MESH: Artificial Intelligence | Medical Informatics Applications | Internet of Things | Computer Security | Privacy
Classification: LCC R859.7.A78 (print) | LCC R859.7.A78 (ebook) | NLM W 26.55.A7 | DDC 610.285—dc23/eng/20230706
LC record available at https://lccn.loc.gov/2023015691
LC ebook record available at https://lccn.loc.gov/2023015692

ISBN: 978-1-032-43879-5 (hbk)
ISBN: 978-1-032-44079-8 (pbk)
ISBN: 978-1-003-37032-1 (ebk)

DOI: 10.1201/9781003370321

Typeset in Times LT Std
by Apex Covantage, LLC

Contents

Preface... xix
Acknowledgments.. xxviii
Editors.. xxix
Contributors xxxiii

Chapter 1   An Overview of AIoMT Applications 1

Han Sun and Yu Chen

    1.1   Introduction 1
           1.1.1   Key Contributions of the Chapter 2
           1.1.2   Chapter Organization 2
    1.2.   Related Work 2
           1.2.1   Sensor Layer 3
           1.2.2   Edge Layer.. 3
           1.2.3   Server Layer 4
           1.2.4   Communication 4
    1.3.   Applications... 5
           1.3.1   Continuous Health Monitoring 7
           1.3.2   Healthcare-Related Prediction 8
           1.3.3   E-Medical Healthcare 9
    1.4.   Case Study: Deep Learning-based Falling Detection for
         Seniors Living Alone... 9
           1.4.1   Related Work 9
           1.4.3   MARS System—Methodology 10
           1.4.4   Experimental Study...13
    1.5.   Challenges and Future Directions 14
           1.5.1   Challenges 14
           1.5.2   Future Directions...15
    1.6   Conclusions...16
    References 16

Chapter 2   Wearable Medical Electronics in Artificial Intelligence
             of Medical Things 21

Wasswa Shafik

    2.1   Introduction 21
           2.1.1   Key Contributions of the Chapter 23
           2.1.2   Chapter Organization 23
    2.2   Wearable Medical Electronics.. 23
           2.2.1   Electronic Sensor Traits 24
    2.3   Electronic Signals in Sensors 26
           2.3.1   Gait Analysis.. 26

	2.3.2	Photoplethysmography	26
2.3.3	Electromyography	27
2.3.4	Auscultation	27

2.4   Challenges of Electronic Devices in the AIoMT 28
    2.4.1   Data Security Threats... 29
    2.4.2   Data Interoperability 30
    2.4.3   Regulatory Challenges 30
    2.4.4   High Infrastructure Costs..31
    2.4.5   Standardization Challenges...31
    2.4.6   Cybersecurity 31
    2.4.7   Device Mobility..31
    2.4.8   Adoption Scale 32
    2.4.9   Advanced Analytics 32
    2.4.10   Trust Maintenance...32
    2.4.11   Data Security...33
    2.4.12   Licensing Challenge..33
2.5   Benefits of the AIoMT..33
    2.5.1   Medical Diagnosis...33
    2.5.2   Medical Treatment 33
    2.5.3   Patient Empowerment 34
    2.5.4   Reduction in Medical Costs 34
    2.5.5   Reduction in Human Error 34
2.6   Challenges of AIoMTs 34
    2.6.1   Privacy Concerns 34
    2.6.2   Missteps and Errors...35
    2.6.3   Data Management and Power Issues 35
    2.6.4   Bias..35
2.7   Limitation of AIoMT...35
2.8   Future Research Direction...36
2.9   Conclusions and Future Scope 36
References 37

Chapter 3   Electronic Devices in the Artificial Intelligence of the
    Internet of Medical Things (AIoMT)..41

Khairul Eahsun Fahim, Kassim Kalinaki, and Wasswa Shafik

3.1   Introduction 41
    3.1.1   Key Contributions of the Chapter 43
    3.1.2   Chapter Organization 43
3.2   Electronic Sensors in the IoMT...43
    3.2.1   Electronic Sensor Traits 43
3.3   Electronic Signals..45
    3.3.1   Gait Analysis...45
    3.3.2   Photoplethysmography 46
    3.3.3   Electromyography 46
    3.3.4   Auscultation..47

3.4 Challenges of Electronic Devices in the AIoMT 49
    3.4.1 Data Security Threats.. 49
    3.4.2 Data Interoperability 49
    3.4.3 Regulatory Challenges 50
    3.4.4 High Infrastructure Costs.. 50
    3.4.5 Standardization Challenges... 50
    3.4.6 Cybersecurity 50
    3.4.7 Device Mobility..51
    3.4.8 Adoption Scale 51
    3.4.9 Advanced Analytics 51
    3.4.10 Trust Maintenance...52
    3.4.11 Data Security..52
    3.4.12 Licensing Challenge 52
3.5 Benefits of the AIoMT Reviewed...52
    3.5.1 Medical Diagnosis..52
    3.5.2 Medical Treatment 53
    3.5.3 Patient Empowerment 53
    3.5.4 Reduction in Medical Costs 53
    3.5.5 Reduction in Human Errors 53
3.6 Challenges of Reviewed AIoMTs..53
    3.6.1 Privacy Concerns 54
    3.6.2 Missteps and Errors.. 54
    3.6.3 Data Management and Power Issues......................... 54
    3.6.4 Bias... 54
3.7 Future Research Direction of IoMT in Healthcare Industry......55
3.8 Conclusions and Future Scope 55
References 56

Chapter 4 Artificial Intelligence of Medical Things for Medical
Information Systems Privacy and Security....................................... 63

Muyideen Abdulraheem, Emmanuel Abidemi Adeniyi,
Joseph Bamidele Awotunde, Agbotiname Lucky Imoize,
Rasheed Gbenga Jimoh, Idowu Dauda Oladipo, and
Peace Busola Falola

4.1 Introduction 63
    4.1.1 The Contributions of the Chapter............................... 65
    4.1.2 Chapter Organization 65
4.2 Related Work 65
4.3 Artificial Intelligence of Medical Things............................... 68
    4.3.1 Healthcare Systems Based on AIoMT 68
4.4 Categories of Security and Privacy of Data Algorithms......... 69
    4.4.1 Data Privacy and Security... 69
    4.4.2 The Internet of Medical Things 71
4.5 Devices Vulnerabilities and Requirements 71
    4.5.1 IoT Attack Surfaces...71

	4.5.2	IoT Vulnerabilities	72
	4.5.3	IoT Security Requirements	73
	4.5.4	Attacks Based on Device Property	76
	4.5.5	Attacks Based on Adversary Location	76
	4.5.6	Attacks Based on Attacks Strategy	76
	4.5.7	Attacks Based on Information Damage Level	77
	4.5.8	Host-Based Attacks	77

4.6   Requirement of Security in Internet of Medical
        Things System 77
        4.6.1 IoMT Security Incidents 77
        4.6.2 IoMT Regulations on Cybersecurity 78
        4.6.3 Security Mechanisms 79
4.7   Internet of Medical Things System Security Solutions 81
        4.7.1 Attribute Based 82
        4.7.2 ECG Based 83
        4.7.3 MAC Based 83
        4.7.4 ECC Based 83
        4.7.5 Machine-Learning Based 84
        4.7.6 PUF Based 85
        4.7.7 Blockchain Based 86
4.8   Challenges and Further Research 87
4.9   Conclusions and Future Directions 88
Acknowledgment 89
References 89

Chapter 5 AIoMT Enabling Real-Time Monitoring of Healthcare
Systems: Security and Privacy Considerations 97

*Joseph Bamidele Awotunde, Agbotiname Lucky Imoize,
Rasheed Gbenga Jimoh, Emmanuel Abidemi Adeniyi,
Muyideen Abdulraheem, Idowu Dauda Oladipo, and
Peace Busola Falola*

5.1   Introduction 97
        5.1.1 Keys Contributions of This Chapter 99
        5.1.2 Chapter Organization 99
5.2   The Applicability of Artificial Intelligence of Medical
        Things in Real-Time Patient Monitoring Systems 100
5.3   AIoMT-Based Real-Time Patient Monitoring Systems
        Architectures 103
5.4   Security and Privacy Concerns of Artificial Intelligence
        of Medical Things in Patient Real-Time Monitoring
        Systems 106
        5.4.1 Concerns in Artificial Intelligence of
               Medical Things in Patient Real-Time
               Monitoring Systems 107

5.5 Security Threats in Artificial Intelligence of
Medical Things Edge Network 109
5.5.1 Security Risks to Integrity 110
5.5.2 Threats to Authentication Security 111
5.5.3 Security Risks to Authorization 111
5.5.4 Security Intimidations to Availability 112
5.5.5 Risks to Security 113
5.5.6 Risks to Privacy 113
5.6 Countermeasure to Artificial Intelligence Medical Things
for Real-Time Patient Monitoring Systems 113
5.6.1 Access Control 114
5.6.2 Identity Authentication 114
5.6.3 Data Encryption 115
5.6.4 Isolation-Based Mechanism 116
5.6.5 Bio-Cryptographic Key Generation 116
5.6.6 Attestation-Based Architecture 116
5.6.7 Blockchain Technology 117
5.6.8 Intrusion Detection Systems 118
5.7 Conclusions and Future Directions 120
Acknowledgment 120
References 121

Chapter 6 AIoMT Concerns 134

*Abasiama Godwin Akpan, Flavious Bobuin Nkubli,
Victoria Nnaemeka Ezeano, and Anayo Christian Okwor*

6.1 Introduction 134
6.1.1 Key Contribution of the Chapter 136
6.1.2 Chapter Organization 136
6.2 AI in Healthcare Ecosystem 136
6.2.1 Measures of AI Trustworthy in Healthcare 137
6.2.2 AI Methods in Healthcare Applications 137
6.2.3 Security Challenges in Healthcare Systems 139
6.3 Concept of IoT and AIoMT 139
6.3.1 Advantages of AIoMT 140
6.3.2 Smart E-Healthcare 141
6.3.3 AIoMT Architecture in Healthcare 142
6.4 Security Concern in AIoMT-Layered Architecture 144
6.4.1 Security Concern in Perception Layer 144
6.4.2 Security Concern in Network Layer 144
6.4.3 Security Concern in Application Layer 145
6.5 AIoMT Technologies 145
6.6 AIoMT Technologies and Applications 148
6.7 Research in AIoMT 148
6.8 The Challenges of AIoMT 149

6.9   AIoMT Concerns..153
        6.9.1   Threats in AIoMT 154
        6.9.2   Security Issues in AIoMT 154
        6.9.3   Malicious Attacks in AIoMT 157
        6.9.4   Privacy Issues in AIoMT.....................................157
        6.9.5   Trust Issues in AIoMT 160
        6.9.6   Accuracy Issues in AIoMT 160
        6.9.7   Authentication Protocols in AIoMTs 160
        6.9.8   Detection Mechanisms for AIoMTs Networks 160
6.10   Conclusion 161
References 161

Chapter 7   Application of Artificial Intelligence of Medical Things
in Remote Healthcare Delivery...169

Manisha Srivastava, Ahmad Tasnim Siddiqui, and Vishal Srivastava

7.1   Introduction 169
        7.1.1   Objectives 171
        7.1.2   Key Contributions of the Chapter 171
        7.1.3   Chapter Organization 171
7.2.   Related Work 172
        7.2.1   AI and IoMT in Healthcare Industry 174
        7.2.2   Other Useful Technologies in Healthcare 175
7.3   Methodology...175
7.4   Architecture of IoMT Framework......................................179
7.5   Applications of AIoMT in Remote Healthcare 180
7.6   The Potential Benefits and Impacts of AIoMT 182
7.7   Challenges in Remote Healthcare Delivery 184
7.8   Limitations of the Study 185
7.9   Conclusions..185
References 185

Chapter 8   Cyberattacks against Artificial Intelligence-Enabled
Internet of Medical Things..191

Adewole Usman Rufai, Ebun Philip Fasina,
Charles Onuwa Uwadia, Aishat Titilola Rufai, and
Agbotiname Lucky Imoize

8.1   Introduction 191
        8.1.1   Major Contributions of the Chapter 193
        8.1.2   Chapter Organization 193
8.2   Related Works...193
8.3   Nature and Types of Cyberattacks 194
        8.3.1   Physical Attacks 194
        8.3.2   Network Attack 200

8.4   Characteristics of Cyberattacks 200
8.5   Targeted Artificial Intelligence-Enabled Internet of
        Medical Things (AIoMTs) Security Aspects 201
        8.5.1   Application Security 201
        8.5.2   Connectivity Security 202
        8.5.3   Device Security 202
8.6   Existing Security Measures in the Medical Domain 202
        8.6.1   Encryption 203
        8.6.2   Access Control 203
        8.6.3   Device Authentication 204
        8.6.4   Software Updates 204
        8.6.5   Network Segmentation 204
        8.6.6   Penetration Testing 204
        8.6.7   Data Backup 205
        8.6.8   Security Training 205
8.7   A Conceptual Framework for AIoMT Security 205
8.8   Methodology 207
        8.8.1   Data Collection 207
        8.8.2   Data Preprocessing 208
8.9   Results and Discussions 210
8.10   Conclusions and Future Scope 213
Acknowledgment 214
References 214

Chapter 9   Cyberattacks against AIoMT Architectures 217

                  Abasiama Godwin Akpan, Fergus Uchenna Onu,
                  Flavious Bobuin Nkubli, Anayo Christian Okwor, and
                  Geofery Luntsi

9.1   Introduction 217
        9.1.1   Contribution of the Chapter 218
        9.1.2   Chapter Organization 219
9.2   Concept of Cyber Security 219
        9.2.1   Cyber Threats 219
        9.2.2   Security Risk 220
        9.2.3   Computer Emergency Response Team (CERT) 220
        9.2.4   Cyber Incident Response Team (CIRT) 220
        9.2.5   Cyber Security Strategy 220
9.3   Review of Related Works 221
9.4   ML for Cyber Security Tasks 223
        9.4.1   AI Applications for Threats Prevention 223
        9.4.2   AI Applications for Threat Detection 223
        9.4.3   AI Applications for Threat Response and Recovery 224
        9.4.4   AI Applications for Active Defense 224
9.5   Functions of Cyber Security Center 225

9.6   AIoMT Model 225
9.7   Nature of Cyberattacks... 226
9.8   Types of Cyberattacks against AIoMT............................. 228
        9.8.1   One-Pixel Attacks 229
        9.8.2   Attacks in AIoMT 229
        9.8.3   Cyberattacks on AIoMT.. 229
        9.8.4   Security Challenges in Healthcare Systems............ 229
        9.8.5   AIoMT Security Trepidation.................................231
9.9   Man-in-the-Middle Attack Mitigation in AIoMT 232
9.10   Intrusive Detecting Systems 232
9.11   Cyberattacks on PACS..233
        9.11.1   Scenario 1: Importing of Patient Information
                  from Storage Space Including Malware 234
        9.11.2   Attack 2: Compromising the Set of Connections
                  in the Clinic 234
        9.11.3   Attack 3: Integration of Malware in Digital
                  Imaging 234
        9.11.4   Attack 4: Interactions in Medical Images and
                  Reports 235
        9.11.5   Attack 5: Exploitation of a Cruel Clinical Images
                  and a System Permeation of Cruel Health Level
                  Information..235
9.12   Conclusion 236
References 236

Chapter 10 Local Differential Privacy for Artificial Intelligence
of Medical Things 241

*Yuichi Sei, Akihiko Ohsuga, J. Andrew Onesimu, and
Agbotiname Lucky Imoize*

10.1   Introduction 241
10.2   Assumption... 243
        10.2.1   Target Scenario.. 243
        10.2.2   Target ML Model 244
        10.2.3   Target Data Type 244
10.3   Related Work 245
        10.3.1   Local Differential Privacy (LDP) 245
        10.3.2   LDP ML Model Generation from Raw Data 246
        10.3.3   ML Model Generation from LDP Data.................. 246
        10.3.4   ML Model Generation with Indirect
                  LDP Access to Raw Data 246
        10.3.5   LDP Synthetic Data Generation 246
        10.3.6   Copula 247
10.4   Decision Tree with LDP Data 248
        10.4.1   Categorical Data.. 248
        10.4.2   Numerical Data 250

10.5   Proposed Algorithm 253
        10.5.1 Outline..253
        10.5.2 Covariance Matrix Generation from LDP Data........253
        10.5.3 CDF Generation from LDP Data 256
        10.5.4 Copula Sample Generation...................................257
10.6   Evaluation 257
        10.6.1 Synthetic Datasets 258
        10.6.2 Experiment with Real Datasets............................259
10.7   Discussion.. 264
        10.7.1 Advantages and Limitations................................. 264
        10.7.2 Comparison of ML Algorithms 264
        10.7.3 Handling High-Dimensional Data 264
        10.7.4 Preprocessing Techniques 265
10.8   Conclusion 265
Acknowledgment... 265
References 266

Chapter 11 Artificial Intelligence of Internet of Medical Things (AIoMT)
            in Smart Cities: A Review of Cybersecurity for Smart
            Healthcare 271

            Kassim Kalinaki, Mugigayi Fahadi, Adam A. Alli,
            Wasswa Shafik, Magombe Yasin, and Nambobi Mutwalibi

11.1   Introduction 271
        11.1.1 Chapter Contributions 272
        11.1.2 Chapter Organization 272
11.2   Applications of AI in Smart Healthcare...........................273
        11.2.1 Surgical Robots 273
        11.2.2 Exoskeletons 274
        11.2.3 Prosthetics 274
        11.2.4 Artificial Organs 274
        11.2.5 Healthcare Automation Robots 274
        11.2.6 Autonomous Identification of Diseases..................275
        11.2.7 Personalized Medicine 275
        11.2.8 Medication Errors...275
        11.2.9 Candidate Identification Meant for Clinical Trials 275
        11.2.10 Cybersecurity 275
        11.2.11 Healthcare Monitoring and Wearables..................276
        11.2.12 AI in Health Fraud Detection.............................276
11.3   Cybersecurity Aspects of AIoMT in Smart Cities 276
11.4   Secure AIoMT Framework for Smart Healthcare in
        Smart Cities 278
11.5   IoMT Attacks, Threats, and Countermeasures for
        Smart Healthcare... 280
11.6   Lessons 284
11.7   Future Directions.. 284

11.8   Conclusion 285
References 285

Chapter 12 Digital Twins in the AIoMT..293

Qian Qu and Yu Chen

12.1   Introduction 293
       12.1.1   Key Contributions of the Chapter 294
       12.1.2   Chapter Organization 294
12.2   Digital Twins in AIoMT: An Overview 295
       12.2.1   An Introduction to Digital Twins 295
       12.2.2   Applications of DT in IoMT 296
12.3   Integrating Digital Twin Technology and AIoMT 299
       12.3.1   System Architecture... 299
       12.3.2   Major Function Blocks 300
12.4   Case Study: DT-AIoMT Enabled Senior
       Safety Monitoring..301
       12.4.1   Hybrid SSA-LSTM Detection and
                Prediction Model 301
       12.4.2   Experimental Study... 302
12.5   Conclusions and Open Challenges 303
References 305

Chapter 13 Artificial Intelligence-Assisted Internet of Medical Things
Enabling Medical Image Processing................................ 309

*Ajimah Nnabueze Edmund, Christopher Akinyemi Alabi,
Oluwaseun Olayinka Tooki, Agbotiname Lucky Imoize, and
Tanko Daniel Salka*

13.1   Introduction 309
       13.1.1   Key Contributions 310
       13.1.2   Chapter Organization 310
13.2   Medical Images and Their Acquisition Techniques...............310
       13.2.1   Radiography (X-ray)...311
       13.2.2   Computerized Tomography (CT) 311
       13.2.3   Magnetic Resonance Imaging (MRI) 311
       13.2.4   Nuclear Medicine Imaging.....................................313
       13.2.5   Ultrasound 313
       13.2.6   Elastography 314
       13.2.7   Photoacoustic Imaging 314
       13.2.8   Echocardiography..314
       13.2.9   Functional Near-Infrared Spectroscopy....................315
       13.2.10 Magnetic Particle Imaging....................................316
13.3   Medical Image Processing 316
       13.3.1   Basic Medical Image Processing Tasks 316
       13.3.2   Quantitative Measurement of Medical Imaging 320
       13.3.3   Image Data Visualization......................................320

13.4   Related Works on AI-Enabled Medical Image Processing 323
13.5   AI-Based Experiment on COVID-19 Detection.....................325
        13.5.1   Proposed Model Description.................................325
        13.5.2   Methodology 325
        13.5.3   Result and Discussion...327
13.6   AIoMT and the Radiologist...328
13.7   Research Advances and Gaps in AI-Based Medical
        Image Processing...330
13.8   Conclusion and Future Direction...331
Acknowledgment.. 331
References 331

Chapter 14 Application of AIoMT in Medical Robotics.................................335

*Aishat Titilola Rufai, Adewole Usman Rufai, and
Agbotiname Lucky Imoize*

14.1   Introduction 335
        14.1.1   Key Contributions of the Chapter 336
        14.1.2   Chapter Organization 337
14.2   Related Work...337
        14.2.1   Medical Robotics System and Applications..............338
        14.2.2   Current Application of Medical Robots....................342
14.3   Concept of AIoMT in Medical Robotics................................343
        14.3.1   How IoMT Works...343
        14.3.2   IoMT Applications 344
        14.3.3   AIoMT System 349
        14.3.4   Technological Concepts for Smart Healthcare
                  Systems...350
        14.3.5   AIoMT in Medical Robotics—Overview 355
        14.3.6   Application of AIoMT in Medical Robotics—
                  Emergence of AIoMRT...356
14.4   Current Limitations of AIoMRT and Future Directions........357
14.5   Learned Lessons...358
14.6   Conclusion 359
Acknowledgment.. 359
References 359

Chapter 15 AIoMT on Intelligent Location and Clustering
of Medical Units.. 365

*Pablo Rodríguez de León, María Dolores Torres Soto,
Aurora Torres Soto, Eunice Esther Ponce de León Sentí, and
Carlos Ochoa Zezzatti*

15.1   Introduction 365
        15.1.1   Key Contributions of the Chapter 366
        15.1.2   Chapter Organization 367

15.2 Related Concepts 367
       15.2.1 Multi-Criteria Decision-Making Methods 367
       15.2.2 Multi-Criteria Decision-Making Methods 367
       15.2.3 TOPSIS 368
       15.2.4 K-means 370
       15.2.5 Haversine's Formula 370
       15.2.6 First Level of Healthcare in Aguascalientes
               State 371
       15.2.7 Territorial Integration, Urban Environment,
               and Community Consultation System
               (SCITEL) 372
15.3 Literature Review 372
15.4 Material and Methods 378
       15.4.1 Conceptual Design 378
       15.4.2 Methodology 378
       15.4.3 Data Collection 379
       15.4.4 SCITEL Data Collection 379
15.5 Results 380
       15.5.1 Processing Clustering Software Framework 380
       15.5.2 Modified K-means Algorithm for Fixed and
               Mobile Centers 381
       15.5.3 New Health Jurisdiction 4 Health Centers
               Distribution 382
       15.5.4 TOPSIS Variables and Process 384
15.6 Discussions 388
15.7 Conclusions 391
References 391

Chapter 16 AIoMT Training, Testing, and Validation 394

Vitalis Afebuame Iguoba and Agbotiname Lucky Imoize

16.1 Introduction 394
       16.1.1 Key Contribution of the Chapter 395
       16.1.2 Chapter Organization 396
16.2 Related Work 396
       16.2.1 The Architectural Design of AIoMT 397
       16.2.2 The Challenges of Big Data in
               AI Applications 399
       16.2.3 The Basic Steps for AI Data Training 403
16.3 AIoMT Training 403
       16.3.1 Challenges of AI Data Training 404
16.4 AIoMT Testing 405
       16.4.1 Challenges of AI Data Testing 405
16.5 AIoMT Validation 406
16.6 Conclusions and Future Scope 407
Acknowledgment 407
References 407

Chapter 17 AIoMT for Medical Image Steganalysis 411

*Oluyemi Paul Adejumo, Aderonke Favour-Bethy Thompson,
and Arome Junior Gabriel*

    17.1   Introduction 411
          17.1.1 Key Contributions of the Chapter 413
          17.1.2 Chapter Organization 414
    17.2   Related Work 414
    17.3   Materials and Methods/Methodology 416
          17.3.1 Data Collection Phase 416
          17.3.2 Pre-Processing Phase 416
          17.3.3 Convolutional Neural Networks Model
                 Training Phase 416
          17.3.4 Activation Function 418
          17.3.5 Pooling Layer 419
          17.3.6 Batch Normalization 419
          17.3.7 Fully Connected Layer 419
          17.3.8 SoftMax Function 419
          17.3.9 Adaptive Momentum Estimate (Adam) 420
    17.4   System Implementation and Evaluation 420
          17.4.1 Dataset Distributions 420
          17.4.2 Training and Validation 421
          17.4.3 Performance Evaluation 421
    17.5   Discussions 422
          17.5.1 Parameter Tuning 425
    17.6   Conclusions and Future Scope 426
    References 426

Chapter 18 Case Studies in AIoMT Applications: A Secure Medical
Cyber-Physical System for the Monitoring and Diagnosis
of Lassa Fever 429

*Adebowale Joseph Adelakun, Boniface Kayode Alese,
Aderonke Favour-Bethy Thompson, and Olufunso Dayo Alowolodu*

    18.1   Introduction 429
          18.1.1 The Chapter Contribution 430
          18.1.2 Chapter Organization 431
    18.2   Review of Related Work 431
          18.2.1 Review of Related Works 431
          18.2.2 Summary of Analysis of Related Work 432
          18.2.3 Research Motivation and Objectives 433
    18.3   Methodology 433
          18.3.1 Proposed Algorithms for the Digital
                 Monitoring of Lassa Fever Contacts 433
          18.3.2 The Proposed AIoMT Framework 434
          18.3.3 The Machine Learning Predictive Model 436

    18.4   The Results and Discussions 439
          18.4.1 Confusion Matrices 439
          18.4.2 ROC Curves 440
          18.4.3 The Performance Result... 440
    18.5   Conclusions.. 440
    References 442

Chapter 19 AIoMT-Assisted Telemedicine: A Case Study of eSanjeevani
                Telemedicine Service in India... 445

Ambili Parathra Sreedharan Pillai

    19.1   Introduction 445
          19.1.1 Key Contributions of the Chapter 446
          19.1.2 Chapter Organization 447
    19.2   Related Work 447
    19.3   Architectural Design of AI-Powered Telemedicine
          System 448
          19.3.1 AIoMT in Brain Tumor Diagnosis........................... 449
    19.4   AI-Powered Conversational Chatbots 455
          19.4.1 Self-Service Kiosks Support for Telemedicine 456
          19.4.2 Robots to Aid AIoMT 456
          19.4.3 Future of Robotics in Telemedicine 456
    19.5   eSanjeevani—A Case Study...458
          19.5.1 Objectives...458
          19.5.2 System Architecture 458
    19.6   Conclusion and Future Directions 459
    Acknowledgment.. 460
    References 460

Index... 465

Preface

The fast-growing number of patients suffering from various ailments has overstretched the carrying capacity of traditional healthcare systems. Often, it becomes challenging to get reliable, accurate, efficient, and adequate medical results using conventional methods of healthcare delivery. In order to address this problem, the Internet of Medical Things (IoMT) was proposed. IoMT accelerates the remote monitoring of medical services and aids early detection of any medical problem in patients. Recently, Artificial Intelligence (AI) application to medical data analysis has remarkably facilitated the treating and diagnosing of critical health issues. Integrating Artificial Intelligence into the Internet of Medical Things has given birth to Artificial Intelligence of Medical Things (AIoMT). AIoMT has ushered a dramatic change in the medical field to orchestrate rapid diagnosis, treatment, and management of health issues suffered by a growing number of patients worldwide.

AIoMT facilitates quick responses to patients' needs more efficiently and effectively. However, there are growing concerns that AIoMT is highly vulnerable to several cyber and malicious attacks due to a lack of robust security and privacy control. In addition, the interconnection of billions of medical devices in AIoMT poses enormous security vulnerabilities leading to unlawful exploitation of patients' medical records. Consequently, malicious intruders could reconfigure medical devices, and patients' lives could be in critical danger. Thus, this could severely impact the rapid deployment, trust, and usage of AIoMT systems.

Additionally, AIoMT requires extensive training and awareness to aid successful implementation. In order to enhance the immunity of AIoMT against cyberattacks, proper security measures must be put in place. The required training skills must be provided to all parties involved in the healthcare ecosystem, and the need for a book that addresses these concerns cannot be overemphasized.

This handbook discusses critical AIoMT security and privacy issues. First, the book critically examines the existing security designs and proffers solutions to revamp the traditional security architecture. Also, the book explores the application of cryptographic and noncryptographic solutions to addressing critical security and privacy concerns in AIoMT devices and systems. These solutions are analyzed and compared in terms of the required resources, computational complexity, and system performance. Next, the book discusses emerging lightweight, provably secure algorithms and protocols to reduce computational overheads and communication costs. Finally, the need to design efficient intrusion detection algorithms and attack prevention techniques to tackle these security concerns are discussed extensively. The book is well structured in nineteen chapters outlined as follows:

Chapter 1 gives an overview of AIoMT applications. The Internet of Things (IoT) refers to intelligent service technologies that process and respond to information in the physical and virtual worlds through interactions between uniquely identified, pervasively deployed devices, machines, objects, people, and even animals. With advances in artificial intelligence (AI), the fifth-generation and beyond (B5G) communications, and biosensors, IoT technology is changing modern life in multiple domains, including transportation, industrial automation, energy response, and healthcare. The Internet of Medical Things (IoMT) aims to create a digital healthcare system in medical and healthcare-related fields, such as data acquisition, situational analysis, patient monitoring, and emergency alert generation. IoMT can notify relevant healthcare service personnel through real-time, continuous monitoring and tracking. Hence, IoMT provides remote patient services and enables rapid assistance from doctors or first responders when an alarm is issued. Another critical application of IoMT is storing data for in-depth analysis. The massive, continuous health-related data collected by the IoMT is essential to analyze an individual's health status and provide better health advice. On the societal side, IoMT allows healthcare organizations access to critical analysis and data-driven insights, accelerating the development of the future healthcare industry. A Multi-sensor Action Recognition-based Senior falling detection (MARS) system is presented as a case study in the chapter, aiming to protect seniors' safety without compromising the privacy of those living alone. In addition, the chapter discusses two major categories of IoMT applications: indoor and outdoor environments, and their advantages and disadvantages. Finally, the chapter highlights open issues in IoMT research and discusses possible future directions.

Chapter 2 presents wearable medical electronics in the artificial intelligence of medical things. The authors noted that the integration of artificial intelligence (AI) and the Internet of Things (IoT) avails the recent development in the medical sector, specifically digital health, referred to as the Internet of Medical Things (IoMT). This development makes it simpler for patients to relax, for health problems to be solved quickly and modestly, for hospital medications to be given right away, and for healthcare to be more personalized. Artificial intelligence and other key support technologies like big data, mobile internet, cloud computing, microelectronics, and others have made processing the collected patient data possible for better insights. This has turned traditional healthcare into an all-around, efficient, and personalized experience. During the recent COVID-19 pandemic, AI medical applications have become more popular worldwide. People who were sick with the virus were saved with the help of intelligent technologies. The AIoMT makes it leisurely to collect, analyze, and make sense of a considerable amount of patient information so that healthcare and well-being monitoring can be done effectively through different electronic devices. The chapter comprehensively surveys several wearable medical electronics in the AIoMT. There has been a focus on the known and commonly used medical devices, such as the electronic signals for AIoMT sensors. In addition, the AIoMT architecture shows how smart sensors can be used to collect, combine, and control data for smart healthcare structures. The chapter reviews the challenges of electronic devices in the AIoMT, like data security threats, data interoperability, and regulatory concerns addressed to improve medical standards of operation for medical personnel, patients, and other medical stakeholders. Finally, open research issues for future research in AIoMT are highlighted.

Chapter 3 explores electronic devices in the Artificial Intelligence of the Internet of Medical Things (AIoMT). The current medical diseases and infections necessitate advanced medical equipment (medical devices) to bridge the gap between existing and predictable diseases. This gap has been bridged by integrating traditional medical settings with artificial intelligence (AI). AI simulates human intelligence processes through machines, exclusively known as smart systems. The global pandemic witnessed a wider acceptance of AI applications in medicine. Intelligent technologies and their associated algorithms in the healthcare domain were used to save the individuals affected by the virus. This technique has produced what is now called the artificial intelligence of medical things (AIoMT), which has made it possible to collect, analyze, and interpret an unprecedented amount of patient information for effective healthcare and well-being monitoring through various electronic devices. Through these medical devices (or medical things), artificial intelligence and other key support technologies such as big data, mobile internet, cloud computing, microelectronics, and others have made it possible to process the collected patient data to provide better insights, thereby transforming the traditional healthcare into an all-round, efficient and personalized experience. The chapter presents a comprehensive survey of several electronic devices in the AIoMT. The identified and commonly utilized medical devices have been highlighted, including electronic signals for AIoMT sensors. The AIoMT architecture demonstrates a comprehensive evolution using smart sensors to accumulate, aggregate, and regulate data for innovative healthcare structures. The chapter reviews the challenges of electronic devices in the AIoMT, like data security threats, data interoperability, and regulatory concerns, among others, that need to be addressed to improve medical standards of operation for medical persons and patients, and other medical stakeholders. Lastly, the chapter highlights open research issues of future research in AIoMT.

Chapter 4 focuses on the artificial intelligence of medical things for medical information systems security and privacy. Artificial intelligence (AI) is a modern approach based on computer research that aims to create algorithms and programs that make machines clever and effective at carrying out jobs that ordinarily require highly educated human intelligence. Deep learning (DL), standard artificial neural networks, fuzzy logic, and speech recognition are all examples of machine learning (ML). These are only a few AI subsets with distinctive capabilities and functionalities, making it easier for humans to intervene in medical assessment, diagnostic devices, and decision-making. The significant difficulties that the healthcare business confronted influence the standard of patient treatment. Maintaining data privacy and security is challenging when such a vast amount of sensitive data is present. Most healthcare equipment is susceptible to hacks, endangering patient data, and derisory management of life-support systems can significantly affect a patient's treatment. In order to address this problem, AI of Medical Thing (AIoMT) is being used to increase the high reliability and effectiveness of the healthcare system. AIoMT carries patient records, contacts, and other clinical records, and devices are packed with clinical data. Even though these ubiquitous and affordable sensing technologies can change reaction therapy into preventive services, safety, and confidentiality problems are frequently a threat. IoMT system administration and security are likewise very challenging. The chapter explores several methods for securing AIoMT devices and ensuring data privacy to address the security concerns militating against using AIoMT to safeguard patients' information.

Chapter 5 discusses AIoMT enabling real-time monitoring of healthcare systems, emphasizing security and privacy. The authors observed that one of the critical elements in determining a person's living standards is access to adequate and high-quality healthcare services. Developed nations work to make their healthcare systems as effective and affordable as possible. Real-time healthcare with medical services is a promising way to speed up disease prediction and treatment while reducing healthcare expenses. In remote monitoring systems, Artificial Intelligence of Medical Things (AIoMT) is becoming increasingly popular daily. Remote monitoring systems include those that monitor things like vehicles or properties, children or pets, parking or fleets management, water and oil leakages, and the energy infrastructure, among others. Hence, it helps in various medical services that can be remotely realized, like chronic disease diagnosis and monitoring, resulting in improved healthcare services and decreased overhead costs. As a result, this chapter reviews the role of AIoMT in advanced healthcare systems. The chapter discusses the opportunities for AIoMT-based applications for real-time monitoring systems. Additionally, the prevalent security and privacy of AIoMT-based real-time monitoring systems are examined. The chapter concludes with probable future advances in AIoMT-based monitoring systems.

Chapter 6 takes a closer look at the proliferating AIoMT concerns. The Artificial Intelligence of Medical Things (AIoMT) and the principal devices uphold valuable data that is a favorite target for adversarial attacks. Hence, healthcare applications require medical data privacy and trusted platforms to handle data efficiently and intelligently. The study focuses on AIoMT concerns like security, privacy, trust, and accuracy. The objective is to present an overview of the core security and privacy controls that must be deployed in modern AIoMT scenery to protect the users. A qualitative review of AIoMT literature was conducted to ascertain key concerns of AIoMT. The review revealed that the AIoMT requires efficient protocol authentication.

Chapter 7 covers the application of artificial intelligence to medical things in remote healthcare delivery. Telemedicine frameworks connect patients with medical specialists or attendants using features including live talk, video conferencing, or regular telephone calls. Clinical expertise will benefit from an image-based AI with high accuracy, enabling them to make the right decisions, diagnose their patients, and deliver medical aids properly and timely. Even when a less experienced practitioner diagnoses the patient, it is still possible to get accurate results. In addition, patients' involvement in decision-making will boost compliance with healthcare services. IoT integrates data analytics and sensors embedded in machines to offer various real-time medical solutions. An IoMT network consists of connected devices that collect vital real-time data. There are many applications of AI and IoMT, such as Electrocardiogram Monitoring (ECG), Glucose Level Detection, Oxygen Saturation Monitoring, Blood Pressure Monitoring, Mental well-being, Chronic Kidney Disease (CKD) monitoring, Wheelchair Management, Smart City and healthcare services, and much more, which are highlighted in the chapter.

Chapter 8 dwells on cyber attacks against artificial intelligence-enabled internet of medical things. The fourth industrial revolution is characterized by cyberspace's ubiquity and its exploitation by criminal elements (hackers) that are ready to compromise cyberspace by engaging in cyber-attacks. Internet of Medical Things (IoMT) describes the aggregation of clinical sensors or devices connected to the internet that collects medical data for real-time monitoring of patients. Making it

AI-enabled provides the Internet of Medical Things (Artificial intelligence enabled internet of medical things (AIoMT)) with the predictive power for a much more efficient treatment of patients. However, the ubiquity of AIoMT makes it vulnerable to cyber-attacks. Furthermore, its safety-critical nature informed the need to make the AIoMT platform secure. Another motivation is the loss of medical data privacy should data leaks occur. In coming up with the potential solutions to Artificial intelligence enabled internet of medical things (AIoMT) vulnerabilities, the small form factor, limitation of memory, power efficiency, and computational capacity of the sensors are taken into cognizance. The chapter explores the nature and various types of cyber-attacks. Various malware attacks are presented, and the various security measures to address the malware are proposed. Also, a new conceptual framework incorporating artificial intelligence and software-defined networking (SDN) was presented, thereby providing holistic mitigation of various threats to the AIoMT system. The proposed framework was simulated with the WUSTL-EHMS-2020 dataset applied to seven machine-learning models. Results indicate that the extreme gradient boosting model outperformed other models with 95.02% accuracy, 98.66% F1 score, and 84.44% AUC score.

Chapter 9 discusses cyber-attacks against AIoMT architectures. AIoMT is a promising technological driver for the contemporary clinical revolution. However, even as these advances guarantee enhanced healthcare services at abridged costs, they also become risky as various linked devices are vulnerable to unlawful exploitation. The chapter presents an inclusive study of the most exploited weaknesses in the existing AIoMT architectures. In addition, the chapter emphasizes the methods for guaranteeing authentication in AioMT networks. Also, the study proposes an intrusion detective system based on ML techniques using networking and authenticating constraints as attributes that distinguish standard congestion from attack congestion. Finally, the study noted that the secured AIoMT system could identify network anomalies and the means for validating patients.

Chapter 10 presents local differential privacy for artificial intelligence of medical things. The collection of medical and personal health data is taking place in diverse locations due to the development of IoT technology. This technology has created possibilities for using medical data for novel services, but maintaining data privacy is a key consideration. Privacy-preserving medical data collection is achievable by applying Local Differential Privacy (LDP) with the addition of noise. However, machine learning (ML) significantly degrades performance when trained on noisy data. The chapter aims to develop an ML model using LDP data, such as decision trees. Instead of applying the machine learning model as is, copulas were used to generate synthetic data that can remove the effects of the noise of LDP. The results of simulations using real and synthetic data confirm that the proposed algorithm was effective for decision trees, deep neural networks, and k-nearest neighbors.

Chapter 11 reviews the artificial intelligence of the internet of medical things in smart cities, focusing on cybersecurity for smart healthcare. As the convergence of AI and the Internet of Medical Things (IoMT) continue to gain momentum, the Artificial Intelligence of the Internet of Medical Things (AIoMT) paradigm has captured the attention of both academia and industry. The potential for AIoMT to revolutionize healthcare is undeniable, with applications such as alleviating the strain on healthcare systems caused by staff shortages, addressing the health challenges of aging populations, and tackling the rising incidence of chronic diseases as global health crises like COVID-19. However, the dynamic nature of AIoMT and its ability to process vast amounts of patient data also make it susceptible to cyberattacks, potentially compromising patient data, threatening lives, and damaging the reputation of medical providers. The chapter offers a comprehensive overview of how AI shapes the health sector in smart cities, including the ecosystem and cybersecurity concerns, identifying the various types of cyberattacks and threats, proposing countermeasures, and exploring future developments in the field.

Chapter 12 considers digital twins in the AIoMT. The fast development of technology has brought us new generations of machines, tools, and devices, enabling the evolution of different technique fields, such as industrial manufacturing, education, entertainment, and healthcare. The Internet of Medical Things (IoMT) is one of the best examples of the evolution aiming to build connections between almost everything in the healthcare domain. With the growing demand in various areas of modern healthcare, new approaches have been introduced to address major concerns like medical monitoring, diagnosis accuracy, service availability, data security, and privacy. For example, the Digital Twins (DT) technology creates a digital replica of a physical object (PO) in virtual space. Leveraging state-of-the-art medical devices, smart cameras, and body sensors, the digital twin of a patient can accurately reflect the medical status. Integrating DT with AIoMT, the logical object (LO) can be used to perform real-time monitoring, future prediction, emergency diagnosis, risk control, and other services. The chapter provides a comprehensive overview of DT technology and its applications in telemedicine and e-health. In addition, taking senior safety monitoring as a case study, the work introduces SafeTwins, which integrates DT, blockchain, NFT, and IoMT technologies. The design rationales and key function blocks are illustrated in detail. A proof-of-concept SafeTwins prototype is implemented and investigated experimentally, highlighting the performance and some key design trade-offs. Finally, the chapter shows some existing challenges and opportunities in this exciting technology field. Hoping more discussions are inspired and more novel insights are sparked in the AIoMT community.

Chapter 13 is on artificial intelligence-assisted internet of medical things enabling medical image processing. The chapter presents a comprehensive discussion of medical image modalities and processing techniques. The importance, requirements, and unique challenges facing medical image processing were discussed elaborately. The work highlights the use of Artificial Intelligence (AI) enabled Internet of Medical Things (IoMT) in tackling the identified limitations in image processing. A data set consisting of 5,860 chest X-ray images was obtained from the Kaggle database, and a pre-trained VGG-16 CNN model was used to detect Coronavirus (COVID-19) disease from X-ray images. A bilateral low-pass filter was applied to filter noise from the images. Results indicate 95% accuracy using the presented AI model, posing significantly higher accuracy compared to results obtained using XGBoot and Random Forest models, which have percentage accuracies of 82 and 77, respectively. Therefore, the VGG-16 CNN model has a comparative advantage over the existing AI model. The proposed AI technique applies to medical diagnostic equipment or expertise shortage scenarios. Furthermore, medical images from remote locations can be transmitted using IoMT and presented for medical analysis. The successful implementation of this technique will enhance the quick detection of diseases such as COVID-19.

Chapter 14 focuses on the application of AIoMT in medical robotics. Medical robotics has been an essential part of the medical field, with various applications ranging from surgical, rehabilitative, and assistive robots. In addition, medical robotics has been used with ground-breaking approaches such as artificial intelligence (AI) and the Internet of Medical Things (IoMT). The chapter identifies the development of medical robotics, the theory behind AIoMT in medical robotics, and current trends of AIoMT in medical robotics.

Chapter 15 considers AIoMT on the intelligent location selection and clustering of medical units in Mexico. The population of patients attended by the health centers of the Institute of Health Services of the State of Aguascalientes (ISSEA) in Mexico is increasing daily. With more than 70,000 patients, 89 health centers are under the responsibility of 3 Health Jurisdictions, and they are currently distributed considering only the municipality they belong to decides the responsible Health Jurisdiction. However, the present distribution does not consider distances, patient population, or type of health center. In order to address this problem, this chapter presents the distribution based on Haversine distance. The geographic point for the location of the new Health Jurisdiction was obtained through the integration of Artificial Intelligence of Medical Things (AIoMT) with the implementation of a modified K-Means algorithm. In addition, comprehensive data were obtained from several geographic point communities using the territorial integration, urban environment, community consultation system (SCITEL), and the Technique for Order of Preference by Similarity to Ideal Solution (TOPSIS). Data analysis helps determine the community in which the new Health Jurisdiction should be established.

Chapter 16 centers on AIoMT training, testing, and validation. The authors noted that the application scope of Artificial Intelligence (AI) continues to widen across many domains, such as the medical field, engineering, and other fields. Artificial intelligence enables the computer to perform tasks that require human intelligence. Such tasks include computer vision which deals with visual image recognition and natural language processing. Specifically, AI application is gaining more popularity, especially in the healthcare industry, due to their suitability for medical imaging and chatbots. Integrating AI into the existing healthcare system will further optimize its outlook. AI models are built with a machine learning (ML) algorithm using robust datasets. The prediction accuracy of the AI-based model depends on the training, testing, and validation data used. The quality of training data and the training acquired by the model is directly proportional to the prediction accuracy. However, AI technology faces challenges, such as the non-existent of the large dataset required for model training (due to the confidentiality and privacy issues associated with medical data), the missing values in the large dataset used for training, poor testing, and validation. This chapter focuses on AIoMT training, testing, and validation to address these issues. The authors remarked that obtaining clean and quality data will help mitigate the problems with AI applications in healthcare, and further research is needed to achieve it.

Chapter 17 captures AIoMT for medical image steganalysis. The authors remarked that the growing usage of images to encrypt information had heightened the need for a resourceful classifier like Convolution Neural Networks (CNN) to detect whether an image is precisely what it appears to be. The exciting level of accuracy in cover/ stego image classification has given rise to a new state-of-the-art application of CNN. However, the need to assess the performance level of CNN and its suitability to handle certain image-type classifications cannot be overstated, due to its dependency on its structural factors, such as the learning aspects of the convolutional filter size and numbers. These architectural design facets encompass the number of layers, the pooling operations, the choice of nonlinearity, and its chronological arrangement. A well-ordered CNN model will augment its practical deployment and advance scientific understanding in image steganalysis. The chapter proposes a JPEG color image steganalysis using a CNN classifier to discriminate between stego images and their cover counterparts. Structurally, a bi-segmental CNN model was used to implement the deep learning aptitude of CNN using Adaptive Momentum (Adam) optimization to enhance its performance. The model is structured to learn important image features while avoiding data loss for decent predictive classification accuracy. Hence, the pooling operation was removed from the second segment. The experimental results show the suitability of the proposed model in terms of its ability to perform image steganalysis with no prior knowledge of the embedding algorithm and rate. A suitable convergence speed through a high learning rate that leads to a robust classification accuracy above average is characterized using the proposed model.

Chapter 18 discusses case studies in AIoMT applications, emphasizing a secured medical cyber-physical system for diagnosing Lassa fever. The study proposed a medical cyber-physical model for monitoring and diagnosing Lassa Fever – a case study of the AIoMT application. The proposed system consists of a wearable sensor for real-time monitoring of suspected Lassa fever patients, a Data Analytic center for classifying and detecting Lassa fever patients, a web-enabled interface for Users and Health Officials, and cloud-based Infrastructure to interconnect all the other components of the system. Real-life data was collected from the Federal Medical center for the training, testing, and validation of the machine learning model utilizing five major algorithms Support Vector Machine (SVM), Naive Bayes (NB), Multilayer perceptron Neural Network (MLP—ANN), Decision Tree, and K Nearest Neighbour (K-NN). The NB was found to have the highest accuracy of 68.7% and precision of 68.6%. SVM had an Accuracy of 65.6%, followed by MLP with an accuracy of 63.8%. Feature ranking was carried out on the dataset and ranked the symptoms of Lassa fever. The system was discovered to be effective in aiding the early detection of Lassa cases. It can potentially improve the Medical diagnostic and eliminate the cumbersome or error-prone nature of manual monitoring of Lassa suspects, which is the current practice. It also serves as the basis for further investigation/implementation of AIoMT applications.

Chapter 19 presents AIoMT-assisted telemedicine using a case study of eSanjeevani telemedicine service in India. The application of digital technologies has been present in the healthcare sector for over a century. However, the widespread COVID-19 pandemic forced people to stay isolated. However, the necessity of health consultations and continuous medicinal support forced people to opt for telediagnosis and telemedicinal services for primary healthcare. The sudden growth of Artificial Intelligence techniques enabled online platforms during the pandemic and increased awareness about how to use these platforms. The AI-powered medical sensors will transmit sensitive health record data over wireless networks. This chapter compares the earlier telemedicine systems with the Telemedicine technology powered by AI and IoT. How can potential machine learning/deep learning algorithms be effectively integrated for affordable and reliable healthcare in AIoMT, and tries to find the answer for how next-generation IoT networks can contribute effectively in healthcare? This chapter presents a comparative study on the limitations of contemporary telemedicine, and the future of AIoMT is presented. This study suggests a case study of a successful national telemedicine service provided by the government of India: eSanjeevani. The AWS cloud-based telemedicine service, eSanjeevani, enables audio-video consultations using an open-source stack. eSanjeevani platform has served more than 83 million people since its inception in 2019 and helps India successfully provide eHealthcare to its citizens.

Agbotiname Lucky Imoize
Gelsenkirchen, North Rhine-Westphalia, Germany

Acknowledgments

I sincerely express my profound gratitude to God for His faithfulness and wisdom in editing this book. This book would not have been possible without the support of the Department of Electrical Engineering and Information Technology, Institute of Digital Communication, Ruhr University Bochum, Germany, and the University of Lagos, Nigeria. I acknowledge the sponsorship from the Nigerian Petroleum Technology Development Fund (PTDF) and the German Academic Exchange Service (DAAD) through the Nigerian-German Postgraduate Program. Special thanks to my beloved wife, Kelly, and our sons, Lucius, Luke, and Lucas. Also, I am indebted to the Deeper Life Bible Church, Essen Region, North Rhine-Westphalia, Germany, for their unwavering support. Last, I sincerely thank CRC Press—Taylor & Francis Group for their editorial support.

Editors

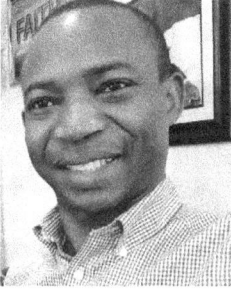

Agbotiname Lucky Imoize (Senior Member, IEEE) received the B.Eng. degree (Hons.) in Electrical and Electronics Engineering from Ambrose Alli University, Nigeria, in 2008 and the M.Sc. degree in Electrical and Electronics Engineering from the University of Lagos, Nigeria, in 2012. He is a lecturer in the Department of Electrical and Electronics Engineering at the University of Lagos, Nigeria. He was, until recently, a research scholar at the Ruhr University Bochum, Germany, under the Nigerian Petroleum Technology Development Fund (PTDF) and the German Academic Exchange Service (DAAD) through the Nigerian-German Postgraduate Program. He was awarded the Fulbright Fellowship as a visiting research scholar at the Wireless@VT Laboratory, Bradley Department of Electrical and Computer Engineering, Virginia Tech., USA, where he worked under the supervision of Prof. R. Michael Buehrer from 2017 to 2018. Before joining the University of Lagos, he was a lecturer at Bells University of Technology, Nigeria. He worked as a core network products manager at ZTE Corporation, Nigeria, and as a Network Switching Subsystem Engineer at Globacom, Nigeria. His research interests cover the fields of 6G wireless communication, wireless security systems, and Artificial Intelligence. He has co-edited four books and co-authored over 150 wireless communication papers in peer review journals and conferences. Imoize is an active reviewer for over 50 international journals and conferences. He is the vice chair of the IEEE Communication Society, Nigeria chapter, a registered engineer with the Council for the Regulation of Engineering in Nigeria (COREN), and a Nigerian Society of Engineers (NSE) member.

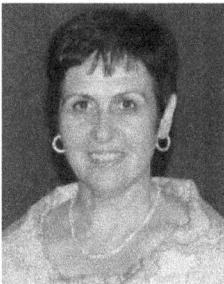

Professor Valentina Emilia Balas is currently a full professor in the Department of Automatics and Applied Software at the Faculty of Engineering, Aurel Vlaicu University of Arad, Romania. She holds a Ph.D. Cum Laude, in Applied Electronics and Telecommunications from the Polytechnic University of Timisoara. Dr. Balas is the author of more than 350 research papers in refereed journals and International Conferences. Her research interests include Intelligent Systems, Fuzzy Control, Soft Computing, Smart Sensors, Information Fusion, Modeling, and Simulation. She is the editor-in-chief of the *International Journal of Advanced Intelligence Paradigms (IJAIP)* and the *International Journal of Computational Systems Engineering (IJCSysE)* and a member of the Editorial Board member of several national and international journals. She is an evaluator expert for national and international projects and Ph.D. Thesis. Dr. Balas is the director of the Intelligent Systems Research Centre at the Aurel Vlaicu University of Arad and the Director of the Department of International Relations, Programs, and Projects at the same university. She served as general chair of the International Workshop Soft Computing and Applications (SOFA) in nine editions organized from 2005–2020, held in Romania and Hungary. Dr. Balas participated in many international conferences as an organizer, honorary chair, session chair, steering, advisory, or International Program Committees member, and keynote speaker. She worked in the interval 2016–2021 on a national project with EU funding support: BioCell-NanoART—Novel Bio-inspired Cellular Nano-Architectures—For Digital Integrated Circuits, 3M Euro from National Authority for Scientific Research and Innovation. She is a member of the European Society for Fuzzy Logic and Technology (EUSFLAT), member of Society for Industrial and Applied Mathematics (SIAM) and a senior member of IEEE, a member of the Technical Committee—Fuzzy Systems (IEEE Computational Intelligence Society), chair of the Task Force 14 in Technical Committee—Emergent Technologies (IEEE CIS), a member in Technical Committee—Soft Computing (IEEE SMCS). Dr. Balas was past vice-president (responsible for Awards) of IFSA—International Fuzzy Systems Association Council (2013–2015), is a joint secretary of the Governing Council of the Forum for Interdisciplinary Mathematics (FIM),—A Multidisciplinary Academic Body in India and recipient of the Tudor Tanasescu Prize from the Romanian Academy for contributions in the field of soft computing methods (2019).

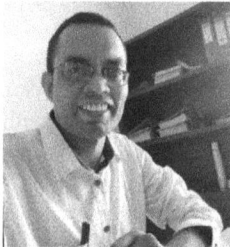

Professor Vijender Kumar Solanki is an associate professor in Computer Science & Engineering at CMR Institute of Technology (Autonomous), Hyderabad, TS, India. He has more than 15 years of academic experience in network security, IoT, Big Data, Smart City, and IT. Before his current role, he was associated with Apeejay Institute of Technology, Greater Noida, UP, KSRCE (Autonomous) Institution, Tamilnadu, India, and Institute of Technology & Science, Ghaziabad, UP, India. He is a member of ACM and a senior member of IEEE. He has attended an orientation program at UGC-Academic Staff College, University of Kerala, Thiruvananthapuram, Kerala & Refresher course at Indian Institute of Information Technology, Allahabad, UP, India. He has authored or co-authored more than 50 research articles published in various journals, books, and conference proceedings. He has edited or co-edited 14 books and Conference Proceedings in soft computing. He received Ph.D. in Computer Science and Engineering from Anna University, Chennai, India, in 2017, and ME, MCA from Maharishi Dayanand University, Rohtak, Haryana, India, in 2007 and 2004 respectively, and a bachelor's degree in Science from JLN Government College, Faridabad Haryana, India in 2001. He is the book series editor of *Internet of Everything (IoE): Security and Privacy Paradigm*, CRC Press, Taylor & Francis Group, USA; *Artificial Intelligence (AI): Elementary to Advanced Practices Series*, CRC Press, Taylor & Francis Group,

USA; *IT, Management & Operations Research Practices*, CRC Press, Taylor & Francis Group, USA; *Bio-Medical Engineering: Techniques and Applications* with Apple Academic Press, USA and *Computational Intelligence and Management Science Paradigm*, (Focus Series) CRC Press, Taylor & Francis Group, USA. He is editor-in-chief of the *International Journal of Machine Learning and Networked Collaborative Engineering* (IJMLNCE) ISSN 2581-3242; *International Journal of Hyperconnectivity and the Internet of Things* (IJHIoT), ISSN 2473-4365, IGI-Global, USA, co-editor *Ingenieria Solidaria Journal* ISSN (2357-6014), associate editor in *International Journal of Information Retrieval Research* (*IJIRR*), IGI-GLOBAL, USA, ISSN: 2155-6377 I E-ISSN: 2155-6385. He has been a guest editor with IGI-Global, USA, InderScience & many more publishers.

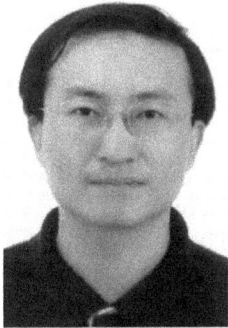

Professor Cheng-Chi Lee received a Ph.D. degree in Computer Science from National Chung Hsing University (NCHU), Taiwan, in 2007. He is currently a distinguished professor with the Department of Library and Information Science at Fu Jen Catholic University. Dr. Lee is currently an editorial board member of *Mathematics, Electronics, International Journal of Network Security, Journal of Computer Science, Cryptography, Future Internet, International Journal of Internet Technology and Secured Transactions, Journal of Library and Information Studies, Journal of InfoLib and Archives*, and guest editor of *Sensors and Electronics*. He also served as a reviewer in many SCI-index journals, other journals, and other conferences. His research interests include data security, cryptography, network security, mobile communications and computing, and wireless communications. Dr. Lee has published over 200 scientific articles in international journals and conferences on the above research fields. He is a member of IEEE, the Chinese Cryptology and Information Security Association (CCISA), the Library Association of The Republic of China, and the ROC Phi Tau Phi Scholastic Honor Society.

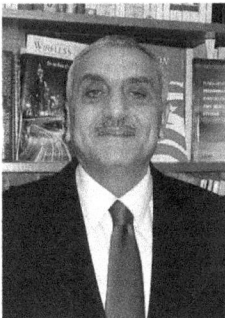

Professor Mohammad S. Obaidat (Fellow of IEEE, Fellow of SCS, and Fellow of AAIA) is an internationally known academic/researcher/scientist/scholar. He received his Ph.D. degree in Computer Engineering with a minor in Computer Science from The Ohio State University, Columbus, USA. He has received extensive research funding and published about Thousand and Two Hundred (1,200) refereed technical articles to date. About half are journal articles, over 100 books, and about 70 book chapters. He is the editor-in-chief of three scholarly journals and an editor of many other international journals. He is the founding Editor-in-Chief of *Wiley Security and Privacy Journal*. Moreover, he is the founder or co-founder of five International Conferences.

Among his previous positions is advisor to the president of Philadelphia University for Research, Development and Information Technology, president and chair of the board of directors of the Society for Molding and Simulation International, SCS, senior vice president of SCS, dean of the College of Engineering at Prince Sultan University, chair, and tenured professor at the Department of Computer and Information Science and director of the MS Graduate Program in Data Analytics at Fordham University, chair and tenured professor of the Department of Computer Science and Director of the Graduate Program at Monmouth University, tenured full professor at King Abdullah II School of Information Technology, University of Jordan, founding dean and professor, College of Computing and Informatics at The University of Sharjah, UAE. He is also The PR of China Ministry of Education Distinguished Overseas Professor at the University of Science and Technology Beijing, China, and an Honorary Distinguished Professor at the Amity University – A Global University. In addition, he is now a distinguished professor at the Indian Institute of Technology-Dhanbad.

He has chaired numerous (Over 180) international conferences and has given numerous (Over 180) keynote speeches worldwide. He has served as ABET/CSAB evaluator and on IEEE CS Fellow Evaluation Committee. He has served as IEEE CS Distinguished Speaker/Lecturer and an ACM Distinguished Lecturer. Since 2004 has been serving as an SCS Distinguished Lecturer. He received many best paper awards for his papers, including ones from IEEE ICC, IEEE Globecom, AICSA, CITS, SPECTS, and DCNET International conferences. He also received Best Paper awards from *IEEE Systems Journal* in 2018 and in 2019 (2 Best Paper Awards). In 2020, he received four best paper awards from *IEEE Systems Journal*. In 2021, he also received the IEEE Systems best paper award. In 2021, he was ranked by Guide2Research as the Number 1 Computer Scientist in UAE in terms of the Number of Publications. He has received many best paper awards from IEEE International Conferences.

He also received many other worldwide awards for his technical contributions, including The 2018 IEEE ComSoc-Technical Committee on Communications Software Technical Achievement Award for contribution to Cybersecurity, Wireless Networks, Computer Networks, and Modeling and Simulation, SCS prestigious McLeod Founder's Award, Presidential Service Award, SCS Hall of Fame—Lifetime Achievement Award for his technical contribution to modeling and simulation and for his outstanding visionary leadership and dedication to increasing the effectiveness and broadening the applications of modeling and simulation worldwide. He also received the SCS Outstanding Service Award. He was awarded the IEEE CITS Hall of Fame Distinguished and Eminent Award. In recognition of his significant scientific contribution, Springer published in Feb 2022 a book honoring his contributions to Computing, Informatics, Networking, and Cybersecurity. It is entitled: *Advances in Computing, Informatics, Networking, and Cybersecurity—A Book Honoring Professor Mohammad S. Obaidat's Significant Scientific Contributions*. He is a fellow of IEEE, a Fellow of SCS, and a Fellow of AAIA.

Contributors

Muyideen Abdulraheem
University of Ilorin
Ilorin, Kwara State, Nigeria

Oluyemi Paul Adejumo
Federal University of Technology
Akure, Nigeria

Adebowale Joseph Adelakun
Federal University of Technology
Akure, Nigeria

Emmanuel Abidemi Adeniyi
Precious Cornerstone University
Ibadan, Nigeria

Abasiama Godwin Akpan
Evangel University
Akaeze, Nigeria

Christopher Akinyemi Alabi
Air Force Institute of Technology
Kaduna, Nigeria

Boniface Kayode Alese
Federal University of Technology
Akure, Nigeria

Adam A. Alli
Islamic University in Uganda
Mbale, Uganda

Olufunso Dayo Alowolodu
Federal University of Technology
Akure, Nigeria

Joseph Bamidele Awotunde
University of Ilorin
Ilorin, Kwara State, Nigeria

Yu Chen
Binghamton University—
    State University of
    New York
Binghamton, New York, USA

Ajimah Nnabueze Edmund
Air Force Institute of Technology
Kaduna, Nigeria

Victoria Nnaemeka Ezeano
Evangel University
Akaeze, Nigeria

Mugigayi Fahadi
Islamic University in Uganda
Mbale, Uganda

Khairul Eahsun Fahim
ZNRF University of Management
    Sciences
Bangladesh

Peace Busola Falola
Precious Cornerstone University
Ibadan, Nigeria

Ebun Philip Fasina
University of Lagos
Lagos, Nigeria

Arome Junior Gabriel
Federal University of Technology
Akure, Nigeria

Vitalis Afebuame Iguoba
Dangote Cement PLC
Obajana, Lokoja, Kogi State,
    Nigeria

Agbotiname Lucky Imoize
University of Lagos
Akoka, Lagos, Nigeria
and
Ruhr University
Bochum, Germany

Rasheed Gbenga Jimoh
University of Ilorin
Ilorin, Kwara State, Nigeria

Kassim Kalinaki
Islamic University in Uganda (IUIU)
Mbale, Uganda

Pablo Rodríguez de León
Benemérita Universidad Autónoma de
   Aguascalientes
Aguascalientes, México

Geofery Luntsi
University of Maiduguri
Maiduguri, Nigeria

Nambobi Mutwalibi
Islamic University in Uganda
Mbale, Uganda

Flavious Bobuin Nkubli
University of Maiduguri
Maiduguri, Nigeria

Anayo Christian Okwor
Evangel University
Akaeze, Nigeria

Idowu Dauda Oladipo
University of Ilorin
Ilorin, Kwara State, Nigeria

J. Andrew Onesimu
Manipal Academy of Higher Education
Manipal, India

Fergus Uchenna Onu
Ebonyi State University
Abakaliki, Nigeria

Akihiko Ohsuga
The University of
   Electro-Communications
Chōfu, Tokyo, Japan

Ambili Parathra Sreedharan Pillai
REVA University
Bangalore, Karnataka, India

Qian Qu
Binghamton University SUNY
Binghamton, USA

Adewole Usman Rufai
University of Lagos
Lagos, Nigeria

Aishat Titilola Rufai
University of Lagos
Akoka, Lagos, Nigeria

Tanko Daniel Salka
Air Force Institute of Technology
Kaduna, Nigeria

Yuichi Sei
The University of
   Electro-Communications
Chōfu, Tokyo, Japan

Eunice Esther Ponce de León Sentí
Benemérita Universidad Autónoma de
   Aguascalientes
Aguascalientes, México

Wasswa Shafik
University Brunei Darussalam
Gadong, Brunei
and
Digital Connectivity Research
   Laboratory (DCRLab)
Kampala, Uganda

Ahmad Tasnim Siddiqui
Babu Banarasi Das University
Lucknow, India

Aurora Torres Soto
Benemérita Universidad Autónoma de
Aguascalientes
Aguascalientes, México

María Dolores Torres Soto
Benemérita Universidad Autónoma de
Aguascalientes
Aguascalientes, México

Manisha Srivastava
Sherwood College of Professional
Management
Lucknow, India

Vishal Srivastava
International Institute of Special Education
Lucknow, India

Han Sun
Binghamton University—State
University of New York
Binghamton, New York, USA

Aderonke Favour-Bethy Thompson
Federal University of Technology
Akure, Nigeria

Oluwaseun Olayinka Tooki
Air Force Institute of Technology
Kaduna, Nigeria

Charles Onuwa Uwadia
University of Lagos
Lagos, Nigeria

Magombe Yasin
Islamic University in Uganda
Mbale, Uganda

Carlos Ochoa Zezzatti
Universidad Autónoma de Ciudad
Juárez
Cuidad Juárez, México

1 An Overview of AIoMT Applications

Han Sun and Yu Chen

1.1 INTRODUCTION

The Internet of Things (IoT) is gaining worldwide acceptance as a new technology that can connect to any network or service anytime, anywhere [1]. It can realize the data exchange between smart devices and the cloud by integrating the existing Internet infrastructure to utilize resources correctly. Thanks to technological processes in communication and hardware, IoT gradually realizes automation in multiple application scenarios, such as traffic congestion control, smart city, security, emergency services, industrial management, and healthcare.

Before the application of IoT in healthcare or medicine, patients and medical staff usually communicated by calling, texting, or face-to-face. In these traditional scenarios, doctors and hospitals cannot track patients' emergencies on time. The lack of smart devices and infrastructure makes it hard to monitor long-term health status. All this has changed after the gradual improvement of the Internet of Medical Things (IoMT). Specifically, the IoMT is the application of the fundamentals, principles, tools, techniques, and concepts of the well-recognized Internet approach, particularly for the medical and healthcare sectors and domains [2]. It can be used in daily healthcare monitoring and save data for future analysis. It can reduce the overall workload and makes timely alarm and long-term tracking possible.

An IoMT-based healthcare application is a collection of smart devices typically includes data collection, Data transmission, and Decision Making. Firstly, health-related data will be collected through sensors such as wearables, remotes, and implants connected to body sensor networks (BSN). Then, the data will be uploaded to the processing center through communication among devices and the cloud for further analysis. With the development of computing and storage capabilities, in some cases, the data will be able to be stored and processed locally. Finally, a data analyzing system can deal with the current situation after receiving data. The system can use the intelligent application to call for help or require other medication suggestions in emergencies. These data will also be stored for long-term health condition analysis.

IoMT can be roughly divided into indoor and outdoor application scenarios [3]. Indoor applications pay more attention to cooperation between multiple devices and store data to prepare for long-term analysis while achieving the short-term goal of timely alerting. Considering the battery and communication limitations of mobile devices, the target of the outdoor application is usually focused on handling emergencies on single devices, such as smart-watch-based falling detection. Although

DOI: 10.1201/9781003370321-1

each application is from a different perspective, the purpose of these applications is to build a more convenient medical system.

1.1.1. KEY CONTRIBUTIONS OF THE CHAPTER

The following are the key contributions of this chapter:

1. This chapter examines some existing IoMT applications, noting their advantages in information fusion, data analysis, and decision making.
2. In general, the significant challenges and prospects of the IoMT to the existing medical field are discussed.
3. Take the seniors' safety as a case study, using deep learning a Multi-sensor Action Recognition-based Senior falling detection (MARS) system is proposed, and the system's effectiveness is proved according to the experiment result.

1.1.2. CHAPTER ORGANIZATION

Section 1.2 presents the background of IoMT by introducing a typical IoMT structure. Section 1.3 shows how IoMT can continuously monitor healthcare information in indoor and outdoor scenarios, including information fusion, data analysis, and decision-making. Section 1.4 demonstrates a case study on senior healthcare monitoring and the application process is presented. Section 1.5 explains the future direction of IoMT applications based on current challenges. Finally, Section 1.6 concludes the chapter.

1.2. RELATED WORK

Although some researchers have proposed a multi-layer structure, the most widely accepted IoMT system is typically a three-layer architecture: the Sensor layer, Edge layer, and Server Layer, as shown in Figure 1.1.

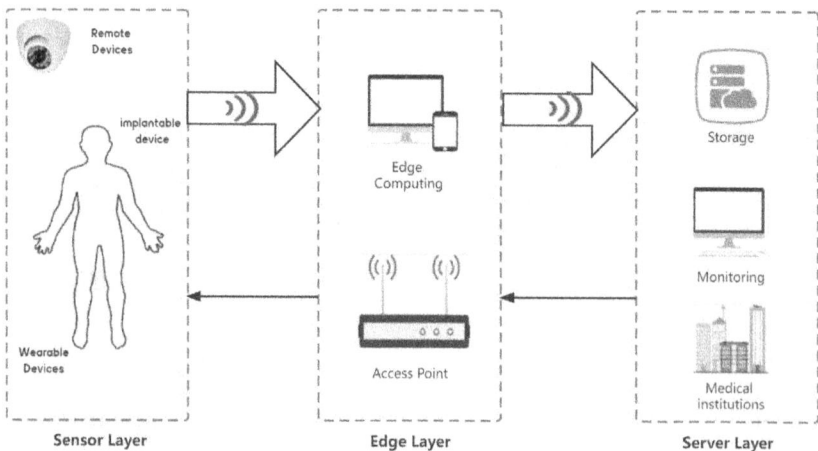

FIGURE 1.1   Illustration of a Three-Layer IoMT Architecture.

1.2.1 SENSOR LAYER

The sensor layer includes various sensors that acquire data from the human body and the environment. These sensors can be divided into three categories according to different acquisition methods:

1. *Remote Sensors*: Sensors that are not in direct contact with the human body, instead, they work remotely to collect the human body and environmental data, such as cameras and room temperature monitoring.
2. *Wearable Sensors*: Sensors attached to the surface of the human body usually have one or more points of contact with the human body. These sensors range from single-purpose, such as electrocardiogram monitoring devices, to multi-purpose, such as smartwatches.
3. *Implantable device*: Sensors placed in the body, such as a pacemaker.

Among these types of sensors, implantable devices are not only rare in number but also require professional doctor assistance, so they are generally not considered. Because it is close to the human body, the data collected by wearable devices will be more accurate, but wearable devices face battery life issues. The balance between continuous battery power and gathering as much data as possible is an issue. Remote sensors usually have a stable power supply, but the distance between the sensors and the human body will reduce the accuracy of the data by including more noise. Therefore, multiple sensors will work collaboratively to acquire data from different angles in real applications. The output of this layer is the collected data, such as the Electrocardiogram (ECG), Electroencephalogram (EEG), photoplethysmographic (PPG), gait, and three-dimensional dynamic data. Table 1.1 shows examples of different sensors for various purposes.

1.2.2 EDGE LAYER

According to the location where the decision-making process is executed, devices at this layer can be divided into two categories: gateway and edge devices for computing.

The traditional approach is to put computing in the cloud. In that case, the second layer usually consists of only a gateway to transmit the pre-processed data to the cloud. These preliminary processes may include noise reduction and adding information such

TABLE 1.1
Sensor Layer

Ref	Year	Sensors Type	Data Type	Category
[4]	2016	Blood Glucose Monitoring	Glycemic	Wearable
[5]	2017	Respiration Sensor	Breathing Rate	Wearable
[6]	2019	ECG sensors & Glucose Monitoring	ECG & Glycemic	Wearable
[7]	2019	Temperature Sensor	Body Temperature	Wearable
[8]	2020	PPG & Heart Rate & ECG	Heart Pulse	Wearable
[9]	2021	Skeleton Image	3DJoint Coordinates	Remote

as location and time [10]. This layer's existence ensures the system's sustainability and the mobility of nodes. Some systems will add functions to this layer to ensure that medical data resume upload when the network connection is interrupted and reconnected [11].

However, with the development of hardware technology, edge devices' increasingly powerful computing and storage capabilities make edge computing achievable [12]. These edge devices can be intelligent terminals, such as a smartwatch, a mobile phone, or an integrated chip for family health. In this design, the edge layer assumes most of the application's functions, and data processing and decision-making are all completed at this layer. Since the output is the decision only, the data transmitted to the next layer will be significantly smaller than the first design. However, the hardware requirement for edge devices will be much higher than for cloud computing.

1.2.3 SERVER LAYER

The server layer, composed of one or more high-performance data centers, centralizes all the data transmitted from the first two layers. Through the analysis of these data, it can realize various functions, including patient control and remote diagnosis [2]. In addition to timely emergency alarms, long-term storage of past health records can help medical staff take the patient's physical condition into consideration. In particular, by placing the computation and decision-making on the edge, the computing resource of the server can be released to support more complex systems, such as the management system of large hospitals [13].

1.2.4 COMMUNICATION

In addition to the three-layer structure, communication is essential so that some structural descriptions will list communication as a separate layer and the architecture is described as a four-layer system [14]. Its first layer collects data by applying Wireless Body Sensor Network (WBSN). The signals, such as ECG collected by the device directly attached to the body, are transmitted to the next layer through the wireless 802.15.6 protocol. The second layer is called the Smart\wireless technology interface tier (tier 2), where all kinds of data are integrated and ready for transmission. The third layer is the infrastructure internet tier, which bridges the edge and server layers. The final tier is the Care-Services tier (tier 4): complete with data storage, analysis, and forward for further service.

The communication or network layer provides various platforms, interface-related services, and data transmission technologies. It uses various communication methods to transmit messages between multiple layers. While ensuring the accuracy of message transmission, it also considers the devices' real-time performance and power consumption. Table 1.2 summarizes the most commonly used protocols for communication. Commonly used communication methods are as follows.

1.2.4.1 Cellular Network

A cellular network, also known as a mobile network, is a mobile communication hardware architecture divided into an analog cellular network and a digital cellular network. By using multiple smaller emitters rather than one large emitter, it is best suited for applications requiring an extremely high data rate. The network technologies based on cellular communication include 3G, 4G, 5G, and GSM. These communication methods can provide a high rate of data exchange when connected to the Internet but require higher power consumption. A GSM module is applied for the communication of multiple sensors and the Arduino is used as the edge device [15].

1.2.4.2   Wi-Fi

Wi-Fi is an acronym referring to the IEEE 802.11x series of standards. It is the most popular wireless communication technology that works with a wide range, which can reach 100 meters indoors. Wi-Fi is more pervasive and easier to deploy than many other communication technologies. What needs to be noted when using Wi-Fi in an IoT environment is its higher power consumption [16]. Furthermore, it is highly susceptible to noise interference and channel blockage. However, due to the higher bandwidth that can be used, Wi-Fi is more suitable for transmitting large data such as audio and video. Especially in the design of Smart-home, wifi is the first choice. With all the sensors being Wi-Fi enabled, the data can be uploaded to the server automatically without human interaction [17].

1.2.4.3   Bluetooth Low Energy

BLE is a personal area network technology designed and marketed by the Bluetooth Special Interest Group [18]. It is intended for emerging applications in healthcare, sports and fitness, security, and home entertainment. Compared to classic Bluetooth, BLE significantly reduces power consumption and cost while maintaining the same communication range. Although these attractive features are obtained at the cost of a lower frequency of data transferring, BLE is promising for healthcare applications because IoMT itself does not require extremely high data exchange rates. Remote Health Monitoring is one of the most common application scenarios for communication among sensors and edge devices [19].

1.2.4.4   Zigbee

Zigbee is a low-speed, short-distance transmission protocol that is applicable to small-scale wireless communication-based control and automation, which saves computer equipment and wired cables between a series of digital devices [20]. It is very safe and efficient and can transfer large amounts of data in a short time. A ZigBee gateway can theoretically connect more than 65,000 devices and form a stable network of more than 100 devices in practical applications [21]. The scale of such a network has far exceeded that of others, which makes it efficient in multiple-sensor fusion. However, Zigbee is less popular than the previous ones, and its promotion in daily use is a problem.

1.3.   APPLICATIONS

With the fast development of hardware equipment and machine learning (ML) technology, the scope of IoMT applications is gradually expanding from personal health management to large-scale hospital management [13]. Not only can the decision be made for both short- and long-term situations, but the corresponding predictions can also be made through data collection and analysis. IoMT can be divided into indoor and outdoor application scenarios in practical applications [3]. Indoor applications can leverage more sensors because devices are connected directly to the power supply. The application can achieve the short-term goal of timely alerting while storing data for long-term analysis through cooperation among multiple devices. Meanwhile, considering the battery and communication constraints of mobile devices, the goals of outdoor applications usually focus on handling emergencies on a single device, such as smart watch-based fall detection. A more detailed application list is shown in Table 1.2.

TABLE 1.2
Application List

Ref	Year	Sensors	Data Type	Purpose
[36]	2015		blood pressure, temperature, and heart rate.	Remote healthcare monitoring
[37]	2015	Smart-phone, wearable sensors	Heart Rate, blood pressure, Body Temperature	Cardiac Status Monitoring
[38]	2016	Mattress	Body weight	Patient Posture to Measure sleep states
[39]	2016	Brain sensors	EEG	Autism patient monitoring
[40]	2016	IMU (Inertial Measurement Unit)	3D-accelerometer	Fall detection
[41]	2017	Temperature sensor, Heart Rate	Heart Rate, Body Temperature	Cardiac Status Monitoring and Alert
[42]	2017		Blood Pressure, Heart pulse	Disease Prediction
[33]	2018	Temperature, Heartbeat, ECG, Accelerometer		Remote healthcare monitoring and prediction
[6]	2019	ECG and continuous Glucose	ECG, Glucose	Type-2 Diabetes monitoring
[24]	2019	Wearable sensors on leg	3D accelerometer	Fall detection
[25]	2019	12-force resistors sensors on pillow	Pressure	Sleep status Monitoring and Seizure control
[28]	2019	EEG	EEG	Seizure Control
[31]	2019	light sensor, PIR motion sensor, microphone, etc		Human Behavior prediction
[43]	2020			Hospital management
[8]	2020	Pulse rate, body temperature, Heartbeat	PPG, Body Temperature, ECG	Remote healthcare monitoring
[35]	2021			Covid-19 first aid treatment
[44]	2021	Chips and nano sensors	Blood pressure, pulse and ECG	Remote healthcare monitoring

TABLE 1.2 *(Continued)*
Application List

Ref	Year	Sensors	Data Type	Purpose
[23]	2021	Camera	Image	Fall detection
[30]	2021	EEG	Brainwave	Emotion recognition and control
[45]	2022	Camera	Body pose Information	Fall Detection
[46]	2022		CT Image	Ovarian cancer distinction
[22]	2022	Flexible biosensor patch	Temperature, blood pressure (BP), ECG	Remote Healthcare monitoring
[32]	2022		EEG	Brain responsiveness in unconscious

1.3.1 Continuous Health Monitoring

Continuous health tracking is the most commonly used and classic application of IoMT, which consists of a wide spectrum from the record and analysis of body data in a healthy state to the state management of chronic diseases can be counted as this category [22].

1.3.1.1 Falling Detections

For seniors, especially those who live alone, even if there is no health problem, falling is a fatal threat, not to mention that most seniors already have disease problems. There is currently much new research on this topic. In an intelligent real-time camera-based fall detection using support vector machines, data can be extracted from surveillance footage by classifying video clips [23]. There are also new advances in fall detection using wearable devices. For example, a recently introduced system can distinguish between daily activities and falls using the three-dimensional acceleration collected by sensors attached to the legs [24].

1.3.1.2 Sleep Monitoring

The focus of sleep detection is not only on sleep quality but, more importantly, the detection of sleep disorders, a common high-incidence health problem [25]. To develop an effective sleep detection system, the first consideration is what kind of physiological signals the system will detect. A unique requirement for sleep detection systems is that most of the sensors are hidden in mattresses or pillows [25] to collect respiratory rate and body movement during sleep as much as possible without affecting sleep quality.

1.3.1.3 Chronic Disease Monitoring

Another application area for continuous health tracking is chronic disease monitoring. Chronic diseases usually refer to conditions that cannot be cured temporarily but can be controlled, such as high blood pressure, low blood sugar, and some heart diseases [6]. Continuation of IoMT assistance will ultimately reduce patient costs and lower the hospital workload. For example, a clear indicator of diabetes is a high level of blood sugar. Therefore, with a blood glucose meter that works continuously 24/7, the system can timely generate an alarm when abnormal blood sugar is detected [26]. At the same time, to exclude the influence of other factors, other signals (e.g., ECG signal) are also introduced into the system for auxiliary analysis [27].

1.3.1.4 Seizure Detections

Seizure is a neurological disorder with recurring seizures caused by sudden electrical disturbances in the brain. Epilepsy detection is a particular case in action recognition. In addition to falling, epilepsy may also cause confusion, memory loss, and other situations that appear to be normal. Currently, the system based on motion recognition cannot make accurate judgments [28]. Thus, more sensors, such as EEG, need to be introduced. The system monitors the patient's condition by continuously processing neural signals acquired from EEG sensors. The aforementioned smart pillow may also be used for epilepsy detection [25].

1.3.1.5 Anxiety Monitoring

The fast pace of modern society makes many people very anxious, and stress has become a common phenomenon in people's daily life. Especially, during the period of the COVID-19 pandemic, preliminary research has shown a slight increase in anxiety disorders among those who recover [29]. Since mental emotions are often reflected in biological data, IoMT is also applied to detect anxiety continuously. One of the most commonly used signals for emotional detection is EEG. Through real-time analysis and upload of EEG signals, the system can detect abnormalities in users and contact them in time [30].

1.3.2 Healthcare-Related Prediction

1.3.2.1 Disease Prediction

Introducing deep learning (DL) technology into IoMT systems is not only for detections but more importantly, machine learning can make predictions for future situations. The health status can be predicted to a certain extent by analyzing the features and patterns from previous data and comparing them with the analysis based on big data [31]. However, the application of prediction encounters more challenges than the application of detection. One of the top concerned issues is the lack of a comprehensive database and the prediction accuracy is based on large-scale data [22]. But it is nontrivial to collect medical data because of many factors, including government rules, insurance policies, and privacy concerns from the patients. Second, each individual's health status is different, and the natural forecast environment still needs many adjustments [32].

Although facing many challenges, there is still progress made in disease prediction [22, 32]. By collecting and checking four biological parameters (body temperature, heartbeat, ECG, and posture), a recently reported system adopts the SVM algorithm to make a prediction and then sends the prediction result together with all the data to the doctor for a final decision [33]. Predictions based on fuzzy theory work well too, as disease outcomes are inherently uncertain [34].

1.3.2.2 Behavior Prediction

Behavior prediction refers to predicting the task action in the future state through the current unfinished action, which is an extension of action recognition research. In the field of IoMT, the purpose of behavior prediction is to warn in advance to avoid greater harm [31].

1.3.3 E-MEDICAL HEALTHCARE

The Covid-19 pandemic has prompted the rapid development of online medical consultations, which not only reduce the delay but also protect both doctors and patients by less contact. Although some diseases still require surgery and actual in-person examination, online consultation can divert people in advance and complete information entry in advance [35]. Drug distribution and reminders can also be incorporated into the smart hospital system through cooperation with the hospital system.

1.4. CASE STUDY: DEEP LEARNING-BASED FALLING DETECTION FOR SENIORS LIVING ALONE

According to the U.S. Census Bureau report, as of 2021, there have been more than 56 million adults over 65 in the United States, accounting for about 16.9% of the national population [47]. As the aging population continues to grow, remote care has become increasingly important for safety. Because of issues such as age and limited mobility, safety is prioritized over health issues such as falls and loss of consciousness [24]. In addition to emergencies such as falls, other specific behavioral manifestations, such as headaches, chest pains, stumbling, vomiting, etc., can also be seen as external manifestations of some chronic diseases [48]. The timely detection and alarm of these abnormal behaviors can not only save lives but also lay the foundation for long-term analysis. Therefore, taking the seniors' safety as a case study, a Multi-sensor Action Recognition-based Senior falling detection (MARS) system is introduced and analyzed in this section.

1.4.1 RELATED WORK

1.4.1.1 Machine-Learning-based Action Detection Methods

From the technical perspective, the current human activity monitoring solutions can be roughly divided into two categories based on the data source: wearable devices and image processing [1].

Falls can be detected by building models based on collected data, which includes falls and regular movements. A data set was collected with 24 test subjects wearing accelerometers, including five young people and 19 older people over 60 years old [49]. In this data set, ten accidental falls were included. Many studies have achieved good results in the action recognition of multi-sensor cooperation [50]. However, the data acquisition is different due to the various sensor locations, which makes the monitoring results of the model inconsistent. It is worth noting that in most of the research, the monitoring is processed offline, which makes the real-time performance of the system unsatisfactory. In addition, the actions that can be recognized are highly constrained by the collected database, which is often limited.

Action recognition based on vision deals with data acquired from cameras located in predetermined places. For example, the living room is usually the most frequently used area in a home environment of everyday activity. Therefore, it is possible to obtain information by installing a camera in the living room in advance. The captured human movements are intelligently analyzed through video or image sequences. In a multi-person action recognition system based on deep learning [51], after combining various algorithms based on an inflected 3D convolutional neural network (3DCNN), the system includes multiple functions such as character recognition, tracking, and action recognition.

1.4.1.2 Skeleton Features Extraction

3D skeleton images can be quickly acquired through depth cameras. Each point of the skeleton image represents the position of the joints of the human body at one moment. Recently, HAR technology based on depth information has developed rapidly in many fields, such as smart homes, games, and human-computer interaction [52]. Skeleton images are less susceptible to appearance factors compared to RGB images.

Human motion information can be represented by a schematic model composed of limbs, a head, and a torso. The parameters of the skeletal image represent the current state of the point, as shown in Figure 1.2. In skeleton-based 3D action representations, actions are collections of 3D position-time sequences. However, HAR processing that relies only on the joint coordinate model might suffer low accuracy because of the differences in the reference frame and recording environment and between different human motion styles [23]. Therefore, many other bone matrix representation methods are introduced. For example, normalization is done based on the length of the shoulders and torso [50], with the new coordinate system centered on the hip joint [53].

1.4.3 MARS System—Methodology

The complete algorithm flow of the proposed MARS system is shown in Figure 1.3. In the Sensor layer, the Kinect V2 camera is set up as the remote sensor. It can directly get skeleton information without any additional processes. After transmitting the skeleton data to the edge device for data processing and decision-making. Finally, the result will be uploaded to the server layer. If there is indeed an emergency, the system will call for help. Otherwise, the data will be stored.

1.4.3.1 3D Skeleton Image Feature Extraction

Instead of 206 bones, the Kinect sensor can build a simplified human skeletal model using 20 keypoint information. As shown in Figure 1.2, 20 points are sufficient to

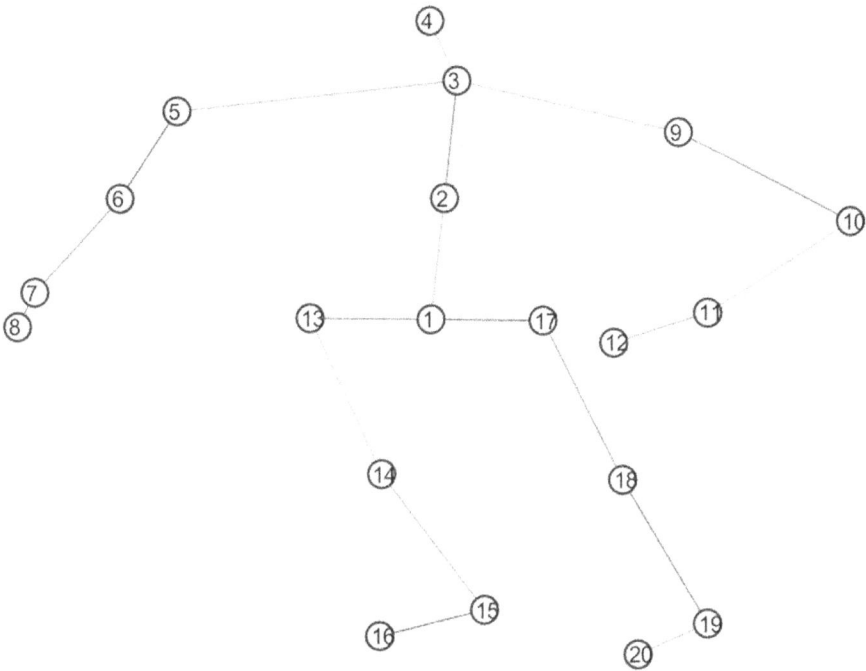

FIGURE 1.2   Figuration of the 20 joints in the skeleton image, The joints are 1. hip center, 2. Middle-spine, 3. shoulder center, 4. Head, 5. Left shoulder, 6. Left elbow, 7. Left wrist, 8. Left-hand, 9. Right-shoulder, 10. Right elbow, 11. Right-wrist, 12. Right-hand, 13.Left-hip, 14. Left knee, 15. Left-ankle, 16. Left-root, 17. Right-hip, 18. Right knee, 19. Right-ankle, 20. Right-foot.

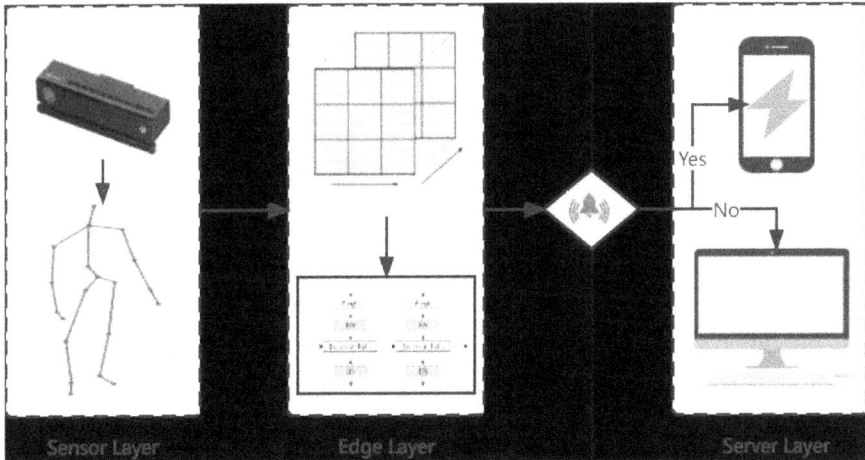

FIGURE 1.3   An overview of the Falling Detection Algorithm.

describe a general human model's motion process in detail. The acquired data is denoted as P (x,y,z), where x and y represent the position of the point in the two-dimensional plane, and the data of z represents the distance from the point to the camera. In the process of action, the part representing the torso remains relatively stable, while the relative motion of the points representing the limbs changes. To better represent the offset of the limb joints relative to the torso and reduce the influence of the z-axis as much as possible, the coordinates of the position points are transferred using the equation:

$$d = p_n - p_{hip} \left(i = 1, 2, 3 ..... n \right) \tag{1.1}$$

This formula calculates the distance from the point (p_n)) other than the hip joint to the hip joint (p_{hip}), thus transforming the entire coordinate system to the center of the hip joint. Another point that may affect the experiment's results is the person's height. The distance between each point will have a gap due to the height difference. In extreme cases, such a gap may cause the system to misjudge an action. Hence, the normalization function is used to correct the data by using the average height of the human body.

1.4.3.2 Independency Recurrent Neural Network-based Action Recognition System

Recurrent Neural Networks (RNN) are a class of deep neural networks that consider the current input and the previous hidden state. To solve the gradient explosion problem of RNN, Independent RNN (IndRNN) [54] has improved the connection layer of simple RNN. The point of independence is that neurons in the same layer do not receive information from their neighbors but only accept hidden information that belongs to themselves at the last T. In IndRNN, neurons do not form a fully-connected layer with each other.

This study uses the IndRNN architecture to complete action recognition. The most significant difference between IndRNN and ordinary RNN is that Hadamard is used in the forgetting function instead of common multiplication. Considering the

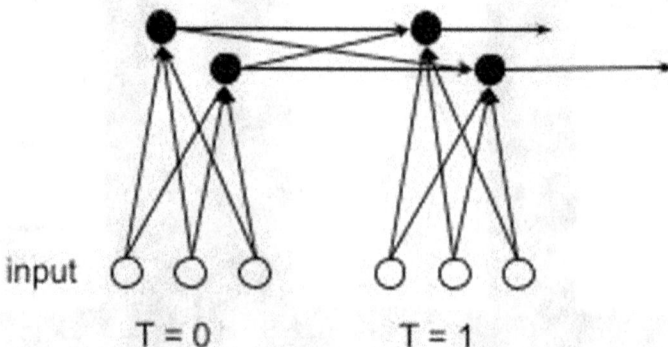

FIGURE 1.4   Difference between Simple RNN and IndRNN

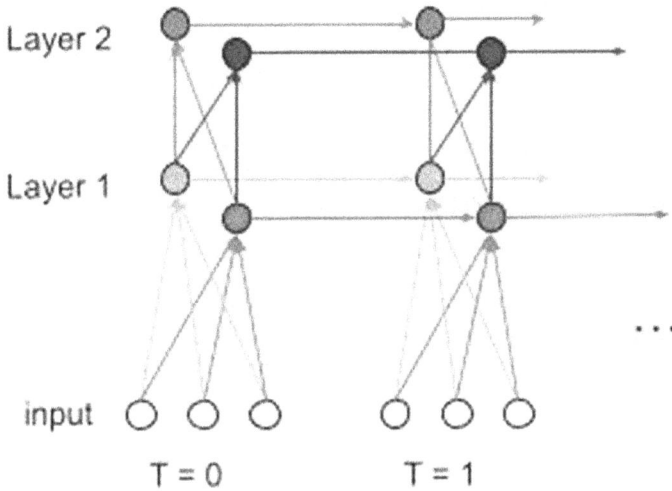

FIGURE 1.4 (Continued)

performance of the Raspberry Pi used as an edge device, only a four-layer IndRNN structure is used this time.

1.4.4 EXPERIMENTAL STUDY

1.4.4.1 Settings

Experimental studies have been conducted to evaluate the proposed action recognition scheme. Training is processed on an Intel i7 NVIDIA GeForce GTX 1080 graphics card under Windows 10. The programming language is python3.8, and PyTorch is used to realize parallel computing.

1.4.4.2 Training Database

The dataset includes 60 actions from 40 subjects. Because three Kinect cameras located in different places were used in the data collection process, each subject's data also included 80 different views. In addition to skeleton data, RGB and depth images can also be used for comparison. The skeleton data contains 3D coordinates of 25 body joints per frame. The last five joints, 21 (spine top), 22 (left-hand tip), 23 (left thumb), 24 (right-hand tip), and 25 (right-hand thumb) are ignored because they represent the end of the limb. It contains too little information to be worth additional consideration.

According to the different division methods, the data sets can be compared from two directions: Based on the subject ID, it can be divided into 40320 training sets and 16560 testing sets, which is called Cross-Subject (CS). On the other hand, based on the camera ID, it can be divided into 37920 for training and 18960 samples for testing, which is called Cross-view (CV). In all datasets, two parts need to be processed separately: there are nine categories of data collected for health-related training that deserve attention and 11 categories that contain multi-person. After removing those categories of multi-person interaction videos, 49 out of 48419 video samples were used for training.

Another advantage of using skeleton images as input is the small data size. After sampling, the skeleton data representing an action is less than 10 Kb. In comparison, the RGB and depth images collected at the same time are 1.88M and 878 Kb, respectively. Almost one percent fewer storage requirements make skeleton images a distinct advantage in edge computing.

1.4.4.3 Results

Table 1.3 compared the proposed MARS system with several other existing methods. Considering that the object of our system is the elderly living alone, only the case of a single skeleton is analyzed in practice. Compared to the results of ST_GCN [55], our accuracy is slightly lower. However, it needs to be considered that the resources in edge computing are limited, and a relatively complex graph convolution process is used [55] to preprocess the data. In smart homes, lightweight but promising motion recognition models should be considered first [9]. The low complexity in feature extraction makes our system suitable for edge computing.

1.5. CHALLENGES AND FUTURE DIRECTIONS

1.5.1 CHALLENGES

Along with the advancement of enabling technologies, the application of IoMT is expanding its influence. There are still many factors restricting the development, such as the lack of standardization among the medical data used in IoMT, how the IoMT itself ensures privacy, etc. At the same time, some non-technical issues are worth considering. For example, research related to medicine requires the participation of many professionals, especially in disease diagnosis.

1.5.1.1 Standardization

The frequency ranges of common biomedical signals are given in Table 1.4.

The frequencies of the various signals used in the system may range from less than ten to several hundred. Therefore, when an application consists of a variety of sensors with different frequencies, synchronization issues need to be considered. No matter which frequency is selected to accommodate, there will be data loss [2]

TABLE 1.3
Results on Database

Algorithm	Year	CV	CS
2-Layer RN[30]	2016	64.1	56.1
2-Layer LSTM[30]	2016	66.8	59.1
ST_GCN[31]	2018	88.84	81.57
4_Layer IndRNN	2021	85.77	80.29
MARS	2022	89.76	79.87

TABLE 1.4
Frequency Ranges of common
Biomedical signals

Signal	Frequency Range (Hz)
PPG	0.5–5
EMG	50–150
Cardiac Auscultation	20–420
Gait Analysis	0–15

1.5.1.2 Security Vulnerability

Security and privacy have always been among the top concerns in the development of IoMT [44]. IoMT handles data that is highly related to personal privacy, and data leaking may cause disastrous consequences to the patients. Data exchange in the application process is carried out through the communication network, so any security issues that may occur in general communication networks also exist in IoMT environments. What makes IoMT security more fatal is that healthcare and telemedicine operations are closely related to personal safety [3]. The authority to handle the reported emergency will determine the life and death of an individual.

1.5.1.3 Medical Image Segmentation and Lack of Database

Machine learning-based IoMT applications require the participation of a large number of professionals and cross-professional corporations. Due to the administration policies and user privacy issues in the telemedicine and e-healthcare domains, health/medical data collection is a non-technologic but significant issue.

1.5.2 FUTURE DIRECTIONS

Despite various challenges and open problems, the performance of IoMT is still remarkable. Research is still in its early stages and there are many directions worth considering:

- *On-Site/Near-Site Solutions.* Due to the limitation of power consumption and computing resources of edge devices, most of the current IoMT applications still put the computing part on the cloud. But solutions that enable the functionality through collaboration between cloud, edge, and fog have begun to grow in recent years [12].
- *Lightweight ML Models.* In continuous monitoring, a local server with a powerful GPU is often the best solution for the high demands of ML [45]. However, lightweight, small, and low-power ML models can optimize the dynamic monitoring problem from another perspective. By reducing the resources required by the model to free up space, the system can cope with more complex requirements.

- *Performance in Resource-Constrained Environments.* Advances in deep learning have made it possible to run under resource constraints [3]. In continuous action recognition, it is worth considering how to obtain better results at low frame rates or resolutions.
- *Novel Applications in the Metaverse Era.* Metaverse is a network of 3D virtual worlds focused on social connections which mainly discusses a persistent and decentralized online 3D virtual environment [56]. It has high performance in remote service, privacy protection, and distributed data storage. Blockchain is considered one of the representative technologies of the Metaverse. In recent years, there have been many IoMT applications based on blockchain, which have discussed data security and distributed storage [34].

1.6   CONCLUSIONS

In this chapter, a detailed review of the start-of-art IoMT application has been represented. By analyzing each layer of a typical IoMT architecture, we sort out the key enabling technologies for IoMT applications. At the same time, a detailed application classification is presented, which shows that the application scenarios of IoMT are vast, ranging from personal health monitoring to prediction and even network-level applications at the social level. Finally, through a case study, we showed an example of the IoMT application for the safety monitoring of seniors living alone. Although IoMT still faces many challenges, including hardware development and security/privacy issues, new technologies, such as the Metaverse, have already opened a promising future for IoMT.

REFERENCES

[1]   Madakam, Somayya, et al. "Internet of things (IoT): A literature review." *Journal of Computer and Communications* 3.05 (2015): 164.
[2]   Ketu, Shwet, and Pramod Kumar Mishra. "Internet of healthcare things: A contemporary survey." *Journal of Network and Computer Applications* 192 (2021): 103179.
[3]   Si-Ahmed, Ayoub, Mohammed Ali Al-Garadi, and Narhimene Boustia. "Survey of machine learning based intrusion detection methods for internet of medical things." *arXiv preprint arXiv:2202.09657* (2022).
[4]   Toschi, E., & Wolpert, H. (2016). Utility of continuous glucose monitoring in type 1 and type 2 diabetes. *Endocrinology and Metabolism Clinics of North America*, 45(4), 895–904.
[5]   Azimi, Hilda, et al. "Breathing signal combining for respiration rate estimation in smart beds." *2017 IEEE International Symposium on Medical Measurements and Applications (MeMeA)*. IEEE, 2017.
[6]   Devarajan, D., Subramaniyaswamy, V., Vijayakumar, V., & Ravi, L. (2019). Fog-assisted personalised healthcare-support system for remote patients with diabetes. *Journal of Ambient Intelligence and Humanized Computing*, 10, 3747–3760. https://doi.org/10.1007/s12652-019-

[7]   Kaur, A., and A. Jasuja. "Health monitoring based on IoT using raspberry pi." *2017 International Conference on Computing, Communication and Automation (ICCCA).* IEEE; 2017, 1335–1340.

[8]   Ruman, Md Raseduzzaman, et al. "IoT based emergency health monitoring system." *2020 International Conference on Industry 4.0 Technology (I4Tech). IEEE, 2020.*

[9]   Wang, Haoran, et al. "Skeleton edge motion networks for human action recognition." *Neurocomputing* 423 (2021): 1–12.

[10] Swayamsiddha, Swati, and Chandana Mohanty. "Application of cognitive internet of medical things for COVID-19 pandemic." *Diabetes & Metabolic Syndrome: Clinical Research & Reviews* 14.5 (2020): 911–915.

[11] Khan, Haider Ali, et al. "IoT based on secure personal healthcare using RFID technology and steganography." *International Journal of Electrical & Computer Engineering (2088–8708)* 11.4 (2021): 3300–3309.

[12] Chen, Jienan, et al. "iRAF: A deep reinforcement learning approach for collaborative mobile edge computing IoT networks." *IEEE Internet of Things Journal* 6.4 (2019): 7011–7024.

[13] Yu, Lei, Yang Lu, and XiaoJuan Zhu. "Smart hospitals based on the internet of things." *Journal of Networks* 7.10 (2012): 1654.

[14] Abdulmohsin Hammood, Dalal, et al. "Body-to-body cooperation in the internet of medical things: Toward energy efficiency improvement." *Future Internet* 11.11 (2019): 239.

[15] Sajjad, Muhammad, Shahryar Shafique Qureshi, and Muhammad Afnan. "IoT based health monitoring system using Arduino Uno." *GSM SIM900D Module and Wifi Module ESP8266* 9 (2018): 16–21.

[16] Pahlavan, Kaveh, and Prashant Krishnamurthy. "Evolution and impact of Wi-Fi technology and applications: A historical perspective." *International Journal of Wireless Information Networks* 28.1 (2021): 3–19.

[17] Linkous, Lauren, Nasibeh Zohrabi, and Sherif Abdelwahed. "Health monitoring in smart homes utilising the internet of things." *2019 IEEE/ACM International Conference on Connected Health: Applications, Systems and Engineering Technologies (CHASE).* IEEE, 2019.

[18] Gomez, Carles, Joaquim Oller, and Josep Paradells. "Overview and evaluation of Bluetooth low energy: An emerging low-power wireless technology." *Sensors* 12.9 (2012): 11734–11753.

[19] Donati, Massimiliano, et al. "A telemedicine service platform exploiting BT/BLE wearable sensors for remote monitoring of chronic patients." *2018 7th International Conference on Modern Circuits and Systems Technologies (MOCAST).* IEEE, 2018.

[20] Alliance, ZigBee. "Zigbee specification: Zigbee document 053474r06 version 1.0." *December 14th (2004).* ZigBee Specification, ZigBee Alliance, http://www.zigbee.org/wp-content/uploads/2014/11/docs-05-3474-20-0csg-zigbee-specification.pdf.

[21] Grigorescu, S. D., et al. "Health monitoring solution using dedicated ZigBee sensor network." *2013 8th International Symposium on Advanced Topics in Electrical Engineering (ATEE).* IEEE, 2013.

[22] Phan, Duc Tri, et al. "A flexible, wearable, and wireless biosensor patch with internet of medical things applications." *Biosensors* 12.3 (2022): 139.

[23] Chen, Yangsen, et al. "Fall detection system based on real-time pose estimation and SVM." *2021 IEEE 2nd International Conference on Big Data, Artificial Intelligence and Internet of Things Engineering (ICBAIE).* IEEE, 2021.

[24] Saadeh, Wala, Saad Adnan Butt, and Muhammad Awais Bin Altaf. "A patient-specific single sensor IoT-based wearable fall prediction and detection system." *IEEE Transactions on Neural Systems and Rehabilitation Engineering* 27.5 (2019): 995–1003.

[25] Siyang, Satetha, Shongpun Lokavee, and Teerakiat Kerdcharoen. "The development of IoT-based non-obstructive monitoring system for human's sleep monitoring." *2019 IEEE International Conference on Consumer Electronics-Taiwan (ICCE-TW).* IEEE, 2019.

[26] Ara, Affreen, and Aftab Ara. "Case study: Integrating IoT, streaming analytics and machine learning to improve intelligent diabetes management systems." *2017 International Conference on Energy, Communication, Data Analytics and Soft Computing (ICECDS).* IEEE, 2017

[27] Sujaritha, M., et al. "An automatic diabetes risk assessment system using IoT cloud platform." *EAI International Conference on Big Data Innovation for Sustainable Cognitive Computing.* Springer, Cham, 2020.

[28] Sayeed, Md Abu, et al. "eSeiz: An edge-device for accurate seizure detection for smart healthcare." *IEEE Transactions on Consumer Electronics* 65.3 (2019): 379–387.

[29] Sundaravadivel, Prabha, Vividha Goyal, and Lakshman Tamil. "i-RISE: An IoT-based semi-immersive affective monitoring framework for anxiety disorders." *2020 IEEE International Conference on Consumer Electronics (ICCE).* IEEE, 2020.

[30] Meng, Weizhi, et al. "Hybrid emotion-aware monitoring system based on brainwaves for the internet of medical things." *IEEE Internet of Things Journal* 8.21 (2021): 16014–16022.

[31] L. Xu and N. Pombo. Human behavior prediction though noninvasive and privacy-preserving internet of things (IoT) assisted monitoring. *2019 IEEE 5th World Forum on Internet of Things (WF-IoT)*, pp. 773–777, 2019.

[32] Nandy, Sudarshan, et al. "IBoNN: Intelligent agent-based internet of medical things framework for detecting brain response from Electroencephalography signal using Bag-of-Neural Network." *Future Generation Computer Systems* 130 (2022): 241–252.

[33] Kamble, Ashvini, and Sonali Bhutad. "IoT based patient health monitoring system with nested cloud security." *2018 4th International Conference on Computing Communication and Automation (ICCCA).* IEEE; 2018.

[34] A. L. Imoize, D. O. Irabor, P. A. Gbadega, and C. Chakraborty, "Blockchain technology for secure COVID-19 pandemic data handling," In *Smart Health Technologies for the COVID-19 Pandemic: Internet of Medical Things Perspectives*, 1st ed., C. Chakraborty and J. J. P. C. Rodrigues, Eds. The Institution of Engineering and Technology, 2022, pp. 141–179.

[35] Sharma, Devansh, Ali Zaid Bin Nawab, and Mansaf Alam. "Integrating M-health with IoMT to counter COVID-19." *Computational Intelligence Methods in COVID-19: Surveillance, Prevention, Prediction and Diagnosis.* Springer, Singapore, 2021. 373–396.

[36] B. Xu, L. Xu, H. Cai, L. Jiang, Y. Luo, and Y. Gu, "The design of an m-Health monitoring system based on a cloud computing platform," Taylor & Francis, 2015.

[37] Kakria, Priyanka, N. K. Tripathi, and Peerapong Kitipawang. "A real-time health monitoring system for remote cardiac patients using smartphone and wearable sensors."

[38] Matar, Georges, et al. "Internet of things in sleep monitoring: An application for posture recognition using supervised learning." *2016 IEEE 18th International Conference on e-Health Networking, Applications and Services (Healthcom).* IEEE, 2016.

[39] Sundhara Kumar, K. B., and Krishna Bairavi. "IoT based health monitoring system for autistic patients." *Proceedings of the 3rd International Symposium on Big Data and Cloud Computing Challenges (ISBCC–16')*. Springer, Cham, 2016.

[40] Chandel, Vivek, et al. "Exploiting IMU sensors for IoT enabled health monitoring." *Proceedings of the First Workshop on IoT-enabled Healthcare and Wellness Technologies and Systems*. 2016, https://doi.org/10.1145/2933566.2933569.

[41] Midhundas Seenia Francis C, and Antony George. Patient monitoring system using raspberry pi. *International Journal of Scientific Research* 6 (2017): 687–689.

[42] Ani, R., et al. "IoT based patient monitoring and diagnostic prediction tool using ensemble classifier." *2017 International Conference on Advances in Computing, Communications and Informatics (ICACCI)*. IEEE, 2017.

[43] Chinmay C., Arij N.A., Intelligent internet of things and advanced machine learning technique for COVID-19, *EAI Endorsed Transactions on Pervasive Health and Technology*, 21(26) 1–14, 2021.

[44] Haque, Rakib Ul, and A. S. M. Hasan. "Privacy-preserving multivariate regression analysis over blockchain-based encrypted IoMT data." *Artificial Intelligence and Blockchain for Future Cybersecurity Applications*. Springer, Cham, 2021. 45–59.

[45] H. Sun and Y. Chen, "Real-time elderly monitoring for senior safety by lightweight human action recognition," *2022 IEEE 16th International Symposium on Medical Information and Communication Technology (ISMICT)*, 2022, pp. 1–6, doi: 10.1109/ISMICT56646.2022.9828343.

[46] Ghazal, Taher M., and Nasser Taleb. "Feature optimization and identification of ovarian cancer using internet of medical things." *Expert Systems* (2022): e12987.

[47] A. on Aging, *A Profile of Older Americans: 2021*. U.S. Department of Health and Human Services, 2021. https://acl.gov/sites/default/files/Aging%20and%20Disability%20in%20America/2019ProfileOlderAmericans508.pdf

[48] Erickson, S. R., B. C. Williams, and L. D. Gruppen. "Relationship between symptoms and health-related quality of life in patients treated for hypertension." *Pharmacotherapy: The Journal of Human Pharmacology and Drug Therapy* 24.3 (2004): 344–350.

[49] Jalal, Ahmad, Md Zia Uddin, and T-S. Kim. "Depth video-based human activity recognition system using translation and scaling invariant features for life logging at smart home." *IEEE Transactions on Consumer Electronics* 58.3 (2012): 863–871.

[50] Aziz, Omar, et al. "Validation of accuracy of SVM-based fall detection system using real-world fall and non-fall datasets." *PLoS One* 12.7 (2017): e0180318.

[51] Carreira, Joao, and Andrew Zisserman. "Quo vadis, action recognition? A new model and the kinetics dataset." *Proceedings of the IEEE Conference on Computer Vision and Pattern Recognition*. IEEE; 2017, pp. 6299–6308.

[52] Jalal, A., M. Z. Uddin, and T.-S. Kim. "Depth video-based human activity recognition system using translation and scaling invariant features for life logging at smart home." *IEEE Transactions on Consumer Electronics* 58.3 (2012): 863–871.

[53] Wei, Ping, et al. "Concurrent action detection with structural prediction." *Proceedings of the IEEE International Conference on Computer Vision (ICCV)*. IEEE; 2013, pp. 3136–3143.

[54] Li, Shuai, et al. "Independently recurrent neural network (IndRNN): Building a longer and deeper RNN." *Proceedings of the IEEE Conference on Computer Vision and Pattern Recognition (CVPR)*. IEEE; 2018, pp. 5457–5466.

[55] Yan, Sijie, Yuanjun Xiong, and Dahua Lin. "Spatial temporal graph convolutional networks for skeleton-based action recognition." *Thirty-Second AAAI Conference on Artificial Intelligence*. 2018, https://doi.org/10.1609/aaai.v32i1.12328.

[56] Shahroudy, Amir, et al. "NTU RGB+ D: A large scale dataset for 3D human activity analysis." *Proceedings of the IEEE Conference on Computer Vision and Pattern Recognition (CVPR)*. IEEE; 2016, pp. 1010–1019.

[57] Petrigna, L., and G. Musumeci. "The metaverse: A new challenge for the healthcare system: A scoping review." *Journal of Functional Morphology and Kinesiology* 7.3 (2022): 63. http://doi.org/10.3390/jfmk7030063. PMID: 36135421; PMCID: PMC9501644.

2 Wearable Medical Electronics in Artificial Intelligence of Medical Things

Wasswa Shafik

2.1 INTRODUCTION

As technology has improved, smart healthcare has changed a lot. It now includes microelectronics, big data, IoT, cloud computing, mobile internet, and mobile health (Nair & Sahoo, 2023). The incorporation of modern medical sensors and different hardware in the health sector has led to the development of a new concept called "IoMT," or sometimes called "the Internet of Health Things," which, along with the aforementioned technologies, has transformed traditional healthcare into a more efficient, all-round, and personalized experience. The global market for smart health is projected to increase by a mean growth rate of 16.2% (Kok, 2023). This creates a dire need for fast, comprehensive, accurate, and intelligent eHealthcare systems, as highlighted by the emergency of global pandemics. Through different medical electronic devices, these systems will be able to collect, analyze, and make sense of a large amount of information about the health and well-being of the patient. Additionally, such systems will provide the means for the periodic management of medical personnel, keeping track of both medical instruments and biological specimens (Bhattarai & Peng, 2023; Deshmukh et al., 2023).

The convergence of IoMT, AI, and big data has added new dimensions to such systems, which are now capable of analyzing the collected data to provide better insights, thereby ushering in a new era in healthcare, such as early-stage chronic disease prediction and personalized and physiological health monitoring systems, among others. Through the IoMT environment, monitoring health can be attained with the aid of numerous wearable medical sensors that record and keep track of patient medical conditions in real time (Shafik et al., 2020; Shafik, 2023). The data produced by such sensors enables medical physicians to reliably and efficiently recognize and respond to critical situations regarding patients to enable them to become more informed regarding their health conditions for future diagnosis and treatment (Mathur et al., 2023). Furthermore, these sensors provide cheaper alternatives to the expensive environment of a hospital as they enable remote detection of abnormalities, evaluation of symptoms, and assessment of the general health of the patients.

The large amount of patient information collected by several devices in the IoMT environment has ushered in new opportunities that leverage the power of AI. Currently known as AI-enabled health, opportunities such as the ability to quickly analyze and interpret patient information, diagnose, and predict future diseases have been reported. Advanced AI techniques have made it possible for medical physicians to remotely track patients' habits and reveal their medical status from the captured data emanating from several sensors along with sensor usage patterns. Through the IoMT environment, AI techniques, for example, support vector machines, random forest, logistic regression, decision trees, k-nearest neighbor, naïve Bayes, and several neural networks have been used for various health-related applications (Irfana Parveen et al., 2023; Narasimharao et al., 2023). Medics, health practitioners, health ministries, and agencies, among others, celebrate and appreciate the integration and application of IoMTs management mainly due to a couple of benefits. Such benefits include patient clinical trials, identification, medication error reduction, personalized medication, and surgery aid.

The IoMT architecture in Figure 2.1 depicts the comprehensive growth of exploiting smart sensors to accumulate data and regulate smart healthcare structures. However, there are notable challenges that face smart healthcare, as discussed. Furthermore, medical institutions rely on internet-based technologies from connected infusion pumps to now telemetry patient monitors, to provide best-in-class patient care. According to (Kok & Setyadi, 2023), they predicted that by 2022, the number of connected medical devices "Things" will reach up to 30 billion. During their study,

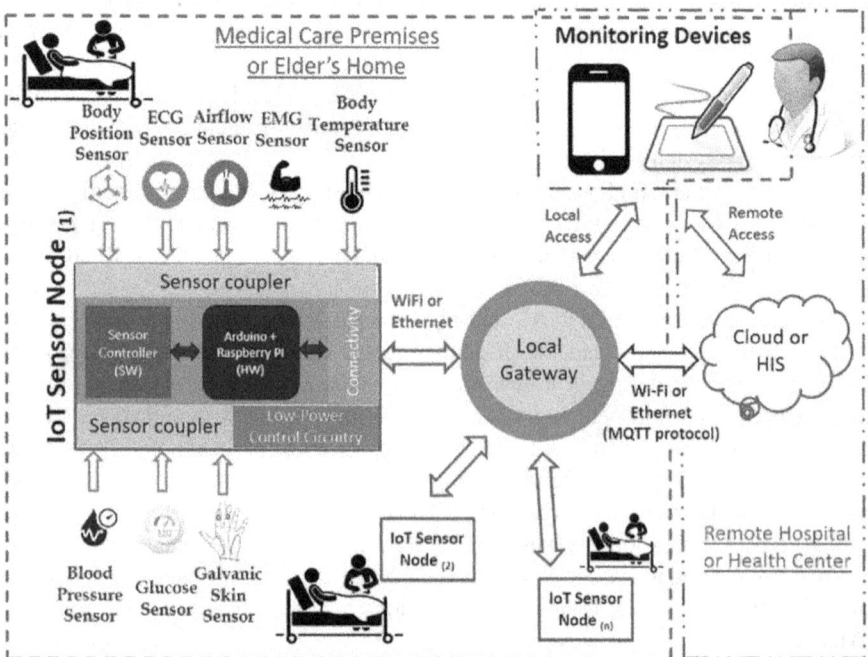

FIGURE 2.1   IoMT architecture with comprehensive growth (Petrellis et al., 2019).

they considered four main health factors that soar with the smart healthcare system, including in homes (like mobile help, vitality, and intelligent clinic, among others), communities (for instance, Xerafy, American Well, and Skytron, among others), clinics, hospitals, and on the body (S. K. Pandey & Pandey, 2023).

Accordingly, it is important for healthcare providers and officials in the healthcare domain to keep track of viral infections to ensure the necessary isolation of patients along with real-time measures to contain infections. In light of current developments, the medical devices that comprise the IoMT and their convergence with AI described earlier have demonstrated tremendous potential in improving the overall health of billions of people worldwide, resulting in improved quality of life (Banday & Bhat, 2023). With the paradigm of AIoMT being new, few studies have been dedicated to detailing the different electronic devices deployed.

2.1.1   KEY CONTRIBUTIONS OF THE CHAPTER

The significant contributions of this chapter are as listed here:

  i. The chapter provides a detailed description of the diverse electronic sensors used in AIoMT in the wider medical industry.
  ii. The different electronic signals transmitted by the different AIoMT sensors are presented.
  iii. The significant challenges and prospects faced in using the identified electronic devices in healthcare have been discussed.
  iv. Some benefits and challenges for the AIoMT are reviewed.
  v. Limitations of AIoMT are presented as well.
  vi. The future research direction of IoMT in the healthcare industry and future scope are depicted.

2.1.2   CHAPTER ORGANIZATION

Section 2.2 presents electronic sensors in IoMT and electronic sensor traits, disposable health sensors, ingestible sensors, patch sensors, connected health sensors, wearables, smart clothing, and implantable sensors. Section 2.3 presents the electronic signals in sensors. Section 2.4 discusses the identified challenges of electronic devices in the AIoMT that include data security threats. Section 2.5 explains the benefits of the AIoMT evaluated. Section 2.6 demonstrates the challenges of evaluated AIoMTs. Section 2.7 demonstrates the future research direction of IoMT in the healthcare industry. Section 2.8 entails the limitation of AIoMT and, lastly, the concluding chapter of AIoMT's future scope is presented in Section 2.9.

2.2   WEARABLE MEDICAL ELECTRONICS

When used in the smart healthcare industry, IoMT combines various processing units with communication technologies, for instance, electronic wireless sensors that remotely monitor patient health status, to enable the prompt transmission of clinical information to healthcare medics (Gupta et al., 2023b). IoMT makes it possible for caregivers to continuously monitor their patient's health, which enhances clinical judgment, lowers patients' medical costs, and ultimately improves patient outcomes. This section presents notable electronic sensor traits related to IoMT applications and presents a brief discussion of the main four commonly used electronic sensor signals.

2.2.1 ELECTRONIC SENSOR TRAITS

As the IoMTs are applied in the medical facility, these electronic sensors show different characteristics, and their contrast causes an impact on the patient. To support its many uses, a plethora of electronic biosensors have been invented and incorporated into the healthcare domain enabled by IoT (Gupta et al., 2023c). Smart home care, clinical diagnostics, preventive medicine, fitness tracking, and a few monitoring services are some of these.

2.2.1.1 Disposable Health Sensors

Diagnostics, patient monitoring, and treatment support are the three main uses for disposable health sensors. The sensors are frequently strip-type, implementable, and ingestible. All these are focused on depending on the patient body nature (Guan et al., n.d.).

2.2.1.2 Ingestible Sensors

The microfabricated integrated circuit for this tiny electronic sensor is made of magnesium, copper, and gold thin layers. As the taken pill enters the stomach, a reaction between the circuit layers and gastric juice occurs. The sensor experiences an electrochemical reaction as a result (Gupta et al., 2023d). The patches of sensors then receive a digital code that denotes the drug type and appropriate dosage along with the time of dosage administration since the sensor is energized by this reaction.

2.2.1.3 Patch Sensors

The patient may monitor their daily activities and medication schedules in appreciation of the transmission of all this data to a smartphone application, which then sends it to the discover portal. Medics and other healthcare professionals can find important data on their patients' daily health reports within the portals to help them choose the most appropriate treatments. By enhancing drug adherence, for instance, authors (Gupta et al., 2023) have reported the Proteus Digital Medicine model, which has transformed the healthcare industry by lowering treatment failure rates and the demand for patient retreatment.

2.2.1.4 Connected Health Sensors

End-use market, electronic sensors, and platform sensors are additional subcategories of connected e-health sensors (Idrees & Khlief, 2023). Wearables, embedded technology, and intrusive sensors are examples of end-use market sensors for IoMT.

2.2.1.5 Wearables

Wearable sensors are continuously worn or put near the human skin to closely keep track of the patient's actions without restricting their usual range of mobility (Gezimati & Singh, 2023). Mobility trackers are an especially well-liked kind of wearable health technology that has several practical uses in other domains such as sports, determining the risk of falling down, and keeping an eye on the senior population, where some devices are demonstrated in Figure 2.2.

2.2.1.6 Smart Clothing

Numerous wearable gadgets have been deployed to measure important aspects of human health in addition to being helpful in encouraging individuals to keep track of daily workouts and sustain a more active and healthier lifestyle. The most typical

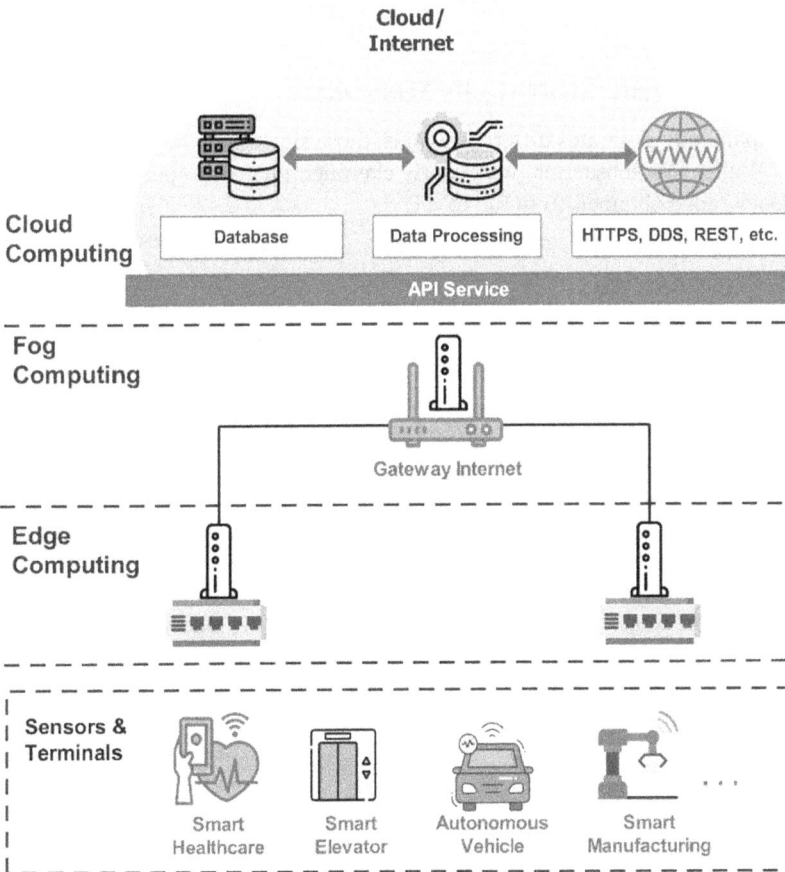

FIGURE 2.2 Current state of computation entailing digital health care (Quy et al., 2022).

of these measurements include electrocardiogram (ECG) and electroencephalogram (EEG) measurements. Body-worn smart gear is one innovative innovation intended to combine wearable sensors with essential health monitoring capabilities (Bhutnal & Moparthi, 2023; Gupta et al., 2023). Compared to current technologies, which frequently only record a small number of physiological data, smart clothing enables people with intermittent illnesses to benefit from several health monitoring systems. Smart clothes substantially decrease the cost of sensors as well, but the efficiency in terms of wireless communication and packet transfer is still not that efficient. A broad review covering almost all aspects and new trends in smart clothes in recent times is listed by Xueli et al., where they listed the mechanisms and the working principle of these devices.

2.2.1.7   Implantable Sensors

Implantable sensors are becoming increasingly popular these days due to low-power technology. A major challenge of these implantable sensors is the sizing, efficient communication, and low power consumption. The efficient transfer of data from these sensors is important in terms of proper working.

2.3   ELECTRONIC SIGNALS IN SENSORS

The human body generates different signals, those signals can be classified based on IoMT. Within this subsection, we majorly classified them into four in terms of their frequency range obtained from the IoMT.

2.3.1   Gait Analysis

Human movements are widely studied, and over the past years, numerous people died due to physical inactivity. Almost 100,000 deaths can be prevented annually if US citizens increase their physical activity by ten minutes each day. That is, gait analysis can play an important role. To keep track of physical activity, proper tracking, monitoring, and measurement are important. It is important to quantitatively assess human locomotion. The most commonly used human locomotion sensing is seen in the step tracker application. Sensors used in this application need to be highly precise, small in weight, user friendly, and easy to use in all environments (Gupta et al., 2023). But further research is needed to figure out the effect of habitual movement on accuracy. An efficient algorithm that is position independent for tracking step counting. It uses five features out of which four are novel and one is derived. Lucian et al. figured out from their experiments that ankle-worn accelerometers and AG have the highest accuracy in terms of counting steps.

2.3.2   Photoplethysmography

Photoplethysmography (PPG) is used for both making biomedical and non-biomedical wearables. This signal is at the center of measuring heart rate variability. In the traditional method, heart rate variability is measured using HRV by means of an electrocardiogram (ECG) signal. To measure the peak-to-peak time interval between cardiac cycles, HRV data were used. HRV analytics can provide a wide range of information to the autonomous nervous system. So, collecting and getting important insights from the HRV data may come in handy (Gupta et al., 2023). However, there are several limitations to acquiring ECG data regarding collecting them at home as requires proper positioning and operation. Trained medical staff are needed to properly position the electrodes in the right position to get proper results, which is sometimes quite unlikely and time consuming. Moreover, some patients complain about other complications such as irritation and itching while going through this process. On the contrary, in the reactance method, the photodiode is placed on the same side as the light source. It measures the intensity of the traveling light. This method is very commonly used in wristband watches. Some of the common devices that use this technique are the pulse oximeter, which is put on the fingertip, and Fitbit watches, respectively (Gupta et al., 2023f). The portability and ease of access features make it very attractive. On top of that, the portability of the sensors and the easy mechanism to capture the PPG signal are making it more popular among mass people.

2.3.3 ELECTROMYOGRAPHY

Through the electromyography (EMG) method, the response of the nerves is measured at the moment electrical stimulation is applied to the nervous system. This stimulation is often referred to as an action potential, and the cumulative addition of the action potential of the motor unit denotes the electromyography signal at the skin surface. Conventionally, there are two techniques to gather the EMG data. One method uses a needle to collect blood samples, and another method is to use an electrode on top of the skin surface (Gupta et al., 2023g). EMG signals acquired from the same muscle but from different sensor locations will result in different results. In most of the common wearable devices, active sensors are used to capture the signal. Usually, three sensors are used in most of these wearables, two of these sensors are metal electrodes, and the rest are used as reference electrodes.

2.3.4 AUSCULTATION

Cardiac patients have to go through cardiac auscultation, in which a physician uses a stethoscope in the first place to diagnose the initial cardiac problems. For there is a dire need for a noninvasive and fast technique to identify the primary cardiac condition. Stethoscope auscultation plays an important role in this. The main heart sound used in medical applications is S1 and S2. S1 signals occur during ventricular contraction, which relates to a QRS complex in ECG. While the cardiovascular system is being analyzed, it is also important to analyze the functions of the lungs. This way, respiratory disorders can easily be identified through lung auscultation. In the case of a physically fit person, lung auscultation doesn't give much information in terms of audible sounds. Wheezing sounds often indicate a lung disease named chronic obstructive pulmonary disease (Nair & Sahoo, 2023). People with this disease often encounter breathing problems. Capturing and detecting these sounds is another important thing. Apart from the anatomy of the heart and lungs, it is vital to understand the anatomy of surface anatomy. People have a misconception that the best sound of auscultation is captured just slightly above the heart, but it is not the case (Kok, 2023). It depends on the direction of the blood flow, and some of the smart wearable devices are demonstrated in Figure 2.3.

Besides the identified electronic sensors, recent medical wearables development showed great potential in accurately and precisely measuring different health-related parameters without the need for a doctor's consultation using the sampled sensors. Although research is ongoing and there is a need to further look into this issue, some IoMTs include epileptic seizure detection, myocardial ischemia monitoring, fatigue detection, physical therapy, wearables, monitoring of sleep apnea, and stress monitoring, among others (Bhattarai & Peng, 2023; Kok, 2023). Both commercial and research items are being investigated in recent studies. But most of the supercomputing personal medical applications are still in the improvement phase.

2.4   CHALLENGES OF ELECTRONIC DEVICES IN THE AIOMT

In contrast to other sectors (IoT applications) where IoT adoption is equally widespread, network managers in the healthcare setup or sector confront difficulties when

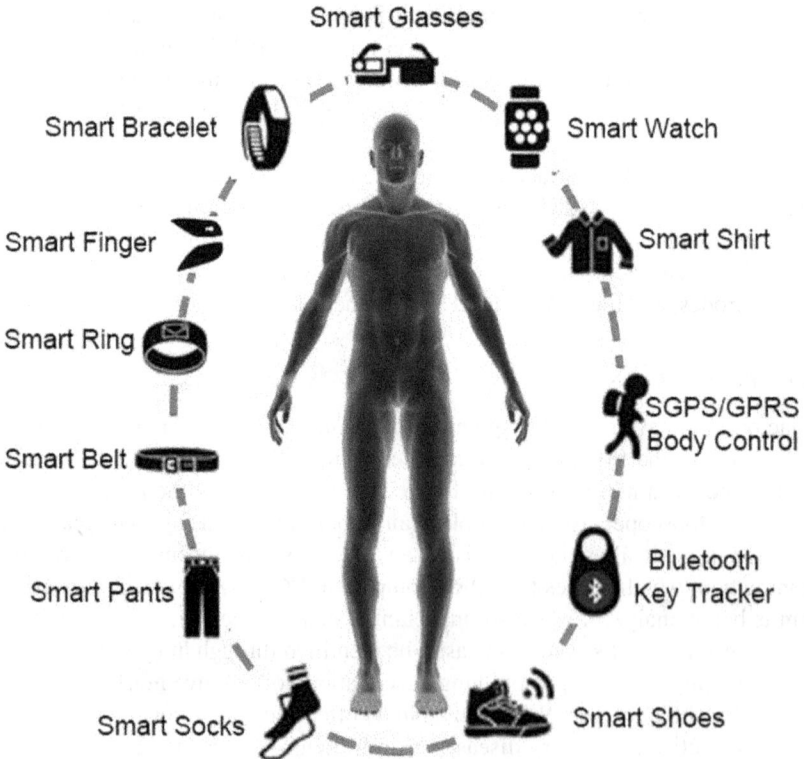

FIGURE 2.3   Sampled wearable medical electronics in IoMTs (Rodrigues et al., 2018).

adopting this IoMT technology. Strict privacy laws, connectivity restrictions brought on by erratic physical settings, and the growing danger of security breaches are just a few of the issues. Not to add that the technology is used in situations where life is at stake (Mathur et al., 2023). Information health technology departments are responsible for ensuring that IoMT equipment is secure, available all the time, and dependable throughout the entire year. While monitoring and safeguarding hundreds, if not thousands, of devices with fewer resources than ever before, these teams are also overworked. Here is a closer look at the top challenges encountered in IoMT applications and some suggestions have been availed (Mathur et al., 2023; Narasimharao et al., 2023). The challenges can be categorized into seven, for instance, data management, interoperability, power consumption, privacy and security of data, cost, efficiency, and environmental impact, among others (as illustrated in Figure 2.4), amidst a few challenges that are not entailed within these categories, which are also discussed.

2.4.1 DATA SECURITY THREATS

Cyber-attacks and medical cyber threats are likely to compromise Medicare data in medical facilities that have not fully encompassed security-based measures in

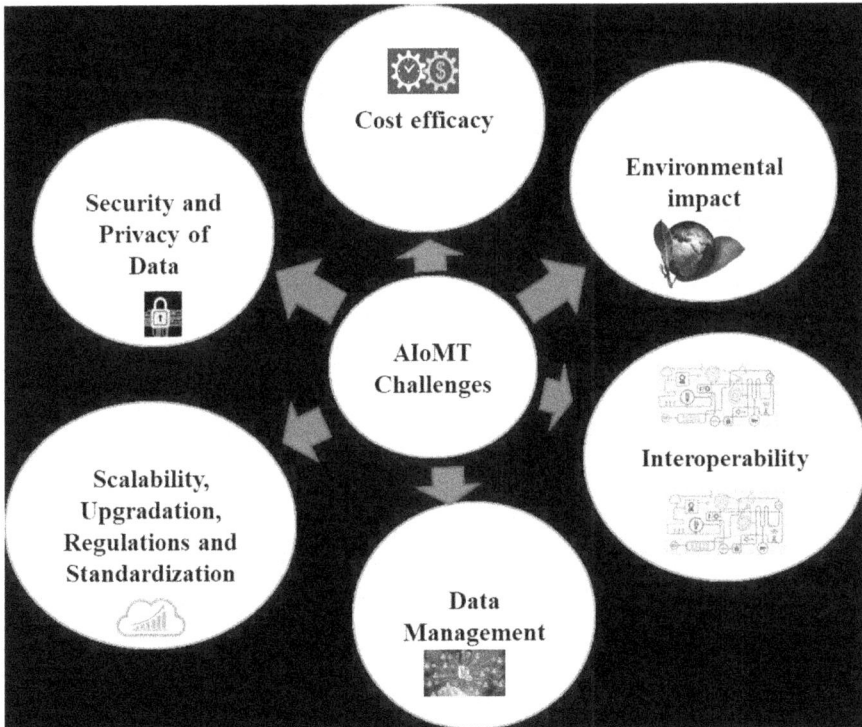

FIGURE 2.4 Summarized AIoMT challenges.

handling patients' data. The danger of exposure is greatly increased when the IoMT data are merged with the existing pool of patient medical data, and the exposure to danger is greatly excavated (Irfana Parveen et al., 2023). In fact, a data breach investigation report presented by Ponemon Institute and Verizon demonstrated that medical data related to personal health information. The likelihood of data breach is more when devices are connected to external systems and to one another. US government data breaches to healthcare in the first five months of 2022 have approximately doubled to the last year (S. K. Pandey & Pandey, 2023).

2.4.2 DATA INTEROPERABILITY

Without a doubt, the more we get data digital, the more the chances to have the data altered mainly in the medical industry. Nevertheless, the majority of data in the medical sector kept in siloed databases, incompatible computer systems, and proprietary software are not interoperable. Consequently, it is complex to exchange, analyze, and realize these kinds of data. This hinders the evolution of medicine since technologies that depend on these data, like big data, AI, and mobile applications, might not be utilized to their extensive capacity (Banday & Bhat, 2023). Therefore, interoperability is a vital component of the anticipated digital advancements in the field of future medicine. Discussion on the ways in which interoperability might facilitate digital transformation in diverse industries, ultimately resulting in global gains in patient health and well-being. From a medical perspective, in case user data originating from a myriad of IoMT devices cannot be aggregated and computationally analyzed to avail medical conclusions that are meaningful and therapeutically applicable, they are useless (Dwivedi et al., 2022). To enable the transmission of patient data to technology users, all devices in the IoMT environment must be compatible with one another along with the payers and providers to fully realize the expected benefits of the technology.

2.4.3 REGULATORY CHALLENGES

Clinical-grade medical "Things" "devices" must have permission and require clearance from national regulators before they may be introduced to the national and international markets. These devices require new regulations from legislators and regulatory agencies that are not familiar enough with how these IoMTs are used (Ding et al., 2023). Those kinds of limitations make the IoMT delayed being used in medical care also due to the limited technological acceptance from those in authority. Christopher M. Butler, Farah Tabibkhoei, Mildred Segura, and Reed Smith LLP shared their insights on the topic and concluded by stressing that even if there is regulatory guidance on the dangers associated with IoMT, compliance criteria are still ambiguous, and there is little relevant legislation or case law. Medical device manufacturers should reduce their exposure to the dangers of cyber vulnerabilities by keeping an eye on regulatory and legal changes pertaining to the IoMT and adhering to best practices.

2.4.4 High Infrastructure Costs

A significant initial outlay is required due to the price of the hardware, specialized IoMT infrastructure, developing consumer-facing applications, and cloud computing. The high infrastructure expenses for IoMT pose a barrier, even though the eventual return on investment is certain. Back in 2015, there were 4.5 billion IoMT devices in operation, and in fact, a Frost and Sullivan report shows that there will be close to 30 billion in less than two years. Deloitte's analysis predicts that by 2022, the IoMT market would be worth $158.1 billion, up from its $41 billion value in 2017 (Chunka et al., n.d.). IoMT also has more wearables, even if that industry is predicted to grow to $29 billion by 2026.

2.4.5 Standardization Challenges

Accreditation of IoMT devices becomes a problem because there are many suppliers and makers of medical devices who are all trying to gain scalability and shorten the time to market for their products. The interoperability of medical devices is impacted by a lack of standardization, which lowers IoMT's overall effectiveness. The issue is being addressed by coalitions and alliances inside the industry, and the sector is receiving substantial assistance from the government.

2.4.6 Cybersecurity

Cybersecurity is a difficult matter that requires knowledge and experience from a variety of professions for comprehension, which the majority of medical persons are not widely informed of. It is comfortable for policy experts and others to become lost in the technical details of cybersecurity, despite the fact that technology measures are an essential component of cybersecurity in the medical sector. In addition, cybersecurity knowledge is usually arranged in silos based on disciplinary boundaries, which lowers the number of insights that can be gained through cross-fertilization (Gupta et al., 2023). This introduction may give connection insight. Importantly, it attempts to leave the reader with two major issues to consider. There is no way to tackle the cybersecurity problem entirely and permanently. Connected medical devices without a doubt, one of the most dangerous IoMT concerns for the medical device business is cybersecurity. Why so? The quality of data transmitted and received by medical devices and the underlying technology are to blame. It can be the patient's personal or financial information, such as the patient's name, date of birth, social security number, and bank account information, among others. In addition to the results of diagnostic trackers, a person's period calendar, or anything else linked to protected health information.

2.4.7 Device Mobility

When employed for therapy, diagnosis, or data handling in IoMT, a device's performance is greatly reduced if it can only be stationary and positioned in one location. Another illustration is a lost network connection, which can turn off any device signaling and have potentially fatal results. Therefore, making IoMT devices functional and mobile is a field to be worked on (Riya et al., 2023). The performance of the gadget is enhanced when the network configuration is replaceable. Once more, it ought to be a secure network switch. To facilitate data gathering and achieve digitalization, remote patient monitoring devices must be mobile and always connected when integrated into the healthcare sector. Several IoMT devices may find it difficult to do this due to constrained network capacity and physical obstructions that cut off wireless signals. Additionally, larger devices could use distinct data formats and connection protocols. The time it takes for these devices to integrate with current IoMT devices may be greatly increased as a result.

2.4.8　Adoption Scale

Scaling is a critical issue for medical technologies. To improve economics and patient outcomes, it is imperative to ensure that Medicare organizations, patients, and professionals recognize the added value of linked medical gadgets. The subject of the IoMT's scalability and wider adoption is still up in the air, even though the industry is expanding and will continue to expand in the future (Khan & Pi, 2023; Salem & Mehaoua, 2023). The additional value of linked medical devices and how they can improve patient outcomes or lower healthcare costs are not understood by all healthcare organizations, professionals, and patients. Limits of governance guidelines and studies demonstrating that IoMT and medical device interconnection are a cost-effective alternative is another impediment. Every medical facility can act at any stage of IoMT integration to make sure the equipment is simple to use and intuitive, as well as to train personnel to develop the skills necessary to maximize the use of the technology (Khan & Pi, 2023). Although the governmental issue is inherently more complex, businesses may present the findings of their own trials, studies, and other research to raise awareness and obtain greater media coverage.

2.4.9　Advanced Analytics

Without efficient algorithms to organize, evaluate, and anticipate potential outcomes, gigabytes of data are useless. It's also important to determine the likelihood of developing a heart failure condition or attack. These instruments not only help preserve the functionality of medical devices and warn in case anything needs a remedy (Muthukaruppankaruppiah et al., 2023). The IoMT can genuinely save lives in this situation. By utilizing cutting-edge algorithms that help to segment and cluster data, identify patterns, and raise alarms about potential hazards, IoT in hospitals, analytics difficulties may be overcome.

2.4.10　Trust Maintenance

To minimize the possibility of subverting the merits that access to data can avail to healthcare technology (Nazir et al., 2023), organizations that innovate mechanisms and services based on the creation and sharing of patient data must ensure openness to patients, the public, and healthcare professionals regarding the utilization of their data.

2.4.11 DATA SECURITY

Over 82% of healthcare firms reported a security breach in the year prior, according to a 2019 Healthcare Information and Management Systems Society poll (Shankar et al., 2023). Hackers are particularly interested in patient health data like electronic medical records and information found in patient databases such as credit card numbers, addresses, and email identifications. These devices repeatedly use outdated software that lacks built-in data security protection because they are primarily utilitarian in design.

2.4.12 LICENSING CHALLENGE

Complicated requirements must be met while incorporating IoMT devices into various medical facilities, compliance standards must be observed, and license approvals must be attained (Shankar et al., 2023; Patra et al., 2023). Even though creating these devices takes time, that is not the only difficulty for IoT service providers in health confront. Regulatory compliance is a sizable obstacle that needs to be overcome.

2.5 BENEFITS OF THE AIOMT

To properly illustrate the benefits, the next section will demonstrate challenges for the AIoMTs; within this subsection, we majorly present them with two benefits and then challenges as detailed subsequently:

2.5.1 MEDICAL DIAGNOSIS

AIoMT aids in a quick and precise medical diagnosis because it is the first step undertaken to treat patient ailments, thereby reducing patient mortality rates. This ultimately leads to improved health and quality of life for individuals. Robots such as the Husky and Veebot have shown great potential in spotting skin tumors accurately and drawing blood, respectively (Wang & Li, 2023). A hundred percent accuracy in the robotic diagnosis of 340 brains using magnetic resonance imaging. Correspondingly, AIoMTs are equipped with the ability to alert medical workers when patients' health deteriorates, as has been shown in this study where doctors were alerted by Google's DeepMind AI system when patients had acute injury of the kidney.

2.5.2 MEDICAL TREATMENT

Because treatment plays an important role in a patient's life, AIoMT has the potential to provide prompt treatment to various patient ailments due to its accuracy, thereby saving lives. In what is now referred to as precision medicine, AIoMT is accelerating the transition from traditional medicine to personalized medicine, targeted treatment, and uniquely composed drugs (Patra et al., 2023). Different AI models have shown great potential in the treatment of COVID-19 as indicated in the studies highlighted. Moreover, with the help of smartphones, AI can aid in prescribing medication to different patients who are unable to physically move to hospital settings. Additionally, robots have achieved tremendous success in rehabilitation and therapy such as the limb-robot rehabilitation system.

2.5.3 PATIENT EMPOWERMENT

AIoMT has the potential to empower individuals to help them make better and more informed health decisions. The large amount of patient data collected by wearable medical devices discussed in the previous section along with the embedded AI helps in analyzing this data, which could alert people with higher risk of becoming ill long before such ailments become serious (Wang & Li, 2023). Doing so allows individuals affected by certain chronic illnesses to better curb their disease, thereby enabling them to live healthier lives through mobile apps. This consequently empowers them and leads to reduced healthcare costs.

2.5.4 REDUCTION IN MEDICAL COSTS

Artificial intelligence is capable of speeding up the creation of life-saving medicines, thereby saving money in medical costs incurred on healthcare delivery systems (Nair & Sahoo, 2023; Narasimharao et al., 2023). AIoMT can optimize medication development in clinical trials, leading to minimization of the time taken to fully certify developed drugs.

2.5.5 REDUCTION IN HUMAN ERROR

The use of AI in the IoMT has shown great benefits in minimizing human errors by medical workers, which saves lives. AIoMT has shown the potential to diagnose patients with a reported 72% more accurate diagnosis compared to the high error rate of medical workers. Without the use of technology in surgical procedures done by medical practitioners, the operation can lead to life-threatening consequences (Mahalakshmi & Lalithamani, 2023). Henceforth, AI plays a vital role in assisting doctors in their surgical procedures due to its simulation of human-made intelligence.

2.6 CHALLENGES OF AIOMTS

Although AI and its convergence with the IoMT have shown tremendous potential to revolutionize healthcare, several technological challenges in their deployment have to be addressed to realize their adaptability and monetization in hospitals/clinics and society in general. This section briefly discusses those challenges.

2.6.1 PRIVACY CONCERNS

There are serious concerns from patients about the large amount of data collected by the different IoMTs. Leakage of such sensitive data through hackers and other means has consequences such as patient blackmail, tarnishing the reputation of health service providers, and the likelihood of loss of lives (R. Pandey et al., 2023). Studies have shown the possibility of AI compromising privacy by predicting the personal information of patients regardless of whether the algorithm has ever been presented with such records. This modus operandi for AI in healthcare may result in lawsuits, especially if the AI's conclusions are made available for public consumption. Hence, the sensitivity of the stored data needs to be protected from unauthorized access and disclosure.

2.6.2 MISSTEPS AND ERRORS

AIoMT systems are not flawless as a patient could be hurt if the wrong treatment is prescribed or if the system fails to detect tumors on a radiological exam, among others. Moreover, if AIoMT systems become popular, a slight error in one has the potential to hurt several (Lee et al., 2023). Additionally, because AI systems work with consumer-facing smart wearable devices and use the data generated by them, those systems may produce invalid results, as indicated in this study using Fitbit trackers.

2.6.3 DATA MANAGEMENT AND POWER ISSUES

The heterogeneity of medical devices running different applications in the AIoMT system creates a data management problem such as storage and incompatible dataset formats created by various legacy third-party systems. Additionally, the large volume of data (big data) generated needs to be stored and analyzed. Hence, the need for scalable and intelligent machine learning algorithms for processing such a large amount of patient data becomes vital. Most devices in the AIoMT have low power capacities, which affect the operational time (Riya et al., 2023). An efficient mechanism capable of increasing the battery power of IoMT devices needs to be envisaged and deployed to increase their operational time.

2.6.4 BIAS

AI-enabled health suffers from the dangers of prejudice and inequality because such systems, by design, learn from the information fed into them leading to the absorption of biases from supplied datasets (Alabdan et al., 2023). Regardless of whether the AIoMT systems are trained on accurate, reliable, and representative datasets, bias will still be reflected, as noted in the study, where an AI system trained on healthcare datasets learns to recommend lower painkiller doses to patients of African-American race. Such a decision is purely based on systemic bias instead of biological traits.

2.7 LIMITATION OF AIOMT

Regardless of the benefits of AIoMTs, there are some limitations that are identified and discussed subsequently. As a result of the ongoing development of technology, business processes in every industry are undergoing continuous change, including medicine. One of these industries experiencing this problem is the healthcare industry. In the coming years, the IoTs, IoMTs, and generally AIoMT will bring countless fabulous opportunities for the healthcare industry. Using IoMT, we are able to derive additional value from the data we acquire. The IoMT improves the effectiveness and quality of the results delivered by various devices. However, there are a few limitations that are encountered in every technological progress, including data privacy concerns, security issues due to the use of wireless medical things, the cost of these AIoMTs, and inaccuracy while handling real-time medical data and operation. It is further noted that these medical developments necessitate training for medical doctors to use applications and structures effectively, and implementation of software by medical analytics can be seen as a limitation as some medical people are not much in operating technology.

2.8 FUTURE RESEARCH DIRECTION

The adoption of AI in the health sector through its convergence with the IoMT is transforming healthcare delivery in aspects such as patient experience, how medical workers practice medicine, and how drugs are being manufactured. Soon, AIoMT is expected to improve the precision of wearable medical devices and their ability to collect, store, and interpret data about patients' health conditions. Consequently, this will allow medical workers to engage with their patients with the help of tele-medicine to achieve improved healthcare service delivery. Overall, the new means of getting healthcare services will drastically reduce the healthcare cost incurred for all groups of patients. Because much of how AI operates is unknown to any layman, the policies and legal frameworks that govern its use, especially in the healthcare sector, will have to be instituted to promote public confidence in its use and protect citizens from any fallout from its irresponsible deployment. Initiatives in that direction have been made by the European Union through its quest to come up with the Artificial Intelligence Act, which is aimed at promoting uniformity in the governance of AI technologies in different sectors, among which include the health sector. The other initiative is the Pan-Canadian AI strategy, which along with the European one, will help the medical community and regulators in monitoring the adoption and explainability of various AI technologies and how their use impacts different contexts in the healthcare industry. Through a combination of standards and regulations, the accuracy, security, reliability, and health use of AI technologies will need to be instituted. This is because AI technologies are capable of learning patterns and modifying their recommendations in ways not envisioned by their creators. This poses regulatory issues, which will need to be addressed as the technology evolves. Adopting a community-led approach by medical workers, technologists, researchers, and other stakeholders is one way that can be adopted to develop standards for data collection and testing of AI-enabled health technologies. AIoMT trends such as chatbot technologies (voice assistants) are seen to revolutionize the healthcare sector with their increased adoption by different healthcare providers. As evidenced by their extensive usage during the COVID-19 global pandemic and other health emergencies, voice assistants such as Google Assistant, Apple Siri, and Amazon Alexa proved very useful in responding to COVID-19-related public questions.

2.9 CONCLUSIONS AND FUTURE SCOPE

Due to its potential to transform the delivery of medical care, the IoMT has rapidly gained the interest of researchers since its inception. They are able to monitor and manage a number of health-related disorders and issues. The IoMT devices allow us to monitor our medical records and take the necessary safety precautions. IoMT plays a significant role in boosting the effectiveness and precision of electronic devices in the medical industry. In this chapter, a comprehensive examination of a range of electronic equipment discovered in the AIoMT has been conducted. For your convenience, the identified and extensively used medical equipment, including electrical signals for AIoMT sensors, are highlighted subsequently. In addition, AIoMT's architecture demonstrates significant development by utilizing intelligent sensors to collect, aggregate, and manage data for intelligent healthcare buildings. In addition, the chapter discusses the challenges that electronic gadgets pose to AIoMT. These challenges include, but are not limited to, threats to data security, interoperability issues, and regulatory concerns. All of these challenges, along with others, must be addressed to improve medical operating standards, not just for medical staff but also for patients and other medical stakeholders. Unanswered research questions that will be the focus of future research in AIoMT are discussed in the conclusion. IoT innovations such as automated medical delivery, connected inhalers and contact lenses, monitoring for Parkinson's disease, monitoring for glucose levels, monitoring for depression and mood, and many others have unquestionably benefited the medical business. Thanks to AIoMT, the patient experience is improved and workflows are optimized. Patients stand to benefit from increased participation and fewer in-person physician appointments. Providers can better assist patients now that they have access to more accurate data, improved diagnostics, and more effective time management. AIoMT will very certainly be supplemented in the future by more innovations that will further streamline the medical profession for practitioners and patients. This chapter is limited in that it cannot cover the many electronic device and AIoMT-related issues that have been raised. This is a restriction. Diverse parties should make a more concentrated effort to develop laws and regulatory frameworks that regulate the deployment of AI in various health situations. Additionally, in order to boost public confidence in the use of AI and IoMT in the healthcare industry, it will be important to seek and implement solutions to the highlighted concerns.

REFERENCES

Alabdan, R., Alruban, A., Hilal, A. M., & Motwakel, A. (2023). Artificial-Intelligence-Based Decision Making for Oral Potentially Malignant Disorder Diagnosis in Internet of Medical Things Environment. *Healthcare*, *11*(1), 113.

Banday, M. T., & Bhat, L. (2023). Towards Building Internet-of-Things-Inclusive Healthcare for Neglected Tropical Diseases. *The Internet of Medical Things (IoMT) and Telemedicine Frameworks and Applications*, 39–75.

Bhattarai, A., & Peng, D. (2023). An Integrated Secure Efficient Computing Architecture for Embedded and Remote ECG Diagnosis. *SN Computer Science*, *4*(1), 1–15.

Bhutnal, V., & Moparthi, N. R. (2023). Internet of Things-Enabled Diabetic Retinopathy Classification from Fundus Images. In *IOT with Smart Systems* (pp. 757–764). Springer.

Chunka, C., Banerjee, S., & Sachin Kumar, G. (n.d.). A Secure Communication Using Multifactor Authentication and Key Agreement Techniques in Internet of Medical things for COVID-19 Patients. *Concurrency and Computation: Practice and Experience*, e7602.

Deshmukh, A., Tyagi, A. K., Hansora, H., & Menon, S. C. (2023). Applications of Distributed Ledger (Blockchain) Technology in E-Healthcare. In *The Internet of Medical Things (IoMT) and Telemedicine Frameworks and Applications* (pp. 248–261). IGI Global.

Ding, X., Zhang, Y., Li, J., Mao, B., Guo, Y., & Li, G. (2023). A Feasibility Study of Multi-mode Intelligent Fusion Medical Data Transmission Technology of Industrial Internet of Things Combined with Medical Internet of Things. *Internet of Things*, 100689.

Dwivedi, R., Mehrotra, D., & Chandra, S. (2022). Potential of Internet of Medical Things (IoMT) Applications in Building a Smart Healthcare System: A Systematic Review. *Journal of Oral Biology and Craniofacial Research*, *12*(2), 302–318.

Gezimati, M., & Singh, G. (2023). Internet of Things Enabled Framework for Terahertz and Infrared Cancer Imaging. *Optical and Quantum Electronics*, *55*(1), 1–17.

Guan, Z., Li, Y., Yu, S., & Yang, Z. (n.d.). Deep Reinforcement Learning-Based Full-Duplex Link Scheduling in Federated Learning-based Computing for IoMT. *Transactions on Emerging Telecommunications Technologies*, e4724.

Gupta, S., Sharma, H. K., & Kapoor, M. (2023a). Application and Challenges of Blockchain in IoMT in Smart Healthcare System. In *Blockchain for Secure Healthcare Using Internet of Medical Things (IoMT)* (pp. 39–53). Springer.

Gupta, S., Sharma, H. K., & Kapoor, M. (2023b). Artificial Intelligence-Based Cloud Storage for Accessing and Predication. In *Blockchain for Secure Healthcare Using Internet of Medical Things (IoMT)* (pp. 157–168). Springer.

Gupta, S., Sharma, H. K., & Kapoor, M. (2023c). Blockchain-Based EHR Storage and Access Control System. In *Blockchain for Secure Healthcare Using Internet of Medical Things (IoMT)* (pp. 131–144). Springer.

Gupta, S., Sharma, H. K., & Kapoor, M. (2023d). Digital Medical Records (DMR) Security and Privacy Challenges in Smart Healthcare System. In *Blockchain for Secure Healthcare Using Internet of Medical Things (IoMT)* (pp. 67–78). Springer.

Gupta, S., Sharma, H. K., & Kapoor, M. (2023e). Introduction to Blockchain and Its Application in Smart Healthcare System. In *Blockchain for Secure Healthcare Using Internet of Medical Things (IoMT)* (pp. 55–65). Springer.

Gupta, S., Sharma, H. K., & Kapoor, M. (2023f). Introduction to Smart Healthcare and Telemedicine Systems. In *Blockchain for Secure Healthcare Using Internet of Medical Things (IoMT)* (pp. 1–11). Springer.

Gupta, S., Sharma, H. K., & Kapoor, M. (2023g). Methodologies for Improving the Quality of Service and Safety of Smart Healthcare System. In *Blockchain for Secure Healthcare Using Internet of Medical Things (IoMT)* (pp. 103–117). Springer.

Idrees, A. K., & Khlief, M. S. (2023). Efficient Compression Technique for Reducing Transmitted EEG Data without Loss in IoMT Networks Based on Fog Computing. *The Journal of Supercomputing*, 1–26.

Irfana Parveen, C. A., Anjali, O., & Sunder, R. (2023). Internet of Things: A Review on Its Applications. *Information and Communication Technology for Competitive Strategies (ICTCS 2021)*, 123–134.

Khan, I. A., & Pi, D. (2023). Explainable Learning Machines for Securing the IoMT Networks. In *The Internet of Medical Things (IoMT) and Telemedicine Frameworks and Applications* (pp. 135–154). IGI Global.

Kok, C. L. (2023). A Low Cost, Power Efficient, Social Distancing Notification Embedded System Based on Intelligent Wireless Sensor Network. In *The Internet of Medical Things (IoMT) and Telemedicine Frameworks and Applications* (pp. 262–275). IGI Global.

Kok, C. L., & Setyadi, Y. (2023). Li-Ion-Based DC UPS for Remote Application. In *The Internet of Medical Things (IoMT) and Telemedicine Frameworks and Applications* (pp. 276–289). IGI Global.

Lee, H. Y., Lee, K. H., Lee, K. H., Erdenbayar, U., Hwang, S., Lee, E. Y., Lee, J. H., Kim, H. J., Park, S. B., & Park, J. W. (2023). Internet of Medical Things-Based Real-Time Digital Health Service for Precision Medicine: Empirical Studies Using MEDBIZ Platform. *Digital Health*, 9, 20552076221149660.

Mahalakshmi, R., Lalithamani, N. (2023). Preventing COVID-19 Using Edge Intelligence in Internet of Medical Things. In: Gupta, D., Khanna, A., Bhattacharyya, S., Hassanien, A.E., Anand, S., Jaiswal, A. (eds) International Conference on Innovative Computing and Communications. Lecture Notes in Networks and Systems, vol 473. Springer, Singapore. (pp. 213–227). https://doi.org/10.1007/978-981-19-2821-5_18

Mathur, G., Pandey, A., & Goyal, S. (2023). Applications of Machine Learning in Healthcare. In *The Internet of Medical Things (IoMT) and Telemedicine Frameworks and Applications* (pp. 177–195). IGI Global.

Muthukaruppankaruppiah, S., Nagalingam, S. R., Murugasen, P., & Nandaamarnath, R. (2023). Human Fatty Liver Monitoring Using Nano Sensor and IoMT. *Intelligent Automation & Soft Computing*, 35(2).

Nair, A. K., & Sahoo, J. (2023). Internet of Things in Smart and Intelligent Healthcare Systems. In *Intelligent Internet of Things for Smart Healthcare Systems* (1st ed.). eBook ISBN9781003326182. CRC Press.

Narasimharao, M., Swain, B., Nayak, P. P., & Bhuyan, S. (2023). Development of Real-Time Cloud Based Smart Remote Healthcare Monitoring System. In *Ambient Intelligence in Health Care* (pp. 217–224). Springer.

Nazir, S., Zhang, Y., & Tianfield, H. (2023). Trusted Federated Learning for IoMT-Solutions and Challenges. In *Federated Learning for Internet of Medical Things: Concepts, Paradigms, and Solutions*. CRC Press.

Pandey, R., Pandey, A., Maurya, P., & Singh, G. D. (2023). Prenatal Healthcare Framework Using IoMT Data Analytics. In *The Internet of Medical Things (IoMT) and Telemedicine Frameworks and Applications* (pp. 76–104). IGI Global.

Pandey, S. K., & Pandey, S. (2023). IoT and Healthcare: Study of Conceptual Framework and Applications. In *The Internet of Medical Things (IoMT) and Telemedicine Frameworks and Applications* (pp. 1–16). IGI Global.

Patra, M. K., Kumari, A., Sahoo, B., & Turuk, A. K. (2023). Smart Healthcare System Using Cloud-Integrated Internet of Medical Things. In *Exploring the Convergence of Computer and Medical Science Through Cloud Healthcare* (pp. 60–83). IGI Global.

Petrellis, N., Birbas, M., & Gioulekas, F. (2019). On the Design of Low-Cost IoT Sensor Node for e-Health Environments. *Electronics*, 8(2), 178.

Quy, V. K., Hau, N. V., Anh, D. V., & Ngoc, L. A. (2022). Smart Healthcare IoT Applications Based on Fog Computing: Architecture, Applications and Challenges. *Complex & Intelligent Systems*, 8(5), 3805–3815.

Riya, K. S., Surendran, R., Tavera Romero, C. A., & Sendil, M. S. (2023). Encryption with User Authentication Model for Internet of Medical Things Environment. *Intelligent Automation & Soft Computing*, 35(1).

Rodrigues, J. J., Segundo, D. B. D. R., Junqueira, H. A., Sabino, M. H., Prince, R. M., Al-Muhtadi, J., & De Albuquerque, V. H. C. (2018). Enabling Technologies for the Internet of Health Things. *IEEE Access*, 6, 13129–13141.

Salem, O., & Mehaoua, A. (2023). Ephemeral Elliptic Curve Diffie-Hellman to Secure Data Exchange in Internet of Medical Things. In *Emerging Trends in Cybersecurity Applications* (pp. 3–20). Springer.

Shafik, W. (2023). A Comprehensive Cybersecurity Framework for Present and Future Global Information Technology Organizations. In *Effective Cybersecurity Operations for Enterprise-Wide Systems* (pp. 56–79). IGI Global.

Shafik, W., Matinkhah, S. M., & Ghasemzadeh, M. (2020). Theoretical Understanding of Deep Learning in UAV Biomedical Engineering Technologies Analysis. *SN Computer Science*, *1*(6), 1–13.

Shankar, N., Nallakaruppan, M. K., Ravindranath, V., Senthilkumar, M., & Bhagavath, B. P. (2023). Smart IoMT Framework for Supporting UAV Systems with AI. *Electronics*, *12*(1), 86.

Wang, J., & Li, X. (2023). Secure Medical Data Collection in the Internet of Medical Things Based on Local Differential Privacy. *Electronics*, *12*(2), 307.

3 Electronic Devices in the Artificial Intelligence of the Internet of Medical Things (AIoMT)

Khairul Eahsun Fahim, Kassim Kalinaki, and Wasswa Shafik

3.1 INTRODUCTION

In the past decade, smart healthcare has undergone a tremendous transformation as a result of advancements in key support technologies that include the Internet of Things (IoT), big data, cloud computing, microelectronics, and mobile internet. The incorporation of modern medical sensors and different hardware in the health sector has led to the development of a new concept called the Internet of Medical Things (IoMT) [1] or Internet of Health Things (IoHT) [2], which along with the aforementioned technologies, has transformed the traditional healthcare into a more efficient, all-round and personalized experience. Between 2020 and 2027, the global market for smart health is projected to increase by a mean growth rate of 16.2%. This creates a dire need for fast, comprehensive, accurate, and intelligent eHealthcare systems, as highlighted by the emergency of global pandemics such as COVID-19 [4]. These systems will be capable of collecting, analyzing, and interpreting an unprecedented amount of patient information for effective health and well-being monitoring through various medical electronic devices [5]. Additionally, such systems will provide the means for the periodical management of medical personnel, keeping track of both medical instruments and biological specimens.

The convergence of Internet of Medical devices (IoMT), AI, and big data has added new dimensions to such systems, which are now capable of analyzing the collected data to provide better insights, thereby ushering in a new era in healthcare, such as early stage chronic disease prediction and personalized and physiological health monitoring systems, among others. Through the IoMT environment, monitoring health can be attained with the aid of numerous wearable medical sensors that record and keep track of the patient medical conditions in real time [4]. The data produced by such sensors enables medical physicians to reliably and efficiently recognize and respond to critical situations regarding patients to enable them to become more informed regarding their health conditions for future diagnosis and treatment.

Furthermore, these sensors provide cheaper alternatives to the expensive environment of a hospital as they enable remote detection of abnormalities, evaluation of
symptoms, and the general health of the patients [3, 5].

The large amount of patient information collected by several devices in the IoMT
environment has ushered in new opportunities that leverage the power of AI. Currently
known as AI-enabled health, opportunities such as the ability to quickly analyze and
interpret patient information, diagnose, and predict future diseases have been reported
[6, 7]. Advanced AI techniques have made it possible for medical physicians to remotely
track patients' habits and reveal their medical status from the captured data emanating
from several sensors along with sensor usage patterns. Through IoMT environment,
AI techniques, for example, support vector machines [8], random forest [9], Logistic
Regression [10], Decision Trees [11], k-nearest neighbor, naïve Bayes [12], and several
neural networks [13] have been used for various health-related applications. Different
medics, health practitioners, health ministries, and agencies, among others, together
celebrate and appreciate the integration and application of IoMTs management mainly
due to a couple of benefits. Such benefits include patient clinical trials, identification,
medication error reduction, personalized medication, and surgery aided, among others.

The IoMT architecture in Figure 3.1 depicts the comprehensive growth of exploiting smart sensors to accumulate data and regulate smart healthcare infrastructure.
However, there are notable challenges that face smart healthcare, as discussed.
Furthermore, medical institutions rely on internet-based technologies from connected infusion pumps to now telemetry patient monitors, to provide best-in-class
patient care [14]. During their study, they considered four main health factors that
soar with the smart healthcare system, including in homes (like mobile help, vitality,
and intelligent clinic, among others), community (for instance, Xerafy, American
Well, and Skytron, among others), in-clinic, in the hospital, and on body.

Accordingly, it is important for Medicare providers and officials in the healthcare
domain to keep track of viral infections to ensure the necessary isolation of patients,
along with real-time measures to contain infections. In appreciation of the current

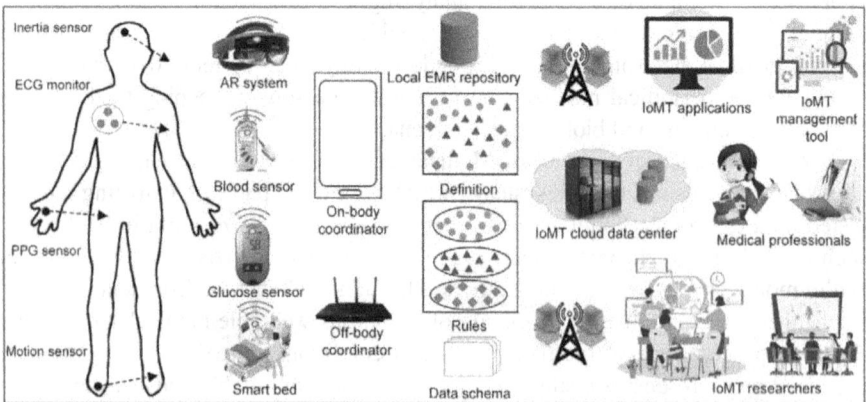

FIGURE 3.1 IoMT architecture with comprehensive growth by exploiting smart sensors to
accumulate data and regulate smart healthcare structure [15].

development, the medical devices that constitute the IoMT and their convergence with AI described earlier have shown tremendous potential in improving the overall health of billions of individuals all over the world, thereby leading to improved quality of life. With the paradigm of AIoMT being new, few studies have been dedicated to detailing the different electronic devices deployed.

3.1.1 Key Contributions of the Chapter

The significant contributions of this chapter are listed next:

  i. The chapter provides a detailed description of the diverse electronic sensors used in AIoMT in the wider medical industry.
 ii. The different electronic signals transmitted by the different AIoMT sensors are presented.
iii. The significant challenges and prospects faced in using the identified electronic devices healthcare have been discussed.
 iv. Some benefits and challenges for the AIoMT are reviewed, and the future research direction of IoMT in the healthcare industry and future scope are depicted.

3.1.2 Chapter Organization

Section 3.2 presents electronic sensors in IoMT and electronic sensor traits, disposable health sensors, ingestible sensors, patch sensors, connected health sensors, wearables, smart clothing, and implantable sensors. Section 3.3 presents the electronic signals in sensors. Section 3.4 discusses the identified challenges of electronic devices in the AIoMT that include data security threats. Section 3.5 explains the benefits of the AIoMT reviewed. Section 3.6 demonstrates the challenges of reviewed AIoMTs. Section 3.7 gives the conclusion and future research direction of IoMT in the healthcare industry.

3.2 ELECTRONIC SENSORS IN THE IOMT

When used in the smart healthcare industry, IoMT combines various processing units with communication technologies, for instance, electronic wireless sensors that remotely monitor patient health status, to enable the prompt transmission of clinical information to healthcare medics. IoMT makes it possible for caregivers to continuously monitor their patient's health, which enhances clinical judgment, lowers patients' medical costs, and ultimately improves patient outcomes. This section presents notable electronic sensor traits as it relates to IoMT applications, and a brief discussion of the main four commonly used electronic sensor signals used are presented.

3.2.1 Electronic Sensor Traits

As IoMTs are applied in the medical facility, these electronic sensors show different characteristics, and their contrast causes an impact on the patient. To support its many uses, a plethora of electronic biosensors have been invented and incorporated into the healthcare domain enabled by IoT. Smart home care, clinical diagnostics, preventive medicine, fitness tracking, and a few monitoring services are some of these.

3.2.1.1 Disposable Health Sensors

Diagnostics, patient monitoring, and treatment support are the three main uses for disposable health sensors. The sensors are frequently strip-type, implementable, and ingestible. All these are focused on depending on the patient body nature [16].

3.2.1.2 Ingestible Sensors

The microfabricated integrated circuit for this tiny electronic sensor is made of magnesium, copper, and gold thin layers. As the taken pill enters the stomach, a reaction between the circuit layers and gastric juice takes place. The sensor experiences an electrochemical reaction as a result [16]. The patches of sensors then receive a digital code that denotes the drug type and appropriate dosage along with the time of dosage administration since the sensor is energized by this reaction.

3.2.1.3 Patch Sensors

The patient may monitor their daily activities and medication schedules in appreciation of the transmission of all this data to a smartphone application, which then sends it to the discover portal. Medics and other healthcare professionals can find crucial data on their patients' daily health reports within the portals to help them choose the most appropriate treatments. By enhancing drug adherence, for instance, authors in [17] have reported the Proteus Digital Medicine model, which has transformed the healthcare industry by lowering treatment failure rates and the demand for patient retreatment.

3.2.1.4 Connected Health Sensors

End-use market, electronic sensor, and platform sensors are additional subcategories of connected e-health sensors [18]. Wearables, embedded technology, and intrusive sensors are examples of end-use market sensors for IoMT.

3.2.1.5 Wearables

Wearable sensors are continuously worn or put near human skin to closely keep track of the patient's actions without restricting their usual range of mobility. Mobility trackers are an especially well-liked kind of wearable health technology that has several practical uses in other domains such as sports, determining risk of falling down, and keeping an eye on the senior population [19].

3.2.1.6 Smart Clothing

Numerous wearable gadgets have been deployed to measure important aspects of human health in addition to being helpful in encouraging individuals to keep track of daily workouts and sustain a more active and healthier lifestyle. The most typical of these measurements include electrocardiogram (ECG) and electroencephalogram (EEG) measurements [20]. Body-worn smart gear is one innovative innovation intended to combine wearable sensors with essential health monitoring capabilities.

Compared to current technologies, which frequently only record a small number of physiological data, smart clothing enables people with intermittent illnesses to benefit from several health monitoring systems. Smart clothes substantially decrease the cost of sensors as well, but the efficiency in terms of wireless communication and packet transfer is still not that efficient. A broad review covering almost all aspects and new trends in smart clothes in recent times is listed by Xueli et al., where they listed the mechanisms and the working principle of these devices [21].

3.2.1.7 Implantable Sensors

Implantable sensors are becoming increasingly popular these days due to low-power technology [22]. A major challenge of these implantable sensors is the sizing, efficient communication, and low power consumption. The efficient transfer of data from these sensors is crucial in terms of proper working, and some devices are demonstrated in Figure 3.2.

3.3 ELECTRONIC SIGNALS

The human body generates different signals, those signals can be classified based on IoMT. Within this subsection, we majorly classified them into four in terms of their frequency range obtained from the IoMT.

3.3.1 Gait Analysis

Human movements are widely studied, and over the past years, numerous people died due to physical inactivity. Almost 100,000 deaths can be prevented annually if

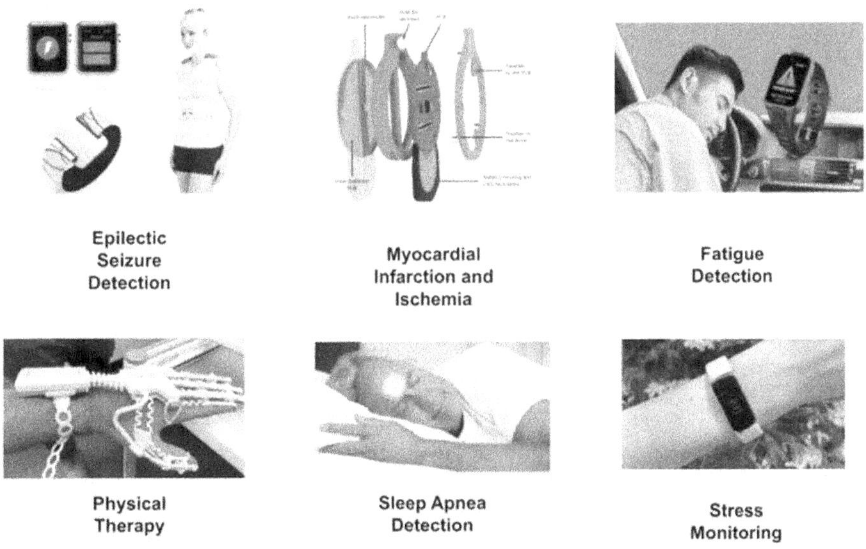

FIGURE 3.2   Summarized IoMT sensors [23–25].

the citizens of the United States increase the level of their physical activity by ten minutes each day. That is, gait analysis can play an important role. To keep track of physical activity, proper tracking, monitoring, and measurement are important. It is important to quantitatively assess human locomotion [26]. The most commonly used human locomotion sensing is seen in the step tracker application. Sensors used in this application need to be highly precise, small in weight, user friendly, and easy to use in all environments. A study conducted by Dillon et al. in [27] found that ankle-worn accelerometers give the best accuracy regarding measuring step counts. But further research is needed to determine habitual movement's effect on accuracy. An efficient algorithm that is position independent for tracking step counting. It uses five features out of which four are novel and one is derived. Lucian et al. figured out from their experiments that ankle-worn accelerometers and AG have the highest accuracy in terms of counting steps.

3.3.2 PHOTOPLETHYSMOGRAPHY

Photoplethysmography (PPG) is used for making both biomedical and non-biomedical wearables. This signal is at the center of measuring heart rate variability. In the traditional method, heart rate variability is measured using HRV by means of an electrocardiogram (ECG) signal. To measure the peak-to-peak time interval between cardiac cycles, HRV data were used. HRV analytics can provide a wide range of information to the autonomous nervous system. So, collecting and getting important insights from the HRV data may come in handy. However, there are several limitations to acquiring ECG data regarding collecting them at home as requires proper positioning and operation. Trained medical staff are needed to properly position the electrodes in the right position to get proper results, which is sometimes quite unlikely and time consuming. Moreover, some patients complain about other complications such as irritation and itching while going through this process [28]. On the contrary, in the reactance method, the photodiode is placed on the same side as the light source. It measures the intensity of the traveling light. This method is very commonly used in wristband watches [29]. Some of the common devices that use this technique are the pulse oximeter, which is put on the fingertip, and Fitbit watches, respectively. The portability and ease of access features make it very attractive. On top of that, the portability of the sensors and the easy mechanism to capture the PPG signal are making it more popular among mass people.

3.3.3 ELECTROMYOGRAPHY

Through the electromyography (EMG) method, the response of the nerves is measured the moment electrical stimulation is applied to the nervous system. This stimulation is often referred to as an action potential, and the cumulative addition of the action potential of the motor unit denotes the electromyography signal at the skin surface. Conventionally, there are two techniques to gather the EMG data. One method uses a needle to collect blood samples, and another method is to use an electrode on top of the skin surface [30]. EMG signals acquired from the same muscle but from different sensor locations will result in different results. In most of the common wearable devices, active sensors are used to capture the signal. Usually, three sensors are used in most of these wearables, two of these sensors are metal electrodes, and the rest are used as reference electrodes.

3.3.4 AUSCULTATION

For there is a dire need for a noninvasive and fast technique to identify the primary cardiac condition. Stethoscope auscultation plays an important role in this. The main heart sound used in medical applications is S1 and S2. S1 signals occur during ventricular contraction, which relates to a QRS complex in ECG [31]. While the cardiovascular system is being analyzed, it is also important to analyze the functions of the lungs. This way, respiratory disorders can easily be identified through lung auscultation. In the case of a physically fit person, lung auscultation doesn't give much information in terms of audible sounds. Wheezing sounds often indicate a lung disease named chronic obstructive pulmonary disease. People with this disease often encounter breathing problems (citation needed here). Capturing and detecting these sounds is another important thing. Apart from the anatomy of the heart and lungs, it is vital to understand the anatomy of surface anatomy. People have a misconception that the best sound of auscultation is captured just slightly above the heart, but it is not the case. It depends on the direction of the blood flow [19].

Besides with the identified electronic sensors, recent medical wearables development showed great potential in accurately and precisely measuring different health-related parameters without the need for a doctor's consultation using the sampled sensors depicted in Figure 3.3. Although research is ongoing and there is a need to further look into this issue, some IoMTs include epileptic seizure detection, myocardial

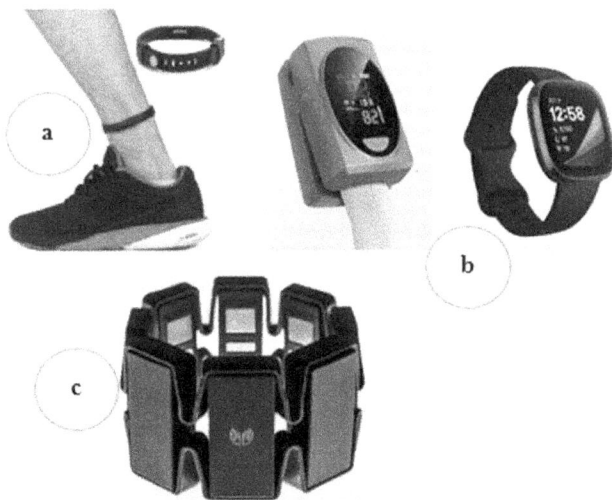

FIGURE 3.3 Sampled electronic sensor in IoMT [32–34].

ischemia monitoring, fatigue detection, physical therapy, wearables, monitoring of sleep apnea, and stress monitoring, among others. Both commercial and research items are being investigated in recent studies. But most of the supercomputing personal medical applications are still in the improvement phase. Thus, Table 3.1 focuses on the recent trends in IoMT research.

TABLE 3.1
Summary of Recent IoMT Application Research

Reference	AIoMT	Feature	Developments
[35]	Insertable Loop Recorder	14 months of monitoring and data logging Weighs 17g	Cardiopulmonary monitoring
[36]	MEMS Blood Pressure Sensor	Implanted using a catheter into the right ventricle of the heart	
[37]	Tele Pulse Oximeter	Measures oxygen in the blood Probes and handheld computers are used to process the data	
[38]	Pulse Graph	Finger-mounted optical sensor acceleration sensor	
[39]	PPG Ring Sensor	Wireless data transmission	
[40]	Phonocardiography	Subcutaneous implantable capsule, biomorph piezoelectric sensor	
[41]	Stress Level	Synchronous measurement of the heart rate	
[42]	Assessment		
[43]	Diabetes Management System	Extract fluids with a patch sensor. Results are extracted and wirelessly sent every 3.8 seconds	Controlling diabetes
[44]	Skin Breakdown Detection	Abnormal stresses are evaluated by monitoring pressure, and humidity	
[45]	Implantable Sensor for Blood Glucose Monitoring	Implantable optical sensor for continuous monitoring of blood glucose	
[23]	Implantable Microcomputer	Consists of a SOC microcontroller, a variable gain amplifier, and large memory capacity	Stimulating muscle and brain activity
[24]	BiCMOS Wireless Simulator Chip	Allows wireless and stand-alone operation. Low power consumption	
[25]	Gastrointestinal Traversable Capsule	Battery-powered sensor integrated silicon device.	
[46]	Given	Small disposable imaging capsule	
[47]	Knee Arthroplasty Monitoring	Inertial measurement unit (IMU) sensors. Low-maintenance remote monitoring	Pre- and post-surgery monitoring
[48]	Hip Prosthesis Monitoring Device	Implantable contains microcontroller, accelerometer, and a transmitter	

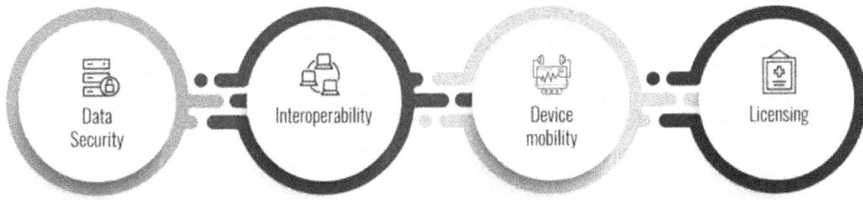

FIGURE 3.4   IoMT challenge classification.

3.4   CHALLENGES OF ELECTRONIC DEVICES IN THE AIOMT

In contrast to other sectors (IoT applications) where IoT adoption is equally widespread, network managers in the healthcare setup or sector confront difficulties when adopting this IoMT technology. Strict privacy laws, connectivity restrictions brought on by erratic physical settings, and the growing danger of security breaches are just a few of the issues. Not to add that the technology is used in situations where life is at stake. Information health technology departments are responsible for ensuring that IoMT equipment are secure, available all the time, and dependable throughout the entire year. While monitoring and safeguarding hundreds, if not thousands, of devices with less resources than ever before, these teams are also overworked. Here is a closer look at the top challenges encountered in IoMT applications and some suggestions have been availed [49, 50]. The challenges can be categorized into four, for instance, data security, interoperability, device mobility, and licensing (as illustrated in Figure 3.4), amidst a few challenges that are not entailed within these categories, which are also discussed.

3.4.1   Data Security Threats

Cyber-attacks and medical cyber threats are likely to compromise Medicare data in medical facilities that have not fully encompassed security-based measures in handling patients' data. In fact, a data breach investigation report presented by Ponemon Institute and Verizon demonstrated that medical data related to personal health information. The likelihood of data breaches is more when more devices are connected to external systems and to one another. US government data breaches to healthcare in the first five months of 2022 have approximately doubled from the last year [51].

3.4.2   Data Interoperability

In a medical perspective, in case user data originating from a myriad of IoMT devices cannot be aggregated and computationally analyzed to avail medical conclusions that are meaningful and therapeutically applicable, they are useless. To enable the transmission of patient data to technology users, all devices in the IoMT environment must be compatible with one another along with the payers and providers to fully realize the expected benefits of the technology. Having interoperability in devices demonstrates three main advantages, improving health experience, higher performance, and better care coordination. Some of the most used instances for interoperability are patient-concentrated care that in return leads to advanced care planning, care coordination, and dental health information exchange [52].

3.4.3 REGULATORY CHALLENGES

Clinical-grade medical "Things" "devices" must have permission and require clearances from national regulators before they may be introduced to the national and international markets [53]. These devices require new regulations from legislators and regulatory agencies that are not familiar enough with how these IoMTs use. Those kinds of limitations make the IoMT delayed being used in medical care also due to the limited technological acceptance from those in authority. These regulations are mainly categorized into three with detailed discussion on every category, for instance [54], the US Food and Drug Administration, legislative and Judicial. Christopher M. Butler, Farah Tabibkhoei, Mildred Segura, and Reed Smith LLP shared their insights on the topic and concluded by stressing that even if there is regulatory guidance on the dangers associated with IoMT, compliance criteria are still ambiguous, and there is little relevant legislation or case law. Medical device manufacturers should reduce their exposure to the dangers of cyber vulnerabilities by keeping an eye on regulatory and legal changes pertaining to the IoMT and adhering to best practices [55].

3.4.4 HIGH INFRASTRUCTURE COSTS

A significant initial outlay is required due to the price of the hardware, specialized IoMT infrastructure, developing consumer-facing applications, and cloud computing. The high infrastructure expenses for IoMT pose a barrier, even though the eventual return on investments is certain [56]. Back in 2015, there were 4.5 billion IoMT devices in operation, and in fact a Frost and Sullivan report shows that there will be close to 30 billion in less than two years. Deloitte's analysis predicts that by 2022, the IoMT market would be worth $158.1 billion, up from its $41 billion value in 2017 [57]. IoMT also has more wearables, even if that industry is predicted to grow to $29 billion by 2026.

3.4.5 STANDARDIZATION CHALLENGES

Accreditation of the IoMT devices becomes a problem because there are many suppliers and makers of medical devices who are all trying to gain scalability and shorten the time to market for their product [58]. The interoperability of medical devices is impacted by a lack of standardization, which lowers IoMT's overall effectiveness. The issue is being addressed by coalitions and alliances inside the industry, and the sector is receiving substantial assistance from the government.

3.4.6 CYBERSECURITY

The quality of data transmitted and received by medical devices and the underlying technology are to blame. It can be the patient's personal or financial information, such as the patient's date of birth, name, social security number, bank account information, etc., in addition to the results of diagnostic trackers, a person's period calendar, or anything else linked to protected health information [59–61].

3.4.7 DEVICE MOBILITY

When employed for therapy, diagnosis, or data handling in IoMT, a device's performance is greatly reduced if it can only be stationary and positioned in one location [62, 63]. Another illustration is a lost network connection, which can turn off any device signaling and have potentially fatal results. Therefore, making IoMT devices functional and mobile is a field to be worked on. The performance of the gadget is enhanced when the network configuration is replaceable. Once more, it ought to be a secure network switch. To facilitate data gathering and achieve digitalization, remote patient monitoring devices must be mobile and always connected when being integrated into the healthcare sector. Large IoMT devices may find it difficult to do this due to constrained network capacity and physical obstructions that cut off wireless signals. Additionally, larger devices could use distinct data formats and connection protocols [64]. The time it takes for these devices to integrate with current IoMT devices may be greatly increased as a result.

3.4.8 ADOPTION SCALE

Scaling is a serious issue for medical technologies. To improve economics and patient outcomes, it is imperative to ensure that Medicare organizations, patients, and professionals recognize the added value of linked medical gadgets [65]. The subject of the IoMT's scalability and wider adoption is still up in the air, even though the industry is expanding and will continue to expand in the future. The additional value of linked medical devices and how they can improve patient outcomes or lower healthcare costs are not understood by all healthcare organizations, professionals, and patients. Limits of governance guidelines and studies demonstrating that IoMT and medical device interconnection are a cost-effective alternative is another impediment. Every medical facility can act at any stage of IoMT integration to make sure the equipment is simple to use and intuitive, as well as to train personnel to develop the skills necessary to maximize the use of the technology. Although the governmental issue is inherently more complex, businesses may present the findings of their own trials, studies, and other research to raise awareness and obtain greater media coverage [66].

3.4.9 ADVANCED ANALYTICS

Without efficient algorithms to organize, evaluate, and anticipate potential outcomes, gigabytes of data are useless. It's also important to determine the likelihood of developing a heart failure condition or attack. These instruments not only help preserve the functionality of medical devices and warn in case anything needs a remedy. The IoMT can genuinely save lives in this situation [67]. By utilizing cutting-edge algorithms that help to segment and cluster data, identify patterns, and raise alarms about potential hazards, IoT in hospitals, analytics difficulties may be overcome.

3.4.10 TRUST MAINTENANCE

To minimize the possibility of subverting the merits that access to data can avail to healthcare technology, organizations that innovate mechanisms and services based on the creation and sharing of patient data must ensure openness to patients, the public, and health care professionals regarding the utilization of their data.

3.4.11 DATA SECURITY

Over 82% of healthcare firms reported a security breach in the year prior, according to a 2019 Healthcare Information and Management Systems Society poll. Hackers are particularly interested in patient health data like electronic medical records and information found in patient databases such as credit card numbers, addresses, and email identifications. These devices repeatedly use outdated software that lacks built-in data security protection because they are primarily utilitarian in design [68].

3.4.12 LICENSING CHALLENGE

Complicated requirements must be met while incorporating IoMT devices into various medical facilities, compliance standards must be observed, and license approvals must be attained. Even though creating these devices takes time, that is not the only difficulty, IoT service providers in health confront. Regulatory compliance is a sizable obstacle that needs to be overcome [69]. Ignoring this problem could increase future risks and costs associated with litigation.

3.5   BENEFITS OF THE AIOMT REVIEWED

To properly illustrate the benefits, the next section will demonstrate challenges for the reviewed AIoMTs, within this subsection, we majorly present them into two benefits and then, challenges as detailed subsequently:

3.5.1 MEDICAL DIAGNOSIS

AIoMT aids in quick and precise medical diagnosis because it is the first step undertaken to treat patient ailments thereby reducing patient mortality rates. This ultimately leads to improved health and quality of life for individuals. Robots such as the Husky and Veebot have shown great potential in spotting skin tumors accurately and drawing blood, respectively [70]. Within the study [71], a 100% accuracy in the robotic diagnosis of 340 brains using magnetic resonance imaging. Correspondingly, AIoMTs are equipped with the ability to alert medical workers when patients' health deteriorates, as has been shown in this study where doctors were alerted by Google's DeepMind AI system when patients had acute injury of the kidney [72].

3.5.2 MEDICAL TREATMENT

Because treatment plays a crucial role in a patient's life, AIoMT has the potential to provide prompt treatment to various patient ailments due to its accuracy, thereby saving lives. In what is now referred to as precision medicine, AIoMT is accelerating the transition from traditional medicine to personalized medicine, targeted treatment, and uniquely composed drugs. Different AI models have shown great potential in the treatment of COVID-19 as indicated in studies [73]. Also, with the help of smartphones, AI can aid in prescribing medication to different patients who are unable to physically move to hospital settings [74]. Authors in [75] have shown great potential in the deployment of AI in the treatment of cancer using IBM's Watson system. Additionally, robots have achieved tremendous success in rehabilitation and therapy such as the limb-robot rehabilitation system [76].

3.5.3 PATIENT EMPOWERMENT

AIoMT has the potential to empower individuals to help them make better and more informed health decisions. The huge amount of patient data collected by wearable medical devices discussed in the previous section along with the embedded AI helps in analyzing this data, which could alert people with higher risks of becoming ill long before such ailments become serious [77]. Doing so allows individuals affected by certain chronic illnesses to better curb their disease, thereby enabling them to live healthier lives through mobile apps. This consequently empowers them and leads to reduced healthcare costs.

3.5.4 REDUCTION IN MEDICAL COSTS

Artificial intelligence is capable of speeding up the creation of life-saving medicines, thereby saving money in medical costs incurred on healthcare delivery systems. AIoMT can optimize medication development in clinical trials leading to minimization of the time taken to fully certify developed drugs [78].

3.5.5 REDUCTION IN HUMAN ERRORS

The use of AI in the IoMT has shown great benefits in minimizing human errors by medical workers, and thus saves lives. AIoMT has shown the potential to diagnose patients with a reported 72% more accurate diagnosis compared to the high error rate of medical workers. Without the use of technology in surgical procedures done by medical practitioners, the operation can lead to life-threatening consequences. Henceforth AI plays a vital role in assisting doctors in their surgical procedures due to its simulation of human-made intelligence [79].

3.6 CHALLENGES OF REVIEWED AIOMTS

Although AI and its convergence with the IoMT have shown tremendous potential to revolutionize healthcare, several technological challenges in their deployment have to be addressed to realize their adaptability and monetization at hospitals/clinics and society in general. This section briefly discusses those challenges.

3.6.1 PRIVACY CONCERNS

There are serious concerns from patients about the huge amount of data collected by the different IoMT. Leakage of such sensitive data through hackers and other means has consequences such as patient blackmail, tarnishing the reputation of health service providers as well as the likelihood of loss of lives. Studies have shown the possibility of AI compromising privacy by predicting the personal information of patients regardless of whether the algorithm has ever been presented with such records [80]. This modus operandi for AI in healthcare may result in lawsuits especially if the AI's conclusions are made available for public consumption. Hence, the sensitivity of the stored data needs to be protected from unauthorized access and disclosure.

3.6.2 MISSTEPS AND ERRORS

AIoMT systems are not very perfect as a patient could be hurt if the wrong treatment is prescribed or if the system fails to detect tumors on a radiological exam, etc. also, if AIoMT systems become popular, a slight error in one has the potential to hurt several. Additionally, because AI systems work with consumer-facing smart wearable devices and use data generated by them, those systems may produce invalid results, as indicated in this study using Fitbit trackers [81].

3.6.3 DATA MANAGEMENT AND POWER ISSUES

The heterogeneity of medical devices running different applications in the AIoMT system creates a data management problem such as storage, incompatible dataset formats created by various legacy IT third-party systems. Additionally, the huge volume of data (big data) generated needs to be stored and analyzed. Hence, the need for scalable and intelligent machine learning algorithms for processing such huge amount of patient data becomes crucial. Finally, most devices in the AIoMT have low power capacities, which affect the operational time [82]. An efficient mechanism capable of increasing the battery power of IoMT devices needs to be envisaged and deployed to increase their operational time.

3.6.4 BIAS

AI-enabled health suffers from the dangers of prejudice and inequality because such systems, by design, learn from the information fed into them leading to the absorption of biases from supplied datasets. Regardless of whether the AIoMT systems are trained on accurate, reliable, and representative datasets, bias will still be reflected, as noted in the study, where an AI system trained on healthcare datasets learns to recommend lower painkiller doses to patients of African-American race. Such a decision is purely based on systemic bias instead of biological traits [83].

3.7 FUTURE RESEARCH DIRECTION OF IOMT IN HEALTHCARE INDUSTRY

The adoption of AI in the health sector through its convergence with the IoMT is transforming healthcare delivery in aspects such as patient experience, how medical workers practice medicine, and how drugs are being manufactured. Soon, AIoMT is expected to improve the precision of wearable medical devices and their ability to collect, store, and interpret data about patients' health conditions. Consequently, this will allow medical workers to engage with their patients with the help of tele-medicine to achieve improved healthcare service delivery. Overall, the new means of getting healthcare services will drastically reduce the healthcare cost incurred for all groups of patients [84, 85]. Because much of how AI operates is unknown to any lay-man, policies and legal frameworks that govern its use, especially in the healthcare sector, will have to be instituted to promote public confidence in its use and protect the citizens from any fallout from its irresponsible deployment. Initiatives in that direction have been made by the European Union through its quest to come up with the Artificial intelligence Act, which is aimed at promoting uniformity in the gover-nance of AI technologies in different sectors, among which include the health sector. The other initiative is the Pan-Canadian AI strategy which along with the European one, will help the medical communities and regulators in monitoring the adoption and explainability of various AI technologies and how their use impacts different contexts in the healthcare industry [86]. Through a combination of standards and regulations, the accuracy, security, reliability, and health use of AI technologies will need to be instituted. This is because AI technologies are capable of learning patterns and modifying their recommendations in ways not envisioned by their creators. This poses regulatory issues, which will need to be addressed as the technology evolves. Adopting a community-led approach by medical workers, technologists, researchers, and other stakeholders is one way that can be adopted to develop standards for data collection and testing of AI-enabled health technologies. AIoMT trends such as chat-bot technologies (voice assistants) are seen to revolutionize the healthcare sector with their increased adoption by different healthcare providers. As evidenced by their extensive usage during the COVID-19 global pandemic and other health emergen-cies, voice assistants such as google assistant, Apple Siri, and Amazon Alexa proved very useful in responding to COVID-19-related public questions [87, 88].

3.8 CONCLUSIONS AND FUTURE SCOPE

The rise of the Internet of Medical Things (IoMT) has demonstrated fast gaining researchers' attention due to its potential to transform the way healthcare is deliv-ered. It allows them to monitor and manage various medical conditions and diseases. With IoMT devices, we can monitor our health records and take necessary precau-tions. IoMT is playing a vital role in the healthcare industry to improve the effi-ciency and accuracy of electronic devices. In this chapter, a comprehensive survey has been done on several electronic devices in the AIoMT. The identified and com-monly utilized medical devices have been highlighted, including electronic signals for AIoMT sensors. Moreover, AIoMT architecture demonstrates a comprehensive evolution using smart sensors to accumulate, aggregate, and regulate data for smart healthcare structures. The chapter further demonstrates a review of the challenges of electronic devices in the AIoMT, for instance, data security threats, data interoperability, and regulatory concerns, among others, which need to be addressed to improve medical standards of operation for not only medical persons but also patients and other medical stakeholders. Lastly, open research issues of future research in AIoMT are highlighted. With wonderful advancements such as automated medical delivery, connected inhalers and contact lenses, Parkinson's disease monitoring, glucose monitoring, depression and mood monitoring, and more, IoT technology has undoubtedly benefited healthcare. AIoMT improves the patient experience and streamlines workflows. Greater involvement and fewer in-person doctor visits benefit patients. Providers now have access to more accurate data, improved diagnosis, and more effective time management. More developments that further streamline the medical profession for both practitioners and patients are certainly to accompany AIoMT in healthcare in the future. This chapter is limited by its inability to address the different challenges pointed out for both electronic devices and AIoMT. As a recommendation for the readers of this chapter, a more concerted effort should be done by different stakeholders in instituting policies and legal frameworks that will regulate the deployment of AI in different health contexts. Also, solutions for the different challenges identified will have to be sought and implemented to promote public confidence in the usage of AI and IoMT in the health sector. Different researchers, students, and other stakeholders keen on this area will find the discussions in this chapter very useful.

REFERENCES

[1]   G. J. Joyia, R. M. Liaqat, A. Farooq, and S. Rehman, "Internet of medical things (IOMT): applications, benefits and future challenges in healthcare domain," *Journal of Communications*, 2017, doi:10.12720/jcm.12.4.240-247.

[2]   H. Kaur, M. Atif, and R. Chauhan, "An internet of healthcare things (IoHT)-based healthcare monitoring system," in *Advances in Intelligent Computing and Communication*, pp. 475–482, 2020, doi:10.1007/978-981-15-2774-6_56.

[3]   G. Muhammad, M. F. Alhamid, and X. Long, "Computing and processing on the edge: smart pathology detection for connected healthcare," *IEEE Networks*, vol. 33, no. 6, pp. 44–49, 2019, doi:10.1109/MNET.001.1900045.

[4]   F. Alshehri and G. Muhammad, "A comprehensive survey of the internet of things (IoT) and AI-based smart healthcare," *IEEE Access*, vol. 9, pp. 3660–3678, 2021, doi:10.1109/ACCESS.2020.3047960.

[5]   M. Nasr, Md. M. Islam, S. Shehata, F. Karray, and Y. Quintana, "Smart healthcare in the age of AI: recent advances, challenges, and future prospects," *IEEE Access*, vol. 9, pp. 145248–145270, 2021, doi:10.1109/ACCESS.2021.3118960.

[6]   J. B. Awotunde, S. O. Folorunso, S. A. Ajagbe, J. Garg, and G. J. Ajamu, "AiIoMT: IoMT-based system-enabled artificial intelligence for enhanced smart healthcare systems," in *Machine Learning for Critical Internet of Medical Things*, Cham: Springer International Publishing, pp. 229–254, 2022, doi:10.1007/978-3-030-80928-7_10.

[7]   A. Alabdulatif, N. N. Thilakarathne, and K. Kalinaki, "A Novel Cloud Enabled Access Control Model for Preserving the Security and Privacy of Medical Big Data", *Electronics (Basel)*, vol. 12, no. 12, p. 2646, Jun. 2023, doi: 10.3390/electronics12122646.

[8]   N. H. Sweilam, A. A. Tharwat, and N. K. Abdel Moniem, "Support vector machine for diagnosis cancer disease: a comparative study," *Egyptian Informatics Journal*, vol. 11, no. 2, pp. 81–92, 2010, doi:10.1016/j.eij.2010.10.005.

[9]   M. Khalilia, S. Chakraborty, and M. Popescu, "Predicting disease risks from highly imbalanced data using random forest," *BMC Medical Informatics and Decision Making*, vol. 11, no. 1, p. 51, 2011, doi:10.1186/1472-6947-11-51.

[10] P. Kaur, R. Kumar, and M. Kumar, "A healthcare monitoring system using random forest and internet of things (IoT)," *Multimedia Tools and Applications*, vol. 78, no. 14, pp. 19905–19916, 2019, doi:10.1007/s11042-019-7327-8.

[11] F. Galbusera, G. Casaroli, and T. Bassani, "Artificial intelligence and machine learning in spine research," *JOR Spine*, vol. 2, no. 1, p. e1044, 2019, doi:10.1002/jsp2.1044.

[12] Y. Shen, Y. Li, H. T. Zheng, B. Tang, and M. Yang, "Enhancing ontology-driven diagnostic reasoning with a symptom-dependency-aware Naïve Bayes classifier," *BMC Bioinformatics*, vol. 20, no. 1, p. 330, 2019, doi:10.1186/s12859-019-2924-0.

[13] S. C. Nwaneri, C. Yinka-Banjo, U. C. Uregbulam, O. O. Odukoya, and A. L. Imoize, "Explainable neural networks in diabetes mellitus prediction," in *Explainable Artificial Intelligence in Medical Decision Support Systems*, 1st ed., A. L. Imoize, J. Hemanth, D.-T. Do, and S. N. Sur, Eds., London: The Institution of Engineering and Technology, 2022, pp. 313–334.

[14] W. Shafik, "A Comprehensive Cybersecurity Framework for Present and Future Global Information Technology Organizations," In *Effective Cybersecurity Operations for Enterprise-Wide Systems*, 2023, (pp. 56–79). IGI Global.

[15] R. U. Rasool, H. F. Ahmad, W. Rafique, A. Qayyum, and J. Qadir, "ECG," *Journal of Network and Computer Applications*, vol. 201, pp. 103332, 2022, doi:10.1016/J.JNCA.2022.103332.

[16] F. Al-Turjman, M. H. Nawaz, and U. D. Ulusar, "Intelligence in the internet of medical things era: a systematic review of current and future trends," *Computer Communications*, vol. 150, pp. 644–660, 2020, doi:10.1016/J.COMCOM.2019.12.030.

[17] R. S. Plowman, T. Peters-Strickland, and G. M. Savage, "Digital medicines: clinical review on the safety of tablets with sensors," *Expert Opinion on Drug Safety*, vol. 17, no. 9, pp. 849–852, 2018, doi:10.1080/14740338.2018.1508447.

[18] M. Haghi, K. Thurow, and R. Stoll, "Wearable devices in medical internet of things: scientific research and commercially available devices," *Healthcare Informatics Research*, vol. 23, no. 1, pp. 4–15, 2017, doi:10.4258/hir.2017.23.1.4.

[19] F. Qureshi and S. Krishnan, "Wearable hardware design for the internet of medical things (IoMT)," *Sensors*, vol. 18, no. 11, p. 3812, 2018, doi:10.3390/s18113812.

[20] Healthwatch, "Smart clothing technology—wearable monitoring solutions," https://healthwatchtech.com/technology/ (accessed July 11, 2022).

[21] X. Nan, X. Wang, T. Kang, J. Zhang, L. Dong, et al., "Review of flexible wearable sensor devices for biomedical application," *Micromachines (Basel)*, vol. 13, no. 9, p. 1395, 2022, doi:10.3390/mi13091395.

[22] B. Sadri, D. Goswami, M. Sala de Medeiros, A. Pal, B. Castro, et al., "Wearable and implantable epidermal paper-based electronics," *ACS Applied Materials & Interfaces*, vol. 10, no. 37, pp. 31061–31068, 2018, doi:10.1021/acsami.8b11020.

[23] C. Diorio and J. Mavoori, "Computer electronics meet animal brains," *Computer (Long Beach Calif)*, vol. 36, no. 1, pp. 69–75, 2003, doi:10.1109/MC.2003.1160058.

[24] M. Ghovanloo, K. Beach, K. D. Wise, and K. Najafi, "A BiCMOS wireless interface chip for micromachined stimulating microprobes," in *2nd Annual International IEEE-EMBS Special Topic Conference on Microtechnologies in Medicine and Biology—Proceedings*, pp. 277–282, 2002, doi:10.1109/MMB.2002.1002330.

[25] A. Astaras, M. Ahmadian, N. Aydin, L. Cui, E. Johannessen et al., "A miniature inte-grated electronics sensor capsule for real-time monitoring of the gastrointestinal tract (IDEAS)," in *Proceedings of the IEEE ICBME Conference*, Piscataway, NJ, 2002.

[26] P. F. Saint-Maurice, B. I. Graubard, R. P. Troiano, D. Berrigan, D. A. Galuska et al., "Estimated number of deaths prevented through increased physical activity among US adults," *JAMA Internal Medicine*, vol. 182, no. 3, pp. 349–352, 2022, doi:10.1001/jamainternmed.2021.7755.

[27] R. McCullagh, C. Dillon, A. M. O'Connell, N. F. Horgan, and S. Timmons, "Step-count accuracy of 3 motion sensors for older and frail medical inpatients," *Archives of Physical Medicine and Rehabilitation*, vol. 98, no. 2, pp. 295–302, 2017, doi:10.1016/J.APMR.2016.08.476.

[28] J. Yoo, Long Yan, Seulki Lee, Hyejung Kim, and Hoi-Jun Yoo, "A wearable ECG acquisition system with compact planar-fashionable circuit board-based shirt," *IEEE Transactions on Information Technology in Biomedicine*, vol. 13, no. 6, pp. 897–902, 2009, doi:10.1109/TITB.2009.2033053.

[29] E. A. Feukeu and S. Winberg, "Photoplethysmography heart rate monitoring," *International Journal of E-Health and Medical Communications*, vol. 12, no. 3, pp. 17–37, 2021, doi:10.4018/IJEHMC.20210501.oa2.

[30] D. I. Rubin, "Needle electromyography: basic concepts," *Handbook of Clinical Neurology*, vol. 160, pp. 243–256, 2019, doi:10.1016/B978-0-444-64032-1.00016-3.

[31] Y. C. Yeh and W. J. Wang, "QRS complexes detection for ECG signal: the difference operation method," *Computer Methods and Programs in Biomedicine*, vol. 91, no. 3, pp. 245–254, 2008, doi:10.1016/J.CMPB.2008.04.006.

[32] FitBit, "Fitness trackers | shop fitbit," www.fitbit.com/global/us/products/trackers (accessed November 7, 2022).

[33] "Finger tip blood Oxygen SpO2 pulse oximeter heart rate monitor USA shipping | eBay," www.ebay.com/itm/154839406575 (accessed November 7, 2022).

[34] Thalmic Labs, "Unveiling the final design of the MyoTM Armband | by Thalmic Labs | thalmic | Medium," https://medium.com/thalmic/unveiling-the-final-design-of-the-myo-armband-10576c0ae95b (accessed November 7, 2022).

[35] J. Qian, "Glucose monitoring in various matrices with near-infrared spectrometry and chemometrics," Doctor of Philosophy (PhD), University of Iowa, 2013.

[36] K. Kalinaki, N. N. Thilakarathne, H. R. Mubarak, O. A. Malik, and M. Abdullatif, 'Cybersafe Capabilities and Utilities for Smart Cities', in Cybersecurity for Smart Cities, Springer, Cham, 2023, pp. 71–86. doi: 10.1007/978-3-031-24946-4_6.

[37] D. Raskovic, "Medical monitoring applications for wearable computing," *The Computer Journal*, vol. 47, no. 4, pp. 495–504, 2004, doi:10.1093/comjnl/47.4.495.

[38] Yutaka Kondo, Katsuyuki Honda, and Keisuke Tsubata, "Development of Seiko Pulse Graph (Part of the sensor)," *The Horological Institute of Japan*, pp. 38–48, 1997.

[39] H. H. Asada, P. Shaltis, A. Reisner, S. Rhee, and R. C. Hutchinson, "Mobile monitoring with wearable photoplethysmographic biosensors," *IEEE Engineering in Medicine and Biology Magazine*, vol. 22, no. 3, pp. 28–40, 2003, doi:10.1109/MEMB.2003.1213624.

[40] L. Torres-Pereira, P. Ruivo, C. Torres-Pereira, and C. Couto, "A noninvasive telemetric heart rate monitoring system based on phonocardiography," in *ISIE '97 Proceeding of the IEEE International Symposium on Industrial Electronics*, pp. 856–859. doi:10.1109/ISIE.1997.648825.

[41] E. Jovanov, A. O'Donnell Lords, D. Raskovic, P. G. Cox, R. Adhami et al., "Stress monitoring using a distributed wireless intelligent sensor system," *IEEE Engineering in Medicine and Biology Magazine*, vol. 22, no. 3, pp. 49–55, 2003, doi:10.1109/MEMB.2003.1213626.

[42] H. G. Kim, E. J. Cheon, D. S. Bai, Y. H. Lee, and B. H. Koo, "Stress and heart rate variability: a meta-analysis and review of the literature," *Psychiatry Investigation*, vol. 15, no. 3, pp. 235–245, 2018, doi:10.30773/pi.2017.08.17.

[43] S. M. H. Yeung, S. J. L. Bakker, G. D. Laverman, and M. H. de Borst, "Fibroblast growth factor 23 and adverse clinical outcomes in type 2 diabetes: a bitter-sweet symphony," *Current Diabetes Reports*, vol. 20, no. 10, pp. 1–9, 2020, doi:10.1007/S11892-020-01335-7/TABLES/3.

[44] J. Morley, E. J. Richter, J. W. Klaesner, K. S. Maluf, and M. J. Mueller, "In-shoe multi-sensory data acquisition system," *IEEE Transactions on Biomedical Engineering*, vol. 48, no. 7, pp. 815–819, 2001, doi:10.1109/10.930906.

[45] J. Zhang, J. Xu, J. Lim, J. K. Nolan, H. Lee, and C. H. Lee, "Wearable glucose monitoring and implantable drug delivery systems for diabetes management," *Advanced Healthcare Materials*, vol. 10, no. 17, p. 2100194, 2021, doi:10.1002/ADHM.202100194.

[46] G. Costamagna, S. K. Shah, M. E. Riccioni, F. Foschia, M. Mutignani et al., "A prospective trial comparing small bowel radiographs and video capsule endoscopy for suspected small bowel disease," *Gastroenterology*, vol. 123, no. 4, pp. 999–1005, 2002, doi:10.1053/GAST.2002.35988.

[47] S. M. Bolam, B. Batinica, T. C. Yeung, S. Weaver, A. Cantamessa et al., "Remote patient monitoring with wearable sensors following knee arthroplasty," *Sensors*, vol. 21, no. 15, p. 51432021, 2021, doi:10.3390/S21155143.

[48] L. Molly, M. Quirynen, K. Michiels, and D. Van Steenberghe, "Comparison between jaw bone augmentation by means of a stiff occlusive titanium membrane or an autologous hip graft: a retrospective clinical assessment," *Clinical Oral Implants Research*, vol. 17, no. 5, pp. 481–487, 2006, doi:10.1111/J.1600-0501.2006.01286.X.

[49] S. Hamid, N. Z. Bawany, A. H. Sodhro, A. Lakhan, and S. Ahmed, "A systematic review and IoMT based big data framework for COVID-19 prevention and detection," *Electronics*, vol. 11, no. 17, p. 2777, 2022, doi:10.3390/ELECTRONICS11172777.

[50] A. Ferrag, I. A. Jayaraj, B. Shanmugam, S. Azam, and G. N. Samy, "A systematic review of radio frequency threats in IoMT," *Journal of Sensor and Actuator Networks*, vol. 11, no. 4, p. 62, 2022, doi:10.3390/JSAN11040062.

[51] M. Adil, M. K. Khan, M. M. Jadoon, M. Attique, H. Song, and A. Farouk, "An AI-enabled hybrid lightweight authentication scheme for intelligent iomt based cyber-physical systems," *IEEE Transactions on Network Science and Engineering*, p. 17, 2022, doi:10.1109/TNSE.2022.3159526.

[52] M. K. Kavita, S. Verma, A. Kumar, M. F. Ijaz, and D. B. Rawat, "ANAF-IoMT: a novel architectural framework for iomt-enabled smart healthcare system by enhancing security based on RECC-VC," *IEEE Transactions on Industrial Informatics*, vol. 18, no. 12, pp. 8936–8943, 2022, doi:10.1109/TII.2022.3181614.

[53] P. Manickam, S. A. Mariappan, S. M. Murugesan, S. Hansda, A. Kaushik et al., "Artificial intelligence (AI) and internet of medical things (IoMT) assisted biomedical systems for intelligent healthcare," *Biosensors (Basel)*, vol. 12, no. 8, p. 562, 2022, doi:10.3390/bios12080562.

[54] www.meddeviceonline.com/doc/the-internet-of-medical-things-raises-novel-compliance-challenges-0001/ (accessed November 11, 2022).

[55] S. Rahmadika, P. V. Astillo, G. Choudhary, D. G. Duguma, V. Sharma et al., "Blockchain-based privacy preservation scheme for misbehavior detection in lightweight IoMT devices," *IEEE Journal of Biomedical and Health Informatics*, pp. 1–13, 2022, doi:10.1109/JBHI.2022.3187037.

[56] F. Pelekoudas-Oikonomou, G. Zachos, M. Papaioannou, J. C. M. de Ree, and G. Ribeiro, "Blockchain-based security mechanisms for IoMT edge networks in IoMT-based

healthcare monitoring systems," *Sensors*, vol. 22, no. 7, pp. 2449, 2022, doi:10.3390/s22072449.

[57] P. Singh, G. S. Gaba, A. Kaur, M. Hedabou, and A. Gurtov, "Dew-cloud-based hierarchical federated learning for intrusion detection in IoMT," *IEEE Journal of Biomedical and Health Informatics*, pp. 1–10, 2022, doi:10.1109/JBHI.2022.3186250.

[58] J. Almalki, W. Al Shehri, R. Mehmood, K. Alsaif, S. M. Alshahrani et al., "Enabling blockchain with IoMT devices for healthcare," *Information*, vol. 13, no. 10, p. 448, 2022, doi:10.3390/info13100448.

[59] Y. Jun, A. Craig, W. Shafik, and L. Sharif, "Artificial intelligence application in cybersecurity and cyberdefense," *Wireless Communications & Mobile Computing*, pp. 1–10, 2021, doi:10.1155/2021/3329581.

[60] F. Shokoor, W. Shafik, and S. M. Matinkhah, "Overview of 5g & beyond security," *EAI Endorsed Transactions on Internet of Things*, vol. 8, no. 30, 2022, doi:10.4108/eetiot.v8i30.1624.

[61] A. A. Alli, K. Kassim, N. Mutwalibi, H. Hamid, and L. Ibrahim, "Secure fog-cloud of things: architectures, opportunities and challenges," in *Secure Edge Computing*, 1st ed., M. Ahmed and P. Haskell-Dowland, Eds., CRC Press, 2021, pp. 3–20.

[62] M. U. Nasir, S. Khan, S. Mehmood, M. A. Khan, A. Rahman, and S. O. Hwang, "IoMT-based osteosarcoma cancer detection in histopathology images using transfer learning empowered with blockchain, fog computing, and edge computing," *Sensors*, vol. 22, no. 14, p. 5444, 2022, doi:10.3390/s22145444.

[63] J. Ktari, T. Frikha, N. ben Amor, L. Louraidh, H. Elmannai, and M. Hamdi, "IoMT-based platform for e-health monitoring based on the blockchain," *Electronics (Basel)*, vol. 11, no. 15, p. 2314, 2022, doi:10.3390/electronics11152314.

[64] C.-H. Yang, Y.-Y. Liu, C.-H. Chiang, and Y.-W. Su, "National IoMT platform strategy portfolio decision model under the COVID-19 environment: based on the financial and non-financial value view," *Annals of Operations Research*, 2022, doi:10.1007/s10479-022-05016-4.

[65] R. Hireche, H. Mansouri, and A.-S. K. Pathan, "Security and privacy management in internet of medical things (IoMT): a synthesis," *Journal of Cybersecurity and Privacy*, vol. 2, no. 3, pp. 640–661, 2022, doi:10.3390/jcp2030033.

[66] I. A. Khan et al., "XSRU-IoMT: explainable simple recurrent units for threat detection in internet of medical things networks," *Future Generation Computer Systems*, vol. 127, pp. 181–193, 2022, doi:10.1016/j.future.2021.09.010.

[67] W. Shafik, S. M. Matinkhah, and F. Shokoor, "Recommendation system comparative analysis: internet of things aided networks," *EAI Endorsed Transactions on Internet of Things*, vol. 8, no. 29, 2022.

[68] J. Srivastava, S. Routray, S. Ahmad, and M. M. Waris, "Internet of medical things (IoMT)-based smart healthcare system: trends and progress," *Computational Intelligence and Neuroscience*, vol. 2022, pp. 1–17, 2022, doi:10.1155/2022/7218113.

[69] A. M. Rahmani and S. Y. Hosseini Mirmahaleh, "Flexible-clustering based on application priority to improve IoMT efficiency and dependability," *Sustainability*, vol. 14, no. 17, p. 10666, 2022, doi:10.3390/su141710666.

[70] S. Yeasmin, "Benefits of artificial intelligence in medicine," in *2nd International Conference on Computer Applications and Information Security*, ICCAIS, 2019, doi:10.1109/CAIS.2019.8769557.

[71] M. F. Siddiqui, A. W. Reza, and J. Kanesan, "An automated and intelligent medical decision support system for brain MRI scans classification," *PLoS ONE*, vol. 10, no. 8, p. e0135875, 2015, doi:10.1371/journal.pone.0135875.

[72] "NHS using Google technology to treat patients—BBC News," www.bbc.com/news/health-38055509 (accessed December 8, 2022).

[73] M. Jamshidi et al., "Artificial intelligence and COVID-19: deep learning approaches for diagnosis and treatment," *IEEE Access*, vol. 8, pp. 109581–109595, 2020, doi:10.1109/ACCESS.2020.3001973.

[74] "How will artificial intelligence change healthcare?" *World Economic Forum*, www.weforum.org/agenda/2015/10/how-will-artificial-intelligence-change-healthcare (accessed December 8, 2022).

[75] S. P. Somashekhar, M. J. Sepúlveda, S. Puglielli, A. D. Norden, E. H. Shortliffe et al., "Watson for oncology and breast cancer treatment recommendations: agreement with an expert multidisciplinary tumor board," *Annals of Oncology*, vol. 29, no. 2, pp. 418–423, 2018, doi:10.1093/annonc/mdx781.

[76] K. Kakhi, R. Alizadehsani, H. M. D. Kabir, A. Khosravi, S. Nahavandi et al., "The internet of medical things and artificial intelligence: trends, challenges, and opportunities," *Biocybernetics and Biomedical Engineering*, vol. 42, no. 3, pp. 749–771, 2022, doi:10.1016/j.bbe.2022.05.008.

[77] S. Vollmer, B. A. Mateen, G. Bohner, F. J. Király, R. Ghani et al., "Machine learning and artificial intelligence research for patient benefit: 20 critical questions on transparency, replicability, ethics, and effectiveness," *BMJ*, vol. 368, 2020, doi:10.1136/bmj.l6927.

[78] J. T. Beck, M. Rammage, G. P. Jackson, A. M. Preininger, I. Dankwa-Mullan et al., "Artificial intelligence tool for optimizing eligibility screening for clinical trials in a large community cancer center," *JCO Clinical Cancer Informatics*, no. 4, pp. 50–59, 2020, doi:10.1200/cci.19.00079.

[79] S. Sunarti, F. Fadzlul Rahman, M. Naufal, M. Risky, K. Febriyanto, and R. Masnina, "Artificial intelligence in healthcare: opportunities and risk for future," *Gaceta Sanitaria*, vol. 35, pp. S67–S70, 2021, doi:10.1016/j.gaceta.2020.12.019.

[80] M. Marwan, A. Kartit, and H. Ouahmane, "Security Enhancement in healthcare cloud using machine learning," *Procedia Computer Science*, vol. 127, pp. 388–397, 2018, doi:10.1016/J.PROCS.2018.01.136.

[81] O. Ore and M. Sposato, "Opportunities and risks of artificial intelligence in recruitment and selection," *International Journal of Organizational Analysis*, vol. 30, no. 6, pp. 1771–1782, 2021.

[82] K. Kakhi, R. Alizadehsani, H. M. D. Kabir, A. Khosravi, S. Nahavandi, and U. R. Acharya, "The internet of medical things and artificial intelligence: trends, challenges, and opportunities," *Biocybernetics and Biomedical Engineering*, vol. 42, no. 3, pp. 749–771, 2022, doi:10.1016/j.bbe.2022.05.008.

[83] Z. Yang, L. Jianjun, H. Faqiri, W. Shafik, A. Talal Abdulrahman et al., "Green internet of things and big data application in smart cities development," *Complexity*, 2021, doi:10.1155/2021/4922697.

[84] R. Dwivedi, D. Mehrotra, and S. Chandra, "Potential of internet of medical things (IoMT) applications in building a smart healthcare system: a systematic review," *Journal of Oral Biology and Craniofacial Research*, vol. 12, no. 2, pp. 302–318, 2022, doi:10.1016/j.jobcr.2021.11.010.

[85] A. L. Imoize, P. A. Gbadega, H. I. Obakhena, D. O. Irabor, K. V. N. Kavitha, and C. Chakraborty, "Artificial intelligence-enabled internet of medical things for COVID-19 pandemic data management," in *Explainable Artificial Intelligence in Medical Decision Support Systems*, 1st ed., A. L. Imoize, J. Hemanth, D.-T. Do, and S. N. Sur, Eds., London: The Institution of Engineering and Technology, 2022, pp. 357–380.

[86] W. Shafik, S. M. Matinkhah, and M. Ghasemzadeh, "Theoretical understanding of deep learning in uav biomedical engineering technologies analysis," *SN Computer Science*, vol. 1, no. 6, pp. 1–3, 2020, doi:10.1007/s42979-020-00323-8.

[87] E. Sezgin, Y. Huang, U. Ramtekkar, and S. Lin, "Readiness for voice assistants to support healthcare delivery during a health crisis and pandemic," *NPJ Digital Medicine*, vol. 3, no. 1, p. 122, 2020, doi:10.1038/s41746-020-00332-0.

[88] A. T. Rufai, K. F. Dukor, O. M. Ageh, and A. L. Imoize, "XAI robot-assisted surgeries in future medical decision support systems," in *Explainable Artificial Intelligence in Medical Decision Support Systems*, 1st ed., A. L. Imoize, J. Hemanth, D.-T. Do, and S. N. Sur, Eds., London: The Institution of Engineering and Technology, 2022, pp. 167–195.

4 Artificial Intelligence of Medical Things for Medical Information Systems Privacy and Security

Muyideen Abdulraheem, Emmanuel Abidemi Adeniyi, Joseph Bamidele Awotunde, Agbotiname Lucky Imoize, Rasheed Gbenga Jimoh, Idowu Dauda Oladipo, and Peace Busola Falola

4.1 INTRODUCTION

Insufficient protection in AIoMT medical systems might have serious negative consequences, such as loss of patient privacy owing to eavesdropping and the slow identification of life-threatening situations incidents due to the interruption of regular AIoMT device processes by Denial of Service (DoS) assaults [1]. In addition, AIoMT devices typically process and store specific captured data some include functionality and patient records capabilities to promote the users' well-being. As a result, AIoMT devices are anticipated to require substantially greater levels of security than standard IoT and computer devices [2.]. However, when designing AIoMT healthcare systems, security and dangers are frequently neglected.

Users' personal information, in particular, must have their privacy carefully protected. However, numerous instances of critical patient health data being compromised on cloud servers from major corporations, such as Facebook and Yahoo [3], raise the issue of whether such information can be secured. In reality, because individual medical information is so treasured on the black market, hostile attackers increasingly focus on medical servers and eHealth systems [4]. Because of this, providers of medical services must take increasingly more control safeguards, which invariably boosts the cost of establishing, running, and sustaining these health treatments.

The development of post-attack measures is just as important as establishing defenses against attacks. Unlike monetary information such as credit card security codes, individual medical information might reflect a person's current health difficulties, which can be swiftly rendered ineffective and useless [5]. The recovery and destruction of stolen data are both difficult and crucial when certain data is taken as a result of a security vulnerability. The number of cyberattacks against medical services has increased, despite the most recent laws and regulations implemented by governments and authorities [6].

The AIoMT is a subset of the Internet of Things (IoT) technology consisting of diagnostic instruments linked to track clinical outcomes. AIoMT healthcare IoT devices blend automated, interfacial sensing, and artificial intelligence based on machine learning to provide clinical surveillance without the intervention of humans. AIoMT technology connects patients and clinicians through medical equipment, allowing remote access for gathering, analyzing, and transferring medical information through a secure server. In addition, AIoMT technology allows wireless surveillance of health indicators, reducing unnecessary hospital delays and, as a result, healthcare expenses.

The AIoMT medical technologies market includes point-of-care (POC) gadgets for use in hospitals or medical centers and portable and in-home individual real-time health surveillance systems [7], for examples POC diagnostic devices are used to obtain diagnostic results while with the patient or close to the patient. In addition, smartphone-integrated devices, smart wristbands, smart fabrics and apparel, and sports watches for activity and fitness tracking are all included in the category of wearable personal health monitoring devices [8].

An on-demand medical examination and the televisit system are two clinical applications where AIoMT enables POC monitoring. These applications can track the unintentional falls of senior citizens. Although elderly adults may ultimately fall, the surroundings can be monitored, and incidents prevented to avoid long-term harm.

AIoMT is now the leading technology for managing patient health data [9]. It primarily serves a variety of purposes in homes, hospitals, and body sensors. The AIoMT environment is constructed using a vast array of medical equipment, sensors, and other things [10]. Additionally, these effective gadgets can potentially cover a specific body surface. The medical sector can readily handle therapeutic records because of the AIoMT system's quick development [11], where the physician assists in the early discovery of problems and effective diagnosis.

Although the evolution of AIoMT applications has been seen in recent years limited to the two issues of security and privacy, as the AIoMT infrastructure contains a vast amount of medical data, it is crucial to managing health data [12]. The AIoMT network illustrates how various attacks can readily be introduced and cause performance degradation. As a result, important data are lost [13]. Insufficient medical equipment or detector permission or verification, a lack of understanding [14] regarding data encryption, an unsecured device interface, etc., make the system insecure. The most important method for creating an efficient AIoMT system is to use authentication measures to secure and protect patient data privacy.

Additionally, ciphertext data is produced using encryption techniques such as Elliptic Curve Cryptography (ECC), and Diffie-Hellman to protect against malicious threats. Blockchain technology has also recently been heavily incorporated in AIoMT applications, improving security performance. However, all of the aforementioned approaches to protecting medical information have their limitations [15].

4.1.1 THE CONTRIBUTIONS OF THE CHAPTER

The primary contribution of this work is as follows:

    i. Present many methods for ensuring the security and privacy preservation of data in AIoMT
   ii. Classify the AIoMT deployment techniques and their future perspectives
  iii. Explain the historical analysis of AIoMT devices and the performance indicators used for validating and monitoring
   iv. Present the research gaps and data security and privacy difficulties in IoMT devices

4.1.2 CHAPTER ORGANIZATION

Section 4.2 presents the related works on the security and privacy of Artificial Intelligence Internet of Medical Things. Section 4.3 discusses AI of Medical Things. Section 4.4 presents the category of security and privacy data algorithms. Section 4.5 discusses the vulnerabilities and requirements of the devices. Section 4.6 presents the security requirement in the internet of medical things system. Section 4.7 discusses the internet of medical things system security solutions. Section 4.8 presents challenges and further research, and finally, Section 4.9 concludes the chapter with future direction.

4.2 RELATED WORK

To secure medical data across the AIoMT infrastructure, [16] investigated the idea of the Crypto-Stego technique. This model was created by assuming the steganographic and cryptographic approaches. Finally, the accurate data needed to assess the performance was gathered. As a result, it has shown to be an effective paradigm and has given superior outcomes in terms of data loss, security, capability, and noticeable quality. For the purpose of protecting the data in the AIoMT platform, in the context of smart transactions, authors in [17] have suggested a consortium-based public blockchain. It has been merged with the Inter Planetary File Systems (IPFS) cluster node, where agreements must authenticate in order to access a client's healthcare data. Additionally, the cluster layer served as a storage layer. Data was securely sent via consortium blocks after authentication. In contrast to previous studies that have been implemented, the suggested method has demonstrated greater security.

The private blockchain technology was created by authors in [18] to keep medical information safe. It developed a decentralized network where a large amount of data will be stored. To ensure data secrecy, the Elliptic Curve Integrated Cryptographic Algorithm was employed to accomplish a twofold encryption procedure. As a result, the performance was evaluated and it was determined that it had reduced transaction time and increased data security. The IoMT platform now includes a blockchain-assisted Secure Data Management Framework (BSDMF) studied by authors in ref. [19] to ensure data transmission through the AIoMT environment. The study was finally completed, and the findings were validated using a variety of metrics, including increased accuracy and precision rates, a higher trust factor, and a shorter response time.

The "Efficient Privacy-preserving outsourced Support Vector Machine (EPoSVM)" for the AIoMT segment has been described by authors in ref. [20]. It has implemented eight secure-based compute procedures to safely train the SVM network. As a result, the prepared data was acquired in a protected method, proving the confidentiality of the medical data while the model was being tested. Therefore, it was clear from the evaluation that the suggested strategy, as opposed to earlier ones, has achieved excellent security and privacy. Authors in ref. [21] hybrid approach for protecting and preserving the data across IoMT was introduced in 2021.

Here, the innovative hybrid paradigm was created by combining "Enhanced On-Demand Vector (EAODV)-enabled routing with Medium Access Control (MAC)." The registration procedure was initially supported for offline hardware. As a result, it has prevented the entry of unauthorized strategies into the system. Following this, the device-related server must communicate the mutual authentication method once the device has started the process. The data reliability and integrity were preserved by modifying the encryption and decryption procedure during the sessions. Finally, the modeling results concluded that the efficiency had increased.

AIoMT platform data preservation hybrid method described by the author in ref. [22] is known as a blockchain-based Distributed Data Storage System (DDSS). Its major goal is to ease some restrictions on characteristics like latency and storage expense. SRAC (Specific Ring Based Access Control) was used to improve the verification of the device admission into the system. Finally, the performance was evaluated, and the results were impressive enough to give an efficient method of data preservation.

Authors in ref. [23] used the ANFIS model in 2021 to manage security for IoMT applications using a blockchain. The fundamental objective of this strategy was to help people go about their everyday lives while protecting them from sick people. The k-nearest neighbor (kNN) was used in this instance to examine performance using an accuracy measure. Authors in ref. [23] introduced the innovative architecture of Mutual Authentication and Key Agreement (MAAKA) based on the features of Provably Secure and Lightweight (PSL), known as PSL-MAAKA for IoMT. In order to complete the authentication process, XOR and hash operations were used, respectively. Additionally, a security study was performed using the random oracle model approach. Finally, it has been demonstrated by the experimental findings that the proposed approach has minimal overhead complexity.

The study introduced the deep learning Encrypting and Decoding Network (DeepEDN) technique for health data protection [24]. In the study, the medical photos were used for testing purposes. The Cycle-Generative Adversarial Network (Cycle-GAN) has been developed and used to learn image-related data. The learning approach's encryption portion also used "Hidden Factors" that might be recovered after decryption. Finally, the performance was confirmed, and the results guaranteed improved system performance and efficiency.

The model of the Efficient Differentially Private Data Clustering technique has been improved by Guan et al. (EDPDCS). K-Means clustering was used in this case to select the first centroid data point and optimize the budget portion for improving accuracy. The smallest and most static values for the privacy budget were taken into consideration throughout the iteration. The efficiency and accuracy were enhanced using the clustering strategy. Finally, an analysis of the performance demonstrated improved data preservation performance.

Over the AIoMT platform, authors in ref. [24] have enclosed a protected and effective system. The main goal of this research was to lessen and avoid the overhead issue among the biosensors it used. Additionally, it was necessary to secure the patient's health records. As a result, the improved system has effectively secured network integrity, biosensor energy usage, minimal delay, and a low packet loss ratio. Authors have studied elliptic curve cryptography with lightweight authentication [25] for the IoMT platform. The AVISPA tool was used to implement it, and standard protocols were used to protect patient data. Because of this, security performance analysis was conducted using formal and informal methods.

In order to make sure the suggested approach has improved the robustness and efficiency of IoMT devices, a comparative analysis was done. The ontology-oriented IoMT Security Assessment Framework (IoMT-SAF) has been suggested for the IoMT industry by authors in ref. [26]. It has recognized the best resolutions that have helped people make enhanced decisions for data security based on customer requirements. Finally, with its performance improvement, it has outperformed. Asymmetric encryption and authorization are used methods that have been framed over the IoMT environment by authors in ref. [27]. Here, distributed symmetric encryption was used to control the transmission mechanism as well as the storage purpose. Additionally, permission and authentication were completed.

As a result, the widespread outcomes have shown it accomplished the anticipated performance. A study in ref. [28] has presented an innovative lightweight authentication method for protecting medical information. The framework suggested in this case was called Lightweight Authentication, Access Control, and Ownership (LACO). The main worry was that the server might change the patient's clinical data if the possession changed. Additionally, the LACO device was created to protect against assaults, including insider threats and denial-of-service attacks (DoS). As a result, the performance outcomes were measured and validated.

Multivariate-Quadratic-Equations (MQ) general populace encryption and the encrypted rainbow concept method have been proven by authors in ref. [29] for use in IoMT applications. This algorithm was used for an end-to-end platform that has shown to be resistant to such attacks. As a result, a few countermeasures were considered to assess the performance. As a result, excellent outcomes were obtained to deliver higher performance. Studies in ref. [30] have impacted hybrid Teaching and Learning Based Optimization (HTLBO) to produce the best results. To identify the security and authentication procedure in this case, the Chinese Remainder Theorem (CRT) was created. Finally, thorough results have shown reduced calculation time and energy costs.

For maintaining the medical data securely, authors in ref. [31] proposed the "Blockchain Enabled Authenticated Key Management Protocol for IoMT (BAKMP-IoMT)." It was incorporated into the AVISPA program, which automates the authentication of network safekeeping procedures and applications and has remarkably resisted numerous outbreaks. Finally, the simulation was run, and the outcomes were verified using a variety of techniques. Therefore, the vast results have demonstrated that it has lessened the stress on computation and communication. In relation to fog nodes, in ref. [32], authors have created new IoMT devices. This model's main goal was to manage patient data privacy and confidentiality. The proposed approach was evaluated using an integration of these models, and its exceptional findings have demonstrated its effective performance.

4.3 ARTIFICIAL INTELLIGENCE OF MEDICAL THINGS

The Artificial Intelligence of Medical Things (AIoMT) is made up of smart medical equipment that are all connected. Handling medical data is the main goal of the AIoMT application. As a result, Figure 4.1 shows an overall diagram of devices, including servers, medical equipment, and IoT devices. Another consideration in data transmission is AIoMT communication, which may be divided into four categories: bodily connections, home area networks, neighborhood area networks, and broad-area networks. The body area network has recently emerged as the preferred method of communication with AIoMT devices. Wearable body sensors are used to collect certain personal health information, which is subsequently communicated over the Internet and shown in the AIoMT application. Three diagrams show the body area network in diagrammatic form.

4.3.1 HEALTHCARE SYSTEMS BASED ON AIoMT

As shown in Figure 4.1, AIoMT -based healthcare systems frequently have three tiers: sensor level, personal server level, and medical server level. Numerous recently proposed IoMT-based healthcare systems, including in ref. [33], have embraced this

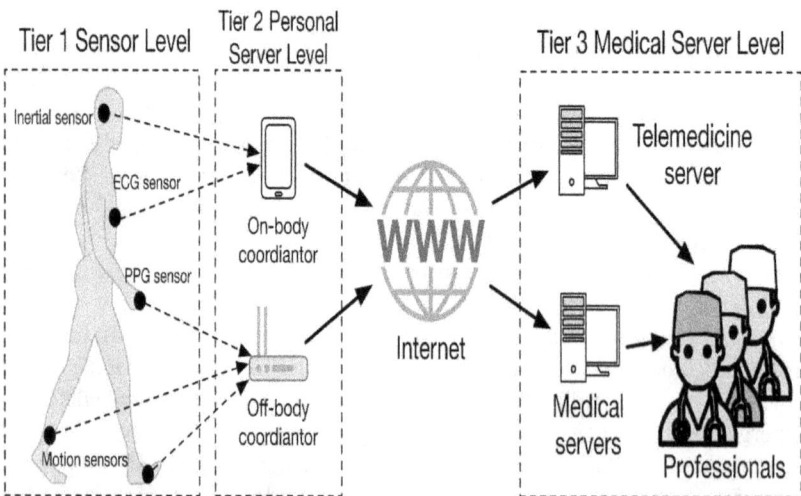

FIGURE 4.1 Architecture of IoMT-based healthcare systems.

architecture. The sensor level, where medical equipment and sensors are situated, creates a local network known as the body sensor network (BSN) [34]. In addition, reduced wireless infrastructure standards such as Bluetooth Low Energy (BLE), Near-Field Communication (NFC), and Radio-Frequency Identification (RFID) are used for mobile technology at the sensing and private server levels frequently used.

Unlike NFC and RFID, which can only support ultra-low power and close-proximity direct interactions, as required by implanted devices, BLE offers a variety of network topologies, including star and mesh. Personal servers can be on-body equipment, such as cell devices, programmers, and tablets, or off-body equipment, such as modems and gateways that will receive the physiological data that the medical devices have acquired. Prior to transferring patient data to centralized medical servers, personal servers are used to process and store patient data locally. When the network connection to the medical servers is severed, the normal operation must be possible on a personal server. Doctors and other medical professionals can remotely access patient data to give patients quick recommendations.

With the patients' permission, algorithms, and computer software for prompt diagnosis and evaluations of the progress of rehabilitation can also be run on the medical platform. In the previous few years, a number of IoMT-based healthcare schemes have been proposed for continuous patient checking. Conversely, many of them, like MobiCare in [35], do not implement any security and privacy protections in their designs or are left out for future studies. The safety of the systems and the confidentiality of patient data have not received as much attention from this research as other design concerns like power consumption and usability have. Healthcare systems based on recently developed IoMT, such as BSN-Care [36], have included encryption and authentication techniques in their designs.

4.4 CATEGORIES OF SECURITY AND PRIVACY OF DATA ALGORITHMS

Over time, algorithms categorization for data security and privacy has improved. The AIoMT platform is explained in this section. To improve system efficiency, a variety of conventional techniques have been applied. The key areas of study are the authentication procedure, encryption and decryption algorithms, and blockchain-based solutions. As a result, the algorithm classification for protecting data privacy in the AIoMT sector is shown in Figure 4.2.

4.4.1 DATA PRIVACY AND SECURITY

In various IoT and IoE architectures, secure communication is essential for preserving data privacy and confidentiality. Data privacy refers to the rules to be followed when collecting, storing, and transferring data to protect the user's personal information. Secure key management [37] and the physically unclonable function [38] can increase security.

Devices based on the Internet of Things are being used more frequently as it becomes a more integral part of our daily lives. As cities continue to grow, it is estimated that 70% of gadgets will be Internet of Things (IoT)-based. By 2025,

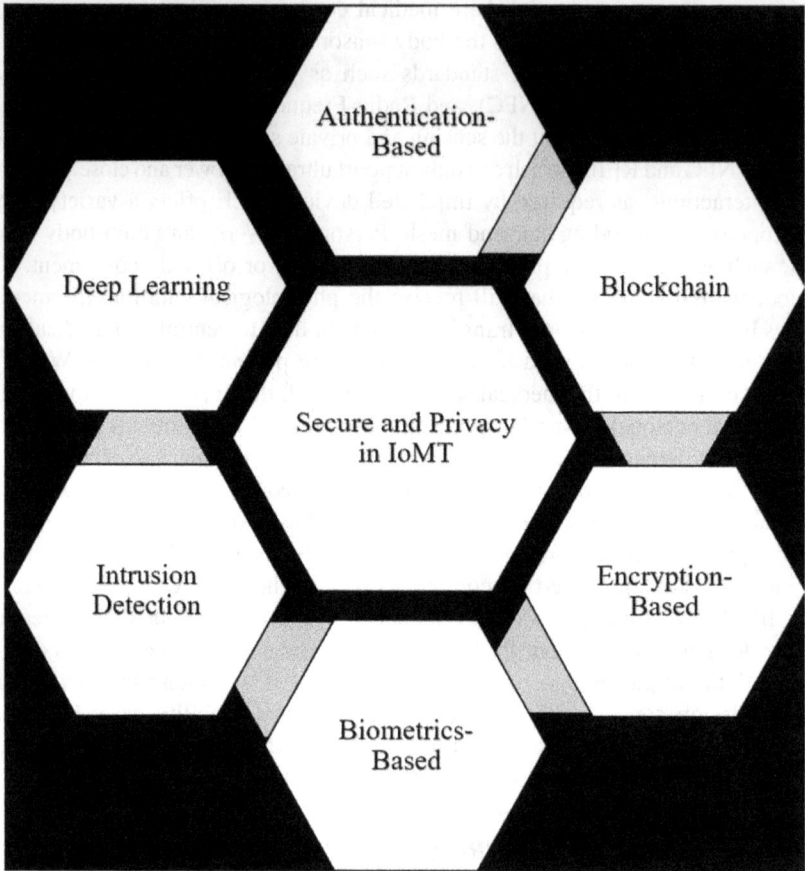

FIGURE 4.2 Secure and privacy-preserving algorithm for AIoMT data.

$14.4 trillion worth of gadgets will be used, according to the author in ref. [39]. M2M traffic is growing; by 2022, it is predicted to make up to 45% of all internet traffic. According to a different estimate, the cost-effectiveness of IoT-based smart healthcare would expand worldwide by $1.1 to $2.5 trillion annually by 2025. By 2025, it is expected to have a $2.7 trillion to $6.2 trillion influence on the world economy [40].

By 2025, 75 billion IoT devices will be linked to the international system. The proliferation of IoT devices is drawing hackers to the global network in an effort to accomplish their objectives. Symantec claims that because of the technology's quick growth and development, cybercriminals are increasingly focusing on IoT.

The number of cyberattacks in 2019 was about 3 billion, up 300% from the previous year [41]. Security is the Internet of Everything's network's biggest concern, according to authors in ref. [41]. *The Network in Everything: Independence and Safety in an Interconnected World. Without an off Switch* by Laura DeNardis examines the dangers and concerns associated with IoE. The book also, in relation to confidentiality, cyber-physical protection, and interoperability, tackles politics, economic expansion, personal freedoms, business strategies, and administration [42].

4.4.2 THE INTERNET OF MEDICAL THINGS

The environment becomes an IoMT when health functions are added to IoT devices. IoMT devices are being used more frequently as a result of technological advancements. Additionally, the COVID-19 condition restricts in-person interactions between patients and physicians. Due to the outbreak, a new age of IoMT for medical therapy has evolved [43]. IoMT is establishing a collection of individuals and health equipment (wireless therapeutic devices and implanted health strategies). It uses wireless connections (Bluetooth, Wi-Fi, third generation, fourth generation, fifth generation, ZigBee, etc.) to interchange medical data with healthcare centers such as physicians, hospitals, and medical professionals [44]. Medical devices now contain intelligence and can measure and report bodily indicators such as blood volume, heart rate, and oxygen saturation, thanks to advancements in microelectronics.

The gadgets can be worn on the body as necklaces, watches, belts, shoes, or clothing [45]. Additionally, IoMT has emerged as the most significant advancement in the medical field since it includes not only the elderly but also all elderly unwell people in continuous monitoring and therapy. Even after healing from COVID-19, some people still experience pain, and IoMT offers emergency care when necessary. Many healthcare institutions use the IoMT system throughout the world to deliver care. However, according to the 2020 CyberMDX research, up to 50% of IoMT equipment is vulnerable to assault. IoMT networks stand out from other systems since they may impact patients' lives and cause privacy issues if authors in ref. [46] reveal their identities. Therefore, the IoMT system's top priority is maintaining security and privacy.

According to research from the significant concepts, a cybersecurity firm compromised a record number of patients' sensitive health information in 2021. Medical records attacks damaged 45 million individuals in 2021, up from 34 million in 2020. According to the analysis, from 14 million in 2018 to 51 million today, there have been three times as many data breaches.

4.5 DEVICES VULNERABILITIES AND REQUIREMENTS

Threats to connected devices come in many forms, and they worsen daily. Low-power devices cannot address the necessities of conventional ways to endorse security. Blocking the intrusion of attackers into devices or networks is crucial for maintaining the device and the network protection privacy of the users. This section will provide examples of potential security threats and their mitigation. Security-restricted IoT networks and devices typically have limited resources, making applying traditional security mechanics difficult.

4.5.1 IoT ATTACK SURFACES

As the variety and quantity of IoT strategies grow, so does the security risk. Furthermore, the growing populace (amount of IoT devices), convolution, heterogeneity, variation, interchange, scalability, movement, position, structure, and item distribution all contribute to a rise in the threat environment of IoT networks (policies, regulator, connectivity, consumer, and facilities). The outbreak surface significantly expands with the diversification and proliferation of IoT devices.

An attack surface is made up of entities and enablers (such as networks and protocols) (i.e., devices, approaches, and data). The degree of connectedness between a system's parts and the regulations that control device access to the system together make up the attack surface. IoT hardware serves as numerous network-building components in an IoT architecture. Different types of assault surfaces must be considered [47]. Possible attack surfaces include administrative interfaces, device/cloud web interfaces, update procedures, mobile apps, system components, gadget software, and storage. An attack surface is a collection of vulnerable points that an attacker can use to enter a system to steal, leak, or manipulate data.

Behind every attack surface, IoT network devices have certain features and functions where a number of security weaknesses are present. After determining the attack surface, it is possible to discover security vulnerabilities and possibly exposed regions that need deep-level protection. From a number of angles, it is clear that the IoT ecosystem security is at risk. Undoubtedly, the overwhelming amount of cyber-attacks available to an assailant to conduct their detrimental actions motivates the creation of efficient security solutions. Additionally, because IoT nodes have limited resources, it is impossible to deploy traditional security measures, endangering the entire network. Excellent illustrations of such dangers include the Mirai botnet and its offshoots, which have the ability to hijack IoT devices and execute destructive DdoS attacks.

4.5.2 IoT VULNERABILITIES

IoT gadgets are all around us and provide users with fantastic experiences. However, IoT device adoption has increased security risks because hackers now access a tremendous amount of data in a globally connected environment. IoT devices will be susceptible to sensitive data leaks in the absence of adequate security measures. IoT and cybercrime are imperceptible to the untrained eye and can affect us anytime.

Furthermore, because of their low cost, low power consumption, and inadequate computational capacity, as well as the heterogeneity and scale of the network, IoT devices are susceptible to attacks and safety issues since they lack the necessary built-in security to combat dangers. IoT devices are susceptible to attacks due to user behavior as well as technical factors. These smart gadgets continue to be in danger for the following reasons [48]:

- *Hardware constraints and limited computational power*: There is very little room for security and data protection to be built into these devices because they are made for specific applications that only need a small amount of processing power.
- *Heterogeneous transmission technology*: Since these devices constantly interact with other heterogeneous devices, it is challenging to implement uniform security procedures and protection mechanisms.

- *The device components are weak*: Insecure or outdated core components can potentially destroy millions of smart devices.
- *Users with a total absence of safety practices*: Due to a lack of confidentiality understanding, electronic phones may be vulnerable to risk regions and assault potential. Many Internet of Things (IoT) strategies allow operators to incorporate third-party programs, which may jeopardize the gadget.
- *Lax physical security*: Unlike internet service data centers, a large portion of IoT components are physically accessible to both users and those with nefarious intentions.

The security vulnerabilities are separated into threats at the software and hardware levels [49]. When a system is attacked at the software level, the goal is to make it malfunction so that the attacker can obtain the needed data, such as a password or credit card number. Software-based outbreaks can be restricted by using a firewall, an up-to-date virus database, and current software. Attackers have many options, including hardware- and software-level attacks.

Developing safe Integrated Circuits (IC) or System-on-Chip (SoC) is necessary to design complete secure hardware. However, it is becoming more difficult due to the manufacturing of integrated Very Large Scale Integration (VLSI) chips, the inclusion of third-party Intellectual Property (IP) cores, and nanoscale design. One mischievous circuit inserted during the production course is all it takes to compromise the system, and designers may not even notice.

Lower-level elements exhibit the opposite traits, while the pyramid's upper parts are more brittle and have less potential influence [50]. Cyber threats, it might be said, aim for more power and possibilities lower down the stack. A system component may have flaws that increase the attack surface and make it vulnerable. For instance, an enemy frequently uses IoT system hardware or software vulnerabilities to get access and carry out their hostile behavior. According to HP, there are severe security flaws in 50% of commercially available IoT devices [51]. As the vulnerabilities previously mentioned potentially reveal delicate facts and abuse the IoT system, avoiding and responding to them is crucial. IoT networks are vulnerable to several types of assaults, making security analysis difficult and necessitating the implementation of foolproof security solutions. However, the enormous amount of data produced by IoT environs is improving the system's overall safety level.

4.5.3 IoT Security Requirements

To secure equipment, one must be aware of the security goals. In the most recent technology, the CIA triad—traditional security targets—is known as confidentiality, integrity, and availability. A collection of guidelines defining requirements for authorized parties with access to information are connected to confidentiality. Integrity is another quality that guarantees dependable services so that IoT devices only receive authorized orders and data. Accessibility guarantees that legitimate objects and people can use IoT functions anytime. The Information Assurance and Security, or IAS-octave, is a broad set of safety objectives that address the shortcomings of the CIA triad [52]. The security goals recommended by the IAS, along with their definitions and acronyms, are listed in Table 4.1 [53].

TABLE 4.1
Security Requirements of Healthcare System

Security Requirements	Confidentiality	Integrity	Nonrepudiation	Availability	Privacy	Auditability	Accountability	Trustworthiness
Abbreviations	C	I	NR	A	P	AU	AC	TW
Definition	The method for keeping on-air and stored in a way private and exclusive so that only authorized entities or people have access to it	The process of ensuring that no data is altered and that correctness is maintained	The procedure by which an IoT scheme validates the authenticity and origin of an activity	The practice of ensuring that services are available to those who require them even if there is a power failure or a malfunction	The process through which an IoT system gains access to private information by adhering to rules and norms	The method through which an IoT scheme observes its own behavior	The process by which operators of IoT systems will be held accountable for their behavior	The process by which an IoT scheme may validate a person's identity and create confidence in a third party

4.5.3.1 IoT Attacks

IoTs are vulnerable to a wide range of serious risks, necessitating the establishment of security frameworks in a number of areas. Recognition, confidentiality, dependability, and non-renunciation are a few examples. This section will go through security threats based on certain attributes.

4.5.3.2 Spoofing Attacks

A hacker spoofing outbreak arises when one gadget or client obtains entrance to an alternative device or individual on a network. The attacker attacks the user gadget in relation to assaulting network hosts, stealing sensitive data, distributing malware, or avoiding contact controls [54]. Spoofing assaults are classified into two types [55]: (i) spoofing in the link layer, where the assailant can counterfeit the whole dialogue between the two parties, and (ii) spoofing at the end-to-end surface, where the assailant can mimic a particular facility.

4.5.3.3 Attacks Based on Access Level

There are two sorts of attacks based on the assailant level of control over the system: proactive and reactive.

- *Active attacks*: In this scenario, the attacker intends to disrupt genuine nodes by forging or tampering with the routing information.
- *Inactive attacks*: The invader typically overhears legitimate transmissions between the spreader and receiver to get the data transmitted.

4.5.3.4 Attacks Based on Transmitting Data

IoT devices use sensors to gather data about their surroundings. These sensors can be exploited to run malware installed on a victim device or inject phony sensor patterns, among other things [56]. Attackers may use unintentional communication channels between peripherals of a device to modify key sensor settings (such as mobility of the gadget, altitude, humidity, intensities, and gravitational pull) or transmit malicious commands. These can be propagated through:

Light Sensors: Data packets can be easily transmitted by revolving on and off a light source when using light sensors.

Magnetic Sensors: The magnetic fields in the vicinity of a magnetic sensor affect its ability to function. It will be impacted if the magnetic fields of the device accessories change. Users' consent is not necessary to transfer data using a magnetic sensor, and it is possible to run discreetly in the background [57]. By altering the attractive field of the device atmosphere, an attacker can create fake magnetic sensor data. This can ultimately result in malware messages being sent. An IoT device can receive trigger signals encoded by an electromagnet, and this message will result in some fluctuations in the device's attractive sensed data. This electromagnetic signal can be used to determine the triggering message by calculating differences.

Audio Sensors: Audio sensors can potentially be used to activate malware in IoT devices. A trigger message can be delivered using this form of audio indicator to bypass the device safekeeping procedures. Microphones in newer IoT devices can recognize audio signals with a frequency substantially lesser than the distinct occurrence series.

4.5.4 ATTACKS BASED ON DEVICE PROPERTY

Low-end and high-end devices are the two groups into which IoT devices are split based on device characteristics. The level of impact that each attack type has on the devices varies. IoT devices may exhibit strange behavior in these assaults or may not function properly [58].

Attacks on high-end device classes: High-end device class attacks are launched against the IoT network by strong devices with lots of computing power. The internet protocol is used between extensive devices and the network. The attacker connects to the IoT network using the high computation capability of strong devices' CPUs, such as laptops and computers, in order to launch an assault from any location at any time [59].

Low-end device class attacks: As implied by the attack name, this type of attack uses little power and energy-consuming equipment to launch an outbreak. The tools employed in this attack have radio links that they can utilize to connect to the outside world. In a smart home system, for instance, a wristwatch may be linked to other sophisticated gadgets such as a clever TV, smartphone, refrigerator, temperature sensor, and observation camera. It can also govern how these devices are set up and run. However, IoT gadgets with minimal power consumption, such as wearable technology, can potentially attack the smart home system [60].

4.5.5 ATTACKS BASED ON ADVERSARY LOCATION

An IoT system can be attacked at any time and from any location by a hacker. Someone can start an attack from both inside and outside [61].

External attacks: The majority of malware, such as worms, Trojan horse infections, phishing, and other similar tactics, are used in remote assaults to acquire users' sensitive information. A hacker can take control of an IoT device anywhere on the IoT network. Without knowing the network design beforehand, the attacker uses a trial-and-error approach to try to get access. He will keep trying till he succeeds.

Internal attacks: A person who is a valid internet or system user, who possesses data rights but purposefully misuses it, or whose access results in abuse is considered an insider threat. In this illustration, the attacker breaches a security IoT border component and uses it to launch dangerous malware on IoT devices. The four types of internal attacks include unintentional actors, psychological assailants, and technological awareness actors, all examples of contaminated performers.

4.5.6 ATTACKS BASED ON ATTACKS STRATEGY

To launch an outbreak, the invader employs an approach that involves installing and running malicious code in an IoT device in order to interfere with the IoT network. The approach of the adversary may be physical or conceptual [62].

Physical attacks: In order to use this technique, the attacker desires to gain entrance to the infrastructure of the IoT network. By altering the instructions or organization of the scheme, the antagonist can disrupt a portion or complete the IoT network.

Logical attacks: Unlike physical attacks, logical attacks don't require physical access. The attacker does not physically harm the gadget; instead, the attacker breaks down the communication route.

4.5.7 ATTACKS BASED ON INFORMATION DAMAGE LEVEL

IoT devices are monitored and collected data by sensors. Attackers can readily alter the information because it is open and fluctuating. It can be separated into six types based on how attackers alter the informational level [63]. This includes Interruption, Eavesdropping, Alteration, Fabrication, and Man-in-the-middle attacks.

4.5.8 HOST-BASED ATTACKS

This type of attack involves the host's hardware, software, and human resources. IoT devices incorporate an operating system and other system software or applications. As a result, IoT devices can be attacked via the IoT system host. It is assumed that the adversary used this exploit to access the victim. The three categories of host-based attacks are assaults that are user-based, software-based, and hardware-based. The attacker compromises these resources, and the IoT network is affected differently by each type of assault.

Software-based attacks: A hacker may compromise software to put an IoT device in a precarious position. By using host-based assaults, an attacker can exhaust the device resources or cause resource buffer overflows.

4.6 REQUIREMENT OF SECURITY IN INTERNET OF MEDICAL THINGS SYSTEM

The data handled by the environment has grown more vulnerable as a result of the widespread adoption of IoMT. If a hacker breaches the environment, valuable personal data will be put at risk if malicious intent is used; in some cases, patient lives may also be. Through study and community assistance, numerous similar vulnerabilities have been discovered. In this section, we'll go over a few of the IoMT environments' weaknesses as well as the safeguards put in place to protect them.

4.6.1 IoMT SECURITY INCIDENTS

In order to build trust and deliver high-quality care, safety and privacy (SNP) are the most important qualities to realize. Even though SNP is a significant issue in all other systems, patients' lives and health depend on the healthcare system, making SNP essentially diverse from other schemes. By defending and securing hardware, software, and data, computer system security aims to secure the CIA triad: (1) confidentiality—safeguarding the privacy of data or resources, (2) reliability—preventing illegal entrance to data and upholding credibility to safeguard data properties, and (3) accessibility—making data accessible whenever needed. Malicious invaders are developing new strategies and methods to breach business security, leading, for instance, to data stealing, altering, or blackmail. IoMT has had a number of security-related problems.

IoMT-deployed healthcare businesses have had at least one security breach in almost 90% of cases. According to different research, 35% of businesses, more than 370 businesses, using the IoMT experienced at least one cybersecurity compromise in 2016. IoMT was the target of 45% of all ransomware attacks in 2017. In IoMT contexts, MEDJACK2 demonstrated the efficacious implementation of ransomware outbreaks, which resulted in data theft. The biggest ransomware outbreak of 2017 infected over 200,000 machines around the globe [64]. The Department of Motherland Security Cybersecurity and Infrastructure Institution alerted all medical facilities and other healthcare institutions in December 2020 of a significant danger to secured health records posed by authorization insecurity discovered across several GE Healthcare equipment. This vulnerability was found by healthcare cybersecurity vendor Cyber MDX. The critical severity rating is 9.8 out of 10.

Another caution was issued in relation to a number of Medtronic MyCareLink (MCL) doctors who could affect clinical data. All versions of the MCL Intelligent Series 25000 Patients Analyzer have 8.8 out of 10 severity-rated flaws that were discovered. According to Forescout Research Labs, 33 security flaws in four open-source TCP/IP stacks affect over 150 companies and millions of MDs.

4.6.2 IoMT Regulations on Cybersecurity

Significant governmental agencies are updating the pre-market cybersecurity standards for MDs to assess, accomplish, and reduce care hazards for customers and patients. For example, the Food and Drug Administration (FDA), a federal organization that oversees and controls the medical sector, monitors security occurrences involving doctors in order to strengthen IMD security and guarantee patient safety. In October 2014, the FDA published guidelines on Premarket Submissions for the Management of Cybersecurity. Based on these principles, suggestions for enhanced security management and risk reduction were produced to ensure that device operations wouldn't be harmed, either intentionally or unintentionally. All manufacturers are urged to abide by the suggestions while creating medical devices in order to protect against cybersecurity flaws.

As an aspect of their program verification and risk assessment process, it was also advised to build a cybersecurity vulnerability and management method. A strong cybersecurity risk-management program should be put in place for both the premarket and postmarket growth stages, according to the draft advice of post-market management from 2016 [65]. A prototype of new pre-market guidelines was released in 2018 and published to propose a fresh kind for connected MDs at Tiers 1 and 2, created on connectivity and the magnitude of the potential harm they could do if confiscated. Centered on that example, 501K Tier 1 MDs should be examined to make sure they adhere to FDA regulations for the plan and threat valuation processes [66].

As a regulatory organization, the FDA pushes medical device producers to create "Trustworthy" products. According to the FDA, trustworthy gadgets are

- Relatively secure from cybersecurity intrusion and compromise. Set a minimum typical for correct functioning, accessibility, and consistency.
- Adhere to generally known security measures at all times;
- Are suitably qualified to carry out their intended functions.

In addition, it suggests a framework resembling that of the normalization organization NIST, suggests novel category guidelines, and asks businesses to provide users with a Cybersecurity Bill of Materials (CBOM). The ISO/IEC TR 27550:20194 guide on security architecture for network life procedures, the NIST revised review of SNP measures (NIST 800-532), and the Privacy Engineering Program (PEP3) were all developed in response to security vulnerabilities [67]. Achieving compliance and putting standards into practice is crucial when it comes to mHealth and uHealth systems. The EU MDR cybersecurity mandate has been delayed till 2021 because of the COVID-19 outbreak. It establishes a "defense-in-depth approach," a system of specifications to guarantee that devices are protected.

4.6.3 SECURITY MECHANISMS

As shown in Figure 4.2, the two main categories of security for any IoT system are security provided by both software and equipment. Mathematical techniques are included in software-based security mechanisms as to when to safeguard the network, and computers depend on software. While it requires time to resolve mathematical problems, extracting the keys will be quicker once quantum CPUs are real [68]. On the other hand, encryption techniques, including elliptic curve cryptography (ECC), public key infrastructure (KPI), and advanced encryption standards (AES) are utilized in hardware-based security solutions. Pre-shared key parameters must be prepared with the server or other procedures beforehand for the former.

Although it has the advantages of low computing complexity and great efficiency, it is unrealistic when many devices are involved and share important parameters. Pre-shared key factors are not necessary for asymmetric practices, on the other hand. Instead, both their private and public keys are used. Here, confidentiality also includes the secrecy of private keys [69].

Device authorization and key distribution are critical in such a device-heavy ecosystem barrier to ensuring secure connectivity for IoT. Additionally, these MDs require little in the way of power, storage, and computing capability. Therefore, numerous scientists are collaborating to develop an authentication scheme to implement security measures. Physically Unclonable Functions are comparatively straightforward architecture (PUFs), a family of distinct hardware encryption primitives that can handle many of the security concerns confronting energy-constrained IoT devices, hence providing a paradigm change in many encryption methods. PUF is a type of hardware-based authentication process (AP) that uses little energy and instantly identifies the legitimate user. In IoMT, as a hardware encryption primitive for verification, PUF offers a physically defined "digital fingerprint." When given an input (challenge), a PUF is a physical item that produces an output (response) that acts as a unique identifier. Integrated circuits have inherent physical diversity, which might offer a system for challenge-response in encryption methods [70].

PUF is, as its name implies, exclusive and cannot be copied because of the subjective and insurmountable effects of the IC manufacturing procedure. Every PUF is distinct. Hence it should always be able to make a challenge-response pair (CPR) at random.

A unique CRP (Cx, Rx) for that PUF is indicated by [71] if Cx is a challenge input to the PUF and Rx is the response generated by the PUF.

$$R_x = PUF\left(C_x\right) \tag{1}$$

PUF does not keep a password or key on the device as conventional security systems do. An assailant cannot utilize PUF to use the MDs due to the lack of memory and the fact that CRPs are unique for each PUF. PUF's primary attributes are uniqueness, dependability, and randomization.

Independence: Every challenge-response pair (CRP) of a PUF must differ from chip to chip. Different PUFs shouldn't produce the same CRP set. The ideal uniqueness value is 50%. Using the hamming distance as a gauge (HD), the variance in answer bits is used to calculate the hamming distance.

Reliability: A PUF must be dependable and capable of producing the same result in response to a specific challenge. A PUF reliability should ideally be 100%.

Randomness: Bits of a response should be required to be random (1s and 0s). The presence of 1s and 0s in a response is anticipated to be equal. This criterion ensures that a PUF randomness is always 100%.

Data networking is a different method for safeguarding SNP (NDN). Data chunks are retrieved using names. It is a suggested internet architecture in which data is transmitted from sensors to servers using the names of the data bits. The network layer uses data names for applications or content to identify the producer. There are two kinds of data packets: interest packets (requests) and data wallets (replies). The name of the requested material is contained in the awareness packet, and the data packet is fetched. The interest packet route is also followed by the data packet [71]. Instead of collecting data from the producer as the current system does, the NDN router caches content to give to the user.

It is hard to determine who is seeking the data since NDN packets lack information on the user. Additionally, security is guaranteed due to the content encryption utilizing a cryptographic signature [72]. As shown in Figure 4.2, the forwarding module consists of three parts: a deferred attention map, a contents storage (CS), and a forwarded interests bases (FIB) (PIT). The CS archives the data. FIB controls the route to the destination. Up until the arrival of the data packet, PIT keeps a database for each interest packet. If the information is missing from the interested packet, collect it from the provider and save it in the CS for possible transfer in the future.

4.7 INTERNET OF MEDICAL THINGS SYSTEM SECURITY SOLUTIONS

According to the literature, this segment will assess security protocols for the IoMT networks that have already been published. The finest of each design is presented through comprehension. In 2016, Chiou et al. created an authentication mechanism in an effort to protect the IoMT system and thwart hackers' attempts to infiltrate it [73]. Unfortunately, as demonstrated by [74], the system developed by Chiou et al. does not completely protect users from security risks and does not conceal the identities of patients. Authors in refs. [74] and [75] communicated the private key via a public network when using private keys for authenticating, by scrambling with additional conditions, the private key was shared. Although the authentication mechanism was enhanced, it still lacks complete security.

According to ref. [76] the system is susceptible to impersonation, hijacked sensor nodes, and leaky verification tables because it lacks privacy, unlinkability, and reliable authentication protocols. The system saved authentication parameters in plaintext, making it possible for a sensor node to be stolen and for an assailant to log in and use the credentials and nonce to start an impersonating assault generation [77]. These problems were resolved by authors ref. [78]. Furthermore, their technology does not keep patient-sensitive information or identification settings in the site directory. It is vulnerable to single-point failure because, during the recordkeeping step, it allocates an intermediary node for communication between the device and the server. It creates a simple authentication system by combining hash and XOR operations. After confirming the intermediary node, date, attributes saved, etc., a session key will be created.

Authors in ref. [79] developed an escrow-free personality aggregated signcryption method to safeguard data transport. A smart health service collects clinical data from numerous devices put on the person's body, encrypts and combines it, and then transfers it to a remote hospital server via smartphones in this setup. After authenticating an entity, a network manager generates partial private keys and master and public keys. The company obtains its secret key using shared from vital security servers, which safeguard and generate a secured secret key. Sensors collect data, timestamps, and summaries after encrypting each piece of information in order to save computing costs. The smartphone combines data from all sensors and uses keys to confirm the validity before sending it to the server. The doctor can use the private key for the sensor to decode the PHI file. Even though an eavesdropping attack is thwarted by the need to compute the security code and use the owner key and hidden keys, it is still vulnerable to attacks like DoS and response.

According to ref. in [80], HERMIT, a benchmarking tool, is improving the performance of a carefully chosen group of ten new IoMT applications while attempting to add more features. Lempel-Ziv compression (LZW) and the Advanced Encryption Standard (AES) also stand in for the compression and security functions, respectively. They concentrate on incorporating security measures and processing IoMT data. The framework provides encryption for data protection for this reason.

According to an approach put out by ref. [81], modules cannot be altered to get a personal shared key, and if successful, they, the trustworthy server, will be able to tell because of a function. The device uses a key pair to encrypt an index and its value before sharing it with the server. Then, with the aid of a key pair and matching the index score, the server decrypts the message.

For IoMT systems, [82] presented a three-factor authentication mechanism that uses password, smart card, and biometrics. A user sends an authentication request message comprising shared keys that have been stored and a function of a random integer. During login, a session key is created using this data. The session key is employed for encryption in the subsequent quick authentication phase. Despite the assertion that there is no storage for verification, it computes a stated computation to verify the session key. The secret server key of a certain server is stored on a client device for authentication. If there is a problem with the specific server, service to the client device will be interrupted.

A group-oriented moment authentication scheme agreement utilizing chaotic maps system was presented by [82]. Complex nonlinear dynamical structures that are chaotic, such as chaotic maps [83], have huge parameter spaces, unbroken data distributions, and semigroup structures. A collection key is only good for a specific amount of time, after which a new key will be needed since only authorized parties can access it. In this work, the therapeutic server notifies application providers and user groups of a time-slot variety and an authentication range. The application provider will finish authentication if it receives the identical authentication token within the allotted period. The group's additional members will be validated with the same authentication token if the group's first member has already been verified. No example of how a group member will distribute an authentication token is provided.

Hash operation and XOR operation-based lightweight approaches were proposed [84]. It employs open channels and has six stages. First, a secure sensor key is shared with the trusted gateway during pre-deployment. The device node and client can register in the entry with the aid of this security key. In order to encode the data gathered by the device node, the device and consumer will ultimately assign a period key with the aid of the gateway.

4.7.1 ATTRIBUTE BASED

Authentication using attribute-based cryptography (ABE) system was put out by [85]. Here, it is necessary to have centralized power as well as attributed control. Users request a ciphertext key for mutual cloud authentication by sending attributes authority-certified private key and conversion key to the public cloud assistance. There are various issues with ABE-based systems. The secret key cannot identify the user; thus, no one will be alerted if a bogus key distribution is carried out. Second, depending on how many attributes are used, the ciphertext increases. In addition, when users decrypt [86], a longer computation time is needed. Due to the high cost of decryption, ABE is incompatible with wearable electronics [87].

According to authors in [88], a security approach involves connecting wearable technology to a server for edge devices located in a local hospital. Mutual authentication is finished by client and server computation of data attributes, including digits and secret codes pseudo-number generation. Here, n parts of the secret key are created to facilitate calculation and sharing. The client device needs to perform a lot of processing and storage, which is inappropriate for IoT devices. Resistance to a few assaults, like DoS, Reply, was not demonstrated.

Authors in [89] put forth attribute-based authenticating relying on a plaintexts policy approach. This approach determines who received the initial key of the trustworthy authorities and the property permission. Because the size of the ciphertext is independent of the number of attributes, different numbers of attributes require the same amount of time to decrypt. The projected method, however, requires a substantial quantity of calculations to confirm the user identity. As a result of the user who was given the proxy key, PHI leakage also occurs.

4.7.2 ECG Based

The author in [90] created an ECG-based authentication scheme where ECG signals are de-noised by the use of singular value decomposition (SVD). The noise will be minimized based on mobility status and pre-defined better classification. Weighted online SVD was used to achieve a de-noised signal in the case of light exercise. For walking and running, it is difficult to calculate the angular distance. It is also difficult to perform various workouts or positions when engaging in various activities. In this study, it is assumed that an attacker cannot access the ECG templates of patients. The user identity is not securely protected, and the computation is time-consuming.

4.7.3 MAC Based

Authors of [91] offer a MAC-based approach in which a gateway gathers data from MDs and saves it on cloud servers. Data will be shared in an encoded format with the help of a reliable expert. In order to establish the source and ensure integrity, MAC is utilized as an authentication technique. The connection involving IoT devices and the IoT gateway is not secure. Additionally, a secure channel must be present for the calculated key to be shared with the IoT gateway.

Authors in [92] proposed a smart card and MD verification technique utilizing public-key encryption. Additionally, it uses MAC is used for verification. The reader device will compute and establish the incorrect k-bit in this approach from a hash function that the server shares. The suggested protocol does not include user anonymity. The author developed a method in which a key source generates a confirmation key and a promising key [93] after demonstrating the security flaw in dedication and MAC-based (for a value rather than a range) verification protocols. The user will use these values to calculate a commitment value and distribute the message. To verify the assurance key, a doctor will decode the partially decrypted material using the confirmation and promise keys.

4.7.4 ECC Based

To reconcile the disparity between mobile device loss attacks and local password verification, fuzzy-verifier and honey-list approaches are deployed. However, this does not protect attacks from the man-in-the-middle. In [94], the authors used a fuzzy-based trust-management strategy to thwart Sybil's attempts. Fuzzy-logic processing uses the trust properties, such as node integrity, receptivity, and compatibility, to assess the value of trust. Fuzzy inference system operations and fuzzy filtering are used for double assessment inspections. The newly introduced fuzzy filter employs two algorithms to assess the ultimate trust value.

The author of [95] also created an authentication mechanism employing ECC and energetic identification with user biometric data (ECG). A physician is assigned three separate random values during the registration period, and a hash function is singed into a smart card to provide an active personality. However, despite its defense in the event of a man-in-the-middle assault, it has not been tested against server imperson-ation. In addition, dealing with ECG-related concerns is necessary, and communica-tion expenses are considerable.

Authors in [96] propose a multi-keyword searchable encryption method based on attributes. The attribute-based cryptography approach utilizes a convergence and symmetric key to protect the data, introducing double verification. Furthermore, a time-division technique is also included and used to verify the validity of shared files' access. To initiate an access request, a user must create a search token, which the user must then, following encryption, decode to retrieve unencrypted, verifying the accuracy of the data from the shared partially decrypted result. In this case, the cloud storage vendor that the client has approved confirms the request's validity. In this approach, the user generates a fake secret key during the registration process and uses it to calculate the real private key. Additionally, most decoding computations are carried out on the cloud side to minimize calculations on the user side.

4.7.5 MACHINE-LEARNING BASED

The authors use eight outsourcing processing techniques that protect your privacy in [97] efficient privacy-preserving support vector machine approach. The proposed protocol's great efficiency and accuracy are achieved through outsourced floating point and integer computations. So that safe and confidentiality computations could be performed, the floating point quantity was standardized into a fixed point number with constant accuracy 2E could be performed on it. The cloud service and providers are given a public-private key combination as well as extra secret keys by an initially trusted authority in this approach, who then becomes inactive.

The amount of trust is assessed using trust parameters like compatibility, reliabil-ity, and packet delivery, according to authors in [98] Method of smart neural network-based reputation monitoring. It features a smart home server designed to calculate patient healthcare sensor trust and locate malicious nodes. After estimating credibil-ity, the intelligent home server gets encoded patient data using ECC and SHA256 and exchanges it with the servers. The decrypted data is shared with the doctors if the server determines that the assessed trust meets the threshold values. Binary output is computed by supervised learning using a multi-layer perceptron neural network with an input layer, two hidden layers, and an output layer. The summing function is used in the first stage to total all calculated model parameters. The second stage uses the range limit to generate a figure representing the trust development criterion assessment. Decreasing the trust level can affect communication and calculation times, which makes it more difficult because the system can detect an on-off assault.

The authors in [99] presented an image deep learning-based cryptography and decryption system encrypting and decrypting medical images. A deep-learning-based image encrypted and decrypted network (DeepEDN) is given to finish the encoding procedure and decode the clinical picture. The basic learning network in this technique is the cycle-generative adversarial network, which transmits from the source site to the destination domain. In order to restore the original image to interpret the picture, the target domain applies a reconstructing structure [100]. The encoding scheme starts to spatially down the sample and encrypts the pictures during the first convolution stage. The key-generation procedure produces random keys for each convolution layer encryption. All the convolutional layer parameters are used to create private keys for encryption. The encryption network forward propagation training procedure continuously updates and improves private keys.

4.7.6   PUF Based

The systems previously mentioned are believed to have hardware security modules, trusted authorities, or key generators installed. The side-channel attack could impact these authentication algorithms since they needed memory location or storage. PUF-based authentication solutions are created to prevent recall storage and defend against side-channel assaults. In [99], authors suggested a component of the PUF-based security protocols for IoMT. In this paper, a combined ring oscillator-based PUF for an authentication scheme was developed. The server verifies individuals by matching CRPs saved in the database. With the replies, the patient device produces in response to challenges from the server. It can withstand client-impersonation assaults but not server-impersonation ones.

Authors in [101] suggested a PUF-based verification method that enables individual nodes and servers to validate each other and is immune to server impersonating assaults. After obtaining the customer pseudo-identity and nonce, the server shares a CRP pair with a derived nonce during the authentication stage. The server checks the subsequent CRP, which the client will share once the client verifies the current CRP. Because two CRPs are employed in each stage, CRP usage is higher. It also sets aside a small number of CRPs for synchronization. The procedure for updating reserve CRPs is not indicated if CRP reserves are spent. Therefore, it does not completely eliminate dependency on storing to buffer CRPs and phony IDs.

The author in [102] also created a man-in-the-middle attack-resistant PUF-based authentication system. As authentication is necessary between the patient and the sink node server, as well as the sink node server and the cloud server, two-factor authentication is considered. Each cluster, an issue, and challenge-specific replies conduct computations using a random nonce. Sadly, it is vulnerable to DoS assaults and difficult calculations. Additionally, the client device will decide which challenge needs to be stored. Unfortunately, the device cannot choose challenges randomly since no strong PUF has a set of CRPs.

4.7.7 BLOCKCHAIN BASED

In order to process medical data, authors in [103] presented a comprehensive framework that takes advantage of edge computation and Ethereum interaction. Three separate channels are considered in this blockchain system for separating different data kinds, such as urgent data, which are distinguished from other forms of data. Earlier, an automatic patient-monitoring system was implemented. Important information was given the first attention possible to ensure the lowest possible latency and will work with a lesser constrained cryptocurrency, or one with fewer validators, by supporting quick reaction. Priority settings and features are extracted for configuration adjustments, and priority is the key focus area in this work.

Health chain, a bitcoin concrete evidence scheme created by authors in [104], encrypts health data for granular access control. There are two sub-blockchains in the Healthchain: Userchain and Docchain. IoT data is encrypted using symmetric encryption with AES. The consortium installs auditing nodes, which act as miners in Docchain and contribute data produced by doctor nodes to the blockchain. If the diagnostic key or IoT key is exposed, the user may always update it by producing and transmitting a second key activity.

Additionally, SHA-256 is used for hashing. For the encryption algorithm, 128-bit AES is used, while 1024-bit RSA is used for asymmetric cryptography and signing. Assuming that the consumers' and physicians' security tokens are both compromised and protected and that the computer power of adversaries is constrained, our approach offers conditional security. To find malicious transactions and malicious nodes, this process entails a third-party audit that creates the hospital's private blockchain [105]. This work uses the PBC and OpenSSL libraries to construct a mechanism for comparing complaints that permits the verification process and produces a session key for future correspondence regarding the disease with comparable symptoms. Physicians from several hospitals can communicate data using proxy re-encryption technology. Physicians will act as deputies to upload data, and the medical center server will add blocks once the data has been verified. Public-private key-based encryption is used in this work. Doctors need patients' permission to view their medical records, and safe communication for transferring encoding keys is not addressed.

Authors in [106] suggested a unique collective-reinforcement-learning method based on blockchain to allocate resources flexibly depending on viewport display, block agreement, and content conveyance requirements. It considers an IoMT scheme in which exclusive Using VR technology and healthcare services are integrated into a 360-degree omnidirectional video. Edge access points (EAPs) can either receive or broadcast VR pieces from the web servers to omnidirectional viewports like authors in [107] directly to the virtual reality device (VD) in order to provide video format and responses.

The pre-prepared stage of authentication uses MAC. The EAP blockchain controller creates M-1 MACs for the non-essential nodes and signs the block during the commit phase. Each non-primary node must verify one MAC of the pre-prepare communication, one block autograph, as well as the signatures of the associated transactions. Secure key exchange among implantable MDs and private servers, as well as individual services and blockchain technology cloud servers, is made possible by the blockchain-based approach created by authors in [108]. The concept uses three criteria to increase security throughout its eight stages of development: (1) passwords that are kept on the device, (2) the user password, and (3) user biometrics. Only during the registration process does it use trusted authority. Both the MD and the private server maintain the hidden key after the initial authentication to be used for further authentication. Data from sensors is sent to a personal server, which uses a secret key to relay the data sent to a remote server. Each cloud provider employs an ECC-based private-public pair of keys, with validation handled by the Ripple Protocols Consensus Mechanism.

Decentralized health records and a service automation system based on smart contracts are provided by a unique secured blockchain architecture created by authors in [109]. In addition to the ECC-based authentication scheme, a distributed selective ring-based access control (SRAC) approach is used to enhance security measures and safeguard patient records' confidentiality. By logically merging edge and cloud computing, it employs hybrid computing. A sub-swarm key-generation mechanism combines locally distributed data storage systems (DDSS) networks to form the main or global DDSS.

The hospital chooses a leader edge device at random to retain a caching of physical access documents on the local machine, the cryptographic pool, and so on. This system uses intelligent connections at the hybridized technology layer to construct business rules for initial client or caregiver decision-making. Then, with the aid of a function, an SRAC algorithm is utilized to verify and regulate access (Read/Write). Added to this framework is a gray list for unapproved devices.

4.8   CHALLENGES AND FURTHER RESEARCH

The difficulties with IoMT data security and privacy are described in this section. Some issues that affect IoMT applications' performance, efficiency, and resilience are readily apparent. Lack of medical equipment standards is the main difficult issue. Scalability, consistency, uncertainty, data integrity, uniformity, and effectiveness are some of the most restrictive elements that reduce the effectiveness of the systems. The difficulties encountered when deploying IoMT devices are outlined subsequently.

i. When patient information is disclosed, medical organizations' status and their patients' health are seriously harmed.

ii. Since these tools are being used in a variety of settings, such as hospitals, nursing homes, and distant care, as well as the patients' lack of security awareness, there is a significant risk that hackers may target patient data in-home care and remote care. Similar to how insiders can readily leak patient health information from the hospital. Therefore, the task is to create an effective authentication and authorization mechanism with the future in mind.

iii. *Data flaws*: Because there are so many medical records, processing the data might be difficult because it is possible to give the wrong patient information out. In order to handle the data effectively, it is driven to improve computer-aided and protected IoMT gadget AI prototypes in the future.

iv. *Accuracy and privacy*: Due to the significant security risks it poses for confidentiality, integrity, and accuracy, medical data can be accessed by a variety of malevolent actors within the IoMT environment. The medical information may be deleted or changed due to hostile incursion. Therefore, an advanced approach, such as an intrusion detection system, must be adopted to ensure data accuracy and confidentiality.

IoMT contributions to the healthcare sector are primarily focused on safeguarding patient privacy and safety. Security procedures, including authentication and authorization schemes, are crucial to stop illegal access to private healthcare information. For this reason, finding a cutting-edge strategy that can guarantee data security throughout its whole path is essential. The results of the review indicate that there are various established methods for securing IoMT devices. However, due to various restrictions, including power, size, implantability, and wearability, typical intelligent gadgets cannot be secured using encryption or machine learning-based security techniques.

To ensure these connected phones' security, confidentiality, and trustworthiness, an effective design solution is necessary to meet all security standards and cover the whole medical business. The analysis of the data from the poll also reveals that the blockchain method, lightweight authentication, and ECC algorithm offer the maximum stages of safekeeping. Impending research should therefore focus on developing intrusion detection systems and effective, lightweight cryptography to defend and maintain data from IoMT devices, enabling the construction of sustainable and power-efficient IoMT devices.

4.9   CONCLUSIONS AND FUTURE DIRECTIONS

IoT technology has the potential to draw the attention of assailants to find holes for getting assistance due to the rapid growth of connecting physical devices with the virtual world. Researchers and business experts constantly work to develop a sturdy system by eliminating weaknesses. Solutions of many kinds are being created. Manufacturers must uphold a common standard in order to make the ecosystem secure and uniform. To do this, regulatory organizations, to overcome systemic deficiencies, organizations such as the FDA and the EU, are developing rules and modifying criteria. Companies must follow the guidelines in order to offer their products to the public. This chapter outlines the IoMT environment, explains how it works, and highlights network dangers. This chapter enhanced security and maintained privacy by thoroughly reviewing the existing security techniques for IoT devices with limited resources.

Additionally, already-used authentication methods were considered, including ABE, ECC, MAC, ML, PUF, and Blockchain. Future research will examine the IoMT potential in the quantum system age, 5G, and beyond. Investigations will also be conducted into recently found security flaws, such as remote manipulation of Intel, AMD, and other encryption techniques by microprocessor manufacturers. Additionally, the cause of the vulnerabilities and potential fixes will be examined.

ACKNOWLEDGMENT

The work of Agbotiname Lucky Imoize is supported in part by the Nigerian Petroleum Technology Development Fund (PTDF) and, in part, by the German Academic Exchange Service (DAAD) through the Nigerian-German Postgraduate Program under grant 57473408.

REFERENCES

[1]   Djenouri, Y., Belhadi, A., Yazidi, A., Srivastava, G., & Lin, J. C. W. (2022). Artificial intelligence of medical things for disease detection using ensemble deep learning and attention mechanism. *Expert Systems*, e13093.

[2]   Meshram, C., Ibrahim, R. W., Meshram, S. G., Imoize, A. L., Jamal, S. S., & Barve, S. K. (2022). An efficient remote user authentication with key agreement procedure based on convolution-Chebyshev chaotic maps using biometric. *The Journal of Supercomputing*, 78(10), 12792–12814.

[3]   Awotunde, J. B., Imoize, A. L., Ayoade, O. B., Abiodun, M. K., Do, D. T., Silva, A., & Sur, S. N. (2022). An enhanced hyper-parameter optimization of a convolutional neural network model for leukemia cancer diagnosis in a smart healthcare system. *Sensors*, 22(24), 9689.

[4]   Awotunde, J. B., Oladipo, I. D., AbdulRaheem, M., Balogun, G. B., & Tomori, A. R. (2022). An IoMT-based steganography model for securing medical information. *International Journal of Healthcare Technology and Management*, 19(3–4), 218–236.

[5]   Ajagbe, S. A., Florez, H., & Awotunde, J. B. (2022, October). AESRSA: a new cryptography key for electronic health record security. In *Applied Informatics: 5th International Conference, ICAI 2022, Arequipa, Peru, October 27–29, 2022, Proceedings* (pp. 237–251). Cham: Springer International Publishing.

[6]   Nifakos, S., Chandramouli, K., Nikolaou, C. K., Papachristou, P., Koch, S., Panaousis, E., & Bonacina, S. (2021). Influence of human factors on cyber security within healthcare organisations: a systematic review. *Sensors*, 21(15), 5119.

[7]   Li, C. T., Weng, C. Y., Chen, C. L., Lee, C. C., Deng, Y. Y., & Imoize, A. L. (2022). An efficient authenticated key agreement scheme supporting privacy-preservation for internet of drones communications. *Sensors*, 22(23), 9534.

[8]   Vijayalakshmi, K., Uma, S., Bhuvanya, R., & Suresh, A. (2018). A demand for wearable devices in health care. *International Journal of Engineering & Technology*, 7(1–7), 1–4.

[9]   Wei, C. C., Chen, C. W., & Hung, L. C. (2022, November). Establish a smart healthcare system with AIoT for Chinese Medicine. In *2022 10th International Conference on Orange Technology (ICOT)* (pp. 1–5). Shanghai: IEEE.

[10] Ogundokun, R. O., Awotunde, J. B., Onawola, P., & Aro, T. O. (2022). LASSO-DT based classification technique for discovery of COVID-19 disease using chest x-ray images. In *Decision Sciences for COVID-19: Learning Through Case Studies* (pp. 407–422). Cham: Springer International Publishing.

[11] Chen, X., He, D., Khan, M. K., Luo, M., & Peng, C. (2022). A secure certificateless signcryption scheme without pairing for internet of medical things. *IEEE Internet of Things Journal*, 10(10), 9136–9147.

[12] Madhu, B., Chari, M. V. G., Vankdothu, R., Silivery, A. K., & Aerranagula, V. (2023). Intrusion detection models for IOT networks via deep learning approaches. *Measurement: Sensors*, 25, 100641.

[13] Rathore, H., Mohamed, A., Al-Ali, A., Du, X., & Guizani, M. (2017, June). A review of security challenges, attacks and resolutions for wireless medical devices. In *2017 13th International Wireless Communications and Mobile Computing Conference (IWCMC)* (pp. 1495–1501). Valencia: IEEE.

[14] Awotunde, J. B., Misra, S., & Pham, Q. T. (2022, November). A secure framework for Internet of medical things security based system using lightweight cryptography enabled blockchain. In *Future Data and Security Engineering. Big Data, Security and Privacy, Smart City and Industry 4.0 Applications: 9th International Conference, FDSE 2022, Ho Chi Minh City, Vietnam, November 23–25, 2022, Proceedings* (pp. 258–272). Singapore: Springer Nature Singapore.

[15] Jain, M., Choudhary, R. C., & Kumar, A. (2016, December). Secure medical image steganography with RSA cryptography using decision tree. In *2016 2nd International Conference on Contemporary Computing and Informatics (IC3I)* (pp. 291–295). Greater Noida: IEEE.

[16] Hasan, K., Chowdhury, M. J. M., Biswas, K., Ahmed, K., Islam, M. S., & Usman, M. (2022). A blockchain-based secure data-sharing framework for software defined wireless body area networks. *Computer Networks*, 211, 109004.

[17] Ismailisufi, A., Popović, T., Gligorić, N., Radonjic, S., & Šandi, S. (2020, February). A private blockchain implementation using multichain open source platform. In *2020 24th International Conference on Information Technology (IT)* (pp. 1–4). Zabljak: IEEE.

[18] Khatiwada, P., & Yang, B. (2022). An overview on security and privacy of data in IoMT devices: performance metrics, merits, demerits, and challenges. *pHealth*, 2022, 126–136.

[19] Rahulamathavan, Y., Phan, R. C. W., Veluru, S., Cumanan, K., & Rajarajan, M. (2013). Privacy-preserving multi-class support vector machine for outsourcing the data classification in cloud. *IEEE Transactions on Dependable and Secure Computing*, 11(5), 467–479.

[20] Awotunde, J. B., Jimoh, R. G., Imoize, A. L., Abdulrazaq, A. T., Li, C. T., & Lee, C. C. (2022). An enhanced deep learning-based deepfake video detection and classification system. *Electronics*, 12(1), 87.

[21] Chakraborty, C., Khosravi, M. R., Ahmed, S. H., & Rodrigues, J. J. (2022). Guest editorial AIoMT-enabled medical sensors for remote patient monitoring and body-area interfacing: design and implementation, practical use, and real measurements and patient monitoring. *IEEE Journal of Biomedical and Health Informatics*, 26(12), 5769–5771.

[22] Chandini, A. G., & Basarkod, P. I. (2022, July). A robust blockchain architecture for electronic health data using efficient lightweight encryption model with re-encryption scheme. In *2022 IEEE International Conference on Data Science and Information System (ICDSIS)* (pp. 1–6). Hassan: IEEE.

[23] Ahmed, W. K., & Mohammed, R. S. (2022, March). Lightweight authentication methods in IoT: survey. In *2022 International Conference on Computer Science and Software Engineering (CSASE)* (pp. 241–246). Duhok: IEEE.

[24] Wong, S. Y., Soh, M. Y., & Wong, J. M. (2021, November). Internet of medical things: brief overview and the future. In *2021 IEEE 19th Student Conference on Research and Development (SCOReD)* (pp. 427–432). Kota Kinabalu: IEEE.

[25] Oladipupo, E. T., Abikoye, O. C., Imoize, A. L., Awotunde, J. B., Chang, T. Y., Lee, C. C., & Do, D. T. (2023). An efficient authenticated elliptic curve cryptography scheme for multicore wireless sensor networks. *IEEE Access*, 11, 1306–1323.

[26] Rana, A., Chakraborty, C., Sharma, S., Dhawan, S., Pani, S. K., & Ashraf, I. (2022). Internet of medical things-based secure and energy-efficient framework for health care. *Big Data*, 10(1), 18–33.

[27] Adeniyi, A. E., Abiodun, K. M., Awotunde, J. B., Olagunju, M., Ojo, O. S., & Edet, N. P. (2023). Implementation of a block cipher algorithm for medical information security on cloud environment: using modified advanced encryption standard approach. *Multimedia Tools and Applications*, 1–15.

[28] Kumar, R. L., Wang, Y., Poongodi, T., & Imoize, A. L. (Eds.). (2021). *Internet of Things, Artificial Intelligence and Blockchain Technology*. Cham: Springer.

[29] Yang, H., & Yang, B. (2017, November). A blockchain-based approach to the secure sharing of healthcare data. In *Proceedings of the Norwegian Information Security Conference* (pp. 100–111). Oslo, Norway: Nisk J.

[30] Shim, K. A., Park, C. M., & Baek, Y. J. (2015). Lite-Rainbow: lightweight signature schemes based on multivariate quadratic equations and their secure implementations. In *Progress in Cryptology—INDOCRYPT 2015: 16th International Conference on Cryptology in India, Bangalore, India, December 6–9, 2015, Proceedings 16* (pp. 45–63). Switzerland: Springer International Publishing.

[31] Ayoade, O. B., Oladele, T. O., Imoize, A. L., Awotunde, J. B., Adeloye, A. J., Olorunyomi, S. O., & Idowu, A. O. (2023). Explainable artificial intelligence (XAI) in medical decision systems (MDSSs): healthcare systems perspective. In *Explainable Artificial Intelligence in Medical Decision Support Systems* (1st ed.). London: United Kingdom.

[32] Shashidhara, R., Nayak, S. K., Das, A. K., & Park, Y. (2021). On the design of lightweight and secure mutual authentication system for global roaming in resource-limited mobility networks. *IEEE Access*, 9, 12879–12895.

[33] Kumar, M., & Chand, S. (2020). A secure and efficient cloud-centric internet-of-medical-things-enabled smart healthcare system with public verifiability. *IEEE Internet of Things Journal*, 7(10), 10650–10659.

[34] Awotunde, J. B., Jimoh, R. G., Folorunso, S. O., Adeniyi, E. A., Abiodun, K. M., & Banjo, O. O. (2021). Privacy and security concerns in IoT-based healthcare systems. In *The Fusion of Internet of Things, Artificial Intelligence, and Cloud Computing in Health Care* (pp. 105–134). Cham: Springer International Publishing.

[35] Muzammal, M., Talat, R., Sodhro, A. H., & Pirbhulal, S. (2020). A multi-sensor data fusion enabled ensemble approach for medical data from body sensor networks. *Information Fusion*, 53, 155–164.

[36] Hussain, A., Ali, T., Althobiani, F., Draz, U., Irfan, M., Yasin, S., Shafiq, S., Safdar, Z., Glowacz, A., Nowakowski, G., & Khan, M. S. (2021). Security framework for IoT based real-time health applications. *Electronics*, 10(6), 719.

[37] Awotunde, J. B., Ajagbe, S. A., Idowu, I. R., & Ndunagu, J. N. (2021). An enhanced cloud-IoMT-based and machine learning for effective COVID-19 diagnosis system. In *Intelligence of Things: Ai-IoT Based Critical-Applications and Innovations* (pp. 55–76). Cham: Springer.

[38] Ahmad, S., Mehfuz, S., & Beg, J. (2022). Cloud security framework and key management services collectively for implementing DLP and IRM. *Materials Today: Proceedings*, 62, 4828–4836.

[39] AbdulRaheem, M., Oladipo, I. D., González-Briones, A., Awotunde, J. B., Tomori, A. R., & Jimoh, R. G. (2022). An efficient lightweight speck technique for edge-IoT-based smart healthcare systems. In *5G IoT and Edge Computing for Smart Healthcare* (pp. 139–162). Academic Press. Elsevier Publisher.

[40] Abiodun, M. K., Awotunde, J. B., Ogundokun, R. O., Adeniyi, E. A., & Arowolo, M. O. (2021). Security and information assurance for IoT-based big data. In *Artificial Intelligence for Cyber Security: Methods, Issues and Possible Horizons or Opportunities* (pp. 189–211). Cham: Springer International Publishing.

[41]   Mohanty, S. P., Yanambaka, V. P., Kougianos, E., & Puthal, D. (2020). PUFchain: a hardware-assisted blockchain for sustainable simultaneous device and data security in the internet of everything (IoE). *IEEE Consumer Electronics Magazine*, 9(2), 8–16.

[42]   Imoize, A. L., Gbadega, P. A., Obakhena, H. I., Irabor, D. O., Kavitha, K. V. N., & Chakraborty, C. (2023). Artificial intelligence-enabled Internet of medical things for COVID-19 pandemic data management. In *Explainable Artificial Intelligence in Medical Decision Support Systems* (p. 357). London: IET.

[43]   Awotunde, J. B., Ajagbe, S. A., & Florez, H. (2022, October). Internet of things with wearable devices and artificial intelligence for elderly uninterrupted healthcare monitoring systems. In *Applied Informatics: 5th International Conference, ICAI 2022, Arequipa, Peru, October 27–29, 2022, Proceedings* (pp. 278–291). Cham: Springer International Publishing.

[44]   Masud, M., Gaba, G. S., Choudhary, K., Alroobaea, R., & Hossain, M. S. (2021). A robust and lightweight secure access scheme for cloud based E-healthcare services. *Peer-to-peer Networking and Applications*, 14(5), 3043–3057.

[45]   Nwelih, E., Isabona, J., & Imoize, A. L. (2023). Optimization of base station placement in 4G LTE broadband networks using adaptive variable length genetic algorithm. *SN Computer Science*, 4(2), 1–21.

[46]   Rasool, R. U., Ahmad, H. F., Rafique, W., Qayyum, A., & Qadir, J. (2022). Security and privacy of internet of medical things: a contemporary review in the age of surveillance, botnets, and adversarial ML. *Journal of Network and Computer Applications*, 103332.

[47]   Omasheye, O. R., Azi, S., Isabona, J., Imoize, A. L., Li, C. T., & Lee, C. C. (2022). Joint random forest and particle swarm optimization for predictive pathloss modeling of wireless signals from cellular networks. *Future Internet*, 14(12), 373.

[48]   Atlam, H. F., & Wills, G. B. (2020). IoT security, privacy, safety and ethics. In *Digital Twin Technologies and Smart Cities* (pp. 123–149). Cham: Springer.

[49]   Dar, A. A., Alam, M. Z., Ahmad, A., Reegu, F. A., & Rahin, S. A. (2022). Blockchain framework for secure COVID-19 pandemic data handling and protection. *Computational Intelligence & Neuroscience*. (pp. 1–12). London, United Kingdom, England: Hindawi Publisher.

[50]   Awotunde, J. B., Misra, S., Ayoade, O. B., Ogundokun, R. O., & Abiodun, M. K. (2022). Blockchain-based framework for secure medical information in internet of things system. In *Blockchain Applications in the Smart Era* (pp. 147–169). Cham: Springer International Publishing.

[51]   Siboni, S., Sachidananda, V., Meidan, Y., Bohadana, M., Mathov, Y., Bhairav, S., Shabtai, A. and Elovici, Y. (2019). Security testbed for internet-of-things devices. *IEEE Transactions on Reliability*, 68(1), 23–44.

[52]   Abdul-Ghani, H. A., Konstantas, D., & Mahyoub, M. (2018). A comprehensive IoT attacks survey based on a building-blocked reference model. *International Journal of Advanced Computer Science and Applications*, 9(3).

[53]   Abdulghani, H. A., Nijdam, N. A., Collen, A., & Konstantas, D. (2019). A study on security and privacy guidelines, countermeasures, threats: IoT data at rest perspective. *Symmetry*, 11(6), 774.

[54]   Firoozjaei, M. D., Mahmoudyar, N., Baseri, Y., & Ghorbani, A. A. (2022). An evaluation framework for industrial control system cyber incidents. *International Journal of Critical Infrastructure Protection*, 36, 100487.

[55]   Salahdine, F., El Mrabet, Z., & Kaabouch, N. (2021, December). Phishing attacks detection a machine learning-based approach. In *2021 IEEE 12th Annual Ubiquitous Computing, Electronics & Mobile Communication Conference (UEMCON)* (pp. 250–255). New York: IEEE.

[56] Tuptuk, N., & Hailes, S. (2018). Security of smart manufacturing systems. *Journal of Manufacturing Systems*, 47, 93–106.

[57] Rufai, A. T., Dukor, K. F., Ageh, O. M., & Imoize, A. L. (2023). XAI robot-assisted surgeries in future medical decision support systems. In *Explainable Artificial Intelligence in Medical Decision Support Systems* (p. 167). London: IET.

[58] Dange, S., & Chatterjee, M. (2019). IoT botnet: the largest threat to the IoT network. In *Data Communication and Networks: Proceedings of GUCON 2019* (pp. 137–157). Singapore: Springer Singapore.

[59] Sei, Y., Ohsuga, A., & Imoize, A. L. (2023). Statistical test with differential privacy for medical decision support systems. In *Explainable Artificial Intelligence in Medical Decision Support Systems* (p. 401). London: IET.

[60] Mohanta, B., & Mohanta, H. C. (2020). Internet of things enables smart home security issue address using blockchain. *Sodha Sarita Journal*, 7(28), 147–153.

[61] Patel, C., & Doshi, N. (2019). Security challenges in IoT cyber world. In *Security in Smart Cities: Models, Applications, and Challenges* (pp. 171–191). Cham: Springer.

[62] Meshram, C., Obaidat, M. S., Imoize, A. L., Bahkali, I., Tambare, P., & Hsiao, K. F. (2022, October). An efficient authentication technique using convolution chebyshev chaotic maps for TMIS. In *2022 International Conference on Communications, Computing, Cybersecurity, and Informatics (CCCI)* (pp. 1–6). Dalian: IEEE.

[63] Mazarr, M. J., Bauer, R. M., Casey, A., Heintz, S. A., & Matthews, L. J. (2019). *The Emerging Risk of Virtual Societal Warfare: Social Manipulation in a Changing Information Environment*. Fort Belvoir, VA: RAND Corporation.

[64] Kotsiuba, I., Skarga-Bandurova, I., Giannakoulias, A., Chaikin, M., & Jevremovic, A. (2019, December). Technique for finding and investigating the strongest combinations of cyberattacks on smart grid infrastructure. In *2019 IEEE International Conference on Big Data (Big Data)* (pp. 4265–4272). Los Angeles, CA: IEEE.

[65] Sadhu, P. K., Yanambaka, V. P., Abdelgawad, A., & Yelamarthi, K. (2022). Prospect of internet of medical things: a review on security requirements and solutions. *Sensors*, 22(15), 5517.

[66] Aliyu, A., Maglaras, L., He, Y., Yevseyeva, I., Boiten, E., Cook, A., & Janicke, H. (2020). A holistic cybersecurity maturity assessment framework for higher education institutions in the United Kingdom. *Applied Sciences*, 10(10), 3660.

[67] Iwaya, L. H., Ahmad, A., & Babar, M. A. (2020). Security and privacy for mHealth and uHealth systems: a systematic mapping study. *IEEE Access*, 8, 150081–150112.

[68] Awotunde, J.B., Folorunso, S.O., Imoize, A.L., Odunuga, J.O., Lee, C.C., Li, C.T., & Do, D.T. (2023). An ensemble tree-based model for intrusion detection in industrial internet of things networks. *Applied Sciences*, *13*(4), 2479.

[69] Ogundokun, R.O., Arowolo, M.O., Misra, S., & Awotunde, J.B. (2022). Machine learning, IoT, and blockchain integration for improving process management application security. In *Blockchain Applications in the Smart Era* (pp. 237–252). Cham: Springer International Publishing.

[70] AbdulRaheem, M., Balogun, G. B., Abiodun, M. K., Taofeek-Ibrahim, F. A., Tomori, A. R., Oladipo, I. D., & Awotunde, J. B. (2021). An enhanced lightweight speck system for cloud-based smart healthcare. In *Applied Informatics: Fourth International Conference, ICAI 2021, Buenos Aires, Argentina, October 28–30, 2021, Proceedings 4* (pp. 363–376). Springer Nature Switzerland AG, Springer International Publishing.

[71] Gope, P., Gheraibia, Y., Kabir, S., & Sikdar, B. (2020). A secure IoT-based modern healthcare system with fault-tolerant decision making process. *IEEE Journal of Biomedical and Health Informatics*, 25(3), 862–873.

[72] Nagasubramanian, G., Sakthivel, R. K., Patan, R., Gandomi, A. H., Sankayya, M., & Balusamy, B. (2020). Securing e-health records using keyless signature infrastructure blockchain technology in the cloud. *Neural Computing and Applications*, 32, 639–647.

[73] Saeed, M. M., Ali, E. S., & Saeed, R. A. (2023). 6 data-driven techniques and security issues in wireless networks. In *Data-Driven Intelligence in Wireless Networks: Concepts, Solutions, and Applications* (p. 107). USA: CRC Press.

[74] Lele, D., Deepti, P., & Gavekar, D. (2022). Advanced technique for causing immediate threats to prevent social engineering attacks. In *Vidya, Advanced Technique for Causing Immediate Threats to Prevent Social Engineering Attacks*, June 9. Rochester, USA.

[75] Mitev, M., Chorti, A., Reed, M., & Musavian, L. (2020). Authenticated secret key generation in delay-constrained wireless systems. *EURASIP Journal on Wireless Communications and Networking*, 2020(1), 1–29.

[76] Xu, Z., Xu, C., Liang, W., Xu, J., & Chen, H. (2019). A lightweight mutual authentication and key agreement scheme for medical internet of things. *IEEE Access*, 7, 53922–53931.

[77] Batra, I., Verma, S., & Alazab, M. (2020). A lightweight IoT-based security framework for inventory automation using wireless sensor network. *International Journal of Communication Systems*, 33(4), e4228.

[78] Awotunde, J. B., & Misra, S. (2022). Feature extraction and artificial intelligence-based intrusion detection model for a secure internet of things networks. In *Illumination of Artificial Intelligence in Cybersecurity and Forensics* (pp. 21–44). Cham: Springer International Publishing.

[79] Omono, A. K., Wang, Y., Xia, Q., & Gao, J. (2021, December). Implicit certificate based signcryption for a secure data sharing in clouds. In *2021 18th International Computer Conference on Wavelet Active Media Technology and Information Processing (ICCWAMTIP)* (pp. 479–484). Chengdu: IEEE.

[80] Aman, A. H. M., Hassan, W. H., Sameen, S., Attarbashi, Z. S., Alizadeh, M., & Latiff, L. A. (2021). IoMT amid COVID-19 pandemic: application, architecture, technology, and security. *Journal of Network and Computer Applications*, 174, 102886.

[81] Dwivedi, A. D., Srivastava, G., Dhar, S., & Singh, R. (2019). A decentralized privacy-preserving healthcare blockchain for IoT. *Sensors*, 19(2), 326.

[82] Qiu, S., Wang, D., Xu, G., & Kumari, S. (2020). Practical and provably secure three-factor authentication protocol based on extended chaotic-maps for mobile lightweight devices. *IEEE Transactions on Dependable and Secure Computing*, 19(2), 1338–1351.

[83] Chen, M., & Lee, T. F. (2021). Anonymous group-oriented time-bound key agreement for internet of medical things in telemonitoring using chaotic maps. *IEEE Internet of Things Journal*, 8(18), 13939–13949.

[84] Awotunde, J. B., Adeniyi, E. A., Ajagbe, S. A., Imoize, A. L., Oki, O. A., & Misra, S. (2023). Explainable artificial intelligence (XAI) in medical decision support systems (MDSS): applicability, prospects, legal implications, and challenges. In *Explainable Artificial Intelligence in Medical Decision Support Systems* (p. 45). London: IET.

[85] Oberko, P. S. K., Obeng, V. H. K. S., & Xiong, H. (2022). A survey on multi-authority and decentralized attribute-based encryption. *Journal of Ambient Intelligence and Humanized Computing*, 1–19.

[86] Li, H., Yu, K., Liu, B., Feng, C., Qin, Z., & Srivastava, G. (2021). An efficient ciphertext-policy weighted attribute-based encryption for the internet of health things. *IEEE Journal of Biomedical and Health Informatics*, 26(5), 1949–1960.

[87] Tian, H., Li, X., Quan, H., Chang, C. C., & Baker, T. (2020). A lightweight attribute-based access control scheme for intelligent transportation system with full privacy protection. *IEEE Sensors Journal*, 21(14), 15793–15806.

[88] Olugbade, S., Ojo, S., Imoize, A. L., Isabona, J., & Alaba, M. O. (2022). A review of artificial intelligence and machine learning for incident detectors in road transport systems. *Mathematical and Computational Applications*, 27(5), 77.

[89] Prathima, S., & Priya, C. (2022). Improved CP-ABE based crypto technique to secure EHRS with access policy-based authentication schemes. *Journal of Pharmaceutical Negative Results*, 2365–2379.

[90] Patro, K. K., Jaya Prakash, A., Jayamanmadha Rao, M., & Rajesh Kumar, P. (2022). An efficient optimized feature selection with machine learning approach for ECG biometric recognition. *IETE Journal of Research*, 68(4), 2743–2754.

[91] Balasamy, K., Krishnaraj, N., Ramprasath, J., & Ramprakash, P. (2022). A secure framework for protecting clinical data in medical IoT environment. In *Smart Healthcare System Design: Security and Privacy Aspects* (pp. 203–234). USA: Wiley Publisher.

[92] Nyangaresi, V. O., Abduljabbar, Z. A., Mutlaq, K. A. A., Ma, J., Honi, D. G., Aldarwish, A. J., & Abduljaleel, I. Q. (2022). Energy efficient dynamic symmetric key based protocol for secure traffic exchanges in smart homes. *Applied Sciences*, 12(24), 12688.

[93] Jiang, Q., Zhang, N., Ni, J., Ma, J., Ma, X., & Choo, K. K. R. (2020). Unified biometric privacy preserving three-factor authentication and key agreement for cloud-assisted autonomous vehicles. *IEEE Transactions on Vehicular Technology*, 69(9), 9390–9401.

[94] Inedjaren, Y., Maachaoui, M., Zeddini, B., & Barbot, J. P. (2021). Blockchain-based distributed management system for trust in VANET. *Vehicular Communications*, 30, 100350.

[95] Mirsaraei, A. G., Barati, A., & Barati, H. (2022). A secure three-factor authentication scheme for IoT environments. *Journal of Parallel and Distributed Computing*, 169, 87–105.

[96] Sun, J., Ren, L., Wang, S., & Yao, X. (2019). Multi-keyword searchable and data verifiable attribute-based encryption scheme for cloud storage. *IEEE Access*, 7, 66655–66667.

[97] Zhang, H., Tong, L., Yu, J., & Lin, J. (2021). Blockchain-aided privacy-preserving outsourcing algorithms of bilinear pairings for internet of things devices. *IEEE Internet of Things Journal*, 8(20), 15596–15607.

[98] Chiba, Z., Abghour, N., Moussaid, K., & Rida, M. (2019). Intelligent approach to build a Deep Neural Network based IDS for cloud environment using combination of machine learning algorithms. *Computers & Security*, 86, 291–317.

[99] Maniyath, S. R., & Thanikaiselvan, V. (2020). An efficient image encryption using deep neural network and chaotic map. *Microprocessors and Microsystems*, 77, 103134.

[100] Sadhu, P. K., Yanambaka, V. P., Abdelgawad, A., & Yelamarthi, K. (2022). Prospect of internet of medical things: a review on security requirements and solutions. *Sensors*, 22(15), 5517.

[101] Shamshad, S., Ayub, M. F., Mahmood, K., Rana, M., Shafiq, A., & Rodrigues, J. J. (2021). An identity-based authentication protocol for the telecare medical information system (TMIS) using a physically unclonable function. *IEEE Systems Journal*, 16(3), 4831–4838.

[102] Chuang, Y. H., & Lei, C. L. (2021). PUF based authenticated key exchange protocol for IoT without verifiers and explicit CRPs. *IEEE Access*, 9, 112733–112743.

[103] Liu, L., Feng, J., Pei, Q., Chen, C., Ming, Y., Shang, B., & Dong, M. (2020). Blockchain-enabled secure data sharing scheme in mobile-edge computing: an asynchronous advantage actor–critic learning approach. *IEEE Internet of Things Journal*, 8(4), 2342–2353.

[104] Xiao, Y., Xu, B., Jiang, W., & Wu, Y. (2021). The HealthChain blockchain for electronic health records: development study. *Journal of Medical Internet Research*, 23(1), e13556.

[105] Du, M., Chen, Q., Chen, J., & Ma, X. (2020). An optimized consortium blockchain for medical information sharing. *IEEE Transactions on Engineering Management*, 68(6), 1677–1689.

[106] Lin, P., Song, Q., Yu, F. R., Wang, D., & Guo, L. (2021). Task offloading for wireless VR-enabled medical treatment with blockchain security using collective reinforcement learning. *IEEE Internet of Things Journal*, 8(21), 15749–15761.

[107] Song, J., Yang, F., Zhang, W., Zou, W., Fan, Y., & Di, P. (2019). A fast FoV-switching DASH system based on tiling mechanism for practical omnidirectional video services. *IEEE Transactions on Multimedia*, 22(9), 2366–2381.

[108] Rahman, M. A., Hossain, M. S., Islam, M. S., Alrajeh, N. A., & Muhammad, G. (2020). Secure and provenance enhanced internet of health things framework: a blockchain managed federated learning approach. *IEEE Access*, 8, 205071–205087.

[109] Egala, B. S., Pradhan, A. K., Badarla, V., & Mohanty, S. P. (2021). Fortified-chain: a blockchain-based framework for security and privacy-assured internet of medical things with effective access control. *IEEE Internet of Things Journal*, 8(14), 11717–11731.

5 AIoMT Enabling Real-Time Monitoring of Healthcare Systems
Security and Privacy Considerations

Joseph Bamidele Awotunde, Agbotiname Lucky Imoize, Rasheed Gbenga Jimoh, Emmanuel Abidemi Adeniyi, Muyideen Abdulraheem, Idowu Dauda Oladipo, and Peace Busola Falola

5.1 INTRODUCTION

Our world is moving closer to becoming a global village due to the emergence of advanced communication technology. Pervasive healthcare is one of the technical solutions to address global health concerns due to the rising healthcare costs and the desire for higher-quality care. The Internet of Things (IoT), a loosely connected network of gadgets, is a result of the ongoing development of various technologies. Several application fields, including smart homes [1–2], wearables [3–5], traffic monitoring [6–8], agriculture [9–11], etc., have already employed IoT concepts. IoT is advancing in m-health, which offers medical care services via mobile devices, including in security-critical systems like medical care services [12–14]. M-health enables dynamic, dispersed healthcare organizations to obtain the appropriate medical information, resulting in more effective and less expensive healthcare services. A subset of IoT known as the "Internet of Medical Things" (IoMT) comprises an agglomeration of interconnected health sensors and gadgets. IoMT can also include networked communication between patients and medical professionals [15–16]. A sensor attached to the patients' bodies records the medical information. The medical professionals performing the diagnosis, monitoring, and therapy receive the collected data.

Users of smart healthcare can handle a variety of medical issues independently. The patient's healthcare costs are reduced because it allows remote patient monitoring and tracking. Additionally, it enables clinicians to provide their services without being restricted by location. Over the preceding ten years, the trend has shifted in favor of smart wearable technology, intelligent buildings, intelligent communities, and a working, intelligent medical system that can enable an elderly being to maintain a healthful life [3]. In today's digital age, communication between people and objects is made possible by the IoT, a fast-expanding interactive paradigm [17–18].

In both homes and hospitals, the AIoMT is utilized to monitor patients remotely. Online patient surveillance in the medical industry may significantly reduce unnecessary trips to health experts, hospital admissions, constant admissions, and health treatment costs by identifying and managing dangerous sicknesses and disorders at an early level [19–20]. Due to the patient's hospital stay up until the end of the therapy, our healthcare system is currently quite expensive. These problems might be resolved with the aid of clever technologies that can remotely monitor patients. By acquiring and sharing real-time patient health data with professionals, the AIoMT lowers healthcare expenses. This makes it possible to address medical conditions before they develop into serious illnesses [21]. There is no doubt that AIoMT will raise people's standards of living. The development of integrated tools can lead to numerous beneficial improvements in consolidated information platform operations, computer processing, and connectivity with a variety of control. Hence, to identify, monitor, and prevent a variety of chronic and viral disorders in the medical field, numerous IoMT-centered digital and wearable devices and applications are needed [22]. Figure 5.1 depicts the application of IoMT-based systems.

All of these applications must be gathered, and data must be handled in actual-time in order to assess them and decide a choice while maintaining the confidentiality of the patients' personal information and the sensitivity of the data. In other places, the global environment demonstrates that security is now more important than ever at the stage of computing structure, particularly for those working with confidential

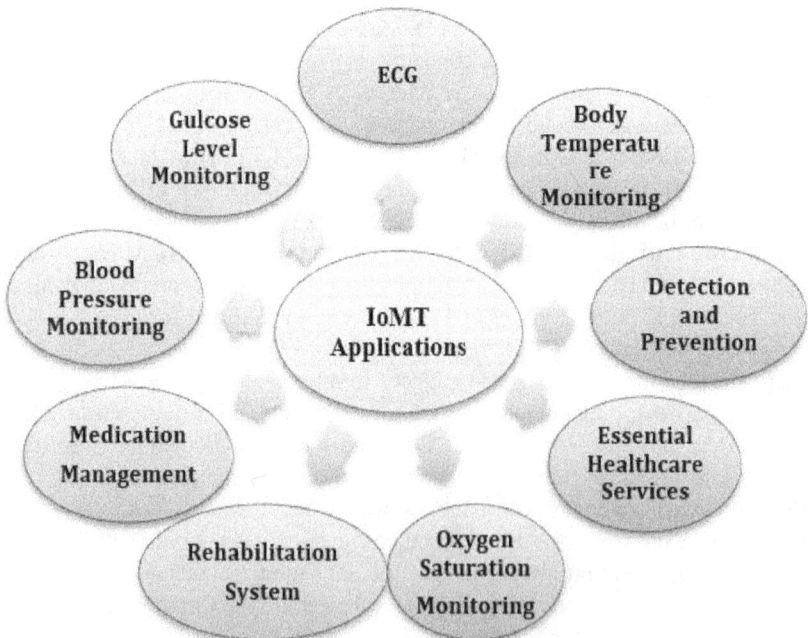

FIGURE 5.1   Applications of Internet of Medical Things (IoMT).

data. Nevertheless, having access to the data is essential. Additionally, architectures must ensure data confidentiality and integrity while resisting distributed assaults like Distributed Denial of Service (DDOS), Man-in-the-Middle (MITM), and Botnets [23–24], which are networks of systems or other gadgets under an attacker's control that use the network to carry out harmful actions against a specific victim. Client-server systems are not vulnerable to this kind of assault because data is duplicated when using distributed architectures. These facts prompted us to reconsider how we create architectural designs and protect data for crucial infrastructures. We can significantly limit the attack surface, thanks to recent technology developments like blockchain [25–26] and, more specifically, smart contracts and confidential computing.

Particularly, the latest innovations in the Internet of Things have sparked the creation of medical equipment with artificial intelligence called the Artificial Intelligence of Medical Things (AIoMT). The safety and confidentiality concerns of such pervasive and inexpensive sensing systems are frequently disregarded, notwithstanding the notion that they have the ability to change the present reactive care to preventative care. As medical equipment collects and processes extremely private personal health data and information, the devices and communications that go with them must be extremely secure to safeguard the privacy of the user. However, the computing power of the smallest AIoMT devices is extremely constrained, and only a few security protocols may be used in such devices. Additionally, given the prevalence of AIoMT devices, the main problems preventing the deployment of AIoMT for medical applications are the difficulty in controlling and assuring guaranteeing the safety of AIoMT systems. Therefore, by giving a broad overview of the most modern techniques, this chapter addressed the safety and confidentiality needs, problems, risks, and future research prospects in the AIoMT systems.

5.1.1 Keys Contributions of This Chapter

The primary contributions of this work are as follows:

  i. Presents applicability of AIoMT application in the real-time patient monitoring system
 ii. Explains the various security and privacy concerns in AIoMT-based applications in the real-time patient monitoring system
iii. Discusses the technologies that can be used to leverage the safety and confidentiality concerns in AIoMT-based systems
 iv. The potential future directions in AIoMT application in real-time patient monitoring systems were presented

5.1.2 Chapter Organization

Section 5.2 presents the applicability of artificial intelligence in medical things in real-time patient monitoring systems. Section 5.3 discusses AIoMT-based real-time patient monitoring systems architectures. Section 5.4 discusses the security and privacy concerns of artificial intelligence of medical things in patient real-time monitoring systems. Section 5.5 presents security threats in artificial intelligence of medical things edge networks. Section 5.6 presents a countermeasure to artificial intelligence medical things for real-time patient monitoring systems, and, finally, Section 5.7 concludes the chapter with future direction.

5.2 THE APPLICABILITY OF ARTIFICIAL INTELLIGENCE OF MEDICAL THINGS IN REAL-TIME PATIENT MONITORING SYSTEMS

Population growth impacts how classical healthcare establishments must provide for the broader public [27]. Despite a strong infrastructure and cutting-edge technology, medical healthcare services are not affordable or widely available to the general populace. Global healthcare costs are increasing as the population ages. China spent more than 4,634 billion yuan in 2016, which is roughly 6.36% of the whole Gross Domestic Product, and 7,231 billion yuan in 2021, which is 7.1% of the total Gross Domestic Product, according to the most recent data [28]. A smart medical device is necessary to inform the audience about their health problems and keep them current on their medical ailment in actual-time in order to solve these challenges. Significant gains in efficiency and care quality are anticipated in the medical sector due to the wide range of AIoMT advances. Recent advancements in microelectronics, materials, and biosensor designs have particularly sparked interest in smart medical gadgets that can be worn or implanted.

Medical sensors are now often utilized in operating rooms, ERs, and intensive care units (ICUs), which provide patient surveillance in actual time. In comparison, the use of device sensors that can be worn makes it possible to provide more individualized care at a lower cost through remote consultation. New applications, including operation guidance, first aid car diagnostics, and other things, will start to arise with the rollout of 5G [29–30]. One of the most significant IoT technologies today is wearable technology [31–32]. In AIoMT-related healthcare systems, wearable devices are at the forefront of every discussion because they have the ability to bring about a significant revolution. They are also considered the best method for tracking, identifying, and monitoring viral and chronic infections in the healthcare industry. Wearable technology, seen as a crucial element of the Internet of Things, enables patients to receive the necessary medical attention when needed [33–34]. Clients have demonstrated a great desire to acquire and wear these gadgets, and they have the capability to significantly alter the quality of human living in the modern day in ways that cannot be fully realized by phones. AIoMT devices with sensors can be used in hospitals to track the deployment of medical staff and equipment [35]. These tools are widely used in the medical sector to observe patients and generate alarms for those who have risky situations.

AIoMT-based medical observation technologies and medical devices that can be worn enable the establishment of "clinics without boundaries," in which health practitioners from various disciplines give medical care services virtually to outpatients. This frees up critical bed spaces for patients who need further care and lowers the financial strain. Additionally, it gives people more ongoing management of their wellness. Remote health monitoring systems were becoming more and more common before COVID-19. The need for wearable medical equipment and smart technology to monitor virtual patients increased during the COVID-19 pandemic

[36–37]. Over the next five years, it is predicted that high requests for the gadgets now on the market are anticipated to rise.

Albeit the use of IoMT innovation in the healthcare industry can assist hospitals in achieving smart healthcare treatment of individuals and smart management of things, resource sharing is challenging due to the relative independence of various medical institutions [38]. The IoMT, which is based on cloud computing, offers sturdy IT fundamental resources and significantly lowers healthcare expenditures. In an effort to boost the effectiveness and caliber of healthcare services, it may not only fulfill the need for bulk storage of health data but also enable healthcare information sharing via cloud platforms [39]. However, relying solely on cloud computing will use up a lot of network communication resources and cause a significant delay, which could endanger patient lives. The capacity of cloud computing to handle data sinks, bringing data processing nearer to the origin instead of outbound data or the cloud, can decrease lag period and provide actual-time and faster medical data processing and evaluation. Edge computing, which makes judicious use of resources on edge devices, lowers reliance on a dispersed or remote centralized server and addresses cloud computing's issues [40]. It results in a more responsive and flexible IT network for hospitals and clinics, allowing patients to get better medical care. Edge computing, however, does not live in a vacuum. Edge computing and cloud computing are joint efforts to create a powerful whole. While edge computing concentrates on the local, cloud computing concentrates on the big picture. The strategic use of edge cloud cooperation will encourage the creation of medical application scenarios more effectively.

The quantity of data that must be analyzed and evaluated will continuously grow along with the rate at which IoMT is adopted. IoMT infrastructures will eventually need to deal with large data. In the realm of IoMT, an AI-based framework is, therefore, unavoidable. The IoMT is increasingly using AI-based techniques for various functions, including patient monitoring, clinical decision support systems, and identifying and predicting potential diseases. The retrieval of patient data has also been made simpler by the widespread use of remote monitoring medical devices, which fall under the IoMT banner. These devices enable continuous monitoring and give healthcare providers instant access to data. In order to create reliable and exact algorithms capable of accurately and quickly diagnosing the condition to avert potentially fatal effects, data must also be well-structured and in huge amounts.

Although AI/ML has the potential to alter healthcare practices and IoMT-integrated medical devices to attain the prospect of commercialization and adaptability in clinics and society, a few technological challenges still need to be addressed. Because AI/ML systems heavily rely on correct data for programming and training the system, the emphasis must be on acquiring a ton of data on high-quality patient training and learning. Another significant problem is the heterogeneity of the data that have been collected. Due to bias and noise in the health records collected from various clinics, there are inconsistencies in the training of AI. Complex ML techniques can be used to homogenize the data sets, improving the accuracy of the clinical diagnosis. Using AI-supported techniques, the field of medicine and surgery will prosper in the future.

Using AIoMT technology, clinicians can now keep an eye on patient health data in real-time. Some groundbreaking investigations have recently examined patient health monitoring using cutting-edge biomedical technologies and an embedded IoMT device. Noninvasive biosensors that enable virtual-time patient surveillance have the potential to raise patient happiness, speed up the delivery of care, promote adherence to treatment, and lead to better health outcomes [41]. For instance, stretchable-material-based sensors can replace traditional techniques that need piercing needles, inflexible circuit boards, terminal connections, and power sources to provide noninvasive and comfortable physiological monitoring [42]. Currently, researchers are using alternative analytes such as saliva, sweat, urine, and tears since noninvasive health monitoring is required.

Due to its accessibility, smartphone-based colorimetric analysis stands out among other cutting-edge new technologies as a suitable platform for noninvasive patient health monitoring. By using intelligent portable devices, colorimetric data may be transformed into digital pictures quickly. A reusable hybrid microfluidic device for colorimetric measurements using a cellphone measurement of typical urine analytes such as glucose, pH, and red blood cells was described by authors in [43]. In order to lower mistakes in smartphone-based colorimetric analysis, authors in [44] proposed a self-referenced portable plasmonic sensing device coupled with an intrinsic standard sample. Furthermore, authors in [45] developed a smartphone application technique and doughnut-shaped reference swatches encircling each detection pad on a colorimetric strip.

Wearable electrochemical sensors now have appealing and adaptable capabilities because of current advances in micro-/nanofabrication, flexible and elastic functional materials, and wireless communications. New possibilities for non-invasive, real-time patient monitoring are made possible by biomarkers in saliva, tears, perspiration, and even breathing out air. For instance, smart contact lenses with integrated glucose sensors, wireless power transfer circuits, and LED pixels were recently reported by authors in [46] to supervise the glucose level in tears. Numerous efforts have been undertaken to create glucose sensors for tears due to the potentially significant benefits of noninvasive and continuous, making them an enticing alternative to blood testing [41]. Although there is still controversy about the relationship between glucose levels in tears and blood glucose levels, this issue is currently being explored. Applying a virtual-time glucose monitoring gadget, for instance, resulted in appreciable increases in glycated hemoglobin levels and a decrease in hypoglycemic occurrences [47], decreasing patients' fear of hypoglycemia and ultimately enhancing their quality of life [48].

Some recently disclosed wearable technologies have employed perspiration detectors to provide continuous, unobtrusive surveillance of biomarkers in sweat [49]. Real-time measurements of patients' metabolites can be obtained via sweat sensors (such as glucose and lactate for muscular exhaustion) [50] plus electrolytes (sodium, potassium, and other trace elements are a few examples) [51]. Similarly, authors in [52] demonstration of an electrochemically improved iontophoresis interface-based platform for automated perspiration extraction and detection. A machine-like stretchable polyethylene terephthalate substrate was patterned with iontophoresis and sensor electrodes in order to create a stable and conformal contact interface. Additionally, authors [53] described an IoT-integrated sweat monitoring system that used a machine-like stretchable sensor array for aggregated in situ perspiration measurement of specifications such as sweat metabolites, electrolytes, and skin temperature.

5.3 AIOMT-BASED REAL-TIME PATIENT MONITORING SYSTEMS ARCHITECTURES

The growth of 5G has boosted data source diversity and accelerated the velocity of big data in medicine [54]. In [55], the authors explained The Institute of Analytics for Health (INAH) in 2021 as a system for scientific and health study that guarantees the ethical and secure use of patient data. Since patient identification is impossible due to double pseudonymization, each data source is, in fact, still in control of its own [55]. To monitor old patients, authors in [56] created a three-tiered structure (sensors, fog, cloud). The correlation of Influxdb, Chronograf, and Kapacitor forms the foundation of the fog layer, and contact with the cloud layer is made possible by a web service. The Druid Indexing Service temporarily saves the information sent to Apache Kafka before ingesting it. In other words, sets containing a few million rows of data are saved on the Hadoop File System by Apache Druid in the form of segments (HDFS). After that, Apache Ambari retrieved the Druid metric sent out to keep track of it, and Druid used Apache Kylin [56]. But with more recent versions of Apache Druid, using Druid without Kylin or, as a substitute, Kylin 4.0 with Parquet is more effective.

The viability of edge-cloud computing in the health industry was demonstrated by authors in [57], who evaluated IoMT design, the design of cloud-based IoMT, and the structure of edge-cloud IoMT. They claimed that while Edge Cloud computing is perfectly suited to 5G, it also poses numerous security risks and confidentiality concerns. The aforementioned will be required at the edge phase, along with distributed intrusion detection, mutual node authentication, hash and encryption algorithm expansion, and communication security protocol development. Additionally, a number of issues still need to be resolved, including the optimization of AI algorithms at the edge phase and cache strategy, and cache update strategy [57]. In [58], the authors suggested the BEdgeHealth decentralized architecture for a cooperative hospital network. This decentralized health architecture incorporates blockchain technology, mobile edge computing, and data exchange for distributed hospital networks. The goal was to lessen the cost of data exchange associated with the current sharing system and the data latency retrieval.

The Things, Fog, and Cloud levels are the three layers that authors in [59] used to develop an architecture to outline upcoming technologies in IoMT. The Things layer comprises sensors, actuators, medical records, and other components. This layer's objective is to gather all information accessible for future treatment. Local routers and gateway equipment employed for safety and data confidentiality make up the Fog layer. Data storing and handling resources are used in the Cloud layer. They demonstrated the potential for using these technologies in IoMT through a few case studies. When attempting to authenticate devices on the network, they employed the Physically Unclonable Function (PUF). To connect the devices without internet connectivity, they employed Software-Defined Networking (SDN). In order to secure data confidentiality and privacy, they lastly adopted the Blockchain [59].

Similarly, authors in [60] introduced the Open mHealth platform that offers a variety of connectors for interacting with healthcare device APIs. The platform automatically converts data from gadgets in Open mHealth or FHIR observations. Scriptr.io manages security intrinsically by applying granular access control rules to activities and stored data. It was recommended by authors in ([61] to link smart contracts with data lakes. The smart contract is divided into three sections. On the blockchain, the initial one, called "Contract Registrar," holds a client ID and identity. Finally, the third "Patient-Provider Interaction Contract" controls the interaction involving patients and medical professionals. The next "Summary Contract" allows patients to ascertain that their medical history is traceable. The data are kept in a data lake apart from the chain. They contend that this mix enables the storage of a range of data.

In [62], the authors provided a classification of safety remedies for IoMT and a characterization of the potential threats. The study states that the security goals for IoMT are data availability, availability, secrecy, integrity, and non-repudiation. It should be noted that, as mentioned by authors in [63], despite the expansion of the IoT, which includes smart clothing, there is still no unified structure capable of linking all intelligent gadgets in intelligent hospitals. However, Nb-IoT can be a viable option by enabling objects to communicate to the web via a very limited bandwidth of 200 kHz by linking straight to the operators' base stations. With this strategy, edge computing is introduced, and [63] created an infusion-monitoring system to track the volume of pharmaceuticals still in the bloodstream and the rate of drug loss in real-time.

The Community Medical Internet of Things (CMIoT) already utilizes IPv6 applications. However, authors in [64] noted that synchronizing the various CMIoT elements is the sole issue that needs to be resolved. In addition, numerous important problems must be solved, such as how to manage IPv6 network routing for the Internet of Things. Assuming the functional criteria are satisfied, they proposed creating a more straightforward protocol message format with their team. This makes it possible to connect the IPv6 network to the physical network more efficiently. Using big data technologies, authors in [65] suggested an architecture for an actual-time health condition forecasting and evaluating system. This design uses a distributed machine learning model on health data incidents streamed through Kafka topics and then ingested into Spark. The author claims their design can do health data insights and stream broadcasting, convey an alarm message to carers, and save the data in a distributed database.

In [66], the authors built an architecture with the dual objectives of identifying and assisting in the treatment of elderly patients with obtrusive sleep apnea (OSA). OSA is a serious sleep anomaly that directly influences living standards. They employed a FOG Computing technique in an intelligent gadget at the network's edge in order to identify the OSA. Batch data are used to accomplish the second goal because they offer descriptive analysis that quantitatively defines the data's actions and are suggestive analyses for the creation of various services. Big Data Tools on Cloud Computing were utilized in this architecture. In Table 5.1, real-time designs for the IoMT are compared for their benefits and drawbacks.

TABLE 5.1
Comparison of Real-Time Architectures for IoMT

Authors	Strength	Gap
Boutros-Saikali, et al., (2018) [60]	They suggested a system built on the scriptr.io system, which offers several connectors for use with the API of medical gadgets.	They solely rely on the scriptr.io platform for their framework and security, which may be a security issue when it comes to protecting user data.
Zhang, et al., (2018) [63]	They suggested a framework for actual-time edge computing for an infusion surveillance platform.	They did not provide a generic architecture that could be used for other use cases; this architecture was created specifically for a given use case.
Liu, et al., (2018) [64]	To resolve the difficulty with the connection between the IPv6 network and the physical network, they suggested creating a new, more straightforward protocol message.	This protocol is not accepted as a standard for dealing with this problem.
Debauche, et al. (2019) [56]	This architecture was created using a variety of free-source parts.	Some of the components utilized today are no longer required (e.g., Apache Druid with Kylin)
Ed-daoudy & Maalmi, (2019) [65]	On transmitting health data occurrences, this architecture applied a distributed ML model.	The accuracy gained from the ML model's training is what determines how accurate the predictions are.
Yacchirema, et al. (2019) [66]	To identify and cure OSA, their architecture made use of big data tools on cloud computing.	This architecture was created primarily to address the OSA issue affecting elderly people.
Sun, et al. (2020) [57]	They claimed that Edge Cloud Computing is ideally suited to 5G after reviewing various IoMT architectures.	That solution has numerous known vulnerabilities, dangers, and privacy concerns.
Girardi, et al. (2020) [61]	Their suggested scheme is to link a Smart Contract to a data lake.	The contract appears to be difficult to comprehend and apply (three sections).
Papaioannou, et al., (2020) [62]	In IoMT, they outlined the security goals.	They failed to give a true use case that included a minimum of one security goal and a potential solution.
Nguyen, et al. (2021) [58]	Blockchain technology is used in this architecture.	This design was created for a hospital that wished to communicate data while minimizing latency securely.
Razdan & Sharma (2022) [59]	They presented an outline of upcoming IoMT technology.	They do not put them to use in a real-world scenario.
Gaur et al., (2015) [67]	Portal for aggregating data from numerous medical facilities for scientific study while protecting patient privacy by double pseudonymization.	Adoption is still subject to approval by medical establishments and ethics bodies.

(Continued)

TABLE 5.1 (*Continued*)
Comparison of Real-Time Architectures for IoMT

Authors	Strength	Gap
Lee et al., (2023) [68]	The paper presents the MEDBIZ platform, which has been put into use and is predicated on the IoMT and supports actual-time digital health services for precision medicine.	Currently, the platform solely supports services in the healthcare industry.
Mohammed & Hasan, (2023) [69]	The study concentrated on virtual surveillance of body temperature, heart rate, and SPO2. In addition, the hardware attached can be utilized to request the patient's position.	Adding additional health parameters to the system, such as ECG, Blood Pressure, Respiratory Rate, Urine Output, Fetal Heart Rate, and others, in response to patient and physician requests.
Yıldırım et al., (2023) [70]	A diabetes prediction model is described for the suggested IoMT framework. The diabetes prediction process is performed on fog using fuzzy logic decision-making and is accomplished on the cloud with SVM, RF, and ANN as ML-based algorithms.	The study is limited to one disease, and future work can extend the framework for diverse healthcare and pandemic applications.
Dahan et al., (2023) [71]	The study introduces an IoMT telemedicine infrastructure for electronic healthcare powered by AI.	Future work on this research can be expanded by using a video-based system.

5.4 SECURITY AND PRIVACY CONCERNS OF ARTIFICIAL INTELLIGENCE OF MEDICAL THINGS IN PATIENT REAL-TIME MONITORING SYSTEMS

The ongoing growth in the number of patients presents new problems for established healthcare systems. The AIoMT was proposed to remedy this issue and to raise the sector's correctness, dependability, efficacy, and efficiency. AIoMT can be considered an advancement and commitment to react to patients' demands more adequately and efficiently. However, AIoMT has a range of problems and difficulties, such as a lack of privacy and safety protections as well as the required education and awareness. In this section, we emphasize the significance of putting the proper safety measures in place to strengthen AIoMT's defenses against cyberattacks. In addition, the subsection examines the primary AIoMT security and privacy concerns and the available security solutions. These technologies include biometrics, blockchain, cryptographic intrusion detection, and authentications. It is significant to highlight that, especially during the emergence of digital healthcare v4.0, the safety controls for AIoMT show a trade-off between the safety level and the system performance [72].

Additionally, AIoMT applications are directly associated with delicate healthcare services because they handle delicate patient data like names, addresses, and medical conditions. Maintaining patient privacy without lowering the security level is the major problem in the AIoMT application. Furthermore, good security and privacy solutions should only involve the bare minimum of computations and resources. AIoMT systems recently became one of the most significant new medical technologies. This technology can produce huge gains by improving the remote monitoring of medical services. Additionally, it can aid in the early detection of any medical problem, protecting the lives and health of people.

Unfortunately, a large number of AIoMT domain's associated medical equipment have security weaknesses that render them susceptible to malicious attack attempts. Such issues might have serious consequences, disrupting (or regulating) medical equipment and impacting patients' lives. These issues must be addressed to keep medical IoT systems' performance and accuracy requirements. Conversely, AIoMT systems are liable to sophisticated assaults due to the widespread utilization of medically sensitive data (like Ransomware) that focus on its primary security features, such as confidentiality, integrity, and privacy. This would have a detrimental effect on the AIoMT systems' reputation, adoption, and widespread use.

In the e-Healthcare space, where intelligent health sensors and gadgets are installed to prolong patients' lives and improve their health, AIoMT systems have become essential. However, as part of planned cybercrimes, this domain was subject to a number of attacks, including botnets that targeted healthcare systems [73–74]. IoT security and privacy issues were explored by authors in [75], although they were not connected to IoMT. Numerous authentication/authorization [76] and intrusion detection [77–78] techniques were offered with little thought to how they might be applied to IoMT in order to ensure a secure IoT environment. Furthermore, the security of healthcare systems has only recently received increased attention. To categorize big data issues and the difficulties in implementing IoMT solutions [79], the authors conducted a broad survey of big data analytics in medicine in [80]. In comparison, research into the merits and demerits of IoT deployment in healthcare devices was done by authors [81] to improve nurses' experiences in hospitals [82]. In this study, we provide a more in-depth, comprehensive, and analytical perspective on the IoMT and healthcare sectors and their relation to the incorporation of cyber-physical systems in the medical sector.

5.4.1 CONCERNS IN ARTIFICIAL INTELLIGENCE OF MEDICAL THINGS IN PATIENT REAL-TIME MONITORING SYSTEMS

Concerns about AIoMT can be divided into four main groups, one of which is voiced by the general public and relates to difficulties with safety, confidentiality, trust, and accuracy.

Security issues: AIoMT devices are vulnerable to a variety of wireless/network assaults since they depend on the usage of available wireless connections. A hacker can collect and eavesdrop on incoming and outgoing data and information because most AIoMT devices either lack security protections by design or because poorly designed authentication security mechanisms are simple for a competent attacker to get over. Due to the inability to recognize and stop such attacks, it is also possible to get illegal access without being noticed. This could lead to higher privileges, the injection of malicious code, or the malware infection of devices. However, AIoMT devices could be taken over (and turned into botnets) and employed in Distributed Denial of Service (DDoS) assaults. The vulnerability of medical systems to botnet or "zombie" attacks, which can result in physical assaults on patients, was demonstrated by authors in [83]. For instance, an assault may reasonably change a medicine dose that might kill the target patient or have severe health effects.

Additionally, terrorists may employ AIoMT devices as a tool for targeted assassination if they were to steal them. In order to prevent being hacked in order to kill him, US Vice President Dick Cheney turned off the wireless functioning of his cardiac implant [84]. Additionally, as stated by authors in [83], IoMT devices might negatively impact patients' psychological well-being since they may frighten them and cause them to experience a heart attack as a result of being surrounded by machines rather than people. To ensure and keep the safety of the Medical-Cyber Physical System (MCPS), as well as other medical systems and equipment, manufacturers of medical equipment must prioritize security as a top priority. To reduce the primary IoMT safety issues, defense against both dormant and aggressive threats is necessary. As a result, suitable security processes and equipment are required.

Privacy issues: Passive assaults, as in traffic analytics, present confidentiality issues due to the risk of acquiring and revealing patient names as well as delicate and personal information. Identifying an attacker's medical information and medical conditions makes this a significant threat to patients. It has grave, potentially fatal consequences for the patients. Another method in which patients' privacy is infringed when hospitals are assaulted is through identity theft. In the vast majority of these actual-life attacks, personal or sensitive information was leaked or otherwise disclosed, resulting in a breach of patients' privacy. Additionally, it calls for the necessity for non-observability, non-linkability, and anonymity. In conclusion, maintaining the confidentiality of private and sensitive medical information is only one aspect of privacy.

Anonymity: When a patient communicates, his identity should be concealed so that he cannot be identified. In other words, passive assaults only have access to your actions and not your identity.

Non-linkability: Passive assaults should not reveal Items of Interest (IoI), such as subjects, messages, events, or activities. This implies that the likelihood of those objects remaining hidden from the attacker's perspective both before and after observation should be the same.

Non-observability: Items of Interest (IoI) that are non-observable are identical to other IoIs of the same category. This implies that messages cannot be separated from random noise (s). In other words, whether a communication has been sent or received by a sender/receiver in a relationship should not be obvious.

Trust issues: Patients' privacy being violated results in significant trust difficulties. Patients are growing weary of the notion of robots taking over human duties (doctors, nurses, and front desk personnel). In light of this, people are warier about having a healthcare robot, machine, or even gadget monitor and manage their medical states [85].

Accuracy issues: This kind of worry has emerged due to the over 144 patients who died in the United States [86] due to unintentional errors brought on by the poor accuracy and diagnosis of medical robots. More than 1,400 patients had partial or permanent injuries as a result of this, and claims of failure showed that more than 8,061 malfunctions had happened in the previous 13 years (2000–2013) [87]. Another illustration is the misdiagnosis of dementia or Alzheimer's in some patients. These instances, together with patient misdiagnosis and incorrect prescriptions, point to devoid of accuracy and precision in the procedures carried out by healthcare robots [88].

As soon as medical devices began to be integrated into IoT systems, AIoMT issues started to appear. The lack of standards is one of the main problems. The authors' detailed discussion of the key IoMT difficulties can be found in [89]. Standardization is crucial for diverse clinical devices to work together and for vendors to implement the proper safety precautions to keep them from being compromised. This would result in higher protection, efficacy, efficiency, scalability, and consistency. In truth, many of these issues are mostly due to IoMT security issues, among other things. Figure 5.2 displays the AIoMT concerns in real-time patient monitoring systems.

5.5 SECURITY THREATS IN ARTIFICIAL INTELLIGENCE OF MEDICAL THINGS EDGE NETWORK

IoT devices in the IoMT edge network have limited resources, which prevents the deployment of resource-intensive encryption methods (the encrypting and decrypting of data), maintaining a significant amount of data privacy and leaving the network open to assaults aimed at compromising the privacy of the stored or shared

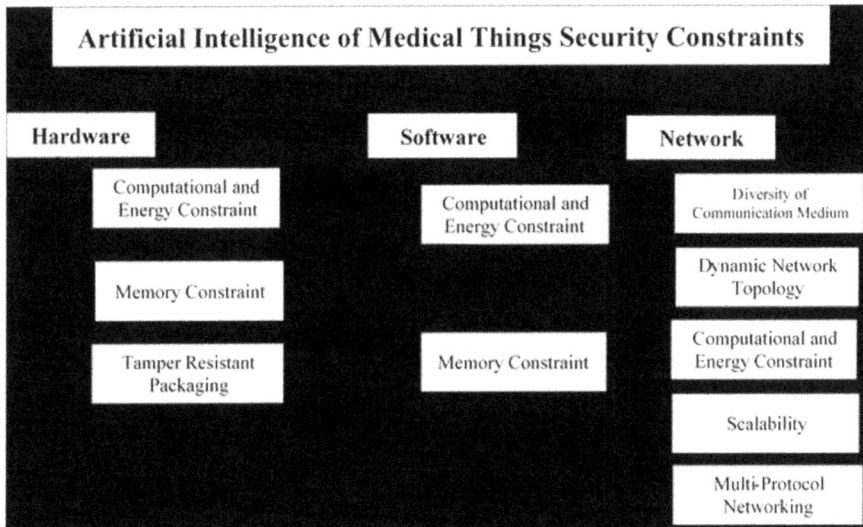

FIGURE 5.2   Security limitations with Artificial Intelligence of Medical Things.

data [90, 91]. By following conversations and reading the information contained in the transmitted packages, an adversary may, for instance, eavesdrop on information being transferred within the IoMT edge network [92]. The enemy has the ability to passively intercept the communication of patient vitals from a gadget sensor that can be worn to an IoMT gateway (such as the patients' smartphone), and gather private information (using traffic analysis, for instance) in need to utilize them wrongfully [93].

Moreover, interrogating assaults, which are a form of impersonation, may jeopardize the confidentiality of data [94]. More specifically, a malicious actor may appear trustworthy and send requests to other entities to disclose users' private information [95].

5.5.1 SECURITY RISKS TO INTEGRITY

A type of attack that has the potential to compromise the authenticity of IoMT edge networks is threatened by a man-in-the-middle (MitM) assault due to the perpetrator's interference in the connectivity involving two sides and the potential for undetected data modification [96]. For example, the IoMT edge network's medical data collection can be transferred to a distant router or retained locally in the local storage of wearable technology. A MitM perpetrator can eavesdrop and alter sent health data during transmission, jeopardizing their authenticity [97–98]. Additionally, the malicious node injection assault is described as the most hazardous physical assault by the authors in [99] since it disrupts the given services and modifies the saved data.

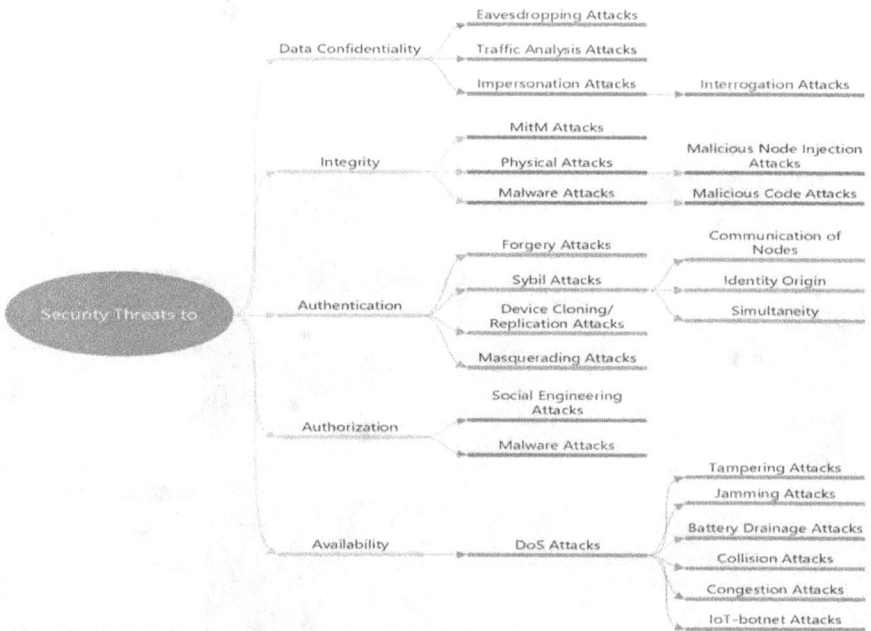

FIGURE 5.3 Categorization of security threats in IoMT edge network.

Physical assaults on the gadgets themselves are another prominent attack method that successfully aims to undermine the integrity of AIoMT devices [100]. For instance, a malicious party with physical access to an AIoMT system could modify its model to affect its behavior. Finally, the absence of portable malware detection tools for IoMT devices enables perpetrators also to hamper the integrity of medical equipment [101]. For example, an attacker can damage the device by running malicious code on an IoMT device and taking advantage of its networking software and hardware's security flaws.

5.5.2 THREATS TO AUTHENTICATION SECURITY

One of the fundamental safety specifications of an IoMT-based medical system is authentication. The standard PKI-based authentication methods are ineffective and cannot be expanded due to the AIoMT devices' ubiquity [102]. Furthermore, adversaries target weak system authentication to access resources depending on people's identities without having legitimate privileges [103]. The most typical authentication process assaults are described in [104–108]. In forgery cyberattacks, the attack's initial phase targets the fabrication of an identity so that the rogue user's identity may be verified. The attacker then sends false data to other entities in an effort to scam them [109]. Sybil attacks, in which an IoMT device assumes many false identities, can also be detrimental since they enable malicious gadgets to mimic other trustworthy gadgets in the AIoMT edge network. For example, the rogue node may be able to establish connections with a number of other AIoMT gadgets in order to increase its influence and possibly trick the platform into making false inferences.

Due to hardware or power limitations, an attacker may engage with a limited amount of Sybil identities at a time, even if they have the technical means to connect with several fake identities simultaneously. Device cloning/replication attacks differ from Sybil attacks because each gadget has only one identity. This kind of assault involves an enemy controlling sensing equipment to extract encrypted data, and it is used to compromise authentication and security goals by making a sizable amount of clones in the network and carrying out other assaults [110]. Since the authorization procedure excludes location-based authentication schemes, the malicious intent to expel devices from the same location is successful [111].

Lastly, AIoMT edge networks may also be the target of impersonating assaults. One of the following two categories may apply to a masquerading attack. By using rogue devices, an adversary either poses as an authorized user to gain access to the services that AIoMT devices offer [112], or an attacker is purportedly disguised as an AIoMT device to deliver false services to users. The last scenario is risky for the medical industry because many patients depend on the AIoMT devices' services for their survival.

5.5.3 SECURITY RISKS TO AUTHORIZATION

Adversaries may target poor authorization procedures on an AIoMT edge network to obtain accessibility to network assets without the proper authorizations. AIoMT systems may be liable to social engineering attacks because of users' lack of security knowledge, according to authors in [113]. As a result, a hostile actor might deceive the AIoMT edge network and pose as a reputable company to gain access to users' medical devices. The patient's life could be in jeopardy if medical gadgets that monitor vital signs are used [114]. Malware attacks may potentially affect the linked AIoMT devices by using their built-in weaknesses, such as holes in authorization systems. The infected AIoMT gadgets can be used as a robot to carry out additional assaults on other AIoMT edge network devices. Hence, the perpetrator can gain entry to network resources or services (like handling of numerous IoMT devices), for instance, a patient's gathered medical information [115].

5.5.4 SECURITY INTIMIDATIONS TO AVAILABILITY

The constraints and drawbacks of the current centralized cloud-based healthcare systems are being overcome by IoT technology, which is being deployed in a growing number of healthcare applications. Unfortunately, the medical systems, where AIoMT gadgets are prevalent, are experiencing resource and computing power limitations [116], posing difficulties in maintaining the services' availability. In reality, the AIoMT edge network's limited resources can make it extremely susceptible to DoS assaults. Several network levels can be subjected to distinct DoS attack types, each impacting the AIoMT edge network differently. Tampering is more specifically defined as the change of sent data that prevents the AIoMT edge network from operating normally. The characteristics of the poor and insecure wireless connectivity in the AIoMT edge network environment make it difficult to identify a tampering attack [117]. Furthermore, jamming attacks use massive amounts of transmitted messages to overwhelm computer or communication resources, preventing IoMT devices from using the services routinely supplied [118].

An AIoMT edge network unavailability renders it immediately ineffective for offering real-time quality healthcare and jeopardizes patient safety. A critical-care individual may not get the attention required in an AIoMT medical alert system, putting their life in danger. This can happen if the AIoMT internet gateway connections are blocked. A battery-draining assault in opposition to the AIoMT gadget that targets the resource-constrained battery usage of the AIoMT device may lead to the same outcome [119]. An adversary that sends the target IoMT device intentionally erroneous or misleading messages can carry out a battery depletion attack [120].

In addition, in collision assaults, data is concurrently transmitted in the same frequency band by two nodes, resulting in an identity mismatch for the recipient. This results in the AIoMT edge network wasting resources by discarding malformed received data packets and retransmitting the identical packets [58]. The huge transmission of pointless messages also contributes to channel congestion attacks, which result in excessive channel traffic and the unavailability of time-related AIoMT services and data [121]. Finally, AIoMT edge network availability can be a target of Distributed Denial of Service (DDoS) attacks. An attacker can overwhelm the target device (like a gateway) with numerous requests using an IoT botnet to overburden it and interrupt the services being offered. It is important to note that due to the limited resources of its devices, the AIoMT edge network in a healthcare system based on AIoMT is more susceptible to DoS assaults than the Cloud platform [122].

5.5.5   Risks to Security

Because AIoMT gadgets rely on public wireless technology, they are vulnerable to network/wireless assaults [123–124]. Because AIoMT devices lack security safeguards due to poor design or insufficient security authentication mechanisms, an attacker may eavesdrop and listen in on inbound and outbound data [125]. Additionally, because the bulk of AIoMT gadgets cannot sense and stop assaults, skilled perpetrators can circumvent security and get patient records without consent [126–127]. Attackers can employ elevated access to penetrate computers with malware or harmful software [128]. The authors' work in [83] demonstrates this since the researchers demonstrate how healthcare equipment is vulnerable to zombie or botnet assaults. For example, an assault might rationally adjust or modify a patient's medicine dose, perhaps fatally affecting their well-being [129]. As a result, because most AIoMT gadgets use blockchain infrastructure, an adversary may find the patient's data on the distributed ledger system [130–131]. Furthermore, medical information in medical procedures is subject to forgery, which might result in erroneous drug control and patient diagnosis, all raising the likelihood of an adverse reaction [132]. As a result of security weaknesses, attackers may send bogus medical warnings and cause high financial costs.

5.5.6   Risks to Privacy

Data collected by AIoMT gadgets may expose sensitive information about a patient's behavior [92]. As noted by the authors in [133], signals transmitted by sensors meant to indicate a patient's status, for example, can expose the computer's medical expertise. Passive assaults, such as traffic analysis, are similar to active attacks in that they allow attackers to spread or acquire patient identities as well as sensitive and confidential data [134–135]. Furthermore, as explained by authors in [105, 136–137], assault by a man-in-the-middle (MitM), for example, might jeopardize the privacy and authenticity of AIoMT networks by tampering with the transmission in order to manipulate the data being sent between entities involved secretly. To jeopardize their confidentiality, for example, the collected medical data may be sent to a remote router where perpetrators could edit and exploit it. Furthermore, professionals like authors in [138–139] have deemed confidentiality and safety issues a serious assault on user confidentiality and data secrecy because unlawful data storage exposes users to authenticity, confidentiality, and data protection risks. This is especially clear since AIoMT gadgets lack a dependable validation method [106, 140]. As a result of the absence of internet connectivity control and data protection, hackers can breach individual privacy through listening.

5.6   COUNTERMEASURE TO ARTIFICIAL INTELLIGENCE MEDICAL THINGS FOR REAL-TIME PATIENT MONITORING SYSTEMS

Although AIoMT systems provide patients and physicians with dependable and efficient healthcare services, they confront significant security problems. Consequently, security is recognized as essential in biomedical research since highly confidential physiology information can quickly be hijacked or exploited over the lifecycle of patient records [20]. Access management, proof of identity, data encryption, blockchain, intrusion detection, isolation-based mechanisms, bio-cryptographic key generation, and attestation-based architecture are the most commonly used ways to guarantee health data security in AIoMT platforms. The use of modern cryptographic and non-cryptographic approaches has now safeguarded wireless communication security.

5.6.1   Access Control

Access control prohibits illegitimate users from gaining access to assets while determining the appropriate degrees of power for approved users [141–142]. When it comes to AIoMT systems, users can limit entry to AIoMT gadgets by setting individual access levels for each individual [143]. It is crucial to emphasize that access control for AIoMT devices can guarantee data confidentiality [144]. This is demonstrated by the scientists of [145], who developed a rudimentary glass-breaking authorization system that incorporates attribute-based and glass-breaking access. Glass-breaking access is set aside for crises, whereas attribute-based access is used for fine-grained access control. According to the researchers, their method is safe and gives highly precise results. A stretchy twofold access control mechanism for an AIoMT information storage system was suggested in a related study by authors in [146]. The researchers claim that their access control system, which is self-adaptive for both urgent and usual circumstances, may eliminate the replication of medical data by employing a smart, secure replication method. A ciphertext strategy based on the attribute-based encryption method was introduced in a different study by authors [147]. The medical attribute values used in this study are concealed by encrypted s-health data (SHRs). The authors effectively handled the patient's confidentiality and health record issues with this access control solution. The research of authors in [148–149] developed a secure data-sharing architecture for AIoMT gadgets that leverages the Slepian Wolf coding method to safeguard patient privacy while preventing insider assaults. The study claims that their proposed framework may function with many cloud servers to give the data.

5.6.2   Identity Authentication

Figures Identity verification is a technique of authenticating a user's identity in order to avert unidentified persons from accessing crucial patient records [150]. In light of this, the researcher of [151] investigated a three-factor verification mechanism for protected message transmission in wireless body area networks in his investigation. The scholars engaged edge servers to advance a robust identity-proof architecture for this system, which leverages data authentication tokens to certify the patients' identity while protecting sensitive physiological parameters. Similarly, authors in [152] presented a key and validation treaty procedure that uses access control machinery to enhance the confidentiality and safety of medical records for patients and providers. However, although addressing modern authentication issues like secure communication, their lightweight authentication and ownership protocol is susceptible to DoS, desynchronization, and traceability attacks.

The authors of [153] created an end-to-end approach for safeguarding AIoMT systems using the session resumption technique and handshake mechanism. According to the authors in [153], their suggested approach can reduce communication latency and overhead by 16% and 26%, respectively. Yet, authors in [154] achieved a 97% assault detection accuracy. This technique is more intriguing because it operates 97% faster than certified-based DTLS schemes, using 2.2 times less RAM and 2.9 times less ROM. The authors introduced a protected IoT system based on access control and privacy-aware aggregate verification machinery in the study in [155]. This system was created using an unspecified certificateless signing structure to safeguard a patient's medical records.

Using a two-way identity authentication approach, another study by authors in [156] proposed a special updating instrument that can be used to update authentication keys and session keys. This technique effectively validates the authenticity and legitimacy of diverse medical sensors. This technique prevents unauthorized users and untrustworthy authentication servers from accessing medical data by using symmetric encryption in conjunction with the elliptic curve encryption techniques. On the other hand, the study of [157] employed a revolving group signature system with elliptic curve cryptography (ECC) to guarantee patient privacy. The authors claim that their study can withstand attacks while offering a number of security enhancements based on the findings.

5.6.3 DATA ENCRYPTION

The encryption process is a safekeeping technology that turns data into code or another shape so that it may only be accessed by those with a secret decryption key [158]. Security experts commonly use this approach since it assures the integrity of patient records, particularly in the biomedical industry [159]. To safeguard network connectivity in AIoMT, researchers such as those in [158, 160] presented a send-receive model approach and key exchange based on AES. The authors also employed homomorphic encryption, which employs a matrix approach to preserve secrecy, and an expert detection method to autonomously analyze the encrypted health information to allow a confidentiality method.

The researchers of [161] proposed a system for protected data gathering that advances the security of data transit and data gathering. According to the research, the suggested platform is built with two techniques: equipment, a compact FGPA approach, and a secret encryption exchange mechanism. Our solution beats previously existing IoT-based medical approaches in regard to performance, with quicker computation times and reduced high-frequency energy usage. The integrity and secrecy of medical data transfers in AIoMT are ensured by a unique D2D-assist data transmission mechanism established by the authors in their study [162]. In accordance with the performance evaluation, the proposed system can outperform existing AIoMT systems in terms of computational and transmission complexity. As a result, it is obvious that a range of encryption approaches may ensure the safety of AIoMT platforms.

Figures medical devices routinely touch the patient's psyche and handle sensitive information. These devices collect important medical-related data from individuals via a wired or wireless communication link. Yet, as transmission technology advanced, enemies began to employ modern methods to augment the hazard of violent and mild assaults. To prevent these assaults, researchers have proposed a variety of cutting-edge defenses that are secure and powerful enough to thwart assaults [92].

5.6.4   ISOLATION-BASED MECHANISM

This monitoring defense policy aims to divide a platform's assets and resources into distinct areas. To characterize the different resource access controls, the researchers of [163] employ a distinct bit at the physical level. To move among the trustworthy and unverified zones in software, distinct system calls or entryways are used. The scientists were able to allocate the safe amount of memory by using the CPU to provide APIs and operation codes. Similarly, the authors' investigation in [164–165] employed hardware primitives to generate function partition. While the shared memory protecting unit (MPU) utilized in these approaches renders them hardware-dependent, a microcontroller registry may be used to ensure that each separated operation can only reach the assigned MPU.

5.6.5   BIO-CRYPTOGRAPHIC KEY GENERATION

The production and transfer of keys is an effective safeguard against intrusions. These approaches rely on physiological properties such as IPI, which is unique and unexpected, making it perfect for encryption [166]. Several practitioners applied such key generation techniques to thwart cyberattacks. To protect the wearable and implanted medical products interaction, the authors of [167], for instance, proposed a bio-cryptographic key management system. This approach generated exceptionally secure encryption techniques by utilizing physiological data from sensors such as an electrocardiogram (ECG), photoplethysmogram (PPG), and heart rate. The researchers of [168] created a heart-beating random binary code (RBS) technique to safeguard interaction between medical equipment. Our technique employed the Hamming Distance measure with a finite monotonic rising sequential-producing mechanism to harvest entropic bits from an ECG based on IPI. The experts state that their approach for producing bio-cryptographic credentials is effective and can recover up to 16 various bits.

5.6.6   ATTESTATION-BASED ARCHITECTURE

Several mitigation strategies have been proposed in the works to prevent run-time attacks on a device's sequence diagram and authenticity, which are often a result of bad programming methods such as system vulnerabilities and bad recall administration. The study, for example, developed Lo-Fat and C-flat schemes that define the hash value built on the path the device traverses [169–170]. This structure employs a prover and a verifier. The prover is a low-end device management software, while the verifier is a remote machine that regulates the flow of a device's application operation. Similarly, the scholars in [171–173] proposed a Hardware-enforced

Control-Flow Integrity (HCFI) and Hardware-Assisted Flow Integrity Extension (HAFIX) based solutions that check each recipient node's label during flow transition. These approaches can detect unusual breaches, such as sequence takeover, soon before they jeopardize security.

5.6.7 BLOCKCHAIN TECHNOLOGY

Blockchain expertise is gradually becoming popular and used in cryptocurrencies, security, trust administration, and immutability. The failure of a few nodes has no impact on the system's robustness in the lack of a third party. The use of digital signatures, data chains, and consensus procedures in operational rules and data documents all contribute to ensuring transparency, nonrepudiation, and confidentiality. The decentralized nature of the blockchain is crucial for developing a contemporary decentralized trust model [123]. A trustworthy cloud computing environment can be built using blockchain [174]. In this scenario, blockchain can also be a potential option to offer security, trust, and authentication services.

Blockchain is a decentralized network system that keeps an ever-growing, tamper-proof data repository using a chain structure of blocks. In multi-party settings, it may provide a new cooperative trust paradigm [175]. Blockchain is also being widely used in the AIoMT due to growing public health awareness [176]. A variety of objects, including people, can be intelligently identified, their positions can be tracked, they can be monitored, and they can be controlled, thanks to the IoT. By linking sensor devices to the network, such as medical wearables, medical microcontrollers, motionless hospital instruments, and health surveillance schemes, the AIoMT uses a variety of patient medical records to provide meaningful data for later treatment [174].

Every day, countless different forms of decentralized medical organizations generate enormous amounts of medical data. The exchange of electronic medical records is necessary since patients must undergo additional testing if they change medical institutions [177]. However, electronic health records (EHRs) contain extremely confidential information regarding diagnosis and treatment [178]. As information escape happens when data is shared across EHRs, maintaining the secrecy and safety of these systems is a critical distress [179].

The special characteristics of cryptocurrency benefits can solve these problems with massive data, including distributed storing and unlinkability. The advantages of combining blockchain and big data are as follows:

1. *Enhancing big data privacy and security*: Blockchain technology's decentralized data storage is appropriate for data exchange between different medical institutions. Its own data encoding technique makes it challenging to allow any unknown individual entrance to the contents.
2. *Enhancing data integrity*: The blockchain model makes it difficult to store information to be altered, ensuring the security and dependability of EMRs.
3. *Fraud avoidance*: Big data now in use cannot address the issue of recording false messages. Blockchain gives medical organizations the ability to assess EMRs that may be false in real-time.

4. *Real-time data analytics*: Medical establishments can perform thorough and methodical real-time diagnoses based on therapeutic data gathered through various channels. The integrity, security, and privacy of each patient record may be ensured by incorporating blockchain expertise with AIoMT schemes [180].

Smart contracts can be employed in the AIoMT space, where it is getting harder to monitor and implement contracts as the number of nodes grows by millions over time [181]. Blockchain can help with this endeavor since it does away with the need for middlemen. The network's brokers or intermediaries, which are used to validate the information and make decisions, need a lot of computation and time. By enabling the participating nodes to cooperate on their behalf, the Blockchain eliminates the need for these middlemen [182]. The main reasons for integrating the Blockchain with AIoMT in e-medical care are to extend the life of sensor nodes by reducing computations, time, and energy. This is mostly used in asset controlling, where smart contracts may be integrated into assets that specify who is in possession of what at any given time. Moreover, algorithmically, a collection of programmable dynamic connections are used in all transactions, depending on the needs. As a result, the devices in the network can operate autonomously and successfully when used in conjunction with the Internet of Medical Things.

Things with a unique address on the Blockchain network can have smart contracts embedded in them. The corresponding code will run whenever environment variables that have been configured take on a value that complies with a smart contract's input requirements. Another way to activate a smart contract is to address a transaction specifically to it [183]. The identical arrays of directives are also carried out on the other chain nodes as it is joined. The chain becomes tamper-proof and irrevocable since each transaction runs independently and cannot be undone once it has been sent [184]. A counter transaction or a hard fork must be carried out in order to undo any transaction. Blockchain-based smart contracts perform best in applications with a high volume of data management transactions. As so much data is being generated and just a small fraction of it is being processed, this situation is suitable for AIoMT-related services [185]. This procedure can be automated with the aid of blockchain, making data execution, processing, and storage quicker and more effective.

5.6.8 INTRUSION DETECTION SYSTEMS

The AIoMT is a paradigm that links patient gadgets and sensors to the whole network and allows them to collaborate to accomplish shared goals, such as cutting-edge home automation. The dispersed and open AIoMT service structure appeals to potential attackers as a tempting target for cyberattacks. Security, therefore, cannot be handled on its own. Every layer of the IoT system needs security included during design and development. AIoMT security worries about threats to human health and life as well as network and data security. As a result, for the AIoMT to be secure and functional, the creation of the AIoMT mechanism need to guarantee security via assault resilience. Also, it's critical to link AIoMT systems with intrusion detection systems (IDS) [186]. IDS aims to monitor and examine network traffic from various resources, find the harmful activity, and report it. It plays a big role in cybersecurity technology. IDS is, in essence, a mechanism used to identify harmful behavior directed at victims using various techniques.

The hacking of AIoMT systems and networks can compromise patient privacy, impede communications, and interfere with the diagnosis of diseases. Because hackers are so skilled, the security risks relating to AIoMT devices and connections are growing. Countless dangerous malware can be the cause of medical device manipulation and illegal internet access to medical records. The method and type of such assaults are evolving quickly, and the current processes are insufficient for identifying malware and conducting the necessary analysis. Most cyberattacks result in DDoS, which prevents authorized users from accessing devices or data. Therefore, spotting any unwanted intrusions into the AIoMT system is crucial.

Authentication, encryption, and intrusion detection are only a few of the security measures that have been established in the past to safeguard IoT systems [187]. An IDS can spot an outbreak by looking at scheme parameters and potential attack indicators or by spotting a change from usual behavior. Bad activities can illegally access cloud servers or steal or manipulate health data by intercepting it while it is being transmitted over wireless media. Moreover, attackers may interfere with the diagnosing process [188]. All of these security breaches have significantly and permanently impacted the environment of AIoMT. An accurate, time-efficient IDS for the AIoMT scheme must be designed to accomplish this.

Scholars have recently concentrated particularly on ML methods for selectively detecting intrusions. Despite the existence of numerous data analysis and statistical approaches for IDS, it is challenging to detect new hostile activity. Yet, ML systems are able to detect dynamic changes in the signatures of these actions. IDS can use ML-based models to identify intrusions at the host and network levels. ML-capable models can even categorize previously discovered hostile behaviors and identify unanticipated activity [189].

Following are a few examples of prior activities undertaken on AIoMT Systems. Several ways have been suggested for creating an IDS over the years. In [198] the authors suggested a cloud-based healthcare system in which only legitimate users were granted authorization. The scheme uses Support Vector Machine techniques to ascertain a patient's condition and the anticipated disease. The system's data mining and discovery processes are ML-based. This work developed a method to combine network flow metrics with biometric data in addition to providing an objective view of malicious behaviors. Authors in [190] suggest a blockchain-based healthcare system architecture. Although it is well known that blockchain technology ensures security, the writers have not looked into or tested the architecture in order to provide any comparison data. Authors in [191] suggested a brand-new medical system for investigation in the Internet of Medical Things field. The researcher worked on the improved Hospital Monitoring System (EHMS) testbed to present the wustl-ehms-2020 database. Man-in-the-middle attacks were the foundation for the suggested dataset. The collection contains patient biometrics and network flow indicators. The k-nearest neighbor approach is the foundation for the cyber security study used by the authors in [192–193]. Authors in [192] tested several attack types using an Indexed Partial Distance search k-Nearest Neighbor (IKPDS), which yields a 99.6% accuracy rate. Authors in [193] demonstrate an accuracy of 85.2% while concentrating primarily on lowering the false alert rate. The research mentioned earlier makes use of an improved version of the KDD Dataset, yet both the dataset and the malicious attack signatures employed date back to 1999.

The most collective method of vulnerability scanning is network intrusion detection (NIDS), which employs network data analytics. Host-based intrusion detection (HIDS) is developed when sensing, and gadget log data are used [194]. Parameters are used in both types of intrusion detection to discover irregularities (unidentified intrusions) and patterns (known assaults) that diverge from typical system activities or sensor data. These detecting systems are almost the same in that an agent collects data and a baseband processor detects and reports intruders. Yet, they differ in the following ways: (i) data source [195], (ii) detection approach [196]: signature-based [141], anomaly-based, and (iii) structure (unified and dispersed) [197]. Signature-based techniques can swiftly discover known attacks but are unable to distinguish novel ones. Anomaly-based, on the contrary, extreme, intrusion detection techniques detect unexpected activity by learning from recent data. They could thus spot novel assaults, albeit with lesser accuracy and greater processing overhead [198–199]. DoS, DDoS, and diverse virus assaults are among the most current threats neutralized by IDSs [200–202].

5.7 CONCLUSIONS AND FUTURE DIRECTIONS

The IoMTs are gradually substituting the conventional healthcare system. However, the development of AIoMT devices and systems has given little consideration to their security requirements. The challenge of adapting conventional safety resolutions to the IoMT system may be one of the primary causes. Attack detection and mitigation have been successfully carried out using AI-based models. In order to overcome the current and future security and privacy challenges with the AIoMT, advanced AI techniques can also be a promising solution. It is essential to comprehend how these tactics may be leveraged to address security and privacy needs while maintaining integrity, operations, and gadget longevity of the AIoMT system due to the current challenges. Therefore, this chapter discussed many layers of AIoMT security and privacy considerations. The chapter identified a number of unresolved security and privacy vulnerabilities that the research community needs to address in order to create a secure and reliable platform for the provision of upcoming AIoMT. We also discussed the practical applications of AIoMTs. Research on AIoMTs will remain to be a prominent topic in the future. There are many complex issues that researchers need to solve. It is important to note that more research should be done to address the issues brought on by the limitations of AIoMT devices to address the dangers that jeopardize the accessibility of the crucial facilities offered by an AIoMT edge system atmosphere.

ACKNOWLEDGMENT

The work of Agbotiname Lucky Imoize is supported in part by the Nigerian Petroleum Technology Development Fund (PTDF) and, in part, by the German Academic

Exchange Service (DAAD) through the Nigerian-German Postgraduate Program under grant 57473408.

REFERENCES

[1]   Elmalaki, S. (2021, May). Fair-iot: Fairness-aware human-in-the-loop reinforcement learning for harnessing human variability in personalized iot. In *Proceedings of the International Conference on Internet-of-Things Design and Implementation* (pp. 119–132). New York: Association for Computing Machinery.

[2]   Sung, W. T., & Hsiao, S. J. (2020). The application of thermal comfort control based on Smart House System of IoT. *Measurement*, 149, 106997.

[3]   Awotunde, J. B., Ogundokun, R. O., Adeniyi, A. E., Ayo, F. E., Ajamu, G. J., Abiodun, M. K., & Ogundokun, O. E. (2022). Cloud-IoMT-based wearable body sensors network for monitoring elderly patients during the COVID-19 pandemic. In *Biomedical Engineering Applications for People with Disabilities and the Elderly in the COVID-19 Pandemic and Beyond* (pp. 33–48). Elsevier, Academic Press.

[4]   Awotunde, J. B., Ajagbe, S. A., & Florez, H. (2022, October). Internet of things with wearable devices and artificial intelligence for elderly uninterrupted healthcare monitoring systems. In *Applied Informatics: 5th International Conference, ICAI 2022, Arequipa, Peru, October 27–29, 2022, Proceedings* (pp. 278–291). Cham: Springer International Publishing.

[5]   Yan, Z., Han, B., Du, Z., Huang, T., Bai, O., & Peng, A. (2021). Development and testing of a wearable passive lower-limb support exoskeleton to support industrial workers. *Biocybernetics and Biomedical Engineering*, 41(1), 221–238.

[6]   Mohammed, K., Abdelhafid, M., Kamal, K., Ismail, N., & Ilias, A. (2023). Intelligent driver monitoring system: An internet of things-based system for tracking and identifying the driving behavior. *Computer Standards & Interfaces*, 84, 103704.

[7]   Imoize, A. L., Hemanth, J., Do, D. T., & Sur, S. N. (Eds.). (2023). *Explainable Artificial Intelligence in Medical Decision Support Systems*. London: IET.

[8]   Yang, X., Liu, G., Guo, Q., Wen, H., Huang, R., Meng, X., . . . & Tang, Q. (2022). Triboelectric sensor array for internet of things based smart traffic monitoring and management system. *Nano Energy*, 92, 106757.

[9]   Tzounis, A., Katsoulas, N., Bartzanas, T., & Kittas, C. (2017). Internet of things in agriculture, recent advances and future challenges. *Biosystems Engineering*, 164, 31–48.

[10]   Hundal, G. S., Laux, C. M., Buckmaster, D., Sutton, M. J., & Langemeier, M. (2023). Exploring barriers to the adoption of internet of things-based precision agriculture practices. *Agriculture*, 13(1), 163.

[11]   Jain, A., Ranjan, N., Kumar, S., & Vishwakarma, S. K. (2023). Internet of things (IoT) in the agriculture sector: Challenges and solutions. In *Sustainable Computing: Transforming Industry 4.0 to Society 5.0* (pp. 69–85). Cham: Springer International Publishing.

[12]   Awotunde, J. B., Ayoade, O. B., Ajamu, G. J., AbdulRaheem, M., & Oladipo, I. D. (2022). Internet of things and cloud activity monitoring systems for elderly healthcare. In *Internet of Things for Human-Centered Design: Application to Elderly Healthcare* (pp. 181–207). Singapore: Springer Nature Singapore.

[13]   Awotunde, J. B., Jimoh, R. G., Ogundokun, R. O., Misra, S., & Abikoye, O. C. (2022). Big data analytics of iot-based cloud system framework: Smart healthcare monitoring systems. In *Artificial Intelligence for Cloud and Edge Computing* (pp. 181–208). Cham: Springer International Publishing.

[14] Subhan, F., Mirza, A., Su'ud, M. B. M., Alam, M. M., Nisar, S., Habib, U., & Iqbal, M. Z. (2023). AI-enabled wearable medical internet of things in healthcare system: A survey. *Applied Sciences*, 13(3), 1394.

[15] Chen, C. M., Liu, S., Li, X., Islam, S. H., & Das, A. K. (2023). A provably-secure authenticated key agreement protocol for remote patient monitoring IoMT. *Journal of Systems Architecture*, 102831.

[16] Awotunde, J. B., Jimoh, R. G., AbdulRaheem, M., Oladipo, I. D., Folorunso, S. O., & Ajamu, G. J. (2021). IoT-based wearable body sensor network for COVID-19 pandemic. In *Advances in Data Science and Intelligent Data Communication Technologies for COVID-19: Innovative Solutions Against COVID-19* (pp. 253–275). Cham: Springer.

[17] Goel, S. S., Goel, A., Kumar, M., & Moltó, G. (2021). A review of internet of things: Qualifying technologies and boundless horizon. *Journal of Reliable Intelligent Environments*, 7, 23–33.

[18] Awotunde, J. B., Ogundokun, R. O., & Misra, S. (2021). Cloud and IoMT-based big data analytics system during COVID-19 pandemic. In *Efficient Data Handling for Massive Internet of Medical Things: Healthcare Data Analytics* (pp. 181–201). Cham: Springer International Publishing.

[19] Haleem, A., Javaid, M., Singh, R. P., & Suman, R. (2021). Telemedicine for healthcare: Capabilities, features, barriers, and applications. *Sensors International*, 2, 100117.

[20] Rajeshwari, B. S., Namratha, M., & Saritha, A. N. (2023). Architecture, current challenges, and research direction in designing optimized, IoT-based intelligent healthcare systems. In *Image Processing and Intelligent Computing Systems* (pp. 223–233). Florida, USA: CRC Press.

[21] Alwan, A., Majdzadeh, R., Yamey, G., Blanchet, K., Hailu, A., Jama, M., . . . & Zaidi, R. (2023). Country readiness and prerequisites for successful design and transition to implementation of essential packages of health services: Experience from six countries. *BMJ Global Health*, 8(Suppl 1), e010720.

[22] Parihar, A., Yadav, S., Sadique, M. A., Ranjan, P., Kumar, N., Singhal, A., . . . & Srivastava, A. K. (2023). Internet-of-medical-things integrated point-of-care biosensing devices for infectious diseases: Toward better preparedness for futuristic pandemics. *Bioengineering & Translational Medicine*, e10481.

[23] Awotunde, J. B., Jimoh, R. G., Folorunso, S. O., Adeniyi, E. A., Abiodun, K. M., & Banjo, O. O. (2021). Privacy and security concerns in IoT-based healthcare systems. In *The Fusion of Internet of Things, Artificial Intelligence, and Cloud Computing in Health Care* (pp. 105–134). Cham: Springer International Publishing.

[24] Awotunde, J. B., Abiodun, K. M., Adeniyi, E. A., Folorunso, S. O., & Jimoh, R. G. (2022, January). A deep learning-based intrusion detection technique for a secured IoMT system. In *Informatics and Intelligent Applications: First International Conference, ICIIA 2021, Ota, Nigeria, November 25–27, 2021, Revised Selected Papers* (pp. 50–62). Cham: Springer International Publishing.

[25] Sakly, H., Said, M., Al-Sayed, A. A., Loussaief, C., Sakly, R., & Seekins, J. (2023). Blockchain technologies for internet of medical things (BIoMT) based healthcare systems: A new paradigm for COVID-19 pandemic. In *Trends of Artificial Intelligence and Big Data for E-Health* (pp. 139–165). Cham: Springer International Publishing.

[26] Awotunde, J. B., Misra, S., Ayoade, O. B., Ogundokun, R. O., & Abiodun, M. K. (2022). Blockchain-based framework for secure medical information in internet of things system. In *Blockchain Applications in the Smart Era* (pp. 147–169). Cham: Springer International Publishing.

[27] Lal, A., Abdalla, S. M., Chattu, V. K., Erondu, N. A., Lee, T. L., Singh, S., . . . & Phelan, A. (2022). Pandemic preparedness and response: Exploring the role of universal health coverage within the global health security architecture. *The Lancet Global Health*, e1675–e1683.

[28]   Liang, W., & Vertinsky, I. (2023). Providing and health medicines access to affordable care for. In *Global Health Security in China, Japan, and India: Assessing Sustainable Development Goals* (pp. 19–45).

[29]   Abdelkader, G., Elgazzar, K., & Khamis, A. (2021). Connected vehicles: Technology review, state of the art, challenges and opportunities. *Sensors*, 21(22), 7712.

[30]   Ibhaze, A. E., Imoize, A. L., & Okoyeigbo, O. (2022, April). A brief overview of energy efficiency resources in emerging wireless communication systems. *Telecom*, 3(2), 281–300. MDPI.

[31]   Aekanth, S. G., & Tillinghast, D. J. (2023). The emergence of wearable technologies in healthcare: A systematic review. *Human-Automation Interaction*, 43–59.

[32]   Etta, V. O., Sari, A., Imoize, A. L., Shukla, P. K., & Alhassan, M. (2022). Assessment and test-case study of Wi-Fi security through the wardriving technique. *Mobile Information Systems*, 2022.

[33]   Singh, S., Sharma, S., Bhadula, S., & Mohan, S. (2023). Industry 4.0 internet of medical things enabled cost effective secure smart patient care medicine pouch. In *New Horizons for Industry 4.0 in Modern Business* (pp. 149–170). Cham: Springer International Publishing.

[34]   Rane, D., Penchala, S., Jain, R., & Chourey, V. (2023). Roles and future of the internet of things-based smart health care models. In *Bio-Inspired Optimization in Fog and Edge Computing Environments* (pp. 223–248). FL, USA: Taylor & Francis Group.

[35]   Patra, M. K., Kumari, A., Sahoo, B., & Turuk, A. K. (2023). Smart healthcare system using cloud-integrated internet of medical things. In *Exploring the Convergence of Computer and Medical Science Through Cloud Healthcare* (pp. 60–83). Pennsylvania, United States, PA: IGI Global Publisher.

[36]   Weinberg, M., Danoff, J. R., & Scuderi, G. R. (2023). Remote patient monitoring following total joint arthroplasty. *Orthopedic Clinics* (pp. 161–168). USA: Elsevier Publisher.

[37]   Umamaheswari, S., Arun Kumar, S., & Sasikala, S. (2023). Expert systems for improving the effectiveness of remote health monitoring in COVID-19 pandemic: A critical review. In *System Design for Epidemics Using Machine Learning and Deep Learning* (pp. 99–121). Cham: Springer.

[38]   AbdulRaheem, M., Oladipo, I. D., González-Briones, A., Awotunde, J. B., Tomori, A. R., & Jimoh, R. G. (2022). An efficient lightweight speck technique for edge-IoT-based smart healthcare systems. In *5G IoT and Edge Computing for Smart Healthcare* (pp. 139–162). United Kingdom: Academic Press.

[39]   Imoize, A. L., Gbadega, P. A., Obakhena, H. I., Irabor, D. O., Kavitha, K. V. N., & Chakraborty, C. (2023). Artificial intelligence-enabled internet of medical things for COVID-19 pandemic data management. In *Explainable Artificial Intelligence in Medical Decision Support Systems* (p. 357). United Kingdom: London.

[40]   Awotunde, J. B., Ijaz, M. F., Bhoi, A. K., AbdulRaheem, M., Oladipo, I. D., & Barsocchi, P. (2022). Edge-IoMT-based enabled architecture for smart healthcare system. In *5G IoT and Edge Computing for Smart Healthcare* (pp. 1–27). United Kingdom: Academic Press.

[41]   Noah, B., Keller, M. S., Mosadeghi, S., Stein, L., Johl, S., Delshad, S., . . . & Spiegel, B. M. (2018). Impact of remote patient monitoring on clinical outcomes: An updated meta-analysis of randomized controlled trials. *NPJ Digital Medicine*, 1(1), 20172.

[42]   Park, J., Kim, J., Kim, S. Y., Cheong, W. H., Jang, J., Park, Y. G., . . . & Park, J. U. (2018). Soft, smart contact lenses with integrations of wireless circuits, glucose sensors, and displays. *Science Advances*, 4(1), eaap9841.

[43]   Jalal, U. M., Jin, G. J., & Shim, J. S. (2017). Paper-plastic hybrid microfluidic device for smart-phone-based colorimetric analysis of urine. *Analytical Chemistry*, 89(24), 13160–13166.

[44]   Wang, X., Chang, T. W., Lin, G., Gartia, M. R., & Liu, G. L. (2017). Self-referenced smartphone-based nanoplasmonic imaging platform for colorimetric biochemical sensing. *Analytical Chemistry*, 89(1), 611–615.

[45] Ra, M., Muhammad, M. S., Lim, C., Han, S., Jung, C., & Kim, W. Y. (2017). Smartphone-based point-of-care urinalysis under variable illumination. *IEEE Journal of Translational Engineering in Health and Medicine*, 6, 1–11.

[46] Chu, M. X., Miyajima, K., Takahashi, D., Arakawa, T., Sano, K., Sawada, S. I., . . . & Mitsubayashi, K. (2011). Soft contact lens biosensor for in situ monitoring of tear glucose as non-invasive blood sugar assessment. *Talanta*, 83(3), 960–965.

[47] Parkin, C. G., Graham, C., & Smolskis, J. (2017). Continuous glucose monitoring use in type 1 diabetes: Longitudinal analysis demonstrates meaningful improvements in HbA1c and reductions in health care utilization. *Journal of Diabetes Science and Technology*, 11(3), 522–528.

[48] Polonsky, W. H., Hessler, D., Ruedy, K. J., & Beck, R. W. (2017). The impact of continuous glucose monitoring on markers of quality of life in adults with type 1 diabetes: Further findings from the DIAMOND randomized clinical trial. *Diabetes Care*, 40(6), 736–741.

[49] Al-omari, M., Liu, G., Mueller, A., Mock, A., Ghosh, R. N., Smith, K., & Kaya, T. (2014). A portable optical human sweat sensor. *Journal of Applied Physics*, 116(18), 183102.

[50] Lee, H., Choi, T. K., Lee, Y. B., Cho, H. R., Ghaffari, R., Wang, L., . . . & Kim, D. H. (2016). A graphene-based electrochemical device with thermoresponsive microneedles for diabetes monitoring and therapy. *Nature Nanotechnology*, 11(6), 566–572.

[51] Gao, W., Emaminejad, S., Nyein, H. Y. Y., Challa, S., Chen, K., Peck, A., . . . & Javey, A. (2016). Fully integrated wearable sensor arrays for multiplexed in situ perspiration analysis. *Nature*, 529(7587), 509–514.

[52] Emaminejad, S., Gao, W., Wu, E., Davies, Z. A., Yin Yin Nyein, H., Challa, S., . . . & Davis, R. W. (2017). Autonomous sweat extraction and analysis applied to cystic fibrosis and glucose monitoring using a fully integrated wearable platform. *Proceedings of the National Academy of Sciences*, 114(18), 4625–4630.

[53] Choi, J., Ghaffari, R., Baker, L. B., & Rogers, J. A. (2018). Skin-interfaced systems for sweat collection and analytics. *Science Advances*, 4(2), eaar3921.

[54] Alabi, C. A., Tooki, O. O., Imoize, A. L., & Faruk, N. (2022, April). Application of UAV-assisted 5G communication: A case study of the Nigerian environment. In *2022 IEEE Nigeria 4th International Conference on Disruptive Technologies for Sustainable Development (NIGERCON)* (pp. 1–5). Lagos: IEEE.

[55] Delsate, T., Lessage, X., Boukhebouze, M., & Ponsard, C. (2021). INAH: The ethical & secure platform for medical data analysis. *ERCIM News*, 126, 20–21.

[56] Debauche, O., Mahmoudi, S., Manneback, P., & Assila, A. (2019). Fog IoT for health: A new architecture for patients and elderly monitoring. *Procedia Computer Science*, 160, 289–297.

[57] Sun, L., Jiang, X., Ren, H., & Guo, Y. (2020). Edge-cloud computing and artificial intelligence in internet of medical things: Architecture, technology and application. *IEEE Access*, 8, 101079–101092.

[58] Nguyen, D. C., Pathirana, P. N., Ding, M., & Seneviratne, A. (2021). Bedgehealth: A decentralized architecture for edge-based iomt networks using blockchain. *IEEE Internet of Things Journal*, 8(14), 11743–11757.

[59] Razdan, S., & Sharma, S. (2022). Internet of medical things (IoMT): Overview, emerging technologies, and case studies. *IETE Technical Review*, 39(4), 775–788.

[60] Boutros-Saikali, N., Saikali, K., & Abou Naoum, R. (2018, April). An IoMT platform to simplify the development of healthcare monitoring applications. In *2018 Third International Conference on Electrical and Biomedical Engineering, Clean Energy and Green Computing (EBECEGC)* (pp. 6–11). Beirut: IEEE.

[61] Girardi, F., De Gennaro, G., Colizzi, L., & Convertini, N. (2020). Improving the health-care effectiveness: The possible role of EHR, IoMT and blockchain. *Electronics*, 9(6), 884.

[62] Papaioannou, M., Karageorgou, M., Mantas, G., Sucasas, V., Essop, I., Rodriguez, J., & Lymberopoulos, D. (2022). A survey on security threats and countermeasures in internet of medical things (IoMT). *Transactions on Emerging Telecommunications Technologies*, 33(6), e4049.

[63] Zhang, H., Li, J., Wen, B., Xun, Y., & Liu, J. (2018). Connecting intelligent things in smart hospitals using NB-IoT. *IEEE Internet of Things Journal*, 5(3), 1550–1560.

[64] Liu, C., Chen, F., Zhao, C., Wang, T., Zhang, C., & Zhang, Z. (2018). IPv6-based archi-tecture of community medical internet of things. *IEEE Access*, 6, 7897–7910.

[65] Ed-daoudy, A., & Maalmi, K. (2019). A new internet of things architecture for real-time prediction of various diseases using machine learning on big data environment. *Journal of Big Data*, 6(1), 1–25.

[66] Yacchirema, D. C., Sarabia-Jácome, D., Palau, C. E., & Esteve, M. (2018). A smart system for sleep monitoring by integrating IoT with big data analytics. *IEEE Access*, 6, 35988–36001.

[67] Gaur, A., Scotney, B., Parr, G., & McClean, S. (2015). Smart city architecture and its applications based on IoT. *Procedia Computer Science*, 52, 1089–1094.

[68] Lee, H. Y., Lee, K. H., Lee, K. H., Erdenbayar, U., Hwang, S., Lee, E. Y., . . . & Youk, H. (2023). Internet of medical things-based real-time digital health service for precision medi-cine: Empirical studies using MEDBIZ platform. *Digital Health*, 9, 20552076221149659.

[69] Ayoade, O. B., Oladele, T. O., Imoize, A. L., Awotunde, J. B., Adeloye, A. J., Olorunyomi, S. O., & Idowu, A. O. (2023). Explainable artificial intelligence (XAI) in medical decision systems (MDSSs): Healthcare systems perspective. In *Explainable Artificial Intelligence in Medical Decision Support Systems* (p. 1). London: IET.

[70] Yıldırım, E., Cicioğlu, M., & Çalhan, A. (2023). Fog-cloud architecture-driven inter-net of medical things framework for healthcare monitoring. *Medical & Biological Engineering & Computing*, 1–15.

[71] Dahan, F., Alroobaea, R., Alghamdi, W., Mohammed, M. K., Hajjej, F., & Raahemifar, K. (2023). A smart IoMT based architecture for E-healthcare patient monitoring sys-tem using artificial intelligence algorithms. *Frontiers in Physiology*, 14, 40.

[72] Olugbade, S., Ojo, S., Imoize, A. L., Isabona, J., & Alaba, M. O. (2022). A review of artificial intelligence and machine learning for incident detectors in road transport sys-tems. *Mathematical and Computational Applications*, 27(5), 77.

[73] Khan, S., & Mailewa, A. B. (2023). Discover botnets in IoT sensor networks: A light-weight deep learning framework with hybrid self-organizing maps. *Microprocessors and Microsystems*, 104753.

[74] Pour, M. S., Nader, C., Friday, K., & Bou-Harb, E. (2023). A comprehensive survey of recent internet measurement techniques for cyber security. *Computers & Security*, 103123.

[75] Kumar, J. S., & Patel, D. R. (2014). A survey on internet of things: Security and privacy issues. *International Journal of Computer Applications*, 90(11).

[76] Sey, D. (2018). A survey on authentication methods for the internet of things. *PeerJ Preprints*, 6, e26474v2.

[77] Mitchell, R., & Chen, I. R. (2014). A survey of intrusion detection techniques for cyber-physical systems. *ACM Computing Surveys (CSUR)*, 46(4), 1–29.

[78] Ayo, F. E., Folorunso, S. O., Abayomi-Alli, A. A., Adekunle, A. O., & Awotunde, J. B. (2020). Network intrusion detection based on deep learning model optimized with rule-based hybrid feature selection. *Information Security Journal: A Global Perspective*, 29(6), 267–283.

[79] Challoner, A., & Popescu, G. H. (2019). Intelligent sensing technology, smart health-
      care services, and internet of medical things-based diagnosis. *American Journal of
      Medical Research*, 6(1), 13–18.
[80] Kuila, S., Dhanda, N., Joardar, S., Neogy, S., & Kuila, J. (2019). A generic survey on
      medical big data analysis using internet of things. In *First International Conference on
      Artificial Intelligence and Cognitive Computing: AICC 2018* (pp. 265–276). Singapore:
      Springer.
[81] Kang, S., Baek, H., Jung, E., Hwang, H., & Yoo, S. (2019). Survey on the demand for
      adoption of internet of things (IoT)-based services in hospitals: Investigation of nurses'
      perception in a tertiary university hospital. *Applied Nursing Research*, 47, 18–23.
[82] Adhikary, T., Jana, A. D., Chakrabarty, A., & Jana, S. K. (2020). The internet of things
      (IoT) augmentation in healthcare: An application analytics. In *ICICCT 2019–System
      Reliability, Quality Control, Safety, Maintenance and Management: Applications
      to Electrical, Electronics and Computer Science and Engineering* (pp. 576–583).
      Singapore: Springer.
[83] Clark, G. W., Doran, M. V., & Andel, T. R. (2017, March). Cybersecurity issues in
      robotics. In *2017 IEEE Conference on Cognitive and Computational Aspects of
      Situation Management (CogSIMA)* (pp. 1–5). Savannah, GA: IEEE.
[84] Peterson, A. (2013). Yes, terrorists could have hacked Dick Cheney's heart. *Washington
      Post*, 21(10), 2013.
[85] Kelly, K. (2012). Better than human: Why robots will—and must—take our jobs. *Wired*.
      www. wired. com/2012/12/ff-robots-will-take-our-jobs/(Accessed 4 August 2014).
[86] Birkmeyer, J. D., Stukel, T. A., Siewers, A. E., Goodney, P. P., Wennberg, D. E., &
      Lucas, F. L. (2003). Surgeon volume and operative mortality in the United States. *New
      England Journal of Medicine*, 349(22), 2117–2127.
[87] Ayala, L., & Ayala, L. (2016). Active medical device cyber-attacks. In *Cybersecurity
      for Hospitals and Healthcare Facilities: A Guide to Detection and Prevention* (pp.
      19–37). Berkeley, CA: Apress.
[88] Sensmeier, J. (2017). Harnessing the power of artificial intelligence. *Nursing
      Management*, 48(11), 14–19.
[89] Hassanalieragh, M., Page, A., Soyata, T., Sharma, G., Aktas, M., Mateos, G., . . . &
      Andreescu, S. (2015, June). Health monitoring and management using Internet-of-Things
      (IoT) sensing with cloud-based processing: Opportunities and challenges. In *2015 IEEE
      International Conference on Services Computing* (pp. 285–292). New York: IEEE.
[90] Hireche, R., Mansouri, H., & Pathan, A. S. K. (2022). Security and privacy manage-
      ment in internet of medical things (IoMT): A synthesis. *Journal of Cybersecurity and
      Privacy*, 2(3), 640–661.
[91] Tabrizchi, H., & Kuchaki Rafsanjani, M. (2020). A survey on security challenges
      in cloud computing: Issues, threats, and solutions. *The Journal of Supercomputing*,
      76(12), 9493–9532.
[92] Hasan, M. K., Ghazal, T. M., Saeed, R. A., Pandey, B., Gohel, H., Eshmawi, A. A., . . . &
      Alkhassawneh, H. M. (2022). A review on security threats, vulnerabilities, and counter
      measures of 5G enabled internet-of-medical-things. *IET Communications*, 16(5), 421–432.
[93] Tang, J., Qin, T., Kong, D., Zhou, Z., Li, X., Wu, Y., & Gu, J. (2023). Anomaly detection
      in social-aware IoT networks. *IEEE Transactions on Network and Service Management*.
      New Jersey, USA: IEEE.
[94] Nehinbe, J. O., Benson, J. A., & Chibuzor, L. (2023). The classification of the investiga-
      tions and punishment for crime syndicates that relate to intrusions against IoT-based
      healthcare systems. In *Blockchain Technology Solutions for the Security of IoT-Based
      Healthcare Systems* (pp. 113–131). United Kingdom: Academic Press.

[95] Ragothaman, K., Wang, Y., Rimal, B., & Lawrence, M. (2023). Access control for IoT: A survey of existing research, dynamic policies and future directions. *Sensors*, 23(4), 1805.

[96] Issa, W., Moustafa, N., Turnbull, B., Sohrabi, N., & Tari, Z. (2023). Blockchain-based federated learning for securing internet of things: A comprehensive survey. *ACM Computing Surveys*, 55(9), 1–43.

[97] Kaushik, K., Singh, V., & Manikandan, V. P. (2023, January). A novel approach for an automated advanced MITM attack on IoT networks. In *Advancements in Interdisciplinary Research: First International Conference, AIR 2022, Prayagraj, India, May 6–7, 2022, Revised Selected Papers* (pp. 60–71). Cham: Springer Nature Switzerland.

[98] Singh, U. K., Sharma, A., Singh, S. K., Tomar, P. S., Dixit, K., & Upreti, K. (2023). Security and privacy aspect of cyber physical systems. In *Cyber Physical Systems* (pp. 141–164). Chapman and Hall/CRC.

[99] Deogirikar, J., & Vidhate, A. (2017, February). Security attacks in IoT: A survey. In *2017 International Conference on I-SMAC (IoT in Social, Mobile, Analytics and Cloud)(I-SMAC)* (pp. 32–37). Palladam: IEEE.

[100] Ghazal, T. M. (2022). Data Fusion-based machine learning architecture for intrusion detection. *Computers, Materials & Continua*, 70(2), 3399–3413.

[101] Rasool, R. U., Ahmad, H. F., Rafique, W., Qayyum, A., & Qadir, J. (2022). Security and privacy of internet of medical things: A contemporary review in the age of surveillance, botnets, and adversarial ML. *Journal of Network and Computer Applications*, 103332.

[102] Munir, K., & Mohammed, L. A. (2018). Biometric smartcard authentication for fog computing. *International Journal of Network Security & Its Applications (IJNSA)*, 10.

[103] Dwivedi, A. D., Singh, R., Ghosh, U., Mukkamala, R. R., Tolba, A., & Said, O. (2021). Privacy preserving authentication system based on non-interactive zero knowledge proof suitable for internet of things. *Journal of Ambient Intelligence and Humanized Computing*, 1–11.

[104] Stojmenovic, I., & Wen, S. (2014, September). The fog computing paradigm: Scenarios and security issues. In *2014 Federated Conference on Computer Science and Information Systems* (pp. 1–8). Warsaw: IEEE.

[105] Alrawais, A., Alhothaily, A., Hu, C., & Cheng, X. (2017). Fog computing for the internet of things: Security and privacy issues. *IEEE Internet Computing*, 21(2), 34–42.

[106] Sun, Y., Lo, F. P. W., & Lo, B. (2019). Security and privacy for the internet of medical things enabled healthcare systems: A survey. *IEEE Access*, 7, 183339–183355.

[107] Riya, K. S., Surendran, R., Tavera Romero, C. A., & Sendil, M. S. (2023). Encryption with user authentication model for internet of medical things environment. *Intelligent Automation & Soft Computing*, 35(1).

[108] Wang, J., & Li, X. (2023). Secure medical data collection in the internet of medical things based on local differential privacy. *Electronics*, 12(2), 307.

[109] Rajasekaran, S. B. (2023). AI and cybersecurity-how AI augments cybersecurity posture of an enterprise. *International Journal of Intelligent Systems and Applications in Engineering*, 11(1), 179–182.

[110] Jeyaselvi, M., Sathya, M., Suchitra, S., Jafar Ali Ibrahim, S., & Kalyan Chakravarthy, N. S. (2022). SVM-Based cloning and jamming attack detection in IoT sensor networks. In *Advances in Information Communication Technology and Computing: Proceedings of AICTC 2021* (pp. 461–471). Singapore: Springer Nature.

[111] Trnka, M., Abdelfattah, A. S., Shrestha, A., Coffey, M., & Cerny, T. (2022). Systematic review of authentication and authorization advancements for the internet of things. *Sensors*, 22(4), 1361.

[112] Makhdoom, I., Abolhasan, M., Lipman, J., Liu, R. P., & Ni, W. (2018). Anatomy of threats to the internet of things. *IEEE Communications Surveys & Tutorials*, 21(2), 1636–1675.

[113] Awotunde, J. B., Chakraborty, C., & Folorunso, S. O. (2022). A secured smart healthcare monitoring systems using blockchain technology. In *Intelligent Internet of Things for Healthcare and Industry* (pp. 127–143). Cham: Springer International Publishing.

[114] Sundas, A., Badotra, S., Bharany, S., Almogren, A., Tag-ElDin, E. M., & Rehman, A. U. (2022). HealthGuard: An intelligent healthcare system security framework based on machine learning. *Sustainability*, 14(19), 11934.

[115] Anusha, R., Vijayashree, J., Jayashree, J., & Yousuff, M. (2023). CPS support IoMT cyber attacks, security and privacy issues and solutions. In *Cyber-Physical Systems for Industrial Transformation* (pp. 157–175). CRC Press.

[116] Nozari, H., Tavakkoli-Moghaddam, R., Ghahremani-Nahr, J., & Najafi, E. (2023). A conceptual framework for Artificial Intelligence of Medical Things (AIoMT). In *Computational Intelligence for Medical Internet of Things (MIoT) Applications* (pp. 175–189). United Kingdom: Academic Press.

[117] Unal, D., Bennbaia, S., & Catak, F. O. (2022). Machine learning for the security of healthcare systems based on internet of things and edge computing. In *Cybersecurity and Cognitive Science* (pp. 299–320). United Kingdom: Academic Press.

[118] Kumbhare, A., & Thakur, P. K. (2022). Security and privacy of biomedical data in IoMT. In *Cognitive Computing for Internet of Medical Things* (pp. 77–104). FL, USA: Chapman and Hall/CRC.

[119] Singh, D., Maurya, A. K., Dewang, R. K., & Keshari, N. (2022). A review on internet of multimedia things (IoMT) routing protocols and quality of service. *Internet of Multimedia Things (IoMT)*, 1–29.

[120] Raymond, D. R., & Midkiff, S. F. (2008). Denial-of-service in wireless sensor networks: Attacks and defenses. *IEEE Pervasive Computing*, 7(1), 74–81.

[121] Butun, I., Österberg, P., & Song, H. (2019). Security of the internet of things: Vulnerabilities, attacks, and countermeasures. *IEEE Communications Surveys & Tutorials*, 22(1), 616–644.

[122] Madhu, B., Chari, M. V. G., Vankdothu, R., Silivery, A. K., & Aerranagula, V. (2023). Intrusion detection models for IoT networks via deep learning approaches. *Measurement: Sensors*, 25, 100641.

[123] Awotunde, J. B., Chakraborty, C., & Folorunso, S. O. (2022). A secured transaction based on blockchain architecture in mobile banking platform. *International Journal of Internet Technology and Secured Transactions*, 12(4), 287–303.

[124] Joshi, A. M., Jain, P., & Mohanty, S. P. (2020, July). Secure-iGLU: A secure device for noninvasive glucose measurement and automatic insulin delivery in iomt framework. In *2020 IEEE Computer Society annual symposium on VLSI (ISVLSI)* (pp. 440–445). Limassol: IEEE.

[125] Dar, A. A., Alam, M. Z., Ahmad, A., Reegu, F. A., & Rahin, S. A. (2022). Blockchain framework for secure COVID-19 pandemic data handling and protection. *Computational Intelligence & Neuroscience*. Volume 2022, Article ID 7025485, 11 pages. https://doi.org/10.1155/2022/7025485

[126] Koutras, D., Stergiopoulos, G., Dasaklis, T., Kotzanikolaou, P., Glynos, D., & Douligeris, C. (2020). Security in IoMT communications: A survey. *Sensors*, 20(17), 4828.

[127] Alsubaei, F., Abuhussein, A., & Shiva, S. (2019). A framework for ranking IoMT solutions based on measuring security and privacy. In *Proceedings of the Future Technologies Conference (FTC) 2018: Volume 1* (pp. 205–224). Springer Nature Switzerland AG: Springer International Publishing.

[128] Fiaidhi, J., & Mohammed, S. (2019). Security and vulnerability of extreme automation systems: The IoMT and IoA case studies. *IT Professional*, 21(4), 48–55.

[129] Sutton, E., Martin, G., Eborall, H., & Tarrant, C. (2023). Undertaking risk and relational work to manage vulnerability: Acute medical patients' involvement in patient safety in the NHS. *Social Science & Medicine*, 115729.

[130] Attaran, M. (2022). Blockchain technology in healthcare: Challenges and opportunities. *International Journal of Healthcare Management*, 15(1), 70–83.

[131] Khezr, S., Moniruzzaman, M., Yassine, A., & Benlamri, R. (2019). Blockchain technology in healthcare: A comprehensive review and directions for future research. *Applied Sciences*, 9(9), 1736.

[132] Huang, X., & Nazir, S. (2020). Evaluating security of internet of medical things using the analytic network process method. *Security and Communication Networks*, 2020, 1–14.

[133] Atamli, A. W., & Martin, A. (2014, September). Threat-based security analysis for the internet of things. In *2014 International Workshop on Secure Internet of Things* (pp. 35–43). Wroclaw: IEEE.

[134] Alsubaei, F., Abuhussein, A., Shandilya, V., & Shiva, S. (2019). IoMT-SAF: Internet of medical things security assessment framework. *Internet of Things*, 8, 100123.

[135] Hatzivasilis, G., Soultatos, O., Ioannidis, S., Verikoukis, C., Demetriou, G., & Tsatsoulis, C. (2019, May). Review of security and privacy for the internet of medical things (IoMT). In *2019 15th International Conference on Distributed Computing in Sensor Systems (DCOSS)* (pp. 457–464). Santorini: IEEE.

[136] Guan, Z., Lv, Z., Du, X., Wu, L., & Guizani, M. (2019). Achieving data utility-privacy tradeoff in internet of medical things: A machine learning approach. *Future Generation Computer Systems*, 98, 60–68.

[137] Treacy, C., Loane, J., & McCaffery, F. (2020). A developer driven framework for security and privacy in the internet of medical things. In *Systems, Software and Services Process Improvement: 27th European Conference, EuroSPI 2020, Düsseldorf, Germany, September 9–11, 2020, Proceedings 27* (pp. 107–119). Springer Nature Switzerland AG: Springer International Publishing.

[138] Sadeghi, A. R., Wachsmann, C., & Waidner, M. (2015, June). Security and privacy challenges in industrial internet of things. In *Proceedings of the 52nd Annual Design Automation Conference* (pp. 1–6). New York: ACM.

[139] Sun, W., Cai, Z., Li, Y., Liu, F., Fang, S., & Wang, G. (2018). Security and privacy in the medical internet of things: A review. *Security and Communication Networks*, 2018, 1–9.

[140] Sagay, A., & Jahankhani, H. (2020). Consumer awareness on security and privacy threat of medical devices. In *Cyber Defence in the Age of AI, Smart Societies and Augmented Humanity* (pp. 95–116). Cham: Springer.

[141] Wang, X., Wang, L., Li, Y., & Gai, K. (2018). Privacy-aware efficient fine-grained data access control in internet of medical things based fog computing. *IEEE Access*, 6, 47657–47665.

[142] Aftab, M. U., Qin, Z., Hussain, K., Jamali, Z., Son, N. T., Van Nam, N., & Van Dinh, T. (2019, September). Negative authorization by implementing negative attributes in attribute-based access control model for internet of medical things. In *2019 15th International Conference on Semantics, Knowledge and Grids (SKG)* (pp. 167–174). Guangzhou: IEEE.

[143] Shanmugam, B., & Azam, S. (2023). Risk assessment of heterogeneous IoMT devices: A review. *Technologies*, 11(1), 31.

[144] Kamalov, F., Pourghebleh, B., Gheisari, M., Liu, Y., & Moussa, S. (2023). Internet of medical things privacy and security: Challenges, solutions, and future trends from a new perspective. *Sustainability*, 15(4), 3317.

[145] Parrend, P., Mazzucotelli, T., Colin, F., Collet, P., & Mandel, J. L. (2018). Cerberus, an access control scheme for enforcing least privilege in patient cohort study platforms: A comprehensive access control scheme applied to the GENIDA project-study of genetic forms of intellectual disabilities and autism spectrum disorders. *Journal of Medical Systems*, 42, 1–19.

[146] Yang, Y., Zheng, X., Guo, W., Liu, X., & Chang, V. (2019). Privacy-preserving smart IoT-based healthcare big data storage and self-adaptive access control system. *Information Sciences*, 479, 567–592.

[147] Zhang, Y., Zheng, D., & Deng, R. H. (2018). Security and privacy in smart health: Efficient policy-hiding attribute-based access control. *IEEE Internet of Things Journal*, 5(3), 2130–2145.

[148] Luo, E., Bhuiyan, M. Z. A., Wang, G., Rahman, M. A., Wu, J., & Atiquzzaman, M. (2018). Privacyprotector: Privacy-protected patient data collection in IoT-based healthcare systems. *IEEE Communications Magazine*, 56(2), 163–168.

[149] Hasan, M. K., Ahmed, M. M., Musa, S. S., Islam, S., Abdullah, S. N. H. S., Hossain, E., . . . & Vo, N. (2021). An improved dynamic thermal current rating model for PMU-based wide area measurement framework for reliability analysis utilizing sensor cloud system. *IEEE Access*, 9, 14446–14458.

[150] Chakraborty, C., Othman, S. B., Almalki, F. A., & Sakli, H. (2023). FC-SEEDA: Fog computing-based secure and energy efficient data aggregation scheme for internet of healthcare things. *Neural Computing and Applications*, 1–17.

[151] Nyangaresi, V. O. (2023). Privacy preserving three-factor authentication protocol for secure message forwarding in wireless body area networks. *Ad Hoc Networks*, 103117.

[152] Aghili, S. F., Mala, H., Shojafar, M., & Peris-Lopez, P. (2019). LACO: Lightweight three-factor authentication, access control and ownership transfer scheme for e-health systems in IoT. *Future Generation Computer Systems*, 96, 410–424.

[153] Moosavi, S. R., Gia, T. N., Nigussie, E., Rahmani, A. M., Virtanen, S., Tenhunen, H., & Isoaho, J. (2016). End-to-end security scheme for mobility enabled healthcare internet of things. *Future Generation Computer Systems*, 64, 108–124.

[154] Moosavi, S. R., Gia, T. N., Nigussie, E., Rahmani, A. M., Virtanen, S., Tenhunen, H., & Isoaho, J. (2015, October). Session resumption-based end-to-end security for healthcare Internet-of-Things. In *2015 IEEE International Conference on Computer and Information Technology; Ubiquitous Computing and Communications; Dependable, Autonomic and Secure Computing; Pervasive Intelligence and Computing* (pp. 581–588). Liverpool: IEEE.

[155] Zhang, Y., Deng, R. H., Han, G., & Zheng, D. (2018). Secure smart health with privacy-aware aggregate authentication and access control in internet of things. *Journal of Network and Computer Applications*, 123, 89–100.

[156] Cheng, X., Zhang, Z., Chen, F., Zhao, C., Wang, T., Sun, H., & Huang, C. (2019). Secure identity authentication of community medical internet of things. *IEEE Access*, 7, 115966–115977.

[157] Dinarvand, N., & Barati, H. (2019). An efficient and secure RFID authentication protocol using elliptic curve cryptography. *Wireless Networks*, 25(1), 415–428.

[158] Adeniyi, A. E., Abiodun, K. M., Awotunde, J. B., Olagunju, M., Ojo, O. S., & Edet, N. P. (2023). Implementation of a block cipher algorithm for medical information security on cloud environment: Using modified advanced encryption standard approach. *Multimedia Tools and Applications*, 1–15.

[159] Oladipupo, E. T., Abikoye, O. C., Imoize, A. L., Awotunde, J. B., Chang, T. Y., Lee, C. C., & Do, D. T. (2023). An efficient authenticated elliptic curve cryptography scheme for multicore wireless sensor networks. *IEEE Access*, 11, 1306–1323.

[160] Attir, A., Naït-Abdesselam, F., & Faraoun, K. M. (2023). Lightweight anonymous and mutual authentication scheme for WBAN. *Computer Networks*, 109625.

[161] Sankaran, K. S., & Kim, B. H. (2023). Deep learning based energy efficient optimal RMC-CNN model for secured data transmission and anomaly detection in industrial IOT. *Sustainable Energy Technologies and Assessments*, 56, 102983.

[162] Azath, H., Gokulraj, J., Surendiran, J., Geetha, D., & Babu, T. G. (2023, January). Security for health information by elliptical curve Diffie-Hellman and improve energy efficiency in WBAN. In *AIP Conference Proceedings* (Vol. 2523, No. 1, p. 020075). Chennai: AIP Publishing LLC.

[163] Costan, V., Lebedev, I. A., & Devadas, S. (2016, August). Sanctum: Minimal hardware extensions for strong software isolation. In *USENIX Security Symposium* (pp. 857–874). Vancouver, BC.

[164] Brasser, F., El Mahjoub, B., Sadeghi, A. R., Wachsmann, C., & Koeberl, P. (2015, June). TyTAN: Tiny trust anchor for tiny devices. In *Proceedings of the 52nd Annual Design Automation Conference* (pp. 1–6).

[165] Koeberl, P., Schulz, S., Sadeghi, A. R., & Varadharajan, V. (2014, April). TrustLite: A security architecture for tiny embedded devices. In *Proceedings of the Ninth European Conference on Computer Systems* (pp. 1–14).

[166] Riya, K. S., Sudhakar, J., Ravichandran, M., Tamilselvi, M., & Sajiv, G. (2022, July). A novel symmetric key compact to reliable connection between sensor nodes using exploitable features of ECG. In *2022 International Conference on Innovative Computing, Intelligent Communication and Smart Electrical Systems (ICSES)* (pp. 1–12). Chennai: IEEE.

[167] Altop, D. K., Levi, A., & Tuzcu, V. (2017). Deriving cryptographic keys from physiological signals. *Pervasive and Mobile Computing*, 39, 65–79.

[168] Pirbhulal, S., Zhang, H., Wu, W., Mukhopadhyay, S. C., & Zhang, Y. T. (2018). Heartbeats based biometric random binary sequences generation to secure wireless body sensor networks. *IEEE Transactions on Biomedical Engineering*, 65(12), 2751–2759.

[169] Dessouky, G., Zeitouni, S., Nyman, T., Paverd, A., Davi, L., Koeberl, P., . . . & Sadeghi, A. R. (2017, June). Lo-fat: Low-overhead control flow attestation in hardware. In *Proceedings of the 54th Annual Design Automation Conference 2017* (pp. 1–6). New York: ACM.

[170] Abera, T., Asokan, N., Davi, L., Ekberg, J. E., Nyman, T., Paverd, A., . . . & Tsudik, G. (2016, October). C-FLAT: Control-flow attestation for embedded systems software. In *Proceedings of the 2016 ACM SIGSAC Conference on Computer and Communications Security* (pp. 743–754). New York: USA.

[171] Christoulakis, N., Christou, G., Athanasopoulos, E., & Ioannidis, S. (2016, March). HCFI: Hardware-enforced control-flow integrity. In *Proceedings of the Sixth ACM Conference on Data and Application Security and Privacy* (pp. 38–49). New York: ACM.

[172] McKeen, F., Alexandrovich, I., Berenzon, A., Rozas, C. V., Shafi, H., Shanbhogue, V., & Savagaonkar, U. R. (2013). Innovative instructions and software model for isolated execution. *Hasp@ isca*, 10(1).

[173] Ghazal, T. M., Afifi, M. A. M., & Kalra, D. (2020). Security vulnerabilities, attacks, threats and the proposed countermeasures for the internet of things applications. *Solid State Technology*, 63(1s).

[174] Adeniyi, E. A., Ogundokun, R. O., Misra, S., Awotunde, J. B., & Abiodun, K. M. (2022). Enhanced security and privacy issue in multi-tenant environment of green computing using blockchain technology. In *Blockchain Applications in the Smart Era* (pp. 65–83). Cham: Springer International Publishing.

[175] Awotunde, J. B., Misra, S., & Pham, Q. T. (2022, November). A secure framework for internet of medical things security based system using lightweight cryptography enabled blockchain. In *Future Data and Security Engineering. Big Data, Security and Privacy, Smart City and Industry 4.0 Applications: 9th International Conference, FDSE 2022, Ho Chi Minh City, Vietnam, November 23–25, 2022, Proceedings* (pp. 258–272). Singapore: Springer Nature Singapore.

[176] Ogundokun, R. O., Arowolo, M. O., Misra, S., & Awotunde, J. B. (2022). Machine learning, IoT, and blockchain integration for improving process management application security. In *Blockchain Applications in the Smart Era* (pp. 237–252). Cham: Springer International Publishing.

[177] Abdulraheem, M., Awotunde, J. B., Jimoh, R. G., & Oladipo, I. D. (2021). An efficient lightweight cryptographic algorithm for IoT security. In *Information and Communication Technology and Applications: Third International Conference, ICTA 2020, Minna, Nigeria, November 24–27, 2020, Revised Selected Papers 3* (pp. 444–456). Springer Nature, Switzerland AG: Springer International Publishing.

[178] Ndzimakhwe, M., Telukdarie, A., Munien, I., Vermeulen, A., Chude-Okonkwo, U. K., & Philbin, S. P. (2023). A framework for user-focused electronic health record system leveraging hyperledger fabric. *Information*, 14(1), 51.

[179] AbdulRaheem, M., Awotunde, J. B., Chakraborty, C., Adeniyi, E. A., Oladipo, I. D., & Bhoi, A. K. (2023). Security and privacy concerns in smart healthcare system. In *Implementation of Smart Healthcare Systems using AI, IoT, and Blockchain* (pp. 243–273). Academic Press.

[180] Qu, Z., Zhang, Z., & Zheng, M. (2022). A quantum blockchain-enabled framework for secure private electronic medical records in internet of medical things. *Information Sciences*, 612, 942–958.

[181] Miller, D. (2018). Blockchain and the internet of things in the industrial sector. *IT Professional*, 20(3), 15–18.

[182] Dobrovnik, M., Herold, D. M., Fürst, E., & Kummer, S. (2018). Blockchain for and in logistics: What to adopt and where to start. *Logistics*, 2(3), 18.

[183] Sharma, A., Tomar, R., Chilamkurti, N., & Kim, B. G. (2020). Blockchain based smart contracts for internet of medical things in e-healthcare. *Electronics*, 9(10), 1609.

[184] Kumar, R. L., Wang, Y., Poongodi, T., & Imoize, A. L. (Eds.). (2021). *Internet of Things, Artificial Intelligence and Blockchain Technology*. Cham: Springer.

[185] Wang, B., Sun, J., He, Y., Pang, D., & Lu, N. (2018). Large-scale election based on blockchain. *Procedia Computer Science*, 129, 234–237.

[186] Gupta, K., Sharma, D. K., Gupta, K. D., & Kumar, A. (2022). A tree classifier based network intrusion detection model for internet of medical things. *Computers and Electrical Engineering*, 102, 108158.

[187] Sharma, M., Pant, S., Kumar Sharma, D., Datta Gupta, K., Vashishth, V., & Chhabra, A. (2021). Enabling security for the industrial internet of things using deep learning, blockchain, and coalitions. *Transactions on Emerging Telecommunications Technologies*, 32(7), e4137.

[188] Zachos, G., Essop, I., Mantas, G., Porfyrakis, K., Ribeiro, J. C., & Rodriguez, J. (2021). An anomaly-based intrusion detection system for internet of medical things networks. *Electronics*, 10(21), 2562.

[189] Rani, A. A. V., & Baburaj, E. (2019). Secure and intelligent architecture for cloud-based healthcare applications in wireless body sensor networks. *International Journal of Biomedical Engineering and Technology*, 29(2), 186–199.

[190] Chakraborty, S., Aich, S., & Kim, H. C. (2019, February). A secure healthcare system design framework using blockchain technology. In *2019 21st International Conference on Advanced Communication Technology (ICACT)* (pp. 260–264). Pyeongchang: IEEE.

[191] Hady, A. A., Ghubaish, A., Salman, T., Unal, D., & Jain, R. (2020). Intrusion detection system for healthcare systems using medical and network data: A comparison study. *IEEE Access*, 8, 106576–106584.

[192] Rao, B. B., & Swathi, K. (2017). Fast KNN classifiers for network intrusion detection system. *Indian Journal of Science and Technology*, 10(14), 1–10.

[193] Shapoorifard, H., & Shamsinejad, P. (2017). Intrusion detection using a novel hybrid method incorporating an improved KNN. *International Journal of Computers and Applications*, 173(1), 5–9.

[194] Gupta, R. K., Chawla, V., Pateriya, R. K., Shukla, P. K., Mahfoudh, S., & Shah, S. B. H. (2023). Improving collaborative intrusion detection system using blockchain and pluggable authentication modules for sustainable smart city. *Sustainability*, 15(3), 2133.

[195] Shamim, N., Asim, M., Baker, T., & Awad, A. I. (2023). Efficient approach for anomaly detection in IoT using system calls. *Sensors*, 23(2), 652.

[196] Dina, A. S., Siddique, A. B., & Manivannan, D. (2023). A deep learning approach for intrusion detection in internet of things using focal loss function. *Internet of Things*, 100699.

[197] Kakandwar, S., Bhushan, B., & Kumar, A. (2023). Integrated machine learning techniques for preserving privacy in internet of things (IoT) systems. In *Blockchain Technology Solutions for the Security of IoT-Based Healthcare Systems* (pp. 45–75). USA: Elsevier Publisher.

[198] Arshad, J., Azad, M. A., Amad, R., Salah, K., Alazab, M., & Iqbal, R. (2020). A review of performance, energy and privacy of intrusion detection systems for IoT. *Electronics*, 9(4), 629.

[199] Rashid, M. M., Khan, S. U., Eusufzai, F., Redwan, M., Sabuj, S. R., & Elsharief, M. (2023). A federated learning-based approach for improving intrusion detection in industrial internet of things networks. *Network*, 3(1), 158–179.

[200] Kalutharage, C. S., Liu, X., Chrysoulas, C., Pitropakis, N., & Papadopoulos, P. (2023). Explainable AI-based DDOS attack identification method for IoT networks. *Computers*, 12(2), 32.

[201] Kaur, J., & Singh, G. (2023). A blockchain-based machine learning intrusion detection system for internet of things. In *Principles and Practice of Blockchains* (pp. 119–134). Cham: Springer.

[202] Panigrahi, R., Borah, S., Pramanik, M., Bhoi, A. K., Barsocchi, P., Nayak, S. R., & Alnumay, W. (2022). Intrusion detection in cyber-physical environment using hybrid Naïve Bayes—Decision table and multi-objective evolutionary feature selection. *Computer Communications*, 188, 133–144.

6 AIoMT Concerns

Abasiama Godwin Akpan, Flavious
Bobuin Nkubli, Victoria Nnaemeka
Ezeano, and Anayo Christian Okwor

6.1 INTRODUCTION

A few years ago, the healthcare ecosystem had witnessed improvements in the areas of emerging technologies and treatment methods [1–3]. Medical services can be improved by incorporating key technologies such as IoT and AI. This improvement offers different opportunities in healthcare delivery. The Internet of Things (IoT) has brought a new wave in the healthcare industry through the connectivity of medical devices [4–6]. These devices gather very useful data to offer further insights into warning signs for doctors or caregivers to deliver remote medical care to patients. AIoMT assists doctors and patients in managing treatments with increased accuracy at reduced costs. Doctors can amass patient records in real-time without visiting the patient [7, 8]. In view of this, AIoMT assists in scrutinizing healthcare information promptly by initiating procedural functions promptly and correctly. Health practitioners deploy smart platforms for continuous monitoring of ailment situations. On the other hand, sick persons can take delivery of medical guidance from medical consultants via automated smart clinical equipment [9, 10]. Artificial intelligence-enabled platforms can intelligently categorize medical data through a flow process from AIoMT sensors to provide the required information related to patients to doctors in a timely manner. The integration of medical devices and requests that are connected to the health care providers via the *super highway (internet)* is branded as *Artificial intelligence of Medical Things (AIoMT)*. The Artificial Intelligence of Medical Things (AIoMT) comprises interconnected medical devices for healthcare monitoring. It ties patients with clinicians through medical devices, allowing remote access to gather, process, and convey medical data over a secured network. AIoMT can lessen hospital visits by linking patients and doctors, permitting the shift of medical data over the Internet. Data gathered from patients, branded as *Electronic Health Record (EHR)*, is available in digital layout. EHRs require a secured structure during transmission and immediately after storage. The AIoMT Healthcare system is presented in Figure 6.1.

The AIoMT segment covers *wearables devices, Implantable devices, Ambient devices, and Stationary devices*. The *wearable devices*—includes ECG, patches for monitoring, BioPatch to check patient's state, insulin pumps, blood monitors, and smart wristbands [11]. *Implantable devices*—includes pacemakers, camera capsules, and cardioverter defibrillators. *Ambient devices*—sensors that change patient's room condition, sensors for motion, sensors for doors, room temperatures, sensors for

DOI: 10.1201/9781003370321-6

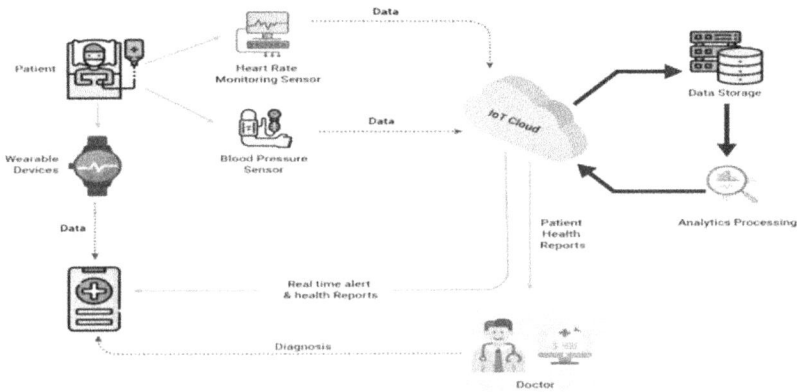

FIGURE 6.1 Adapted AIoMT healthcare system [7].

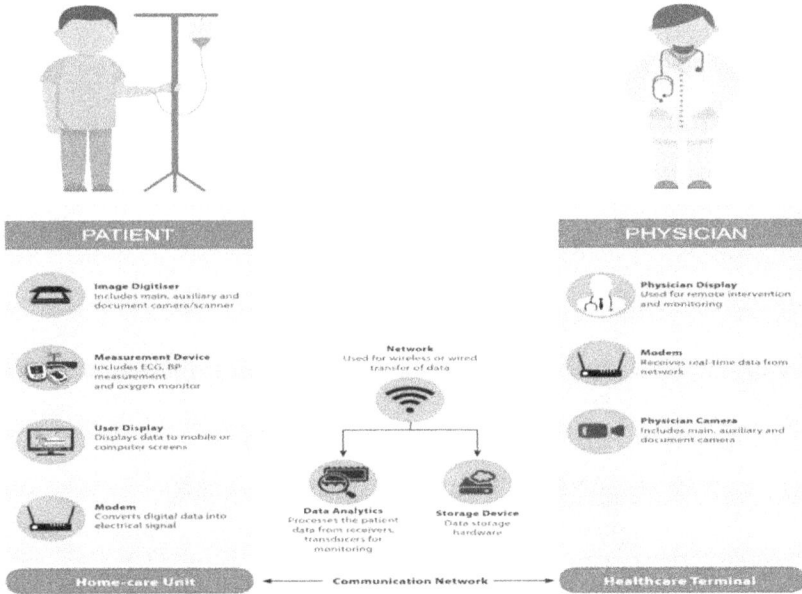

FIGURE 6.2 Adapted AIoMT components [7].

vibration, and sensors for pressure. *Stationary devices*—devices for monitoring the home and devices for surgery.

The expansion of the Internet and the craving for distributed intelligence in a sensor-based network have ignited several issues in managing huge health data collected by diverse healthcare monitoring systems [1–3]. *The artificial intelligence of medical things (AIoMT)* is a potential improvement of an Internet of Medical Things (IoMT) that merges medical sensors and the Internet of Things [4–6]. Figure 6.2 presents the adapted AIoMT components in a typical healthcare ecosystem.

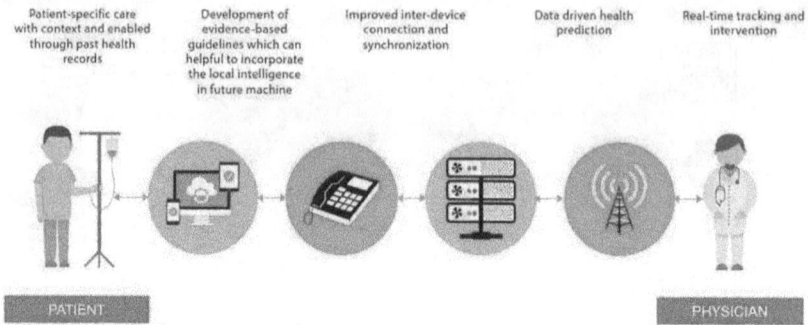

FIGURE 6.3   AIoMT impact [7].

AIoMT know-how is important in recommending possible treatments and thwarting extra harm through remote monitoring by clinicians and self-monitoring [7, 8]. AIoMT is mainly functional for ailment detection [4, 9, 10]. Figure 6.3 shows the impact of AIoMT in the healthcare ecosystem.

6.1.1   KEY CONTRIBUTION OF THE CHAPTER

The following are the significant contributions of this chapter:

   i. Integration of enhanced AIoMT technologies
  ii. Provision of AI methods in healthcare applications
 iii. Highlight of AI measurement of trustworthiness
 iv. Introduction of key security issues in AIoMT-layered architecture
  v. Examination of authentication protocols and detection mechanisms for AIoMT networks

6.1.2   CHAPTER ORGANIZATION

This chapter is presented in sections as follows: Section 6.1 explains the Artificial intelligence of medical things (AIoMT). Section 6.2 reviews AI concepts in the healthcare ecosystem. Section 6.3 explains the concept of IoT and AIoMT. Section 6.4 presents security issues in AIoMT-layered architecture. Section 6.5 presents emerging AIoMT technologies and their applications. Section 6.6 discusses AIoMT concerns. Section 6.7 presents authentication protocols in AIoMT. Section 6.8 explains detection mechanisms for AIoMTs networks. Section 6.9 dwells on AIoMT concerns, and Section 6.10 summarizes the entire study.

6.2   AI IN HEALTHCARE ECOSYSTEM

AI is a smart tool applying various methods to harness vast data for real-time computation and superior forecast. In healthcare, discovering innovative medicines requires numerous clinical trials and approvals by authorities. AI advances precise decisions and aids in hunting for improved medication. ML advancement in AI training pre-existing datasets and improving its decision-making accuracy is a huge gain in healthcare. AI advancement comprises algorithms that build intelligent systems for resourceful tasks routine [12, 13]. The applications of AI in analytic radiographic tasks are experiencing broad valuation [12]. In [14], AI shows remarkable exactness and accuracy in identifying irregularities in imaging and guarantees an enhanced lesion region exposure and classification [15]. AI models in diagnosis and disease treatment are robust [16, 17]. By using AI, detailed outcomes are achieved from Clinical Decision Support System (CDSS). Applying CDSS is extremely efficient in improving the diagnostic processes, reducing the occurrence of idle diagnoses, such as misdiagnosis, and allowing patients timely and appropriate medical treatment [18]. Insider intelligence reported that ML has the latent to produce data-driven clinical decision support (CDS) for clinicians [19]. They asserted their opinion based on the following examples:

  i. Ability to pinpoint treatments for cancer patients by IBM Watson.
  ii. Ease of collection, storage, and access to data through Google Cloud's Healthcare app
  iii. Prediction of outcomes of hospital visitations using the Google Healthcare app
  iv. The application programming interface (API) that helps clinicians makes informed decisions

6.2.1 MEASURES OF AI TRUSTWORTHY IN HEALTHCARE

The field of AI cannot be fully dependable [21]. There are several procedures promoting trusted AI utilization in healthcare as numerated by Refs. [21–25].

  i. *Superiority of information report*: Many health care records need modification through research. Hence, information value and the process of data gathering are significant since it permits the acceptance of the result.
  ii. *Information rationale*: This is the actual understanding of the information which can be validated by leveraging an external source.
  iii. *Regulation*: Various methods to regulate AI subsist. The first stage is making sure AI-defined platforms assemble required rules and conditions, though it is difficult to obtain an entire chain of certifiable conditions that assure AI devices are based on ethics, law, and vigor.

6.2.2 AI METHODS IN HEALTHCARE APPLICATIONS

The ranges of AI methods in medical applications include *ML, DL, and reinforcement learning* as listed by Ref [13]. ML is separated into *supervised learning* and *unsupervised learning*.

TABLE 6.1

AI Algorithms and Its Areas of Usage in Healthcare

S. no.	Citations	AI Algorithms	Usage in Healthcare
1.	[26]	SVM	• Imaging biomarker in neuro-psychiatric
2.	[27]		disorders
			• Human-computer interaction
3.	[28]		• Diagnosing of cancer
4.	[29]		• Alzheimer's detection at early stage
5.	[30]		• Checking of heart disease
6.	[31, 32]		• Forecasting of surgical site disease
7.	[33, 34] [35]		• Checking of glucose
8.	[36]		• Surgical treatment
9.	[37]		• Supervision of epidemic resources
10.			• Supervising healthcare system
11.	[38–40]	NN	• Analysis of cancer ailment
12.	[41]		• Classifying Parkinson's illness
13.	[30]		• Medical imaging on cardiac diseases
14.	[42, 43]		• Alzheimer's detection at early stage
15.	[44]		• Usage of medical sensors
16.	[45, 46]		• Forecasting of diabetes patients
17.	[44]		• Human-computer interaction
18.	[43, 44]		• Supervision of epidemic resources•
19.	[43]		Pattern recognition of human organs
20.	[40]	NB	• Forecasting of ailment
21.	[42, 32]		• Clinical analysis
22.	[46]		• Analysis of device performance
23.	[3, 37, 38]		• Supervision of epidemic resources
24.	[32]	kNN	• Checking of glucose on patients
25.	[28]		• Supervision of epidemic resources
26.	[29, 33]		• Forecasting of ailment
27.	[28]		• Diagnosis of ailment based on computer
28.	[23, 26]		• Forecasting of cardiac ailment
29.	[28, 30]		• Checking system in healthcare
30.	[32]	DT	• Checking of glucose on patients
31.	[34, 35]		• Surgical operation
32.	[27, 28]		• Clinical analysis
33.	[42]		• Analysis of device performance
34.	[37]		• Checking system in healthcare
35.	[43, 44]	RF	• Forecasting of ailment
36.	[37]		• Checking system in healthcare
37.	[30]		• Forecasting of cardiac ailment

TABLE 6.1 *(Continued)*
AI Algorithms and Its Areas of Usage in Healthcare

S. no.	Citations	AI Algorithms	Usage in Healthcare
38.	[30]	Logistic	• Medical imaging on cardiac diseases
39.	[32]	Regression	• Checking of glucose on patients
40.	[36]		• Supervision of epidemic resources
41.	[37, 46]		• Checking system in healthcare

6.2.3 SECURITY CHALLENGES IN HEALTHCARE SYSTEMS

Wael and Nidal posited that cyberattacks on critical healthcare systems could not be less [11]. Nevertheless, security concerns weaken AIoMT connectivity, as argued by researchers are listed by Owida et al. [49]. The list includes:

i. Exploitation of information—the hacker modifies or deletes information on patients' records, which can intimidate patient life.
ii. Records of patients accessed by personnel can be a source for blackmail.
iii. Non-compliance to standards by providers of health devices might ease the hijacking process of patients' information.
iv. Adoption of the internet via public access in healthcare services exposes the entire healthcare network to intruders.
v. Most AIoMT sensors are integrated with wireless networks, hence exposed to wireless safety issues.
vi. Lack of standard safety measures among providers of healthcare devices.
vii. AIoMT devices are constrained by resources. Hence, applications of encryption keys are not appropriate.
viii. DOS and DDoS attackers overflood healthcare servers with a large amount of traffic.

6.3 CONCEPT OF IOT AND AIoMT

IoT structure is composed of net-centric devices connected through systems of virtual ecosystems. Information gathered by devices and sensors is passed straight to the huge cloud storage services, then, data is clean for further analysis. Additional software and applications are needed to aid in the imaging, analysis, and supervision of the data. Figure 6.4 presents various wireless interlinked devices. Recently, 5G/6G has become universal in AIoMT as a result of high speed and low latency value.

Internet of Things (IoT) links several devices, users, databases, etc., in an incorporated way. AIoMT intends to ease medical services. Sahshanu and Sachin [47] considered the Artificial intelligence of medical things (AIoMT) as a blend of medical devices with the Internet of Things (IoT). They argued that AIoMTs bring opportunities for healthcare delivery in which clinical devices are linked and supervised across the *supe-highway*;

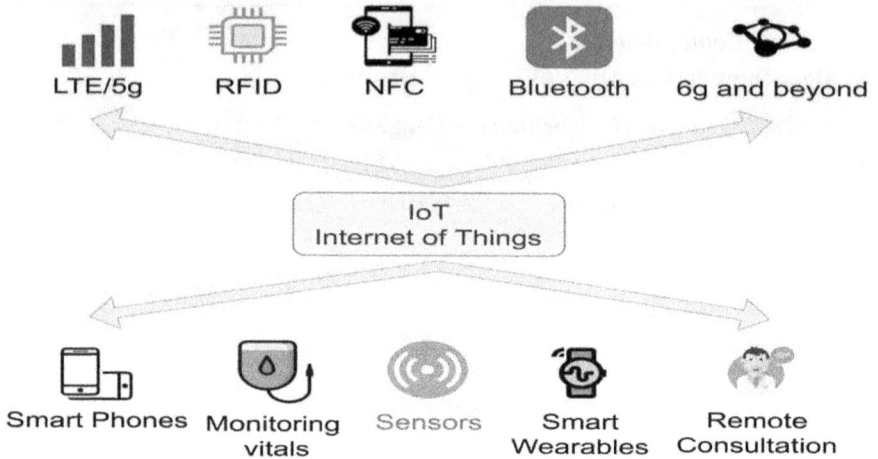

FIGURE 6.4 IoT enabling technologies and devices [47].

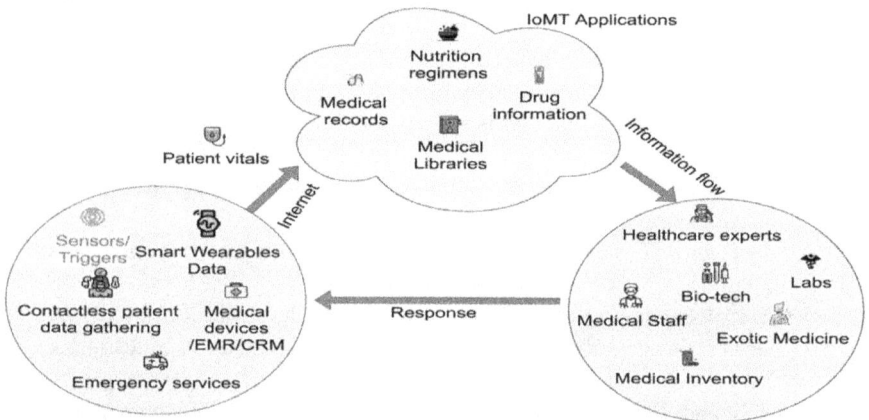

FIGURE 6.5 Adapted intelligence of medical things [47].

facilitating improved patient care. In Figure 6.5, we present AIoMTs in which important health information are assembled through network sensing equipment for transmission to AIoMT platform via the *super-highway*. Also, critical health information passes to the physicians while feedback is sent to the patients.

6.3.1 ADVANTAGES OF AIoMT

The Artificial Intelligence of Medical Things (AIoMT) is considered helpful in many ways. Ghada et al. outlined the advantages of AIoMT [20]. The merits include the following:

   i. Enhanced responses to clinical demands
   ii. Lessening access cost in healthcare

    iii. Provision of quick audience to responses
    iv. Raising quantity in terms of treatments
     v. Giving healthcare professionals better understandings of the patient's condition
    vi. Augmentation of patient care
   vii. Improvement in the quality of life
   vii. Improvement patient knowledge
   vii. Automatic responses to vital changes in patient
  viii. Easiness
    ix. Real-time managing of ailment
     x. Simplicity in usage
    xi. Clinical procedures promptly
   xii. Administration of aging healing progress

6.3.2 SMART E-HEALTHCARE

The foundation of smart healthcare infrastructure is built on intelligent computerized components supported by AI and ML to advance patient care and to include new abilities. Typical examples of computerized healthcare include *remote robot surgery, telehealth, and telemedicine*. Remote robot surgery achieves surgery via decisions by the physician remotely. Tele-health offers nonmedical services remotely, while tele-medicine offers healthcare services at remote sites. Figure 6.6 presents a healthcare system where incoming data from several channels is initially assembled remotely and forwarded to the EHR. Information collected is ordered in format via machines or signal receptors by means of known information format through which individuals can make entries. The system becomes easy to access through other platforms like the Customer Relational Management application. The CRM harnesses devices for information analysis and also assigns information to a known target in the healthcare ecosystem.

    The fundamental records and information from EHR device are processed and forwarded to the Customer Relational Management application to create extra activation for the patients and physicians in the healthcare system. The patients get outgoing

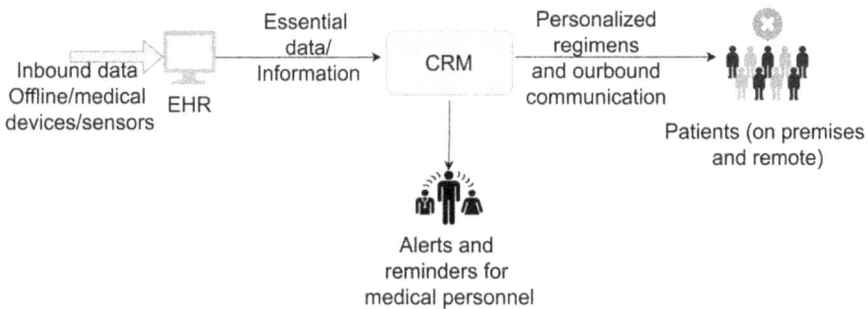

FIGURE 6.6 Adapted smart e-healthcare system [47].

signals from the hospitals and physicians through customized health routines. The healthcare professionals with other allied workers, receive alerts on calls and signals from the application within the system.

6.3.3 AIoMT ARCHITECTURE IN HEALTHCARE

In the AIoMT structural design, healthcare professionals can converse directly via the switches connecting the layer of thing and layer of fog and via restricted dispensation servers at the layer of fog [48]. The structural design for AIoMTs consists of three layers, namely:

   i. *Things layer:* This layer is composed of patients, sensors, actuators, devices for monitoring health information, controlling drugs, routine nutrition creator, etc. A layer of things is openly linked to professionals in healthcare. Information emanating from the components, such as wearables devices, patient-monitoring information, and remote care information, is gathered at the things layer. The equipment employed in this layer ought to be securely positioned to guarantee integrity in the data set.
   ii. *Fog layer:* This layer links the external storage facility and the layer of things. This level is composed of restricted systems and communication linkage machines of a thinly dispersed internet structure. Restricted dispensation rule tied together via lesser level equipment for speedy retort to the client. The collections of storage are needed for administering the control of security, integrity, and confidentiality of the system. Access machines in the fog level are in charge of rerouting information starting from the collections of storage utilities to the next layer called *cloud layer* for advanced processing.
   iii. *Cloud layer:* This layer is composed of information storage space and computation capabilities in terms of the information processed and is obtained for decision processing based on the level. The cloud layer guarantees huge medical and healthcare capabilities to handle administrative and prompt operations with no difficulty. This layer is composed of cloud assets in terms of services where the information generated from the medical networking applications stores analytical works and performs operations considered essential. Figure 6.7 presents the operational services within layers in AIoMT.

Hireche et al. illustrated the AIoMT structure, where the *perception layer* is composed of *sensors and actuators* with entities that recognize and examine fundamental patient signs [84]. The *network layer* is the middle layer that aids the transferring process of medical information to the *application layer* for processing, analyzing, and storing. Figure 6.8 presents various levels in three-layered structure as posited by Ref. [84].

   i. Layer of perception

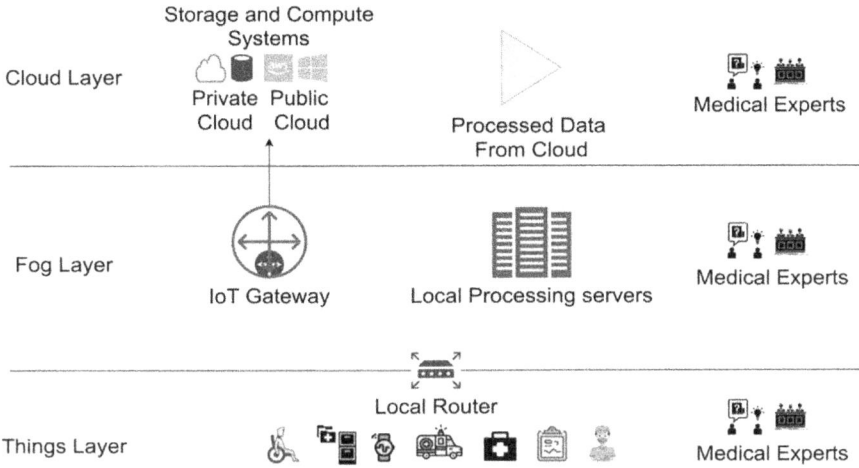

FIGURE 6.7 Adapted operations within layers in AIoMT [47].

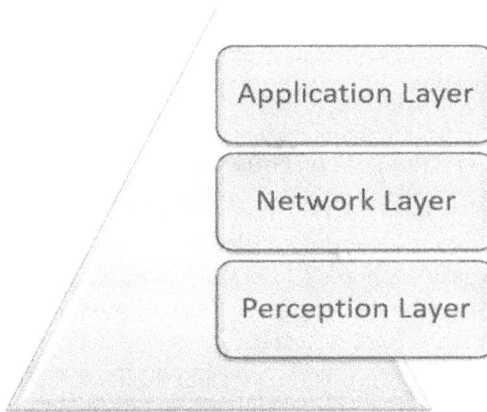

FIGURE 6.8 Modified AIoMT architecture [116].

The layer comprises diverse types of information sensors, such as Radio Frequency Identification (RFID), Barcodes, and other sensor platforms. The main aim of the perception layer is the identification of exceptional objects with the collected information received through the assistance of individual sensors in the network. These individual network sensors comprise sensor networks, smart cards, and Radio Frequency Identification (RFID).

ii. Network layer

The aim of the network level is to broadcast data collected via the lowest layer, i.e., *perception layer* to an information system via any reliable super highway network, such as internet and mobile networks. This comprises digital systems, equipment, and connected or connectionless networks.

iii. Application layer

The application layer recognizes diverse useful applications of Internet of Things as a result of the requirement of the clients. Typical examples include diverse types of utilities, such as automated residence, automated location, automated haulage, and automated sickbay. This also includes applications, linkages, and intelligent devices [49, 11].

6.4   SECURITY CONCERN IN AIOMT-LAYERED ARCHITECTURE

From the AIoMT architectural layers in Figure 6.8, the first layer, the *perceptual layer*, collects information, for example, the RFID and sensor-based signals. Key security concerns at this stage (layer) include external network attacks, for example, *DOS*. The layer of the *network has* to do with achieving safe connectivity for data between the first and second levels with early information processing. Key concern issues in the networking layer of AIoMT are significant since attacks like *man-in-the-middle* can pose threats. The topmost layer is the *application layer*, which takes care of user's needs. Furthermore, the distribution of information is the main attribute of the application layer, and this poses serious security concerns in AIoMT.

6.4.1   SECURITY CONCERN IN PERCEPTION LAYER

AIoMT apprehension at this level considers systems that cannot offer safety and key information to the sensor-based systems. The main reasons for such could be sensor-based devices' inadequate energy and delicate safety capabilities [84]. In this layer, the RFID system has critical threat issues, which include leaking of information, MitM threats, interference, replica threats, and trailing of information. In addition, the security threats in the layer of perception are mainly traffic threats, DOS threats, point replication threats, confined access node threats, and forwarding threats. Key AIoMT safety concerns of equipment at this level are categorized as *security of terminal* and *sensing-based* security concerns.

6.4.2   SECURITY CONCERN IN NETWORK LAYER

This layer primarily includes system nodes and connected or connectionless networks with full security concerns. The network layer experiences security issues such as *data confidentiality, accessing information illegitimately, eavesdropping of information, DoS threat, MitM threat, and malware threat.* A lot of devices in the network layer assemble data from various sources, with information having huge, multisource, and heterogeneous attributes. Key threats flooding the layer of the network are selectively listed:

i. *Selective Forwarding:* The threat involves compromising network terminals or malicious point flooded through the hacker by forwarding false messages through false path.

ii. *HELLO flood attack:* The attacker terminal, which is an illegal terminal in the network, is flooded with the *hello request* to a legitimate terminal. It causes network traffic jamming by forwarding unsolicited messages.

iii. *Sybil attack:* The threat targets fault-tolerant protocols, for example, complex routing, dispersed storage space, and network layout protection. The way out of the threat is to avert any person starting a Sybil threat to be authenticated or encrypted.

iv. *ACK spoofing:* In the case of ACK spoofing threat, rival terminal takes off the ACK by changing false signals to adjacent terminal.

v. *Sinkhole attack:* Sinkhole threat creates selective forwarding exceptionally uncomplicated.

6.4.3 SECURITY CONCERN IN APPLICATION LAYER

This plane affords data authentication, reliability, and privacy. Safety measures concerns in the plane involve distorting data and eavesdropping. In this plane, it coordinates the duty of managing signal jamming or information through the assistance of layered utilities. Targeted threats on the plane aim at cracking legitimate requests and deluging this task, which eventually triggers DoS.

6.5 AIoMT TECHNOLOGIES

Recent advances have sharpened the need for more secure approaches in AIoMT. Sahshanu and Sachin attest that AIoMT has recently witnessed drastic technological improvements [47]. They listed such technologies to lude:

10. i. *Blockchain:* A distributed block of ledger-like connections of computational terminals within sets of connections. The contributions of AIoMT have escalated safety awareness, especially in grid computing. Invariably, block chaining presents means to numerous safety concerns coming from contributing units of e-health [50]. An illustration of a wide variety of these units on the technology is presented in Figure 6.9. The essence of this technology is to find a means to assemble structures and to divide them into lesser units [51].

The units can be incorporated with devices that are appropriate within AIoMT support. The resulting system is distributed and allows decentralization of control in the network [52]. The gain of integrating blockchain structures is the trust it offers, whereas the invasion of health information is high [53]. Security of the technology is high, and it offers the ability to achieve decentralization of data accord, reliability, and suppleness to any form of threats or attacks. The major objectives of setting up this architecture are summarized by Ref. [53].

i. To provide secured clinical records via a trusted platform
ii. To implement flexible access for viewing clinical information
iii. To set up control points for all clinical information
iv. To present distributed data that are precise, reliable, and apt

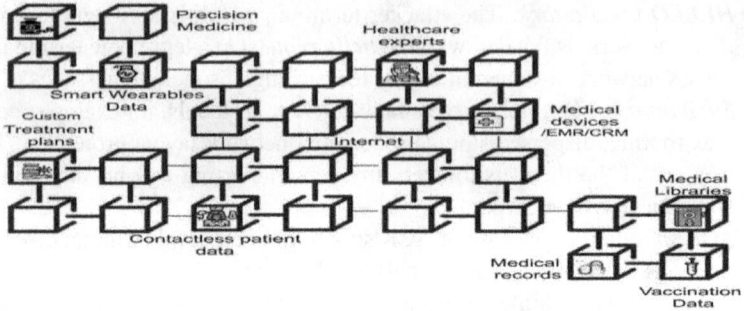

FIGURE 6.9   Application of blockchain in AIoMTs [47].

    v. To implement a visible structure for any possible change
   vi. To provide a means for unauthorized access detection

The initial step of block addition requires the sequence of getting EMR from the server. The algorithmic function to perform the needed routine is stated herewith.

1:   *function Load_File (file)*
2:   *interpret get (file)*
3:   return *interpret*
4:   end function

Adding a block (clinical information or EMR) into the chain, experts must connect to the structure. The algorithmic function to perform the needed routine is stated herewith. The input function is the patient *(n)*.

1: *function Add_block (n)*
2: *connect [Insert arrow] blockchain*
3: *individual [Insert arrow] subscribe(individual)*
4: *interpret [Insert arrow] Upload_File(n.Clinical info)*
5: *block [Insert arrow] generate_block (interpret, timestamp, individual)*
6: *outcomes [Insert arrow] broadcast(block)*
7: *if (outcomes are ok)*
8: *if (block is similar in the chain)*
9: *attach_block_in_Chain()*
10: *show (Block is attached successfully in similar chain)*
11: *else*
12: *attach_block_in_Fork()*
13: *present (Block is attached successfully as a fork in similar chain)*
14: *else*
15: *reject_block()*
16: *show (Block is rejected)*
17: *end function*

ii. *PUF Technology:* The technology creates distinctive biometric features for susceptible rudiments in AIoMT. The distinctive fingerprints emanated from disparity in the production of several equipment. The biometric features are solely for furtive key production (i.e., cryptographic keys) for protecting devices and information within AIoMT since netcentric devices are always under threats and attacks [54]. Figure 6.10 presents the actual planning of these strategies and the fundamental structures the equipment are built on. Also, it is important to note that PUF machines exist in the *thing layer*, as shown in the map. These machines display a critical role in the validation of AIoMT machines [55].

iii. *AI in IoMT:* Accuracy in medication demands sophisticated medical examination and must be customized routines based on a swift delivery point in time [56]. AI becomes a reference point in this scheme since it offers synchronized and coordinated ways in shaping innovative means of handling definite circumstances as a result of notable and real-time data. Several aspects of healthcare can be improved through the application of AI capabilities [57]. These entail methods for conceptualizing AI classifiers, for example, the computerization of information pertaining to patients, arranging patient visits based on scheduled time, deciding laboratory tests, and planning patients' clinical routines, treatments, and operations. The AI classifying agents could be trained in clinical decision-supporting procedures. In case of nondigital classifiers, natural language processing tool proffers a solution in the form of a technique to haul out facts from any formless data set in the system [58]. The resultant formats are laboratory information, assessment records, functioning records, and any other related patients' discharge record [59]. Figure 6.11 presents various platforms of *AI, ML,* and *NLP* in IoMTs.

iv. *SDN:* Networking components of AIoMTs are segregated into *data plane* and *control plane.* Data plane sends data in the direction of its destination, whereas *control plane* handles critical routines permitting the former to

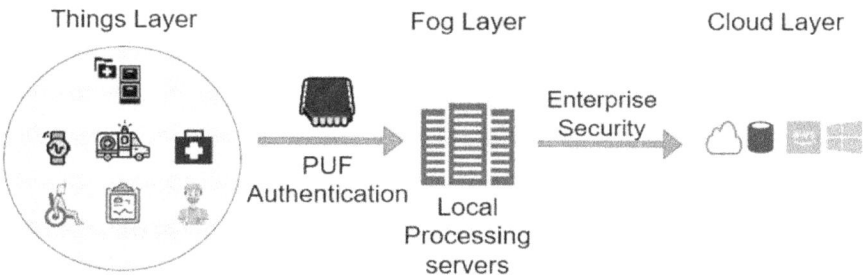

FIGURE 6.10   Adapted PUF in AIoMT [47].

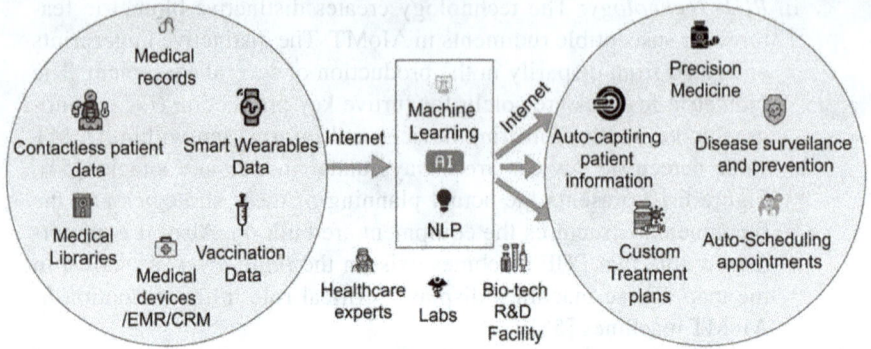

FIGURE 6.11 AI-enabled IoMTs [47].

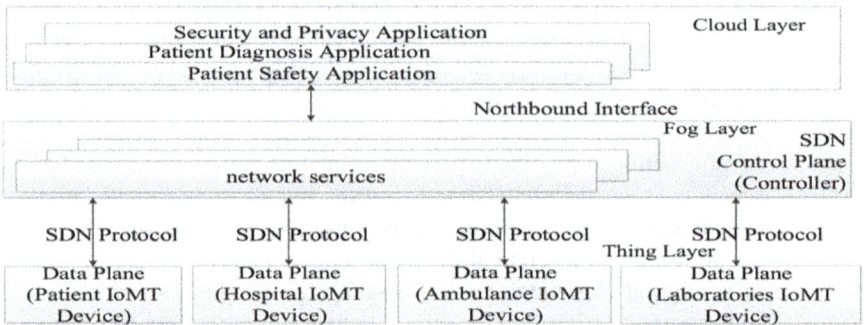

FIGURE 6.12 SDN-enabled IoMTs.

send resolutions [60, 61, 62]. Software-Defined Networking presents a typical means of communicating across the *data plane* and *control plane*. An illustration of typical SDN protocols includes *OpenFlow, Open vSwitch Database Management protocol, and OpenFlow Configuration protocol* [56]. Figure 6.12 presents the SDN enabled AIoMTs.

6.6   AIoMT TECHNOLOGIES AND APPLICATIONS

The utilization of receptive gadgets for collecting clinical information has greatly improved over the years. Recently, clinical information such as electrocardiogram, temperature of the body, pressure of the blood, timing of the heartbeat, and pulsation has changed the accurateness of information, creating a better way of attending to patients and improving healthcare services [63, 64, 65]. Clinical receptive gadgets for monitoring ailments have equally changed the narrative in clinical practice swiftly.

6.7   RESEARCH IN AIoMT

Current review of relevant research literatures in AIoMT shows that in the nearest future vast clinical data and their applicable techniques will unveil.

TABLE 6.2
Technologies in AIoMT

Citations	Tools	Attributes	Purpose
[66]	Artificial intelligence and machine learning	Scrutiny	Clinical examination
[67]	Artificial intelligence	Accurateness	Testing of coronavirus disease
[68]	Recurrent neutral Networks	Lost information	Hepatocellular carcinoma
[69]	Machine learning	Exact	Brain tumor
[70]	Artificial intelligence	Machine learning precision cardiovascular	Artificial intelligence
[71]	Artificial intelligence	Neutral networks	Spectrum distribution
[72]	Machine learning	Block chaining precision	Defense stress stage
[73]	Block chaining	Verification	All
[74]	Block chaining defense	Trusted electronic health record	Block chaining defense
[75]	Block chaining	Defense	Health electronic record
[76]	Cryptography	Defense	Clinical record
[77]	Physical unclonable function	Trust	Host sketching
[78]	Physical unclonable function	Security	Secure sensing
[79]	Physical unclonable function	Validation	mHealth
[80]	Soft-defined networks	Precision	Used for all purposes
[81]	Soft-defined networks	Virtual reality haptic attributes	Training in surgery
[82]	Soft-defined networks	Efficiency	Supervising health routine
[83]	Soft-defined networks	Flowing of network data	Used for all purposes

6.8 THE CHALLENGES OF AIoMT

Challenges in the domain of AIoMT are attributed to several factors. Also, the desire to reduce the barrier between clinicians, patients, and clinical services becomes imperative in this domain. The challenges may be caused by innovative reforms such as:

i. Defense challenges
ii. Confidentiality
iii. Bandwidth constraints
iv. Optimizing device hardware
v. Interoperability
vi. Central processing unit capability
vii. Computer storage
viii. Growth of software and its flexibility
ix. Exchange of routing information
x. Network resources accessibility
xi. Demand for clinical know-how
xii. Confidentiality of information
xiii. Controlling devices due to varieties
xiv. Scalability, size of information, and efficiency

TABLE 6.3

Related Research Literatures in AIoMT

Citations	Architecture	Techniques	Purpose	Performance
[84]	Neurological linkage with dental records for disorders examination	Optimization using NN	Presenting higher model for IoDT	Precision: 97.4%
[85]	ECG signals were assembled and linked with Firebase cloud via Net apps	Improved CNN	To forecast epileptic seizures with precision prompting clinicians	Precision: 98.4%
[86]	Gathering of patient's health history, such as BP, heart pain, and cholesterol	ANFIS	Identifying major attributes of ML-based chest ailment based on forecasting model	Precision: 99.67%
[87]	Machines collection of clinical information, for example, pulsation, chest rate, and pressure of blood via medical wearable devices	DNN	Recommending an innovative replica via hybrid modified water wave	F-measure: 97.2–99.3%
[88]	Collection of information for blood diseases, such as leukemia	DenseNet and ResNet were used	Recommending a précised model for leukemia patients	Precision: 99.5–100%
[89]	Edging infrastructural platforms were recommended	mNet classification	Assisting patients via alert whenever they stop eating	Precision: 87.9–98%
[90]	Detectors were positioned on individual palms to gather health data	DNN	Assisting individuals to stop stressing the body	Precision: 98.3–99.8%
[91]	Ensemble learning-based cyber threats detection was recommended	DT, RF and Naïve Bayes	Detecting cyber threats swiftly	Finding rate: 99.99% Precision: 97.45%
[92]	NN data trained visibly	NN	Health monitoring platform for aging	Precision: 95.6%
[93]	Integration of smart robotic agents for coronavirus testing and finding	DNN	Coronavirus testing and finding in remote locations	No report
[94]	ECG signals were collected and processed via Intel Galileo board	SVM	Providing remote health access to patients	Precision: 99.2%
[95]	ToN-IoT data was used in the testing	Swarm-NN	Identifying threats and attacks during clinical record transfer	Precision: 99.7%
[96]	Data were sent to the cloud for replica forecasting	Fuzzy logic was used	Creating vagueness in a cloud-based medical diagnosis	Precision: 97%

Ref	Description	Application	Model	Outcome
[97]	Connection of sensors to human body via heterogeneous data points	Provision of data mining over different medical data via AI	CNN	Precision: 98%
[98]	Encryption for cloud-based medical image categorization	Provision of proficient and safe analysis of clinical images	Fuzzy CNN	F-measure: 99%
[99]	Microcontrollers with wearable sensors using a DNN architecture	Provision of Protective means for injuries among contestants	DNN	No report
[100]	Chest X-ray imaging transmitted to the cloud via confined devices. Load calculation done and result forwarded	Provision of detection for pneumonia in kids	SVM	Precision: 97.47% F1-score: 97.56%
[101]	Arduino Uno microcontrollers were used to gather clinical information from the Clinical repositories	Assisting patients in remote areas via a proficient platform	NN	Precision: 99.98%
[102]	Hardware comprising of a BAN with elastic on-body natural bioelectronics sensors and actuators	Promoting two signals between the body and the cloud	NN	Precision: 40.7–99.6%
[103]	Information gathered via pulse rate sensor and temperature sensor	Detecting fall to reduce damage with a medical appointment	Multilayer NN	Sensitiveness: 96.5%, Exactness: 98.4%, Precision: 96.3%
[104]	Information gathered via CT-scan, X-ray machines, and RT-CPR, were transmitted to the cloud for coronavirus analysis	Providing IoT-based ML models for coronavirus analysis	RF, SVM Naive Bayes	Precision: 97%
[105]	Dataset presented by the WHO was used with 22 inputs and 1 logical outcome coronavirus examination	Providing protected wireless computation via IoT for corona virus analysis	SVM, ANN, kNN	Accurateness and exactness: 97.5%
[106]	Neutral network was projected and experimented on clinical records prone to adversarial attack scenarios	Perceiving threats or attacks on clinical records	DBN	Precision was reported to be 98%
[107]	Clinical information was gotten from the repository severs	Treating heart ailment early via analysis	DNN	Precision: 99.08%

(Continued)

TABLE 6.3 (Continued)
Related Research Literatures in AIoMT

Citations	Architecture	Techniques	Purpose	Performance
[108]	Application of replica to mHealth records	CNN	To apply QoS to patients via IoMT	Precision: 95–96% for a range of cases
[109]	IoMT-based status data mining architecture comprising of an IoT network, such as ECG sensing devices and electro-dermal actions	CNN	Forecasting human state based on IoMT and wearable devices	Precision: 97.6%
[110]	Application of improved solution for segmenting clinical image	Fuzzy C-means and ANN	Reviewing and contrasting routine detection of brain tumor via MRI	Precision: 98.7%
[111]	Development of AI-based platform for retrieving bio-medical information from dispersed sensors	DL	Examining the relationship between various bio-medical information to identify and analyze diseases	Precision: 96.7%

xv. Predictive models to evaluate ailment
xvi. Performance of software in clinical diagnostic plans
xvii. Healthcare intelligence
xviii. Processing task in real time
xix. Prediction of system performance
xx. Lesser energy consumption
xxi. Information incorporation
xxii. Varied and unstructured information

The activities of AIoMT components are influence by computing capability constraints, such as electrical energy, throughput and space for storage. Consequently, safety clarifications are required through the mastication of the capabilities of AIoMT. The yearning for efficient self-protective means for services, devices, and methods becomes a serious issue for interacting systems [112]. Several safety concerns hinder the activities of AIoMT architectures. Majorly among the security hindrances in AIoMT architecture as listed by Ref. [20] are:

i. Attacks based on spoofing
ii. XSS-Cross-site scripting
iii. Attacks due to replay
iv. Eavesdropping
v. Wireless overcrowding
vi. Attacks based on camouflaging
vii. Worm
viii. Attacks due to man-in-the-middle
ix. Buffer overflow
x. dOS and DDOS

AIoMT critical components negatively exaggerated through such threats are *privacy*, *reliability*, and *authenticity* of the system. Providing security solutions to address these concerns and guarantee safety in AIoMT services is crucial. The information and other components of AIoMT services must be critically safeguarded from cyber threats and attacks as hacking any single component could afford the right to unauthorized usage of critical healthcare data. Cryptographic safety provisions can gain massive trust above AIoMT, given that the interface connects individual and therapeutic things, where critical therapeutic details are collectively shared transversely on set of connections (networks) that attackers may hijack effortlessly if any of the connected machines is penetrated. Hence, there must be well-defined safety structural design installed with a shared universal set of network rules as diverse machines are linked via the AIoMT layout.

6.9 AIOMT CONCERNS

AIoMT concerns aim to ensure that medical records exhibit the CIA concept of *Confidentiality, Integrity,* and *Availability* [20].

i. *Confidentiality in AIoMT:* Privacy is measured as important safety principles. The notion of data privacy emanates from the sole need for safety in communication within the AIoMTs and to guarantee solitary access to clients through permission. Hence, AIoMT clients can be grouped into a variety of groups, for example, *individual, device, task, in-object,* and *out-object.* Privacy in AIoMT is the fundamental task involving clients or organizing procedures associated with client information. Take, for example, in AIoMT, patient's records can never be through illegal units whenever privacy is considered. As a result, every record tag and classification record in the radio frequency identifications is converted into code especially to prevent unauthorized access prior to the period of changing from one state to another [20].

ii. *integrity in AIoMT:* AIoMT is controlled or determined by the sensitivity of the data exchanged from individual machines to another machine. Based on this, information must stay unaltered and unchanged by any illegal individual or unit throughout the changeover session. Take for instance, in clinical schemes, remote patient checks require trust checks by the system in order to sustain patient receptive data precisely. Reliability can be sustained through end-to-end encrypted defense, where information flow is proscribed via the use of *firewall or fault detection processes.*

iii. *Availability in AIoMT:* The major anticipation of AIoMT is that the *flow of data, mechanisms, operations,* and *tools* ought to be exceptional in condition, ease of use, and capability by the client as soon as there is a demand and on time. A typical example is the monitoring devices deployed in healthcare would probably enclose advanced accessibility rations.

6.9.1 THREATS IN AIoMT

AIoMT threat concerns, typical methods, and mitigating channels are listed in Table 6.4.

6.9.2 SECURITY ISSUES IN AIoMT

In ensuring the safety of AIoMT set of connections arrangement, it is tremendously imperative to remove several possible risks to facilitate safety measures against any form of attack and violation of the safety of clinical information. AIoMT know-how is known to be a famous demanding expertise across emerging clinical processes [20]. Safeguarding several levels of safety AIoMT platforms is demanding, since cyberattacks damage incorporated systems [20]. Alteration inserted into any clinical records, by means of leaking, may well intimidate the patient's safety. AIoMT critical infrastructural attacks include:

i. *Spying:* This type of attack on the set of connections within AIoMT is termed *eavesdropping.* Generally, this is achieved whenever critical information is stolen from any proprietary system in clinical settings.

TABLE 6.4

AIoMT Threat Concerns in AIoMT

Threats	Typical methods	Mitigating channels
Self-directed AI	Devices that are closed—loop can maliciously distort information in patient's records	• Execute device audit • Replication of high-risk situation
Reduce Bluetooth power	Attacking Bluetooth stack rules in paired machines	• Cryptographic keys • Update OS regularly • Turn off Bluetooth at idle state
Convergent cloud	Attacks on the weak safety measures in cloud	• Update cloud security • Critical assets auditing • Integration of IDS • Data encryption • Backup critical data • Isolate critical networking infrastructures
Edging processes	Interfacing edging processes to cloud pose a risk	• Point-to-point connections should be afforded • Authenticate direct connections • Dedicated links should be deployed for critical systems
AIoMT diversity	State of dissimilar elements encourages novel hacking	• Extrapolation threats scene during modeling • Monitoring and managing critical infrastructures • End user's agreement implementation
OTS elements	Usage of off-the-shelf modules in AIoMT triggers maximal target for hackers	• Required standards for OTS should be implemented • Safety assessment of critical components should be done promptly
Physical landscape	Hackers exploit nodes via stealing of concealed AIoMT	• Build AIoMT with unparalleled identification and trackers • AIoMT critical assets should be made accountable
Retrofitting	Security weaknesses in obsolete devices can be a point for compromising the entire system	• Enacting laws on duration of critical infrastructures usage • Risk analysis should be carried out on legacy systems to reduce device structures

(Continued)

TABLE 6.4 *(Continued)*
AIoMT Threat Concerns in AIoMT

Threats	Typical methods	Mitigating channels
Quantum computing	Computational requirements would turn some cryptographic devices not useful	• Encrypted algorithm to increase crypto-key parameters. • Migrating critical infrastructures to quantum-safe encrypted level • Develop integrated quantum encrypted methods as safety means

The involvement of this type of attack is basically a result of weaker AIoMT connections within the participatory units, such as client-server connections. Strategy used includes pickup equipment, passwords that are weak, networks that are open, and transmitting links.

ii. *Interception of data:* Hackers interrupt clinical records and forward patients' records to unknown destinations at any point in time, allowing unauthorized persons to sniff into the protocol resolution address files that permit connectivity within the AIoMTs. Once entry is illegally made into the ARP, the hackers penetrate clinical records without permission and acquire encrypted keys.

iii. *Attack through flooding:* This is an overcrowding of the AIoMT network traffic in order to bring down critical clinical infrastructures with the view to lessen system assets through flooding and infusing means through deceitful records and falsification of calls.

iv. *Attacks through birthday:* Relying on fragile *hashes*, especially in password utilization, possibly will create a means for exploiting system vulnerability, making it easier to access healthcare records with no permission. The most excellent resolution to guard the AIoMTs would be to apply secure hash algorithm methods.

v. *Attacks by worms:* This is the most hazardous and disparaging form of malicious code experience within AIoMTs—self-reproductive in nature devoid of individual interference through linked machines, taking opportunity of loopholes in machine capabilities. Virtually all terminals on the network are affected leading to information loss and possible harm on the patient's health. It combines other threats such as botnets/ransomware activating its spreading capabilities across networks of AIoMT.

vi. *Attacks by dictionary:* Prevalent of any cyber threats through this form is by having access to clinical records devoid of permission. This is a typical case of less or no rigorous defense countermeasures on AIoMT.

vii. *Attacks by replay:* In this attack, a typical hacker signals AIoMT components by way of altering or modifying communication to forward false requests to other AIoMT devices. Also, capturing and pilfering broadcasting clinical data is possible via a means of redirecting information to unknown destinations. At the end, severe material harm may be experienced by connected AIoMT terminals.

viii. *Attack by black-nursing:* Internet control message protocol threats are directed toward the central processing unit of computers and firewalls prompted by the denial of service threats averting clinical experts and clients from conveying network congestion across the LAN.

ix. *Attack through Brute Force:* This kind of threat typically involves guessing system security login information, encrypted keys, or hidden application sites. Hackers crack likely keywords to penetrate AIoMT networks for unauthorized functions by acquiring clinical records or patient identification. This threat involves nearly all beleaguered AIoMT apparatus. Also, brute forcing attacks are not restricted to remote clinical sensing of patients.

x. *Attacks by malicious scripting injection:* Incorrect scripting on scheme may provide a phony updating of records, where criminally minded elements may choose to imitate a genuine backup server within the system. The outcome is that the intruder can have accessible right into the AIoMT machines without permission. Table 6.3 presents summarized features of adversarial attacks on AIoMT.

6.9.3 MALICIOUS ATTACKS IN AIoMT

Trending adversarial attacks, defense techniques, causes, and possible threats are listed in Table 6.5.

6.9.4 PRIVACY ISSUES IN AIoMT

Malware can be utilized to explore weaknesses of existing AIoMT infrastructures via the weaknesses in the hardware, networking layers, or the system application/OS [113]. Ghada et al. posited that the safety concerns associated with any protective mechanism in client information are to be used by AIoMTs in active, dispersed, mixed, and organized networks of extensive AIoMT components that recommended terminals to be independent, having the capabilities to classify the safety threats and dealing with the threats via prejudiced and preliminary techniques [20]. Furthermore, several threats are avoidable through the identification of characteristics specifically based on machine usage. Ghada et al. discussed several information-related issues based on safety, confidentiality, vigorous, and the roomy set of connections that requires trust [20]. They opined that some encrypted techniques checkmate most of the AIoMT concerns effectively and efficiently. The *provable information possessions, attribute-based encrypted principles*, and *advanced encrypted principles* were the sole techniques envisaged in promoting the reliability of clinical information. Such procedures commence through the deployment of asymmetric-encrypted protocol and the AES to encryption of information in several formats [20].

The proportion of inside threats to outside threats at all times remains lofty. An enormous effort and methodological know-how are needed in order to attack AIoMT infrastructures externally. Hence, it entails less effort for AIoMT to be attacked from the inside

TABLE 6.5

Malicious Attacks in AIoMT

Adversarial attacks	Defense techniques	Causes	Possible threats
Ransomware	Anti-malicious code, knowledge-based approach through awareness and avoidance of private data	Usage of weak means of authentication, extortion from ransomware	Privacy, reliability, validation, and accessibility
Spyware	Updating of system applications, such as OS and updated antivirus	A definite host required	Privacy, reliability, validation, and accessibility
Trojan horse	Updating physical system components regularly, deploying intrusive detecting system	Indiscriminate software downloads and hidden software updating internally	Privacy, reliability, validation, and accessibility
Viruses	Anti-virus solutions, penetration tester-based approach	Breach/failure of defense network	Privacy, reliability, validation, and accessibility
Botnet	Penetration tester-based approach, intrusive detecting system, and anti-malicious code	Exploitation of AIoMT logical weaknesses	Privacy, reliability, validation, and accessibility
Rootkit	Effective configuration of system, managing system authentication, intrusive detecting system, and patch update	Operating system kernel exploitation and root attributes	Validation
Worm	Intrusive detecting system and anti-malicious code and anti-virus solutions	Breach failure of defense network	Privacy, reliability, validation. and accessibility

with the help of stakeholders. An access control mechanism to secure clinical information of patient's records against internally generated attacks is proposed by Ref. [114].

It allows only legitimate users, that is, authorized patients and doctors to communicate despite the fact of physical boundaries. The proposed model implements authorization in combination with permissions and roles instead of roles only for medical staff. It removes the discrepancies in the existing access control models. The proposed model ensures communication among doctors and patients in a secure, private, and efficient manner. The model is demonstrated by using mathematical modeling along with implementation examples. The proposed model outperformed in comparison with state-of-the-art access control models.

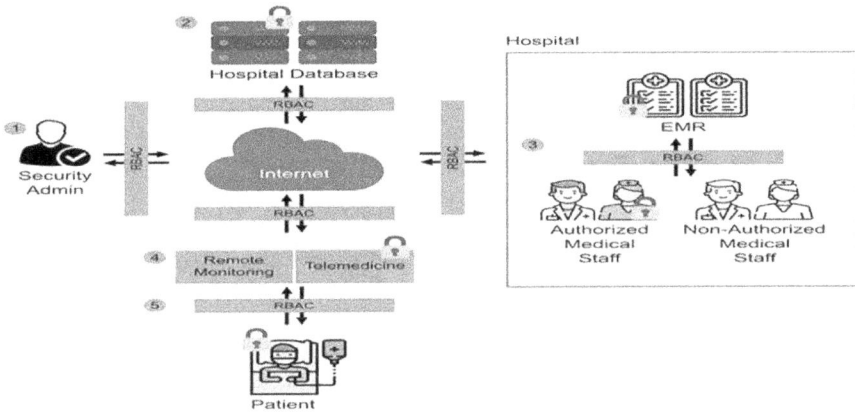

FIGURE 6.13 Defense access control representation [113].

TABLE 6.6
Relative Study of Access Control Model

Model	Merits	Limitations
MAC	A safety expert has overall control over access. Hence, *mandatory access control* offers stiff safety measures.	• No division of task in mandatory access control • Least privilege principle. • Authenticated and reliable components are implemented.
DAC	In discretionary access control, ACL is the determinant for accessing records which are based on validation of the person using it.	• Establishments with huge data experience low scalability.
RBAC	In role-based access, control is rich having tight security of big and complex organizations, thereby reducing cost and complexity.	Across extended administrative domain of an organization.
ABAC	Additional parameters are added in ABAC that includes resource data, requested data, dynamic data of attributes, that is, machine IP, access time, and so on.	ABAC only implements confidentiality or scalability of data at one time.
MDPAC	The proposed model implements access control on the basis of conflicting permissions and roles.	Applicable to three levels of role hierarchy only.

6.9.5 TRUST ISSUES IN AIoMT

The AIoMT assembles connecting terminals via the *superhighway* offering clinically associated services to patients. System connectivity based on trusted devices provides the needed health care services making clinical procedures and managing clinical processes effectively and efficiently irrespective of the isolated locality. The application of XAI model can create trust via outcomes that are explainable or interpretable [115]. The composition of AIoMT comprises the digital and physical scene in order to improve the examination and treatment of patients' ailment accurately advancing their performance and fitness state remotely. Based on this, links to clinically linked terminals become a determinant factor in the patients' health and clinicians. Block chaining approach is a key solution for a trusted AIoMT. Recently, mounting curiosity is focused on the provision of a secured clinical-data-driven management based on block-chaining approaches. This approach is considered by experts as tempered-proven distributing blocks that proffer means for the safety of the AIoMT documenting all transactions of AIoMT digital communication.

6.9.6 ACCURACY ISSUES IN AIoMT

The interaction processes in AIoMT can be under attack based on the distortion of critical information by hackers or possibly will be distorted by a variety of influences above individual management, including the breakdown of proprietary systems. The techniques to make certain that *exactness* and uniqueness of information involve techniques such as *Checksum and Cyclic Redundancy Check*. These are simple fault detective processes that are an integral part of the AIoMT information. Furthermore, uninterrupted synchronization of information for backing up functions and attributes such as *version control*, which sustains the restoration of altered files can guarantee the reliability of information.

6.9.7 AUTHENTICATION PROTOCOLS IN AIoMTs

In achieving safety and resolving issues associated with radio frequency identification detection in AIoMT, Ghada et al. anticipated *NLA schemes* for radio frequency identification detective procedures that demand some safety protocol, for example, *untraceability, onward privacy, pliability to imposture attacks, conflict to desynchronization attacks*, and *valid access* [20].

6.9.8 DETECTION MECHANISMS FOR AIoMTs NETWORKS

Ghada et al. argued against different types of malicious attacks, the organization of the AIoMT platforms, and their functions. They endeavored to categorize the safety procedural implementation in AIoMT [20]. A proportional revision was performed based on the existing design for detecting and preventing malicious agents in AIoMT. The desirable target was on the diverse features of malicious recognition in AIoMT.

6.10   CONCLUSION

In this chapter, we provided an overview related to Artificial Intelligence of Medical Things (AIoMT) and presented AIoMT architecture. The most essential aspect of AIoMT is the connectivity it offers as systems are linked based on the network and are used in monitoring the patient with the help of remote sensors, assembling data, and forwarding patient's data to concerned parties. With all the advantages of AIoMT infrastructures in healthcare ecosystem, its weaknesses call for concern. For this reason, this chapter focused on a number of AIoMT concerns, such as security, accuracy, and trust. This chapter has identified and technically addressed these issues by discussing and comparing various methods of threat mitigation in AIoMTs. In the future, we hope to develop threat model for strategies, build safety mechanisms, and conduct investigations into the key security of AIoMT.

REFERENCES

[1]   P. M. Kumar, C. S. Hong, F. Afghah, G. Manogaran, K. Yu, Q. Hua, and J. Gao, "Clouds proportionate medical data stream analytics for internet of things-based healthcare systems", *IEEE Journal of Biomedical and Health Informatics*, vol. 15, no. 26, pp. 973–982, 2021.

[2]   H. Ma, and X. Pang, "Research and analysis of sport medical data processing algorithms based on deep learning and internet of things", *IEEE Access*, vol. 11, no. 8, pp. 139–143, 2019.

[3]   R. F. Mansour, A. El Amraoui, I. Nouaouri, V. G. Díaz, D. Gupta, and S. Kumar, "Artificial intelligence and internet of things enabled disease diagnosis model for smart healthcare systems", *IEEE Access*, vol. 9, no. 5, pp. 451–459, 2021. http://doi.org/10.1109/ACCESS.2021.3066365

[4]   Y. Kumar, A. Koul, R. Singla, and M. F. Ijaz, "Artificial intelligence in disease diagnosis: A systematic literature review, synthesizing framework and future research agenda", *Journal of Ambient Intelligence and Humanized Computing*, vol. 5, no. 11, pp. 1–28, 2022.

[5]   S. Nandy, M. Adhikari, S. Chakraborty, A. Alkhayyat, and N. Kumar, "IBoNN: Intelligent agent-based internet of medical things framework for detecting brain response from electroencephalography signal using bag-of-neural network", *Future Generation Computer Systems*, vol. 13, no. 7, pp. 241–252, 2022.

[6]   P. D. Singh, G. Dhiman, and R. Sharma, "Internet of things for sustaining a smart and secure healthcare system", *Sustainable Computing: Informatics and Systems*, vol. 3, no. 3, pp. 100–106, 2022.

[7]   R. Kishalaj, "AI enabled internet of medical things", *International Journal of Creative Research Thoughts (IJCRT)*, vol. 9, no. 12, pp. 579–602, 2021.

[8]   A. S. Adly, and M. S. Adly, "Approaches based on artificial intelligence and the internet of intelligent things to prevent the spread of COVID-19: Scoping review", *Journal of Medical Internet Research*, vol. 22, no. 8, pp. 191–204, 2022.

[9]   A. F. Alrefaei, Y. M. Hawsawi, D. Almaleki, T. Alafif, F. A. Alzahrani, and M. A. Bakhrebah, "Genetic data sharing and artificial intelligence in the era of personalized medicine based on a cross-sectional analysis of the Saudi human genome program", *Scientific Reports*, vol. 12, no. 1, pp. 1–10, 2022.

[10] C. Guo, J. Zhang, Y. Liu, Y. Xie, Z. Han, and Yu, J, "Recursion enhanced random forest with an improved linear model (RERF-ILM) for heart disease detection on the internet of medical things platform", *IEEE Access*, vol. 8, no. 5, pp. 9247–9256, 2022.

[11]   T. Wael, and T. Nidal, "A survey on security threats in the internet of medical things (IoMT)", *Journal of Theoretical and Applied Information Technology*, vol. 100, no. 10, pp. 3361–3371, 2022.

[12]   O. Ohad, J. Brenard, and L. Deepak, "Artificial intelligence in medical imaging: Switching from radiographic pathological data to clinically meaningful endpoints", *Viewpoint*, vol. 2, no. 2, pp. 486–488, 2022.

[13]   P. Manickam, S. A. Mariappan, S. M. Murugesan, S. Hansda, A. Kaushik, R. Shinde, S. P. Thipperudraswamy, "Artificial intelligence (AI) and internet of medical things (IoMT) assisted biomedical systems for intelligent healthcare", *Biosensors*, vol. 12, no. 5, pp. 62–70, 2022.

[14]   H. E. Kim, H. H. Kim, and B. K. Han, " Changes in cancer detection and false— positive recall in mammography using Artificial intelligence: A retrospective, multi— reader study", *Lancet Digital Health*, vol. 2, no. 1, pp. 138–148, 2020.

[15]   J. M. Kwon, S. Y. Lee, and K. H. Jeon, " Deep learning—based algorithm for detecting aorticstenosis using electrocardiography", *Journal of the American Heart Association*, vol. 9. no. 1, pp. 47–53, 2020.

[16]   K. H. Abdulkareem, M. A. Mohammed, A. Salim, M. Arif, O. Geman, D. Gupta, and A. Khanna, "Realizing an effective COVID-19 diagnosis system based on machine learning and IOT in smart hospital environment", *IEEE Internet of Things Journal*, early access, January 11, 2021, http://doi.org/10.1109/JIOT.2021.3050775

[17]   A. A. Mutlag, M. K. Abd Ghani, N. Arunkumar, M. A. Mohammed, and O. Mohd, "Enabling technologies for fog computing in healthcare IoT systems", *Future Generation Computer Systems*, vol. 90, pp. 62–78, 2019.

[18]   J. P. Queralta, T. N. Gia, H. Tenhunen, and T. Westerlund, "Edge-AI in LoRa-based health monitoring: Fall detection system with fog computing and LSTM recurrent neural networks", *In 2019 42nd International Conference on Telecommunications and Signal Processing (TSP)*, Budapest, Hungary, pp. 601–604, 2019. doi: 10.1109/TSP.2019.8768883

[19]   Insider Intelligence. *Use of AI in the Healthcare and Medicine is Booming*. eMarketer Analyst Webinar, 2022.

[20]   S. Ghada, H. Ghada, and K. Reham, "Modern study on internet of medical things (IOMT) security", *IJCSNS International Journal of Computer Science and Network Security*, vol. 21, no. 8, pp. 254–266, 2021.

[21]   M. Sendak, M. Elish, M. Gao, J. Futoma, V. Ratliff, and V. Nichols, "The human body is a black box supporting clinical decision-making with deep learning", *Proceedings of the 2020 Conference on Fairness, Accountability, and Transparency*, vol. 6, no. 7, pp. 99–109, 2020,

[22]   A. Markus, J. Kors, and P. Rijnbeek, "The role of explainability in creating trustworthy artificial intelligence for health care: A comprehensive survey of the terminology, design choices, and evaluation strategies", *Journal of Biomedical Informatics*, vol. 11, no. 3, pp. 1–11, 2021.

[23]   US Food and Drug Administration. *Proposed Regulatory Framework for Modifications to Artificial Intelligence/Machine Learning (AI/ML)—Based Software as a Medical Device (SAMD)*. Published: January, 2020. www.fda.gov/media/122535/download.

[24]   N. Cortez, "Digital health and regulatory experimentation at the FDA", *Yale Journal of Law & Technology*, vol. 2, no. 1, 2019, pp. 21–25.

[25]   A. Malhi, S. Knapic, and K. Främling, "Explainable agents for less bias in human-agent decision making", *In International Workshop on Explainable, Transparent Autonomous Agents and Multi-Agent Systems. EXTRAAMAS 2020. Lecture Notes in Computer Science. Springer: Cham. vol. 12175, pp. 129–146. https://doi.org/10.1007/978-3-030-51924-7_8

[26] C. Martin-Isla, V. M. Campello, C. Izquierdo, Z. Raisi-Estabragh, B. Baeßler, S. E. Petersen, and K. Lekadir, "Image-based cardiac diagnosis with machine learning: A review", *Frontiers in Cardiovascular Medicine*, vol. 7, no. 1, pp. 231–239, 2020.

[27] M. Shokrekhodaei, D. P. Cistola, R. C. Roberts, S. Quinones, "Non-invasive glucose monitoring using optical sensor and machine learning techniques for diabetes applications", *IEEE Access Biosensors*, vol. 9, no. 12, pp. 25–29, 2022.

[28] F. Galbusera, G. Casaroli, and T. Bassani, "Artificial intelligence and machine learning in spine research", *JOR Spine*, vol. 10, no. 2, pp. 53–59, 2019.

[29] M. Chang, J. A. Canseco, K. J. Nicholson, N. Patel, and A. R. Vaccaro, "The role of machine learning in spine surgery: The future is now", *Frontiers in Surgery*, vol. 7, no. 5, pp. 54–57, 2020.

[30] M. Goswami, and N. J. Sebastian, "Performance Analysis of Logistic Regression, KNN, SVM, Naïve Bayes Classifier for Healthcare Application During COVID-19", *In Innovative Data Communication Technologies and Application*, Raj, J. S., Kamel, K., Lafata, P., Eds. Springer Nature: Singapore, pp. 645–658, 2022.

[31] P. Kaur, R. Kumar, and M. Kumar, "A healthcare monitoring system using random forest and internet of things (IoT)", *Multimedia Tools and Applications*, vol. 7, no. 8, pp. 19905–19916, 2021.

[32] D. Ardila, A. P. Kiraly, S. Bharadwaj, B. Choi, J. J. Reicher, L. Peng, D. Tse, M. Etemadi, W. Ye, and G. Corrado, "End-to-end lung cancer screening with three-dimensional deep learning on low-dose chest computed tomography", *Nature Medicine*, vol. 2, no. 5, pp. 954–961, 2021.

[33] W. Muhammad, G. R. Hart, B. Nartowt, J. J. Farrell, K. Johung, Y. Liang, and J. Deng, "Pancreatic cancer prediction through an artificial neural network", *Frontiers in Artificial Intelligence*, vol. 2, no. 2, pp. 23–30, 2019.

[34] F. Ramzan, M. U. G. Khan, A. Rehmat, S. Iqbal, T. Saba, A. Rehman, and Z. Mehmood, "A deep learning approach for automated diagnosis and multi-class classification of Alzheimer's disease stages using resting-state FMRI and residual neural networks", *Journal of Medical Systems*, vol. 44, no. 37, pp. 104–110, 2020.

[35] K. Pang, X. Song, Z. Xu, X. Liu, Y. Liu, L. Zhong, Y. Peng, J. Wang, J. Zhou, and F. Meng, "Hydroplastic foaming of grapheme aerogels and artificially intelligent tactile sensors", *Science Advances*, vol. 6, no. 3, pp. 40–45, 2020.

[36] T. Hayasaka, A. Lin, V. C. Copa, L. P. Lopez, R. A. Loberternos, L. I. M. Ballesteros, Y. Kubota, Y. Liu, A. A. Salvador, and L. Lin, "An electronic nose using a single graphene FET and machine learning for water, methanol, and ethanol", *Microsystems & Nanoengineering*, vol. 6, no. 50, pp. 67–75, 2020.

[37] J. J. Khanam, and S. Y. Foo, "A comparison of machine learning algorithms for diabetes prediction", *ICT Express*, vol. 7, pp. 432–439, 2021.

[38] Y. T. Kwon, H. Kim, M. Mahmood, Y. S. Kim, C. Demolder, and W. H. Yeo, "Printed, wireless, soft bioelectronics and deep learning algorithm for smart human-machine interfaces", *ACS Applied Materials & Interfaces*, vol. 12, pp. 49398–49406, 2020.

[39] A. K. Kaushik, J. S. Dhau, H. Gohel, Y. K. Mishra, B. Kateb, N. Y. Kim, and D. Y. Goswami, "Electrochemical SARS-CoV-2 sensing at point-of-care and artificial intelligence for intelligent COVID-19 management", *ACS Applied Bio Materials*, vol. 3, pp. 7306–7325, 2020.

[40] A. Esteva, K. Chou, S. Yeung, N. Naik, A. Madani, A. Mottaghi, Y. Liu, E. Topol, J. Dean, and R. Socher, "Deep learning-enabled medical computer vision", *Digital Medicine*, vol. 4, no. 5, pp. 45–52, 2021.

[41]   Y. Shen, Y. Li, H. T. Zheng, B. Tang, and M. Yang, "Enhancing ontology-driven diagnostic reasoning with a symptom-dependency aware Naïve Bayes classifier", *BMC Bioinform*, vol. 20, pp. 30–36, 2019.

[42]   N. A. Fauziyyah, S. Abdullah, and S. Nurrohmah, "Reviewing the consistency of the naïve bayes classifier's performance in medical diagnosis and prognosis problems", *AIP Conference Proceedings*, vol. 30, pp. 22–42, 2020.

[43]   S. Uddin, I. Haque, H. Lu, M. A. Moni, and E. Gide, "Comparative performance analysis of K-nearest neighbour (KNN) algorithm and its different variants for disease prediction", *Scientific Reports*, vol. 12, pp. 56–62, 2022.

[44]   D. Rahmat, A. A. Putra, and A. W. Setiawan, "Heart Disease Prediction Using K-Nearest Neighbor", *In Proceedings of the 2021 International Conference on Electrical Engineering and Informatics (ICEEI)*, Kuala Terengganu, Malaysia, IEEE: Kuala Terengganu, Malaysia, vol. 23, pp. 1–6, 2021.

[45]   T. Ooka, H. Johno, K. Nakamoto, Y. Yoda, H. Yokomichi, and Z. Yamagata, "Random forest approach for determining risk prediction and predictive factors of type 2 diabetes: Large-scale health check-up data in Japan", *BMJ Nutrition, Prevention & Health*, vol. 4, pp. 140–148, 2021.

[46]   K. Fawagreh, and M. M. Gaber, "Resource-efficient fast prediction in healthcare data analytics: A pruned Random Forest regression approach", *Computing*, vol. 102, pp. 1187–1198, 2020.

[47]   R. Sahshanu, and S. Sachin, "Internet of medical things (IoMT): Overview, emerging technologies, and case studies", *IETE Technical Review*, vol. 39, no. 4, pp. 775–788, 2022. http://doi.org/10.1080/02564602.2021.1927863

[48]   V. S. Naresh, S. S. Pericherla, P. S. RamaMurty, and S. Reddi, "Internet of things in healthcare: Architecture, applications, challenges, and solutions", *Computer Systems Science and Engineering*, vol. 35, no. 6, pp. 411–421, 2020.

[49]   H. A. Owida, J. I. Al-Nabulsi, N. M. Turab, F. Alnaimat, H. Rababah, and M. Y. Shakour, "Autocharging techniques for implantable medical applications", *International Journal of Biomaterials*, vol. 10, no. 8, pp. 20–21, 2021.

[50]   V. S. Naresh, S. S. Pericherla, P. S. RamaMurty, and S. Reddi, "Internet of things in healthcare: Architecture, applications, challenges, and solutions", *Computer Systems Science and Engineering*, vol. 35, no. 6, pp. 411–421, 2020.

[51]   P. J. Taylor, T. Dargahi, A. Dehghantanha, R. M. Parizi, and K. K. Raymond Choo, "A systematic literature review of blockchain cyber security", *Digital Communications and Networks*, vol. 6, no. 2, pp. 147–156, 2020.

[52]   Q. Wang, X. Zhu, Y. Ni, L. Gu, and H. Zhu, "Blockchain for the IoT and industrial IoT: A review internet things", *Special Issue of the Elsevier IoT Journal on Blockchain Applications in IoT Environments*, vol. 10, pp. 100–108, 2020.

[53]   N. Dilawar, M. Rizwan, F. Ahmad, and S. Akram, "Blockchain: Securing internet of medical things (IoMT)", *International Journal of Advanced Computer Science and Applications*, vol. 10, pp. 1–10, 2019.

[54]   A. Shamsoshoara, A. Korenda, F. Afghah, and S. Zeadally, "A survey on physical unclonable function (PUF)-based security solutions for internet of things", *Computer Networks*, vol. 18, no. 3, pp. 107–113, 2020.

[55]   P. Harvey, O. Toutsop, K. Kornegay, E. Alale, and D. Reaves, "Security and privacy of medical internet of things devices for smart homes", *2020 7th International Conference on Internet of Things: Systems, Management and Security (IOTSMS)*, Paris, France, pp. 1–6, 2020. doi: 10.1109/IOTSMS52051.2020.9340231

[56]   Z. Ahmed, K. Mohamed, S. Zeeshan, and X. Dong, "Artificial intelligence with multifunctional machine learning platform development for better healthcare and precision medicine", *Database*, vol. 10, pp. 10–15, 2020.

[57] S. Sharma, "Towards artificial intelligence assisted software defined networking for internet of vehicles", in *Intelligent Technologies for Internet of Vehicles, Internet of Things*, N. Magaia et al., Eds. Cham: Springer, 2021. https://doi.org/10.1007/978-3-030-76493-7_6

[58] S. Lalmuanawma, J. Hussain, and L. Chhakchhuak, "Applications of machine learning and artificial intelligence for Covid-19 (SARS-CoV-2) pandemic: A review", *Chaos Solitons Fractals*, vol. 139, p. 110059, 2020.

[59] A. Sedik, M. Hammad, F. E. Abd El-Samie, B. B. Gupta, and A. A. Abd El-Latif, "Efficient deep learning approach for augmented detection of coronavirus disease", *Neural Computing and Applications*, vol. 5, 2021, pp. 1–18, 2021.

[60] H. Turabieh, A. Abu Salem, and N. Abu-El-Rub, "Dynamic L-RNN recovery of missing data in IoMT applications", *Future Generation Computer Systems*, vol. 89, pp. 575–583, 2019.

[61] S. R., Khan, M. Sikandar, A. Almogren, I. Ud Din, A. Guerrieri, and G. Fortino, "IoMT-based computational approach for detecting brain tumor", *Future Generation Computer Systems*, vol. 109, pp. 360–367, 2020.

[62] A. Kilic, "Artificial intelligence and machine learning in cardiovascular health care", *The Annals of Thoracic Surgery*, vol. 109, no. 5, pp. 1323–1329, 2020.

[63] H. Song, J. Bai, Y. Yi, J. Wu, and L. Liu, "Artificial intelligence enabled internet of things: Network architecture and spectrum access", *IEEE Computational Intelligence Magazine*, vol. 15, no. 1, pp. 44–51, 2020.

[64] L. Rachakonda, A. K. Bapatla, S. P. Mohanty, and E. Kougianos, "Sayopillow: A blockchain-enabled, privacy-assured framework for stress detection, prediction and control considering sleeping habits in the IoMT", *Transactions on Emerging Telecommunications Technologies*, vol. 21, pp. 112–121, 2020.

[65] F. Fotopoulos, V. Malamas, T. K. Dasaklis, P. Kotzanikolaou, and C. Douligeris, "A blockchain-enabled architecture for IoMT device authentication", In *2020 IEEE Eurasia Conference on IoT, Communication and Engineering (ECICE)*, Yunlin, Taiwan, vol. 5, pp. 89–92, 2020. doi: 10.1109/ECICE50847.2020.9301913

[66] S. Lalmuanawma, J. Hussain, and L. Chhakchhuak, "Applications of machine learning and artificial intelligence for Covid-19 (SARS-CoV-2) pandemic: A review", *Chaos Solitons Fractals*, vol. 139, pp. 110–115, 2020.

[67] A. Sedik, M. Hammad, F. E. Abd El-Samie, B. B. Gupta, and A. A. Abd El-Latif, "Efficient deep learning approach for augmented detection of coronavirus disease", *Neural Computing and Applications*, vol. 12, pp. 1–18, 2021.

[68] H. Turabieh, A. Abu Salem, and N. Abu-El-Rub, "Dynamic L-RNN recovery of missing data in IoMT applications", *Future Generation Computer Systems*, vol. 89, pp. 575–583, 2019.

[69] S. R. Khan, M. Sikandar, A. Almogren, I. Ud Din, A. Guerrieri, and G. Fortino, "IoMT-based computational approach for detecting brain tumor", *Future Generation Computer Systems*, vol. 109, pp. 360–367, 2020.

[70] A. Kilic, "Artificial intelligence and machine learning in cardiovascular health care", *The Annals of Thoracic Surgery*, vol. 109, no. 5, pp. 1323–1329, 2020.

[71] H. Song, J. Bai, Y. Yi, J. Wu, and L. Liu, "Artificial intelligence enabled internet of things: Network architecture and spectrum access", *IEEE Computational Intelligence Magazine*, vol. 15, no. 1, pp. 44–51, 2020.

[72] C. Esposito, A. De Santis, G. Tortora, H. Chang, and K. K. Choo, "Blockchain: A panacea for healthcare cloud based data security and privacy?", *IEEE Cloud Computing*, vol. 5, no. 1, pp. 31–37, 2019.

[73] F. Girardi, G. De Gennaro, L. Colizzi, and N. Convertini, "Improving the healthcare effectiveness: The possible role of EHR, IoMT and blockchain", *Electronics*, vol. 9, no. 6, pp. 884–891, 2020.

[74] M. Noura, "Efficient and secure cryptographic solutions for medical data", Theses, Univ. Bourgogne Franche-Comté, July 2019.

[75] V. P. Yanambaka, A. Abdelgawad, and K. Yelamarthi, "PIM: A PUF based host tracking protocol for privacy aware contact tracing in crowded areas", *IEEE Consumer Electronics Magazine*, vol. 2, pp. 1–1, 2021.

[76] H. Ma, Y. Gao, O. Kavehei, and D. C. Ranasinghe, "A PUF sensor: Securing physical measurements", *IEEE PerCom Workshops*, vol. 7, pp. 648–653, 2019.

[77] M. Masud, G. Singh Gaba, S. Alqahtani, G. Muhammad, B. B. Gupta, P. Kumar, and A. Ghoneim, "A lightweight and robust secure key establishment protocol for internet of medical things in COVID-19 patients care", *IEEE Internet of Things Journal*, vol. 6, pp. 1–1, 2020.

[78] S. Liaqat, A. Akhunzada, F. S. Shaikh, A. Giannetsos, and M. A. Jan, "SDN orchestration to combat evolving cyber threats in internet of medical things (IoMT)", *Computer Communications*, vol. 160, pp. 697–705, 2020.

[79] J. Cecil, A. Gupta, M. Pirela-Cruz, and P. Ramanathan, "An IoMT based cyber training framework for orthopedic surgery using next generation internet technologies", *Informatics in Medicine Unlocked*, vol. 12, pp. 128–137, 2019.

[80] Z. Askari, J. Abouei, M. Jaseemuddin, and A. Anpalagan, "Energy efficient and realtime NOMA scheduling in IoMT-based three-tier WBANs", *IEEE Internet of Things Journal*, vol. 9, pp. 1–1, 2021.

[81] S. Badotra, D. Nagpal, S. Narayan Panda, S. Tanwar, and S. Bajaj, "IoT-enabled healthcare network with ^{S}DN", in *2020 8th International Conference on Reliability, InfocomTechnologies and Optimization (Trends and Future Directions) (ICRITO)*, Noida, India, vol. 5, pp. 38–42, 2020. doi: 10.1109/ICRITO48877.2020.9197807

[82] M. Hashem, S. Vellappally, H. Fouad, M. Luqman, and A. E. Youssef, "Predicting neurological disorders linked to oral cavity manifestations using an IoMT-based optimized neural networks", *IEEE Access*, vol. 8, pp. 190722–190733, 2020.

[83] L. Xu, X. Zhou, Y. Tao, L. Liu, X. Yu, and N. Kumar, "Intelligent security performance prediction for IoT-enabled healthcare networks using an improved CNN," *IEEE Transactions on Industrial Informatics*, vol. 18, no. 3, pp. 2063–2074, 2022. doi: 10.1109/TII.2021.3082907

[84] R. Hireche, H. Mansouri, and A. S. K. Pathan, "Security and privacy management in internet of medical things (IoMT): A synthesis", *Journal of Cybersecurity and Privacy*, vol. 2, no. 2, pp. 640–661, 2022. https://doi.org/10.3390/jcp2030033

[85] B. P. Prathaban, R. Balasubramanian, and R. Kalpana, "ForeSeiz: An IoMT based headband for Real-time epileptic seizure forecasting", *Expert Systems*, vol. 18, no. 8, pp. 116–123, 2022.

[86] I. V. Pustokhina, D. A. Pustokhin, D. Gupta, A. Khanna, K. Shankar, and G. N. Nguyen, "An effective training scheme for deep neural network in edge computing enabled internet of medical things (IoMT) systems", *IEEE Access*, vol. 8, pp. 107112–107123, 2020.

[87] N. Bibi, M. Sikandar, I. Ud Din, A. Almogren, and S. Ali, "IoMT-based automated detection and classification of leukemia using deep learning", *Journal of Healthcare Engineering*, vol. 6, no. 4, pp. 164–172, 2020.

[88] L. Rachakonda, S. P. Mohanty, and E. Kougianos, "iLog: An intelligent device for automatic food intake monitoring and stress detection in the IoMT", *IEEE Transactions on Consumer Electronics*, vol. 66, pp. 115–124, 2020.

[89] L. Rachakonda, S. P. Mohanty, and E. Kougianos, "Stress-lysis: An IoMT-enabled device for automatic stress level detection from physical activities", *IEEE International Symposium on Smart Electronic Systems (iSES)*, pp. 204–205, 2020.

[90] P. Kumar, G. P. Gupta, and R. Tripathi, "An ensemble learning and fog-cloud architecture-driven cyber-attack detection framework for IoMT networks", *Computer Communications*, vol. 16, no. 6, pp. 110–124, 2021.

[91] M. F. Khan, T. M. Ghazal, R. A. Said, A. Fatima, S. Abbas, M. A. Khan, G. F. Issa, M. Ahmad, and M. A. Khan, "An IoMT-enabled smart healthcare model to monitor elderly people using machine learning technique", *Computational Intelligence and Neuroscience*, vol. 24, pp. 248–257, 2021.

[92] N. Naren, V. Chamola, S. Baitragunta, A. Chintanpalli, P. Mishra, S. Yenuganti, M. Guizani, "IoMT and DNN-enabled drone-assisted Covid-19 screening and detection framework for rural areas", *IEEE Internet of Things Magazine*, vol. 4, pp. 4–9, 2021.

[93] S. Mishra, H. K. Thakkar, P. K. Mallick, P. Tiwari, and A. Alamri, "A sustainable IoHT based computationally intelligent healthcare monitoring system for lung cancer risk detection", *Sustainable Cities and Society*, vol. 72, pp. 103–117, 2021.

[94] S. Nandy, M. Adhikari, M. A. Khan, V. G. Menon, and S. Verma, "An intrusion detection mechanism for secured IoMT framework based on swarm-neural network", *IEEE Journal of Biomedical and Health Informatics*, vol. 5, pp. 1–1, 2021.

[95] I. Ullah, H. Y. Youn, and Y. H. Han, "Integration of type-2 fuzzy logic and Dempster–Shafer theory for accurate inference of IoT-based healthcare system", *Future Generation Computer Systems*, vol. 124, pp. 369–380, 2021.

[96] K. Medhi, M. M. Arifuzzaman, and M. H. Iftekhar, "An approach to handle heterogeneous healthcare IoT data using deep convolutional neural network", In P. K. Bora, S. Nandi, S. Laskar (Eds.), *Emerging Technologies for Smart Cities*. Singapore: Springer, pp. 25–31, 2021.

[97] J. Deepika, C. Rajan, and T. Senthil, "Security and privacy of cloud- and IoT-based medical image diagnosis using fuzzy convolutional neural network", *Computational Intelligence and Neuroscience*, vol. 8, no. 2, pp. 661–674, 2021.

[98] X. Wu, C. Liu, L. Wang, and M. Bilal, "Internet of things-enabled real-time health monitoring system using deep learning", *Neural Computing and Applications*, vol. 5, no. 2, pp. 456–461, 2021.

[99] J. V. Chagas, D. A. Rodrigues, R. F. Ivo, M. M. Hassan, V. H. de Albuquerque, and P. P. Filho, "A new approach for the detection of pneumonia in children using CXR images based on an real-time IoT system", *Journal of Real-Time Image Processing*, vol. 18, no. 5, pp. 1099–1114, 2021.

[100] K. Hameed, I. S. Bajwa, N. Sarwar, W. Anwar, Z. Mushtaq, and T. Rashid, "Integration of 5G and block-chain technologies in smart telemedicine using IoT", *Journal of Healthcare Engineering*, 2021, vol. 5, no. 3, pp. 881–891.

[101] A. Armgarth, S. Pantzare, P. Arven, R. Lassnig, H. Jinno, E. O. Gabrielsson, Y. Kifle, D. Cherian, T. Arbring Sjöström, G. Berthou, J. Dowling, T. Someya, J. J. Wikner, G. Gustafsson, D. T. Simon, and M. Berggren, "A digital nervous system aiming toward personalized IoT healthcare", *Scientific Reports*, vol. 11, no. 7, pp. 75–82, 2021.

[102] M. Golec, R. Ozturac, Z. Pooranian, S. S. Gill, and R. Buyya, "iFaaSBus: A security and privacy based lightweight framework for serverless computing using IoT and machine learning", *IEEE Transactions on Industrial Informatics*, vol. 5, no. 3, pp. 11–17, 2021.

[103] S. Manimurugan, S. Al-Mutairi, M. M. Aborokbah, N. Chilamkurti, S. Ganesan, and R. Patan, "Effective attack detection in internet of medical things smart environment using a deep belief neural network", *IEEE Access*, vol. 8, no. 7, pp. 77396–77404, 2020.

[104] Z. Al-Makhadmeh, and A. Tolba, "Utilizing IoT wearable medical device for heart disease prediction using higher order Boltzmann model: A classification approach", *Measurement*, vol. 147, pp. 106–115, 2021.

[105] R. Patan, G. S. Pradeep Ghantasala, R. Sekaran, D. Gupta, and M. Ramachandran, "Smart healthcare and quality of service in IoT using grey filter convolutional based cyber physical system", *Sustainable Cities and Society*, vol. 59, no 10, pp. 102–110, 2020.

[106] M. G. R. Alam, S. F. Abedin, S. I. Moon, A. Talukder, and C. S. Hong, "Healthcare IoT-based affective state mining using a deep convolutional neural network", *IEEE Access*, vol. 7, no. 3, pp. 189–202, 2019.

[107] T. Vaiyapuri, A. Binbusayyis, and V. Varadarajan, "Security, privacy and trust in IoMT enabled smart healthcare system: A systematic review of current and future trends", *International Journal of Advanced Computer Science and Applications*, vol. 12, no. 7, pp. 678–685, 2021.

[108] R. Jeba Kumar, J. Roopa Jayasingh, and D. B. Telagathoti, "Intelligent transit healthcare schema using internet of medical things (IoMT) technology for remote patient monitoring", *Internet of Medical Things, Springer*, vol. 6, no. 7, pp. 17–33, 2021

[109] R. Alizadehsani, D. Sharifrazi, N. H. Izadi, J. H. Joloudari, A. Shoeibi, J. M. Gorriz, S. Hussain, J. E. Arco, Z. A. Sani, and F. Khozeimeh, "Uncertainty-aware semi-supervised method using large unlabeled and limited labeled COVID-19 data", *ACM Transactions on Multimedia Computing, Communications, and Applications (TOMM)*, vol. 17, pp. 1–24, 2021.

[110] A. G. Akpan, F. B. Nkubli, V. N. Ezeano, A. C. Okwor, M. C. Ugwuja, U. Offiong, In Ist edited book by: Agbotiname Lucky Imoize, D. Jude Hemanth, Dinh-Thuan Do & Samarendra Nath Sur, "XAI for medical image segmentation in medical decision support systems", *The Institution of Engineering and Technology (IET)*, pp. 137–165, 2022. http://doi.org/10.1049/PBHE050E

[111] Y. Djenouri, A. Belhadi, A. Yazidi, G. Srivastava, and J. Chun-Wei Lin, "Artificial intelligence of medical things for disease detection using ensemble deep learning and attention mechanism", *Expert Systems*, Wiley, 2022. http://doi.org/10.1111/exsy.13093

[112] J. J. Tom, and A. G. Akpan, "Cyberspace: Mitigating against cyber security threats and attacks", *International Journal of Engineering Research & Technology (IJERT)*, vol. 11, no. 11, pp. 327–332, 2022.

[113] A. G. Akpan, J. O. Ugah, and V. N. Ezeano, "Leveraging on cyber security for digital economy: Analysis of emerging cyber security threats and attacks", *International Journal of Scientific & Engineering Research*, vol. 13, no. 7, pp. 663–674, 2022.

[114] M. A. Habib, C. M. Nadeem Faisal, S. Sarwar, M. A. Latif, F. Aadil, M. Ahmad, R. Ashraf, and M. Maqsood, "Privacy-based medical data protection against internal security threats in heterogeneous internet of medical things", *International Journal of Distributed Sensor Networks*, vol. 15, no. 9, pp. 1–12, 2019. http://doi.org/10.1177/1550147719875653

[115] A. G. Akpan, F. B. Nkubli, V. N. Ezeano, A. C. Okwor, M. C. Ugwuja, U. Offiong. In Ist edited book by: Agbotiname Lucky Imoize, D. Jude Hemanth, Dinh-Thuan Do & Samarendra Nath Sur, "XAI methods for precision medicine in medical decision support systems", *The Institution of Engineering and Technology (IET)*, pp. 471–487, 2022. http://doi.org/10.1049/PBHE050E

[116] D. Oladimeji, "An intrusion detection system for internet of medical things", M.Sc. Dissertation in Computer Science, Dalhousie University, Halifax, Nova Scotia, 2021.

7 Application of Artificial Intelligence of Medical Things in Remote Healthcare Delivery

Manisha Srivastava, Ahmad Tasnim Siddiqui, and Vishal Srivastava

7.1 INTRODUCTION

The Internet of Medical Things (IoMT) is gaining universal recognition as well as making it possible to monitor, diagnose, forecast, and prevent communicable diseases. AI of medical Things (AIoMT) comes into existence with the introduction of AI into the Internet of Medical Things (IoMT) [1]. Artificial intelligence (AI), big data, and the Internet of Things (IoT) are all related areas for creating better-personalized healthcare systems. Utilizing interconnected wearable sensors and networks, AI and IoMT can be useful in the medical sector to control diseases effectively. This is called AIoMT. Infectious disease epidemiology is exploring the potential benefits of the Internet of Things (IoT) [2]. The AIoMT combines healthcare gadgets and applications with human resources and data management applications to create an innovative way of interacting. Among the cloud-based IoT, administrations are data transfer and information exchange, investigation, report authentication, clinical cleanliness sensitivity, patient monitoring, and much more. This technology can revolutionize the way medical services work while rewarding a massive number of patients with excellent treatment and more satisfaction, especially during infective disease testing, diagnosis, treatment, and observation. It is easier to interpret data when using AI-based data analytics, and it reduces the amount of time required to analyze data performance. Data can be visualized for better explanation and understanding [3].

Due to the increase in the patient, traditional healthcare system is facing lots of challenges. To overcome all the challenges and complications, IoMT was developed. IoMT is also responsible to handle the accuracy, privacy, and productivity of the health sector [4]. Physicians have been able to provide patients with appropriate recommendations with the use of a wearable and wireless AI-based system. The IoMT has been analyzed extensively in the medical field, resulting in a significant decrease in healthcare costs when diagnosing a patient. Decision-making has also improved, which resulted in better and more reliable treatment. With the Internet of Medical

Things, big data can be generated through the use of sensors and wearable devices for vital physiological and biophysical parameters observation, and data analytics can be performed on these data in other medical decision-making process systems [5–7]. By connecting devices, implementing AI-powered analytics, remotely monitoring patients, and utilizing robotics, telemedicine is transforming healthcare delivery. It is possible to access high-quality care, increase clinical efficiency, and improve access to care through telemedicine systems. With the support of a diverse ecosystem of hardware and software manufacturers, Intel facilitates scalable telemedicine. The entire world has changed due to the COVID-19 epidemic, and healthcare is one of them. As a result of this outbreak, providers were unexpectedly forced to find a way to treat and remotely monitor their patients to prevent the further spread of the disease. IoMT came into the picture and provided better support to the providers. As a result, patients stay more in touch with their providers, clinicians and specialists are easier to reach, and high-risk environments are avoided by both patients and providers [8].

To help patients self-administer treatments, an IoT-based system is able to capture data in real time. It is apparent that the healthcare system of developing countries is rapidly changing due to increased life expectancy during the 1990s, and infectious diseases also impacted a lot [5–7]. With the support of the Internet of Things, entire remote healthcare systems can be made available; they can be as simple as measuring blood pressure (BP) or as sophisticated as sending updates about specific organs within a person's body or even implants. Patients can monitor their vitals at home and send results to their doctors for analysis using wearables and other medical devices. Wearable medical devices are able to track patient vitals the whole day and will transfer and upload data to the cloud for easy, ongoing monitoring, both by the patient and by the healthcare professionals. Patients with chronic illnesses may benefit from this level of monitoring and may even avoid needing to go to an urgent care facility or emergency visits [9, 10]. In telemedicine, artificial intelligence is also improving the ability to take a patient's history by dynamically tweaking questions based on their reactions. The use of artificial intelligence-based tools can offer personalized medication reminders as well as suggest routine health checks based on personal monitoring data [8]. There is a growing interest in artificial intelligence and machine learning in the healthcare industry [11]. Unlike AI techniques like deep learning, explainable AI (XAI) uses machine learning (ML) to explain models and make decisions [12].

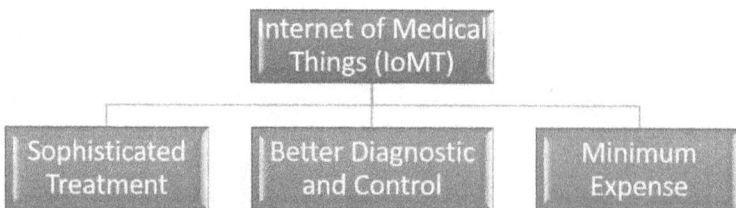

FIGURE 7.1 Major advantages of IoT.

Many IoMT applications of AI are available, which involve machine learning (ML) and natural language processing (NLP) in telehealth care. Accurate medication requires superior diagnostics and personalized treatments with quick delivery time. The AI is making it realistic by providing real-time solutions that establish new treatment pathways based on historical and current data. Personalized medication reminders and routine condition checks can be recommended by AI-powered tools based on personal monitoring data [13].

In the latest consequence, IT has opened new ways for advancement in our lives. Among these technologies, IoT with the combination of AI is an emergent technology that offers enhanced and realistic solutions in the health sector, e.g., keeping medical records appropriately, devices amalgamation, disease causes, and sampling [14].

IoT helps to provide various services in healthcare. IoMT offers an extensive range of services. Some of the important services provided by IoMT are Community Health Care, Pediatric Services, Emergency Health Care, Ambient-assisted Living, Drug Reaction, and m-Health.

IoT also supports the development of IoMT applications. IoMT offers a broad range of applications (Apps). Some of the vigorously used applications of IoMT are BP Monitoring, Glucose Level Detecting, Temperature Monitoring, Rehabilitation, ECG Monitoring, Wheelchair Management, Cognitive Computing, and many more.

7.1.1. OBJECTIVES

- Background study of telemedicine and healthcare applications
- Review of the earlier and modern telemedicine system
- A concurrent study of modish telemedicine systems
- Exploring possible benefits and impacts of AioMT

7.1.2. KEY CONTRIBUTIONS OF THE CHAPTER

The following are the important contributions of the chapter:

- The chapter examines some important applications in the medical sector.
- The potential benefits and impact of IoMT have been discussed.
- Architecture of IoMT has been examined.

7.1.3. CHAPTER ORGANIZATION

Section 7.2 presents the related works on the AI-enabled system, IoT and IoMT, and AioMT in the healthcare industry. Section 7.3 presents the methodology used. Section 7.4 is about the architecture of the IoMT framework, Section 7.5 discusses the applications of AioMT in remote healthcare, Section 7.6 presents the potential benefits and impacts of AioMT, Section 7.7 talks about Challenges in Remote Healthcare Delivery, Section 7.8 talks about the limitations of this study, and finally, Section 7.9 concludes the chapter with future direction.

7.2. RELATED WORK

The purpose of this section is to investigate various existing models that are being developed and implemented using AI, IoT, and IoMT in healthcare. Recent years have seen that the concept of IoT has been used extensively in almost every space of healthcare. Many proposed systems have been introduced and frameworks were offered to serve the health sector. Lots of research and innovation have been done during COVID-19.

It is estimated that a significant impact on the healthcare sector will come from IoT and health technologies within the coming decade [15]. Some important works have been mentioned here:

Jung and Agulto [16] suggested a method for monitoring and tracking pandemics using virtual IoT devices. In addition, this system makes it possible for anyone to monitor and track COVID-19 patients from anywhere in the world in real time. As part of its ongoing monitoring program, the CDC installs COVID-19 VioT (virtual Internet of Things) on the smartphones of people who need to be monitored. The goal of this platform is to provide various secret keys to everyone in order to assure authentication and confidentiality.

Mohammed et al. [17] recommended an IoT-based smart helmet that has a fixed thermal imaging system on it. It detects COVID-19 by analyzing its thermal properties. The smart helmet includes a thermal camera with the arrangement of IoT to observe the screening practice to acquire real-time data. Furthermore, the model is also furnished with facial detection, which shows personal details instantly. The anticipated model has been greatly lauded in the medical systems and would be helpful for the deterrence of COVID-19 increase.

Singh et al. [18] summarized the benefits of employing the IoT for slashing the cost of healthcare. The explorational analysis defined and argued the 12 most important products of IoT to tackle the COVID-19 epidemic.

According to Darwish et al. [19], a Cloud IoT-Health design integrates IoT with Cloud Computing in the medical sector. The research emphasized the challenges encountered by the incorporation along with the current developments in Cloud IoT-Health. The hurdles are characterized by three levels: (i) communication and networking, (ii) technology, and (iii) intelligence.

According to Siriwardhana et al. [20], there is a need to deploy IoT and 5G technologies in order to effectively fight the coronavirus pandemic. The authors also provide some use case circumstances with their challenges and explain how IoT and 5G could facilitate creative approaches to overcome this pandemic in various fields. Likewise, a thorough overview of technologies such as IoT, AI, UAVs, 5G, and blockchain being developed to combat pandemics is presented.

Siddiqui [21] highlighted that when medical consultation is needed for a chronic disease emergency, telehealth monitoring can support remote communities in receiving care in time. In remote areas, it is regarded as an important method of reforming the healthcare system. It can be most effectively used in public healthcare facilities. Improving the quality of health services demands improved accessibility of health statistics. AI-enabled systems can utilize this data to improve medications.

A study by Hussain et al. [22] emphasized the significance of applying artificial intelligence to fight against coronavirus and other diseases. An analysis of several intelligence methodologies suited to different types of medical data was presented in the research study. Also, neural systems and edge-significant learning have been categorized into SVMs (Support Vector Machines) in the present AI technique for clinical data analysis.

An IoMT-SAF, short for Internet of Things Security Assessment Mechanism, has been proposed by Alsubaei et al. [23]. It has been proposed that ontological-based techniques would ensure security in the IoMT environment. It helped participants to select and measure accessible security decisions created for their security, safety, and privacy necessities. It additionally assisted in the process of decision-making.

A proposed blockchain-based private communication framework by Wazid et al. [24] was for drone-assisted healthcare in an IoT-enabled situation and to tackle various threats. A variety of performance parameters were measured to prove the efficacy of their access control, validation, verification, and key management schemes.

According to Camara et al. [25], implantable medical devices (IMDs) can treat patients and constantly monitor their health reports remotely. They also argued about the security, safety, and privacy threat connected to by means of IMDs.

Several methods have been proposed by Merabet et al. [26], which could be used in IoT-based healthcare systems. These include Machine-to-Machine (M2M) and Machine-to-Cloud (M2C) systems. Additionally, they introduced two protocols, the M2C verification protocol, and the M2M verification and validation protocol.

Sundaravadivel et al. [27] in their study argue that a market worth 350 billion dollars is predicted for IoT-based smart healthcare by 2025. Healthcare is increasingly adopting smart medicines and smart radio frequency identification (RFID) cabinets, both of which tap into the Circular Economy (CE) and the Internet of Things (IoT) [26].

Lalmuanawma et al. [28] demonstrated the applications of AI/ML for healthcare. To increase the accuracy of the diagnosis and investigation process for COVID-19 patients, advanced ML and AI solutions are used in conjunction with "radio imaging" technology, which follows a similar approach to blood sample analysis, computed tomography (CT), and X-rays.

In their research, Sedik et al. [29] used a deep learning-based method that has been developed to examine COVID-19 patients through X-rays and CT scans, and the technique has been proven to be 100% accurate.

V. Iguoba and A. L. Imoize [30] argue about psychological factors. According to them, an explanation of healthcare systems from a psychological perspective is very relevant.

According to Frost & Sullivan, the healthcare industry is expected to save over $150 billion by 2025 as a result of artificial intelligence (AI) and cognitive computing. Currently, medical data is becoming increasingly complex and is requiring the use of these technologies to handle the complication and progress of medical data. Using AI in healthcare, providers are able to improve patient outcomes by integrating genomic, clinical, financial, and behavioral data in real-time.

7.2.1 AI AND IoMT IN HEALTHCARE INDUSTRY

IoMT with AI includes machine learning (ML) and natural language processing (NLP) in the preventive medical system. For the system to work, advanced diagnostic testing and tailored treatments must be developed promptly. Through the use of real-time analytics, artificial intelligence can identify new corridors for treating certain conditions that are established on historical and current data. AI solutions can be used to modify the various characteristics of the healthcare ecosystem. NLP technology is capable of extracting information from these unstructured data points. This type of unstructured data can appear as lab reports, operative transcripts, physical assessment notes, and another clearance-related patient information. In particular, these will include artificial intelligence techniques for creating classifiers that will automate the process of capturing patient details, creating a schedule of patient meeting slots, and treatment plans, and the determination of lab tests, medications, and surgical treatments [31].

The use of artificial intelligence (AI) in healthcare is widespread, especially for disease prediction, which enables physicians to diagnose patients' conditions more accurately, such as diabetes [32], and for robotic surgery [33]. Using complex analysis algorithms, this technology makes inferences and predicts medical diagnoses based on data collected by IoT. For periodic control, IoT, and analysis purposes, AI will combine to make connected healthcare monitoring devices intelligent. Nanotechnology and AI-supported approaches combined together with IoMT are crucial for emerging novel healthcare results, involving nanomedicines and nanorobotics.

With progress in cloud computing and the ability to process huge amounts of data, AI/ML has shown potential in observing cardiac electrophysiology and cardiac imageries. AI and ML are competent and processed on data collected from IoMT devices, for example smartwatches, smartphones, and medical imaging in order to enhance disease diagnosis, predict aftereffects, and characterize unusual illnesses.

IoMT is rapidly gaining significance as AI and its supported technologies, including Deep Learning (DL), Machine Learning (ML), Natural Language Processing (NLP), and Computer Vision (CV), grow. As a result of all the aspects of AI listed earlier, all autonomous actions in AI-assisted surgery are based on AI [34].

Panesar and Ashkan et al. argued how the internet and mobile platforms, commanded by AI, can furnish surgical skills remotely. Surgical robots can be guided to carry out surgeries, where proper resources are absent or inaccessible, for example, in space or in areas affected by environmental disasters or wars [35].

To train the system, five input columns are used: age, pregnancy, BMI (body mass index), sugar, and sugar and insulin levels. To evaluate the data set, ML algorithms such as Random Forest, Neural Network, Decision Tree, and k-nearest neighbor (kNN) with secret tiers were used.

7.2.2 OTHER USEFUL TECHNOLOGIES IN HEALTHCARE

Here is a brief introduction to the application of AI methodologies to the medical IoT. It will be important for several technologies to play a role in empowering smart hospices. Some of the technologies are as follows:

Big Data Analytics: Digital prescriptive maintenance (DPM) can be implemented in smart hospitals by utilizing analytics to gain actionable insights. Big data analytics can be used to inspect electronic health records (EHRs) and hospital systems, manage community health research data, and reduce re-hospitalization.

Blockchain: Using blockchain solutions, users can manage and share health records and patient health samples with specific residents. The blockchain network will facilitate the smooth and seamless payment of claims by insurance companies, hospitals, and patients. Blockchain technology plays a vital role in ensuring the security of the system and preventing data leaks. Data stored on this platform is protected. Hospitals, pharmacies, and other health sectors can benefit from this by sharing data securely and by increasing their market potential, so all health sectors can be brought together [36].

5G Networking: It consists of five generations of cellular technology designed to reduce latency, improve speed, and make wireless services more flexible. The 5G network is more flexible and faster than the 4G network. 5G networking provides a theoretical speed of up to 20 Gbps as compared to 4G only 1 Gbps. In addition, 5G promises to provide lower latency, making business applications and other digital experiences such as self-driving cars and online gaming better. Using 5G technology, healthcare providers will be able to regularly monitor vital symptoms such as pulse rate and blood pressure via connected devices [37].

7.3 METHODOLOGY

During the course of this study, systematic reviews of the literature published in apparent international conferences and journals by the foremost publisher's databases, such as IEEE Xplore, PubMed, Google Scholar, and ScienceDirect, have been crawled. An initial literature search was conducted in IEEE Xplore and PubMed using the keywords "IoMT", "AIoMT", and "IoMT in Healthcare." We chose these electronic databases because they are famous databases for IoT and medical studies. The screening results in IEEE have revealed 6,151 papers, and those in PubMed have revealed 2,192; however, duplicate publications were excluded from the results few journal articles remained in IEEE's database and PubMed after applying filtration to articles published from 2017 to 2022.

We also searched within ScienceDirect for the period of 2017–2022 and it returned 2,643 results for "AI Enabled Internet of Medical Things." We excluded a few irrelevant papers from our screening process.

The initial search based on the inclusion criteria produced 8,343 articles. However, after filtering by title and abstract, excluding duplicate articles, and taking into account full-text accessibility, a total of 2,385 articles were found relevant. We have

TABLE 7.1

AI Algorithm Applications in Medical Sector with Their Advantages and Disadvantages

AI Algorithms	Applications in Medical Disciplines	Benefits	Drawbacks
Support Vector Machine (SVM)	• Biomarker imaging in neural and mental ailments [38] • Human Machine Interaction [39] • Cancer treatment [40] • Initial discovery of Alzheimer's disease [41] • Heart examination [42] • Forecasting surgical place infection [43] • Diabetes observation [44] • Surgical procedure [45–47] • Epidemic resource management [48] • Healthcare monitoring system [49]	Highly precise, meeting a solution to a difficulty, solving complications, adequate scaling of multiresolution data, and a minimum sample size is required.	Selecting the suitable kernel function is essential, to the obligation of longer training time for big data sets, and high analytical costs.
Neural Network (NN)	• Cancer identification and treatment [50–53] • Detecting Parkinson's disease [54] • Image-based cardiovascular observation [42] • Alzheimer's ailment [55, 56] • Surgical procedure [45–47] • Sensor apps [57, 58] • Diabetes forecasting [59] • Human-machine interface [60] • Managing epidemic resources [61] • Computer vision [62]	Effectual, quick, and compliant algorithm. Computes output without programming, constantly learns, and enriches. Widely applicable and suitable for multitasking. It can function with nonlinear and complex databases.	Extensive training time and bulky data sets are necessary. Excessive hardware costs and needs long and problematic programs. Understanding and alteration are difficult because of the BlackBox nature. Disposed to overfitting. Excessive data reliance may produce incorrect outcomes.

Naïve Bayes (NB)	• Ailment forecast [63] • Health diagnosis [64, 65] • Systems administration [65] • Managing epidemic resources [49]	Easy accomplishment, high learning, and categorization speed. Able to manage overfitting, disorderly data, and missing quantities. Able to forecast the category of a test dataset. Helpful for resolving multi-class projection troubles.	Inclined for the non-ideal training set. Difficulty in implementing regressions and co-dependent properties. Not appropriate for complicated glitches.
k-nearest neighbor (kNN)	• Sugar level tests for diabetes [44] • Epidemic resource administration [48] • Ailment forecast [66] • Computer-assisted diagnosis [67] • Heart ailment forecast [68] • Healthcare observation system [49]	Easy procedure. No postulations for the aspects and results of the dataset. Effective against disorderly data and handling large data. Steady performance, rapid learning pace, and good overfitting administration.	Time-consuming, and sensitive to local data. Average accuracy, slow classification rate. Poor management of correlated data
Decision Tree (DT)	• Sugar level tests for diabetes [28] • Surgical procedure [15, 50] • Medical diagnosis [55] • Systems performance management [55] • Healthcare observation technique [39]	Rapid, efficient, and straightforward to understand and decode. Can operate on an enormous variety of data types. High computational learning, and categorization rate.	Complicated estimations, time and mathematically costly. Weak in controlling overfitting, incorrect, and correlated data. Incompetent at execution of regression and has average precision.

(Continued)

TABLE 7.1 (Continued)
AI Algorithm Applications in Medical Sector with Their Advantages and Disadvantages

AI Algorithms	Applications in Medical Disciplines	Benefits	Drawbacks
Random Forest (RF)	• Disease predicting [59, 60] • Healthcare supervising system [39] • Heart ailment forecast [27]	Good for managing corrupt data. High categorization pace. Good for controlling huge and diverse databases. Defining qualities automatically. Input feature regularization is not important.	The composite work function, and hassles in finishing. Moderate accurateness, gradual learning pace, poor control of absent values. Disposed to overfitting. The appropriate clarity of depth and number of trees is important.
Logistic Regression (LR)	• Image-based heart monitoring [27] • Sugar level tests for diabetes [28] • Epidemic resource management [38] • Healthcare observing system [39, 61]	Simple implementation and elucidation. Good working out efficacy. Outputs are well synchronized and classified. Experimental parameter tweaking is not required. Excellent accuracy for easy data sets.	Thumps to solve non-linear barriers. Imagines linearity in reliant and independent variables. Organized to overfitting for high dimensional datasets. Extremely reliant on parameters and characteristics.

used AND and OR logic keywords in the search criteria of the articles. In addition, this systematic review also considered significant articles within the references of the selected articles.

7.4 ARCHITECTURE OF IOMT FRAMEWORK

As the internet has been integrated and inhabited into our daily lives, we have seen IoMT applications and systems emerge.

Typically, IoMT systems work in these key layers that integrate various devices, tools, and technologies, detecting sensors, and systems that are all linked through electrical and electronic connections and wireless links. The structure and performance of every layer are illustrated in Figure 7.2 given next [69]:

Perception layer: A perception layer of the IoMT consists of data sources such as health monitors, smart devices, and mobile applications, which encompass sensors, for example, infrared sensors, medical instruments, radio frequency identification (RFID) cameras, smart device sensors, and global positioning systems (GPS). By using a robust, wireless, or wired network broadcast framework, which functions as the high-level performing transportation medium, sensing systems recognize changes in an environment; recognize objects, locations, longitudes and latitudes (magnitudes), demographics, etc.; and transform statistics into digital signals [69].

Gateway layer: As previously described, networks provide communication and storage of information between sensors and gateways. In addition to RFID, Bluetooth, wireless sensor networks, low-power Wi-Fi, Zigbee, and mobile communications [70]. Communication can also be short-range, such as with RFID, wireless

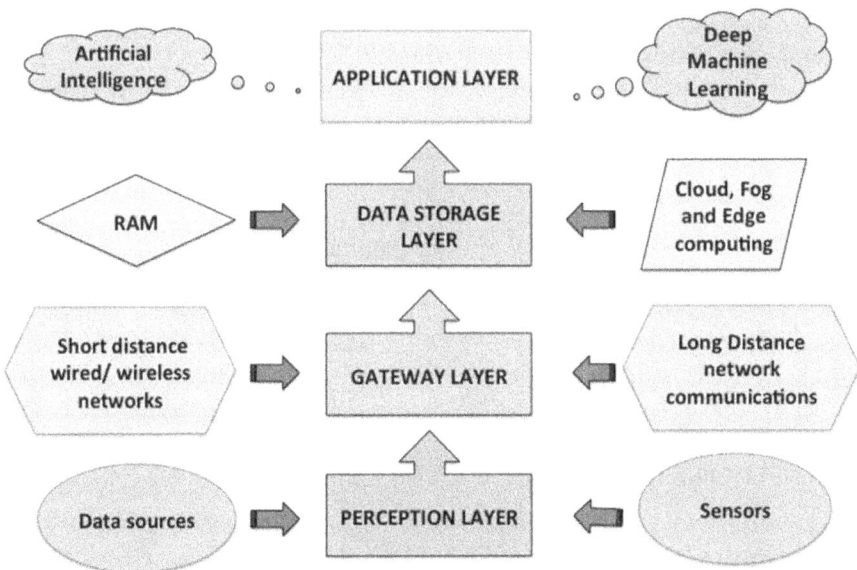

FIGURE 7.2 Layer architecture of IoMT Framework [70].

sensor networks, and cloud computing. Applications of IoMT can be boosted and become major factors in healthcare growth as a result of the colossal communication potential [71].

Data storage layer: Management services, security controls, process modeling, and device management tools must be able to work at a rapid pace to process massive raw data in order to extract relevant information. Data management, data analysis, and user management are all incorporated into this management/application layer [70].

Application or service layer: The application layer functions primarily for interpreting data and delivering services tailored to applications. Using AI and deep machine learning (DML), the application layer comprehends the EMR data and monitors trends and variations in the scrutinization of data on a daily or weekly basis to make judgments concerning diagnosis and cure [70].

7.5 APPLICATIONS OF AIOMT IN REMOTE HEALTHCARE

As we move forward with each passing day, the future of healthcare is slowly taking shape. As the IoT becomes more widespread, a variety of healthcare solutions will be enabled, each bringing with it its own set of benefits. By redefining the space where devices interconnect with people and healthcare solutions are delivered, the Internet of Things is undoubtedly renovating the healthcare industry. With the advancements in the diagnostic and curative sectors, it has never been more pertinent to recognize that we humans keep a close eye on medical developments.

With the adoption of IoMT and associated technology, some complications associated with remote intensive care, telehealth, telemedicine, robots, and sensors have been resolved. In spite of this, mass adoption of the technology appears challenging due to considerations such as data privacy and security, management and control of large amounts of data, flexibility, and upgrades.

The transformation of an outdated healthcare system into one that is smart and modified is recognized by the dawn of modern medical devices geared around IoMT-based technologies. Coronavirus has expanded the use of many standing IoMT-based devices. The COVID-19 event has spawned an incalculable number of devices that were explicitly created for the event. There are many benefits associated with IoMT in healthcare for patients, physicians, patient families, hospitals, and insurance companies also. Individuals and their families living alone are impacted significantly.

Figure 7.3 shows various types of IoMT healthcare services and applications.

Some of the services provided are Ambient Assisted Living (AAL), Community Healthcare (CH), Children's Health Information (CHI), Adverse Drug Reaction (ADR), Wearable Device Access (WDA), and Semantic Medical Access (SMA) [72].

APPLICATIONS OF THE INTERNET OF THINGS IN HEALTHCARE

Researchers have created a framework for managing health data sources like EHRs and medical images using analytical applications for healthcare systems [73]. A service-based approach is used in application development that sick people and other users require, regardless of their use of applications. Accordingly, services are

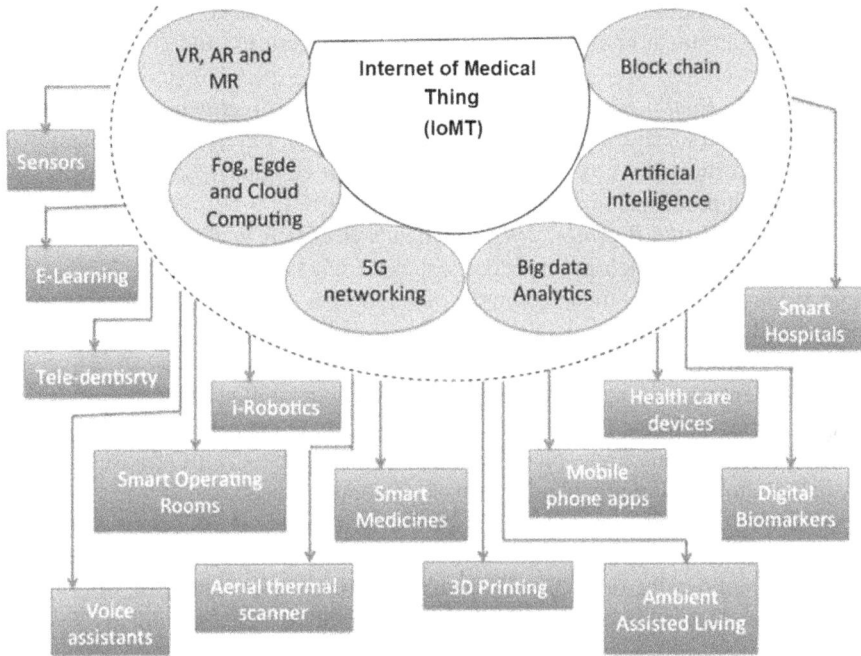

FIGURE 7.3 IoMT and related technologies [70].

developed in response to the developer's offerings, while applications are developed in response to the user's needs [73].

Glucose Level Sensing: The metabolic disease diabetes is symbolized by persistently high blood glucose (sugar) levels. Medication timing, meal planning, and activity planning can be made easier by monitoring blood glucose levels [69].

Electrocardiogram Monitoring: A simple pulse rate, the basic pace, and a diagnosis of arrhythmias, cardiac or myocardial ischemia, and prolonged QT periods are all included in the inspection of the electrocardiogram (ECG), i.e., the activity of the heart recorded by electrocardiography sometimes also known as the cardiac monitor.

Medication Management: There is a serious risk to public well-being from noncompliance in the medication market, as well as a huge financial loss caused by this problem. AIoMT presents some promising solutions for tackling this problem [73].

BP and Body temperature Monitoring: In order to make IoT-based blood and BP monitor, a KIT meter and an NFC (Near Field Communication) cellphone are combined. Combining the tools optimizes blood pressure measurement. And for body temperature measurement, combining a thermometer with an IoT channel is the key to this technology. RFID nodes are used in IoT systems to measure body temperature and transmit data.

Oxygen Saturation Monitoring: In this technology, the oximeter is attached to IoT using either Bluetooth or the Internet to make sure the transfer of instantaneous data between the patient and medical experts.

Imminent Healthcare: Medical reception becomes easier and more secure with the deployment of IoT-based amenities, architectures, and application software [73].

Children's Health Information (CHI): A vital part of growing understanding around children's health is educating the community as well as children themselves and their families about the needs of children with emotional, social, ethical, and mental health problems.

Electronic Health Record (EHR): A patient's electronic health record (EHR) is a digital replication of their paper record. An electronic health record (EHR) is a real-time, patient-centric documentation that makes access to information instantaneous, secure, and available for everyone with authorization.

Remote Patient Monitoring: The most common application of IoT devices is remote patient monitoring. It is expected that IoT devices will be able to collect patient health metrics collected from a medical facility without the patient being physically present, including pulse rate, blood pressure, fever, and more. This removes the need for patients to travel to providers or to pick up items themselves [73].

Adverse Drug Reaction (ADR): Adverse drug reaction (ADR) refers to damage caused by medication. Through the use of barcodes or NFC-enabled devices, the terminal identifies the drug. Based on this information, an intelligent information system determines whether a drug is harmonious with the patient's allergy synopsis and electronic health testimony [73].

Ingestible Sensors: The process of collecting data from the human body is usually messy and time-consuming. Nobody enjoys having a camera or other devices stuck in their digestive area. Through the use of ingestible sensors, information can be collected in a much less invasive manner from the digestive and other systems. They can determine PH levels in the stomach, for example, or locate the source of internal bleeding.

Point-of-Care Devices: Equipment used outside the laboratories for diagnosis [74].

It is essential that the devices are small enough to be swallowed easily. Furthermore, they must be safe to ingest, as well as able to liquefy or pass through the body easily. Numerous companies are working on digestible sensors that meet these criteria.

An IoT gadget accumulates patient data and the information is sent to the application where healthcare specialists and patients can access it. To recommend treatments or generate alerts, algorithms may analyze the data. Healthcare professionals may be alerted if a patient's heart rate falls unusually low, for instance, by an IoT sensor. There are IoMT devices that are very popular and beneficial. Some eminent IoMT devices in healthcare are Systematic Insulin Delivery, Swallowable Sensors, Sensor-enabled Nebulizers, Connected Catheters, Smart Medication Dispensers, and Parkinson's House.

7.6 THE POTENTIAL BENEFITS AND IMPACTS OF AIOMT

Despite having access to healthcare facilities in the poorest and most remote locations, traditional healthcare is experiencing technologically advanced and connected products that are putting a paradigm shift in motion as a result of digital transformation in consumers' hands. As a result of the evolving new drifts in technologies, the Internet of Medical Things is becoming increasingly widespread and capable of observing, diagnosing, predicting, and preventing transmissible ailments. IoMT, artificial intelligence (AI), and big data all play important roles in designing a better healthcare system, thanks to their major contributions. AIIoMT, which brings together AI and the Internet of Things, enables appropriate control of diseases by utilizing interconnected wearable sensors and networks. AIIoMT combines healthcare devices and their applications with human resource and data revolution systems to create an innovative way of connecting the two. When offering healthcare to all groups of patients without favoritism to the rich or the poor, the AI-IoMT strategy should be investigated to see if it can achieve a positive outcome in defying progressive diseases. By analyzing the relationship between the measured signals and the sample parameters, AI/ML can extract hidden information from IoMT devices. Measurement time, signal strength, sensitivity, and specificity can also be improved through AI techniques.

The IoMT and AI are bridging this gap and creating new avenues for improving India's current healthcare system on the basis of cost, efficacy, efficiency, and approachability. A fully connected ecosystem is being created by intelligent sensors, enabling remote or home healthcare to become mainstream. It is essential for IoMT to integrate sensors, AI, big data, and blockchain as well as provide multiple benefits to patients.

Some of the key benefits are as follows [74]:

Improved Patient Care: A better treatment outcome can be achieved with improved patient care.

Lowered Per-Patient Costs: As per the study by Deloitte, US healthcare expenditure will touch $8.3 trillion thru 2040. There are, however, solutions that can reduce this number with the use of the Internet of Medical Things.

Improved Patient Experience: The patient experience becomes even more important as healthcare moves toward value-based care. Patients' outcomes are improved by IoMT, patient visits are reduced, and doctor-patient communication is improved.

Reduced Burden on Practitioners: The Internet of Medical Things helps practitioners overcome burnout, which is experienced by almost 80% of them.

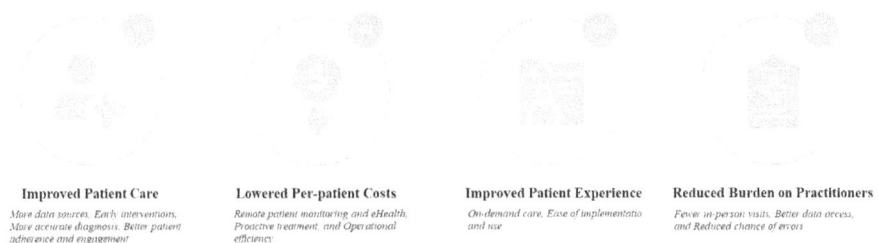

Improved Patient Care	Lowered Per-patient Costs	Improved Patient Experience	Reduced Burden on Practitioners
More data sources. Early interventions. More accurate diagnosis. Better patient adherence and engagement	Remote patient monitoring and eHealth. Proactive treatment. and Operational efficiency	On-demand care. Ease of implementatio and use	Fewer in-person visits. Better data access. and Reduced chance of errors

FIGURE 7.4   Key benefits of IoMT [74].

7.7 CHALLENGES IN REMOTE HEALTHCARE DELIVERY

The implementation of remote healthcare systems is not an easy task. There are many challenges to be overcome, ranging from infrastructure, operations, management, standards, legal, awareness, and acceptability. To achieve the true goal of remote healthcare, we must focus on other factors in addition to security and privacy. Some of the challenges are given as follows:

- There is a lack of adequate infrastructure.
- There is no proper integration between legacy healthcare systems and traditional healthcare systems.
- There is a shortage of healthcare professionals with specialized skills.
- Medical devices used in remote health care do not have enough service centers.
- The lack of a legal framework that defines the roles and responsibilities of each stakeholder, as well as legal action in the event of non-compliance.
- Absence of trust. A tendency for people to resist changes and be hesitant to trust new services exists by nature.
- Health monitoring equipment is unfamiliar to most patients.
- Identifying those patients who should be given priority to monitor remotely.
- Lack of inclusive and national policies and regulations concerning remote healthcare.
- Lack of global standards for equipment and file formats for storing and analyzing health data. Interoperability is, therefore, complicated.

Other Challenges:

- *Security challenges*: As a result of the large network of linked devices and the sensitive nature of the data, cyberattacks and security threats are more likely to occur. A growing number of devices will increase the risk of a network breach. The sensitive data of a person is involved, so security is an essential factor. Hospitals maintain enormous amounts of data, including prescriptions, bills, medical records, and claim settlements [36].
- *Interoperability*: It is imperative that IoMT devices transmit and use data efficiently in the network in order for it to be effective.
- *Rise in temperature*: In the IoMT device, the antennas absorb radiation and the circuitry consumes power, which causes the temperature to rise. As a result of the increase in temperature, tissue and other organs of the user under observation may be damaged. It is therefore essential to consider transmission and power consumption in IoMT devices [75].
- *Scaling capabilities*: The progression of any technology depends on how highly it is scaled. Health bodies need to use medical devices to their utmost potential so that they can push value-added results.

To overcome all the remote patient monitoring challenges, there needs to be a specific and effective AI-based remote monitoring management system that can help in decision-making. By using the system, healthcare organizations can become more efficient and patients can receive the care they need, no matter where they are.

7.8   LIMITATIONS OF THE STUDY

In this study, we used both centralized and distributed databases whose input data was based on Digital Device input data. These database systems must be protected from physical tampering, internet-based software attacks, network-based attacks, and hardware-based attacks. Another concern is data privacy, especially since IoT devices are being used in more sensitive industries, like healthcare. It can assist in making cities and homes smarter by allowing them to be controlled via mobile phones. It enhances security and offers personal protection. When we automate our processes, we save a lot of time. The information is easily accessible, even if we are far away from our actual location, and it is updated frequently.

7.9   CONCLUSIONS

As a result of modern technology being used in healthcare systems, global health challenges are being solved in a more equitable manner, allowing both the poor and rich to benefit from medical services. Most telemedicine frameworks utilize live chat, video conferencing, or regular telephones to communicate with specialists or attendants. As infectious diseases increase and medical costs rise, healthcare systems in developing countries are becoming increasingly ineffective. We should be thankful for modern technological equipment growth, which has given considerable development in the health sector. A unique therapy can be developed for every patient by using IoMT. This allows caregivers to create therapies tailored to their specific needs and characteristics. Furthermore, AIoMT-based medical systems are formed on a feedback loop, which means feedback is automatically repeated for better patient outcomes. Patients have benefitted from AI and IoT-based systems by receiving real-time treatment and creating a social forum for assistance. This chapter presents a system enabling AI-based IoMT in the healthcare domain. With the availability of applications like ECG Monitoring, Glucose Level Sensing, Oxygen Level Monitoring, BP Monitoring, and smartphone healthcare solutions, we are able to monitor patients and share their vitals quickly and accurately. These applications are blessings to the patients. The use of IoMT system-enabled, AI-based models in healthcare systems is challenging for a number of reasons, e.g., data security and privacy. Some other challenges include interoperability, confidentiality, and resource management. To fully benefit from AIoMT models in healthcare systems, it is urgent to address these problems. In the future, we need to work more on the privacy and security of AIoMT-based systems.

REFERENCES

[1] A. L. Imoize, P. A. Gbadega, H. I. Obakhena, D. O. Irabor, K. V. N. Kavitha, and C. Chakraborty (2022). "Artificial intelligence-enabled internet of medical things for COVID-19 pandemic data management". In A. L. Imoize, J. Hemanth, D.-T. Do, and S. N. Sur (eds.), Explainable Artificial Intelligence in Medical Decision Support Systems, 1st ed. The Institution of Engineering and Technology, pp. 357–380.

[2]   J. B. Awotunde, S. O. Folorunso, S. A. Ajagbe, J. Garg, and G. J. Ajamu (2022). "Chapter 10 AiIoMT: IoMT-based system-enabled artificial intelligence for enhanced smart healthcare systems". In F. Al-Turjman and A. Nayyar (eds.), Machine Learning for Critical Internet of Medical Things. Springer Nature, 2022, pp. 229–254.

[3]   D. V. Dimitrov (2016). "Medical internet of things and big data in healthcare". Healthc Inform Res, 22(3), pp. 156–163.

[4]   S. A. Wagan, J. Koo, I. F. Siddiqui, et al. (2022). "Internet of medical things and trending converged technologies: A comprehensive review on real-time applications". J King Saud Univ—Comp Inf Sci. https://doi.org/10.1016/j.jksuci.2022.09.005.

[5]   P. Kaur, R. Kumar, and M. Kumar (2019). "A healthcare monitoring system using random forest and internet of things (IoT)". Multimed Tools Appl, 78(14), pp. 19905–19916.

[6]   F. E. Ayo, J. B. Awotunde, R. O. Ogundokun, S. O. Folorunso, and A. O. Adekunle (2020). "A decision support system for multi-target disease diagnosis: A bioinformatics approach". Heliyon, 6(3), e03657.

[7]   I. D. Oladipo, A. O. Babatunde, J. B. Awotunde, and M. Abdulraheem (2021). "An Improved hybridization in the diagnosis of diabetes mellitus using selected computational intelligence". Commun Comp Inf Sci, 2021(1350), 272–285.

[8]   The Future of Telemedicine Technology with IoT and AI—Intel (n.d.). "Intel". www.intel.com/content/www/us/en/healthcare-it/telemedicine.html. Accessed on: 10/10/2022.

[9]   B. Fong, A. C. M. Fong, and C. K. Li. (2010). Telemedicine Technologies: Information Technologies in Medicine and Telehealth. John Wiley & Sons. https://doi.org/10.1002/9780470972151

[10] I. Antohe, M. Floria, and E. M. Carausu (2017). "Telemedicine: Good or bad and for whom?". 2017. E-Health and Bioengineering Conference (EHB), Sinaia, pp. 49–52. https://doi.org/10.1109/EHB.2017.7995358

[11] O. B. Ayoade et al. (2022). "Explainable artificial intelligence (XAI) in medical decision systems (MDSSs): Healthcare systems perspective". In A. L. Imoize, J. Hemanth, D.-T. Do, and S. N. Sur (eds.), Explainable Artificial Intelligence in Medical Decision Support Systems, 1st ed. The Institution of Engineering and Technology, pp. 1–43.

[12] J. B. Awotunde, E. A. Adeniyi, S. A. Ajagbe, A. L. Imoize, O. A. Oki, and S. Misra (2022). "Explainable artificial intelligence (XAI) in medical decision support systems (MDSS): Applicability, prospects, legal implications, and challenges". In A. L. Imoize, J. Hemanth, D.-T. Do, and S. N. Sur (eds.), Explainable Artificial Intelligence in Medical Decision Support Systems, 1st ed. The Institution of Engineering and Technology, pp. 45–90.

[13] S. Razdan and S. Sharma (2021). "Internet of medical things (IoMT): Overview, emerging technologies, and case studies". IETE Tech Rev. https://doi.org/10.1080/02564602.2021.1927863

[14] M. Javaid and I. H. Khan (2021). "Internet of things (IoT) enabled healthcare helps to take the challenges of COVID-19 pandemic". J Oral Biol Craniofacial Res, 11(2), pp. 209–214.

[15] A. A. Aljabr and K. Kumar (2022). "Design and implementation of internet of medical things (IoMT) using artificial intelligent for mobile-healthcare". Measurement Sens. https://doi.org/10.1016/j.measen.2022.100499.

[16] Y. Jung and R. Agulto (2020). "A public platform for virtual IoT-based monitoring and tracking of COVID-19". Electronics, 10(12), (Basel) 2021.

[17] M. N. Mohammed, et al. (2020). "Novel COVID-19 detection and diagnosis system using IOT based smart helmet". Int J Psychosoc Rehabil, 24(7), pp. 2296–303.

[18] R. P. Singh, M. Javaid, A. Haleem, and R. Suman (2020). "Internet of things (IoT) applications to fight against COVID-19 pandemic". Diabetes Metab Syndr Clin Res Rev, 14(4), pp. 521–524.

[19] A. Darwish, A. E. Hassanien, M. Elhoseny, A. K. Sangaiah, and K. Muhammad (2019). "The impact of the hybrid platform of internet of things and cloud computing on health-care systems: Opportunities, challenges, and open problems". J Ambient Intell Humaniz Comput, 10(10), pp. 4151–4166.

[20] Y. Siriwardhana, G. De Alwis, G. Gur, M. Ylianttila, and M. Liyanage (2020). "The fight against COVID-19 pandemic with 5G technologies". IEEE Eng Manag Rev. https://doi.org/10.1109/EMR.2020.3017451.

[21] A. T. Siddiqui (2022). " Successful conditions in implementing telehealth sup-port to remote areas". In Mamta Mittal and Gopi Battineni (eds.), Information and Communication Technology (ICT) Frameworks in Telehealth, Springer. https://doi.org/10.1007/978-3-031-05049-7.

[22] A. A. Hussain, O. Bouachir, F. Al-Turjman, and M. Aloqaily (2020). "AI techniques for COVID-19". IEEE Access, 8, pp. 128776–128795.

[23] F. Alsubaei, A. Abuhussein, V. Shandilya, and S. Shiva (2019). "IoMTSAF: Internet of medical things security assessment framework". Internet of Things, 8, p. 100123.

[24] M. Wazid, B. Bera, A. Mitra, A. K. Das, and R. Ali (2020). "Private blockchain-envisioned security framework for AI-enabled IoT-based drone-aided healthcare ser-vices". In DroneCom '20: Proceedings of the 2nd ACM MobiCom Workshop on Drone Assisted Wireless Communications for 5G and Beyond, London, September 25, 2020, ACM, pp. 37–42.

[25] C. Camara, P. Peris-Lopez, and J. E. Tapiador (2015). "Security and privacy issues in implantable medical devices: A comprehensive survey". J Biomed Inform, 55, pp. 272–289.

[26] F. Merabet, A. Cherif, M. Belkadi, O. Blazy, E. Conchon, and D. Sauveron (2020). "New efficient M2C and M2M mutual authentication protocols for IoT-based healthcare appli-cations". Peerto-Peer Netw Appl, 13(2), pp. 439–474.

[27] P. Sundaravadivel, E. Kougianos, S. P. Mohanty, and M. K. Ganapathiraju (2017). "Everything you wanted to know about smart health care: Evaluating the different technologies and components of the internet of things for better health". IEEE Consum Electron Mag, 7, pp. 18–28.

[28] S. Lalmuanawma, J. Hussain, and L. Chhakchhuak (2020). "Applications of machine learning and artificial intelligence for Covid-19 (SARS-CoV-2) pandemic: A review". Chaos Solit Fractals, 139, p. 110059.

[29] A. Sedik, M. Hammad, F. E. Abd El-Samie, B. B. Gupta, and A. A. Abd El-Latif (2021). "Efficient deep learning approach for augmented detection of coronavirus disease". Neural Comput Appl, 2021, pp. 1–18.

[30] V. Iguoba and A. L. Imoize (2022). "The psychology of explanation in medical deci-sion support systems". In A. L. Imoize, J. Hemanth, D.-T. Do, and S. N. Sur (eds.), Explainable Artificial Intelligence in Medical Decision Support Systems, 1st ed. The Institution of Engineering and Technology, pp. 489–506.

[31] S. Razdan and S. Sharma (2021). "Internet of medical things (IoMT): Overview, emerg-ing technologies, and case studies". IETE Tech Rev. https://doi.org/10.1080/02564602.2021.1927863.

[32] S. C. Nwaneri, C. Yinka-Banjo, U. C. Uregbulam, O. O. Odukoya, and A. L. Imoize (2022). "Explainable neural networks in diabetes mellitus prediction". In A. L. Imoize, J. Hemanth, D.-T. Do, and S. N. Sur (eds.), Explainable Artificial Intelligence in Medical Decision Support Systems, 1st ed. The Institution of Engineering and Technology, pp. 313–334.

[33] A. T. Rufai, K. F. Dukor, O. M. Ageh, and A. L. Imoize (2022). "XAI robot-assisted surgeries in future medical decision support systems". In A. L. Imoize, J. Hemanth, D.-T. Do, and S. N. Sur (eds.), Explainable Artificial Intelligence in Medical Decision Support Systems, 1st ed. The Institution of Engineering and Technology, pp. 167–195.

[34] R. C. Deo (2015). "Machine learning in medicine". Circulation, 132, pp. 1920–1930. https://doi.org/10.1161/CIRCULATIONAHA.115.001593.

[35] S. S. Panesar and K. Ashkan (2018). "Surgery in space". Br J Surg, 105, pp. 1234–1243. https://doi.org/10.1002/bjs.10908.

[36] R. L. Kumar, Y. Wang, T. Poongodi, and A. L. Imoize, Eds. (2021). Internet of Things, Artificial Intelligence and Blockchain Technology, 1st ed. Springer Nature.

[37] Cisco (n.d). "What is 5G?". www.cisco.com/c/en/us/solutions/what-is-5g.html Accessed on: 18/12/2022.

[38] G. Orru, W. Pettersson-Yeo, A. F. Marquand, G. Sartori, and A. Mechelli. (2012). "Using support vector machine to identify imaging biomarkers of neurological and psychiatric disease: A critical review". Neurosci Biobehav Rev, 36, pp. 1140–1152. https://doi.org/10.1016/j.neubiorev.2012.01.004.

[39] D. Farina, I. Vujaklija, M. Sartori, T. Kapelner, F. Negro, N. Jiang, K. Bergmeister, A. Andalib, J. Principe, and O. C. Aszmann. (2017). "Man/machine interface based on the discharge timings of spinal motor neurons after targeted muscle reinnervation". Nat Biomed Eng, 1, p. 25. https://doi.org/10.1038/s41551-016-0025.

[40] N. H. Sweilam, A. A. Tharwat, and N. K. Abdel Moniem. (2010). "Support vector machine for diagnosis cancer disease: A comparative study". Egypt Inform J, 11, pp. 81–92. https://doi.org/10.1016/j.eij.2010.10.005.

[41] L. Khedher, J. Ramírez, J. M. Górriz, A. Brahim, and F Segovia (2015). "Early diagnosis of Alzheimer's disease based on partial least squares, principal component analysis and support vector machine using segmented MRI images". Neurocomputing, 151, pp. 139–150. https://doi.org/10.1016/j.neucom.2014.09.072.

[42] C. Martin-Isla, V. M. Campello, C. Izquierdo, Z. Raisi-Estabragh, B. Baeßler, S. E. Petersen, and K. Lekadir (2020). "Image-based cardiac diagnosis with machine learning: A review". Front Cardiovasc Med, 7, p. 1. https://doi.org/10.3389/fcvm.2020.00001.

[43] C. Soguero-Ruiz, W. M. E. Fei, R. Jenssen, K. M. Augestad, J.-L. R. Álvarez, I. M. Jiménez, R.-O. Lindsetmo, and S. O. Skrøvseth (2015). "Data-driven temporal prediction of surgical site infection". In Proceedings of the AMIA Annual Symposium Proceedings, American Medical Informatics Association, San Francisco, CA, 14–18 November 2015, p. 1164.

[44] M. Shokrekhodaei, D. P. Cistola, R. C. Roberts, and S. Quinones (2021). "Non-invasive glucose monitoring using optical sensor and machine learning techniques for diabetes applications". IEEE Access, 9, pp. 73029–73045. https://doi.org/10.1109/ACCESS.2021.3079182.

[45] D. A. Hashimoto, G. Rosman, D. Rus, and O. R. Meireles (2018). "Artificial intelligence in surgery: Promises and perils". Ann Surg, 268, pp. 70–76. https://doi.org/10.1097/SLA.0000000000002693.

[46] F. Galbusera, G. Casaroli, and T. Bassani (2019). "Artificial intelligence and machine learning in spine research". JOR Spine, 2, p. e1044. https://doi.org/10.1002/jsp2.1044.

[47] M. Chang, J. A. Canseco, K. J. Nicholson, N. Patel, and A. R. Vaccaro (2020). "The role of machine learning in spine surgery: The future is now". Front Surg, 7, p. 54. https://doi.org/10.3389/fsurg.2020.00054.

[48] M. Goswami and N. J. Sebastian (2022). "Performance analysis of logistic regression, KNN, SVM, Naïve Bayes classifier for healthcare application during COVID-19". In J. S. Raj, K. Kamel, and P. Lafata (eds.), Innovative Data Communication Technologies and Application. Vol. 96. Springer Nature, pp. 645–658.

[49] P. Kaur, R. Kumar, and M. Kumar (2019). "A healthcare monitoring system using random forest and internet of things (IoT) Multimed". Tools Appl, 78, pp. 19905–19916. https://doi.org/10.1007/s11042-019-7327-8.

[50] E. Svoboda (2020). "Artificial intelligence is improving the detection of lung cancer". Nature, 587, pp. S20–S22. https://doi.org/10.1038/d41586-020-03157-9.

[51] N. Khosravan and U. Bagci (2018). "S4ND: Single-shot single-scale lung nodule detection". In Proceedings of the International Conference on Medical Image Computing and Computer-Assisted Intervention, Granada, Spain, 16–20 September 2018, pp. 794–802.

[52] D. Ardila, A. P. Kiraly, S. Bharadwaj, B. Choi, J. J. Reicher, L. Peng, D. Tse, M. Etemadi, W. Ye, and G. Corrado (2019). "End-to-end lung cancer screening with three-dimensional deep learning on low-dose chest computed tomography". Nat Med, 25, pp. 954–961. https://doi.org/10.1038/s41591-019-0447-x.

[53] W. Muhammad, G. R. Hart, B. Nartowt, J. J. Farrell, K. Johung, Y. Liang, and J. Deng (2019). "Pancreatic cancer prediction through an artificial neural network". Front Artif Intell, 2, p. 2. https://doi.org/10.3389/frai.2019.00002.

[54] T. J. Hirschauer, H. Adeli, and J. A. Buford (2015). "Computer-aided diagnosis of Parkinson's disease using enhanced probabilistic neural network". J Med Syst, 39, p. 179. https://doi.org/10.1007/s10916-015-0353-9.

[55] S. Sarraf, D. D. DeSouza, J. Anderson, and G. Tofighi (2017). "DeepAD: Alzheimer's disease classification via deep convolutional neural networks using MRI and fMRI". BioRxiv, p. 070441. https://doi.org/10.1101/070441.

[56] F. Ramzan, M. U. G. Khan, A. Rehmat, S. Iqbal, T. Saba, A. Rehman, and Z. Mehmood (2020). "A deep learning approach for automated diagnosis and multi-class classification of Alzheimer's disease stages using resting-state fMRI and residual neural networks". J Med Syst, 44, p. 37. https://doi.org/10.1007/s10916-019-1475-2.

[57] K. Pang, X. Song, Z. Xu, X. Liu, Y. Liu, L. Zhong, Y. Peng, J. Wang, J. Zhou, and F. Meng (2020). "Hydroplastic foaming of graphene aerogels and artificially intelligent tactile sensors". Sci Adv, 6, p. eabd4045. https://doi.org/10.1126/sciadv.abd4045.

[58] T. Hayasaka, A. Lin, V. C. Copa, L. P. Lopez, R. A. Loberternos, L. I. M. Ballesteros, Y. Kubota, Y. Liu, A. A. Salvador, and L. Lin (2020). "An electronic nose using a single graphene FET and machine learning for water, methanol, and ethanol". Microsyst Nanoeng, 6, p. 50. https://doi.org/10.1038/s41378-020-0161-3.

[59] J. J. Khanam and S. Y. Foo (2021). "A comparison of machine learning algorithms for diabetes prediction". ICT Express, 7, pp. 432–439. https://doi.org/10.1016/j.icte.2021.02.004.

[60] Y. T. Kwon, H. Kim, M. Mahmood, Y. S. Kim, C. Demolder, and W. H. Yeo (2020). "Printed, wireless, soft bioelectronics and deep learning algorithm for smart human-machine interfaces". ACS Appl Mater Interfaces, 12, pp. 49398–49406. https://doi.org/10.1021/acsami.0c14193.

[61] A. K. Kaushik, J. S. Dhau, H. Gohel, Y. K. Mishra, B. Kateb, N.-Y. Kim, and D. Y. Goswami (2020). "Electrochemical SARS-CoV-2 sensing at point-of-care and artificial intelligence for intelligent COVID-19 management". ACS Appl Bio Mater, 3, pp. 7306–7325. https://doi.org/10.1021/acsabm.0c01004.

[62] A. Esteva, K. Chou, S. Yeung, N. Naik, A. Madani, A. Mottaghi, Y. Liu, E. Topol, J. Dean, and R. Socher (2021). "Deep learning-enabled medical computer vision". NPJ Digit Med, 4, p. 5. https://doi.org/10.1038/s41746-020-00376-2.

[63] M. Langarizadeh and Ighbeli (2016). "Applying naive bayesian networks to disease prediction: A systematic review". Acta Inform Medica, 24, p. 364. https://doi.org/10.5455/aim.2016.24.364-369.

[64] Y. Shen, Y. Li, H. T. Zheng, B. Tang, and M. Yang (2019). "Enhancing ontology-driven diagnostic reasoning with a symptom-dependency-aware Naïve Bayes classifier". BMC Bioinform, 20, p. 330. https://doi.org/10.1186/s12859-019-2924-0.

[65] N. A. Fauziyyah, S. Abdullah, and S. Nurrohmah (2020). "Reviewing the consistency of the Naïve Bayes classifier's performance in medical diagnosis and prognosis problems". AIP Conf Proc, 2242, p. 30019.

[66] S. Uddin, I. Haque, H. Lu, M. A. Moni, and E. Gide (2022). "Comparative performance analysis of K-nearest neighbour (KNN) algorithm and its different variants for disease prediction". Sci Rep, 12, p. 6256. https://doi.org/10.1038/s41598-022-10358-x.

[67] C. Li, S. Zhang, H. Zhang, L. Pang, K. Lam, C. Hui, and S. Zhang (2012). "Using the K-nearest neighbor algorithm for the classification of lymph node metastasis in gastric cancer". Comput Math Methods Med, 2012, p. 876545. https://doi.org/10.1155/2012/876545.

[68] D. Rahmat, A. A. Putra, and A. W. Setiawan (2021). "Heart disease prediction using K-nearest neighbor". In Proceedings of the 2021 International Conference on Electrical Engineering and Informatics (ICEEI), Kuala Terengganu, Malaysia, 12–13 October 2021, Kuala Terengganu, Malaysia: IEEE, 2021, pp. 1–6.

[69] P. Sethi and S. Sarangi (2017). "Internet of things: Architectures, protocols, and applications". J Electric Comput Eng, pp. 1–25. https://doi.org/10.1155/2017/9324035. 9324035.

[70] R. Dwivedi, D. Mehrotra, and S. Chandra (2021). "Potential of internet of medical things (IoMT) applications in building a smart healthcare system: A systematic review". J Oral Biol Craniofac Res, 12(2), pp. 302–318. https://doi.org/10.1016/j.jobcr.2021.11.010.

[71] S. Li, L. D. Xu, and S. Zhao (2018). "5G internet of things: A survey". J Ind Inf Integr. https://doi.org/10.1016/j.jii.2018.01.005.

[72] S. M. R. Islam, D. Kwak, M. H. Kabir, M. Hossain, and K. S. Kwak (2015). "The internet of things for health care: A comprehensive survey". IEEE Access, 3, pp. 678–708. https://doi.org/10.1109/ACCESS.2015.2437951.

[73] M. Alshamrani (2022). "IoT and artificial intelligence implementations for remote healthcare monitoring systems: A survey". J King Saud Univ—Comp Inf Sci, 34, pp. 4687–4701. https://doi.org/10.1016/j.jksuci.2021.06.005.

[74] A. Burak (2022). "How IoMT (Internet of Medical Things) transforms healthcare industry". Relevant Software. https://relevant.software/blog/develop-iomt-solution/#Benefits_of_IoMT_for_healthcare. Accessed on: 19/12/2022.

[75] J. Srivastava, S. Routray, S. Ahmad, and M. M. Waris (2022). "Internet of medical things (IoMT)-based smart healthcare system: Trends and progress". Comput Intell Neurosci, 2022, Article ID 7218113, 17 pages. https://doi.org/10.1155/2022/7218113.

8 Cyberattacks against Artificial Intelligence-Enabled Internet of Medical Things

*Adewole Usman Rufai, Ebun Philip Fasina,
Charles Onuwa Uwadia, Aishat Titilola Rufai, and
Agbotiname Lucky Imoize*

8.1 INTRODUCTION

The Internet of medical things (IoMT) is the Internet of Things (IOT) of the medical domain. It is a network of medical devices made up of medical devices implantable in humans and wearable devices. It is technology characterized by medical devices connected to the patient with the objectives of providing real-time monitoring and crucial decision-making over the Internet by healthcare professionals. IoMT is made up of implantable medical devices (IMDs) and the Internet of wearable devices (IoWDs) [1]. Furthermore, advances in artificial intelligence (AI) have made the artificial intelligence-enabled Internet of medical things (AIoMT) much more powerful as it provides healthcare at a lower cost and better performance. AIoMT technology assists in reducing hospital stays and their associated costs. Moreover, the extent of medical information generated by a AIoMT is in the realm of big data. In healthcare, the privacy and safety of patient data are crucial. Data aggregated by these medical devices are eventually transferred for cloud storage via the Internet. This portends a great concern as patients' data are at risk of cyberattacks.

In Ghubaish et al. [1], the IoMT system architecture is made of four layers. These layers indicate the transition from the data collection stage (sensor layer) to the gateway, cloud, and visualization layers for the physician to take action. The sensor layer: this is the data collection layer. It consists of IMDs and IoWDs that collect patients' biometrics. The data collected are aggregated to the second layer via Bluetooth, wifi, and radio frequency (RF) spectrum dedicated for IMDs. Gateway layer: artificial intelligence-enabled Internet of medical things (AIoMT) sensors are constrained by processing and storage capabilities, hence the need to transfer data to this layer. The patients' smartphone or a dedicated access point with preprocessing and short-term

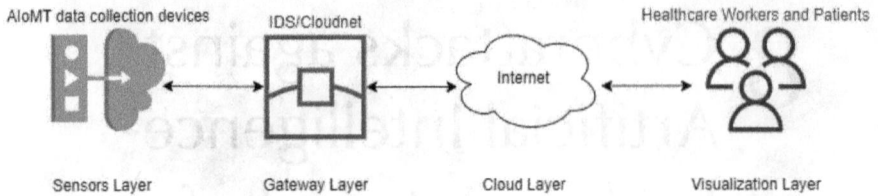

FIGURE 8.1 Artificial intelligence-enabled internet of medical things (AIoMT) system architecture. (Adapted from Ghubaish et al. [1].)

data storage will in turn transmit the data to the cloud. In Figure 8.1, the gateway layer is tweaked by the use of edge technology to allow for low latency and more computational power at the edge of the artificial intelligence-enabled Internet of medical things (AIoMT) system.

The three critical principles of confidentiality, integrity, and availability (CIA) are central security requirements for any system. However, the requirement for artificial intelligence-enabled internet of medical things (AIoMT), as posited by Belkhouja et al. [2], is from the acronym CIANA and other requirements: confidentiality, integrity, availability, non-repudiation, authentication, authorization, and anonymity.

Despite the ubiquity and usefulness of AIoMT, researchers have identified major issues that characterize AIoMT. These include patients' privacy, data security, interoperability, and regulatory issues, among others. AIoMT devices aid in the collection of patients' data with are incorporated into an electronic health records system. This system serves as a decision support system for healthcare professionals [4].

Thus, the transmission of patients' data through the Internet has made patients' data or electronic health record (EHR) vulnerable to various cyberattacks. These concerns are critical since they can lead to wrong diagnosis and treatment and threaten human lives [5]. AIoMT requires an interdisciplinary approach to achieve a robust healthcare system. There is a need for all stakeholders to collaborate in addressing the various challenges discussed earlier bedeviling the AIoMT domain. However, the data obtained from AIoMT devices are mostly big data and are subsequently analyzed with artificial intelligence techniques, such as machine learning (ML) and deep learning (DL).

ML algorithms process large amount of data. These ML algorithms can be used to obtain insights from patients' information, thus giving medical professionals recommendations for decisions. The integration of AI and IoT is to perform real-time analysis of data to assist clinicians in decision-making. Thus, AI has found applications in various areas of the medical field, such as drug discovery, disease prediction, patient diagnosis, disease management, and robotic surgery. Although ML algorithms can be used for threat detection and malware analysis, they also pose cybersecurity risks, which can be described as expanding existing cyber threats and creating new cyberattacks [6]. Thus, ML techniques can be an enabler of cyberattacks. Therefore, due to the complexities of IoT systems, their heterogeneity, and the connection of different devices, they are prone to various security attacks.

8.1.1 Major Contributions of the Chapter

The following are the significant contributions of this chapter:

i. The chapter investigates, highlights, and reports recent advances and countermeasures on cyberattacks against the artificial intelligence-enabled internet of medical things.
ii. We categorize and classify the nature and types of cyberattacks by devising a taxonomy.
iii. We outline the characteristics of cyberattacks.
iv. We propose a framework for AIoMT's security.
v. We simulate the intrusion detection part of the framework.

8.1.2 Chapter Organization

Section 8.2 presents the related works on cyberattacks against the AI-enabled internet of medical things. Section 8.3 discusses nature and types of cyberattacks. Section 8.4 explains characteristics of cyberattacks. Section 8.5 targets the security aspects of the artificial intelligence-enabled internet of medical things (AIoMT). Section 8.6. presents existing security measures in the medical domain. Section 8.7 is a conceptual framework for artificial intelligence-enabled internet of medical things (AIoMT) security. Section 8 discusses the methodology for the simulation. Section 8.9 shows results and discussions. Section 8.10 concludes the chapter with future directions.

8.2 RELATED WORKS

The adaptation of artificial intelligence in detecting and predicting cyberattacks in the Internet of medical things has been an area of active research over the years. Various techniques have been proposed as countermeasures against cyberattacks, these include the use of cryptography, blockchain, machine learning, deep learning, and so on.

Bhatia et al. [7] presented a secure incremental proxy re-encryption for e-healthcare. The proposed system is on a pairing-free lightweight incremental proxy re-encryption scheme without certificates.

Hassan et al. [8] investigated recent advances in edge computing and proposed schemes for the successful deployment of edge computing to Internet of Things (IoT). This is to solve the power and computational limitation of IoT devices and the data collection stage. However, due to the dynamic nature of the IoT environment and the arrays of IoT devices, the edge of a network might be vulnerable to attacks. To mitigate this, security controllers can be deployed at the edge servers.

Hyun et al. [9] proposed the development of an interface to network security functions (NSF) architecture to enable efficient and flexible security service provisioning in cloud-based environments and the integration of (NSF) and Software Defined Network (SDN). However, the work is constrained by lack of standard interfaces to manage the security role sets of the NSFs and a lack of a standard method to describe the capabilities of the NSFs.

Hatzivasilis et al. [11] introduced an overview of the core security and privacy countermeasures to safeguard users and stakeholders of IoMT. The work considered the security of devices, connectivity, and the cloud. However, no security was suggested at the edge of the cloud. Our work incorporates the security of edge devices as well as interface security.

Sengupta et al. [13] came up with the classification of attacks based on the object of vulnerability (devices, network, software, or data), the review of each attack, and the proposal of countermeasures concerning IoT. However, due to security loopholes in blockchain, there exists a need to design adaptable and dynamic blockchain-based security framework, ranging from high-end services to low-powered IoT devices. Incorporating fog-based AIoMT architecture to reduce latency and computational overhead is also crucial.

Bout et al. [6] identified and discussed the advantages of the elaboration of machine learning (ML) attacks and the possible countermeasures already elaborated in the literature. However, few of the works are tested in real applications.

Yanquig et al. [15] built an intrusion detection system using a deep belief network. The work improved on the Euclidean distance method of the density peak clustering algorithm (DPCA) and the use of the kernel function to project original features into high-dimensional kernel space to better cluster nonlinearity in separate traffic data [17, 18].

In Inayat et al. [23], exploration and identification of the application of semi-supervised ML and advanced deep learning (DL) methods for the detection of cyberattacks in IoT systems and devices were considered. The authors resolved the gap between the feature selection method and various datasets used for cyberattack detection in IoT systems and devices. However, scalability issues of detection methods exist when addressing security protocols, and data security was not covered.

Mothukuri et al. [21] used federated learning approach for anomaly detection for IoT attacks by deploying gated recurrent units (GRU).

Table 8.1 summarizes related works in this study.

8.3   NATURE AND TYPES OF CYBERATTACKS

In this section, we will discuss different features of Cyberattacks. Authors of [6, 27, 28] have classified cyberattacks in IoT into four categories which are listed next:

8.3.1   PHYSICAL ATTACKS

Physical attacks occur on the physical device itself; this type of attack occurs where IoT devices lack proper security, that is, devices that are easily accessible to anyone. Thus, attackers can tamper with these IoT devices and extract sensitive information from these devices. In addition, attackers target important aspects of IoT systems such as power consumption, memory, or network connection. The majority of these physical attacks can eventually lead to a Denial-of-service (DoS) [6]. Authors of [29] describe DoS as any incident that limits the network's ability to carry out its intended purpose. In addition, a man-in-the-middle attack requires physical access

TABLE 8.1
Summary of Related Works

Reference	Work Done	Methodology	Contributions	Gaps	Remark
Lu et al. [3]	IoT Cybersecurity	Review	Proposed a four-layered architecture for IoT Taxonomy of attacks in IoT among others	No implementation	
Bhatia et al. [7]	"A secure incremental proxy re-encryption for e-healthcare data sharing in mobile cloud computing"	Cryptography	Proposal of a pairing-free incremental proxy re-encryption scheme		
Hassan et al. [8]	Importance of edge computing in IoTs	Survey	Investigation of recent advances in edge computing from an IoT perspective. Major schemes for the successful deployment of edge computing in IoT	Due to the dynamic nature of the IoT environment and the arrays of IoT devices, the edge of a network might be vulnerable to attacks	Security controllers can be deployed at the edge servers
Hyun et al. [9]	"Interface to Network Security functions for Cloud-based Security Services"	Design of a novel architecture and implementation on two security services scenarios	Development of an I2NSF architecture to enable efficient and flexible security service provisioning in cloud-based environments. Integration of I2NSF and SDN (Software Defined Network)	Lack of: 1) Standard interfaces to manage the security role sets of the NSFs 2) Lack of standard method to describe the capabilities of the NSFs	The proposed architecture Incorporating SDN can be implemented using open-source software
Sun et al. [10]	ANN Framework for Gait-based Biometrics	Biometric cryptosystem approach (BCS)	Proposal of a novel BCS approach for sensing wireless communications for implantable healthcare devices using gait signal energy variations and an ANN framework		

(Continued)

TABLE 8.1 (Continued)
Summary of Related Works

Reference	Work Done	Methodology	Contributions	Gaps	Remark
Hatzivasilis et al. [11]	"Overview of the core security and privacy countermeasures to safeguard users and stakeholders of IoMT"	Review state-of-the-art solutions in IoMT	The study can serve as a guide for IoMT applications within the context of a circular economy	The work considered the security of devices, connectivity, and the cloud. No security is suggested at the edge of the cloud	Our work incorporates the security of the edge devices as well as the interface security
Dai et al. [12]	The work investigates the integration of Blockchain and IoT	A survey of the state-of-the-art	Proposal of the BCoT architecture	Privacy leakage was possible with blockchain transactions. Scalability issues abound with large-scale IoMTs	
Sengupta et al. [13]	"Blockchain Solutions for IoT and IIoT"	Survey	Classification of attacks based on the object of vulnerability (devices, network, software, or data) review of each attack, and the proposal of countermeasures concerning IoT	Due to Security loopholes in Blockchain there exist the need to design adaptable and dynamic blockchain base security framework ranging from high-end services to low-powered IoT devices	Incorporating fog-based AIoMT architecture to reduce latency and computational overhead
Yaacoub et al. [14]	"Securing the Internet of Medical Things systems"	Survey	IoMT systems are presented based on their communication types, device types, and applications. Concerns and risks are presented and evaluated through a proposed qualitative risk analysis method	The major issue in the artificial intelligence-enabled internet of medical things (AIoMT) is that of standardization	
Yanquig et al. [15]	"Building Intrusion Detection System (IDS) using Deep Belief Networks"	ML methodology	The work improved on the Euclidean distance method of the density peak clustering algorithm (DPCA) and the use of the kernel function to project original features into high-dimensional kernel space to better cluster nonlinear in separate traffic data		

(Continued)

Alzahrani et al. [16]	"Presentation of a novel patient monitoring protocol whose security properties are validated by Body area Network logic-based formal analysis"	The use of a network model comprising a system model and an attack model	Lightweight patient-healthcare authentication protocol in wireless body area networks	More work is needed on the efficiencies in the authentication protocol for WBAN	
Ghubaish et al. [1]	"Advances in Internet of Medical Things System Security"	Comprehensive review	The study proposed a security framework that uses some of the features of those techniques for IoMT systems. This framework covers IoMT system security during data collection, transmission, and storage		
Sun et al. [34]	On edge-Cloud Computing and AI in IoTs	Comprehensive review	Incorporation of AI, cloud computing, and edge computing in IoT	Resources limitations and energy consumption are the banes of edge computing. Due to these malicious attacks are possible at the edge. Improvement in symmetric and asymmetric encryption algorithms will be necessary.	AI
Tahsien et al. [18]	"ML-based Solutions for the Security of IoT"	Survey	Presentation of different ML techniques and their application to address various IoT attacks. Possible challenges/limitations in ML-based security of IoT Systems and their perspective research directions	Scalability issues abound with ML solutions	
Alennizi et al. [19]	"Security and Privacy Issues in Cloud Computing"	Survey	Provision of a framework to address the security and privacy concerns of Cloud Computing and the provision of countermeasures to solve these concerns	The work addresses only Cloud Security leaving the other aspects like devices, interface, and connectivity security	

TABLE 8.1 (Continued)
Summary of Related Works

Reference	Work Done	Methodology	Contributions	Gaps	Remark
Avinashiappan [20]	Internet of Medical Things	Review	IoMT System Architecture Taxonomy on device types and IoMT attack types	No, emphasize on the holistic Security of interface, application, and data	
Bout et al. [6]	"Identify and discuss the advantages of the elaboration of ML attacks and the possible countermeasures already elaborated in the literature"	Survey	Provision of detailed state-of-the-art existing surveys on IoT security. ML in IoT and ML-based security Solutions on IoT networks Description of attacks based on ML algorithm integration	Few of the works are tested in real applications	
Suzen et al. [22]	"Protection of the Privacy of IoT-Based Health Records using Blockchain Technology"	Arduino Nano was used in retrieving data from sensors and sent to a raspberry pi access point (RAP)	Safe patient monitoring model. Pulse and galvanic skin responses were used to obtain the data to be used in the proposed model	More work needs to be done on improving the data security and privacy of blockchain networks	
Inayat et al. [23]	"Learning-Based methods for Cyber Attacks Detection in IoT Systems"	Survey	Exploration and identification of the application of semi-supervised ML and advanced DL methods for the detection of cyberattacks in IoT systems and devices Resolving the gap between feature selection method and various datasets used for cyberattack detection in IoT systems and devices	Scalability issues of detection methods when addressing security protocols Data security is not covered	
Manickan et al. [24]	Development of AI and IoMT Systems for Intelligent Healthcare	Comprehensive survey	Comprehensive analysis and taxonomy of AI and IoTM in enhancing the performance of point-of-care (POC) devices used in healthcare	The work is limited to the review at the devices level	

Reference	Title/Focus	Method	Description	Limitation
Maqsood [25]	Gait Recognition System using Deep learning	Deep CNN-based intelligence model	Development of automated surveillance systems blocking attackers' access using reinforcement learning (RL)	
Razdan et al. [26]	Proving an overview of IoMT	Survey and presentation of case studies.	Presented a cloud-fog architecture for IoMTs. Proposed PUF, blockchain, AI, and SDN-based mapping for e-healthcare	AI accountability to IoMTs is still work-in-progress. There are concerns about the efficiency of AI applications
Belkhouja et al. [2]	Data encryption for implantable medical device	Cryptography	Proposed role-based encryption scheme using the CIANA principle.	The work is restricted to implantable medical devices
Sadhu, et al. [38]	Security Requirements and Solutions	Comprehensive review	Exploration of the AIoMT ecosystem and the address of the various challenges and the suggestion of solutions	Largely a survey with no implementation
Bibusayyis, et al. [39]	"Comparison of machine learning (ML) algorithms for intrusion detection"	Machine learning	Investigation of five ML algorithms and the identification of the best ML approach	No deep learning algorithm is considered
Shahid, et al. [40]	Addresses data protection and privacy issues	Review	Provision of recommendations to improve the security and privacy of IoMT implementation	No implementation
Dwivedi et al. [41]	Building a smart health care system	A systematic review	Identification of the challenges faced in the mass adoption of IoMT	No implementation
Nayak et al. [42]	Intelligent framework for IoMT	Hybridization of Bayesian optimization and extreme learning machine	Provision of a novel framework for IoMT security	Our work will validate the proposed conceptual framework

to the IoMT device. Other examples of such attacks include node tampering, physical damage, and node jamming.

8.3.2 NETWORK ATTACK

Network attacks occur during the transmission of information over a network or between communication devices. For example, distributed denial of service (DDoS) attacks occur in the network and cloud storage in healthcare systems. DDoS is one of the most popular cyberattacks within the IoMT network layer [30]. Also, the replay attack is used to capture communication packets, which then send the same packet repeatedly [31]. Few studies highlight ways to mitigate the risk of cyberattacks. Although [30] highlights a new approach to detecting DDoS, more research need to be done to find ways to accurately detect and minimize the risks of cyberattacks. Other classifications include software attacks and encryption attacks (Table 8.2).

8.4 CHARACTERISTICS OF CYBERATTACKS

In identifying and classifying cyberattacks, it is instructive to understand their characteristics. Yaacoub et al. [14] posited that any attack can be classified based on its

TABLE 8.2
Types of Cyberattacks that Fall under Various Categories

Physical Attack	Network Attack	Software Attack	Encryption Attack
Physical damage	Replay attack	Virus and worms	Side channel attack
Node tampering	Routing attack	Trojan social horse	Cryptanalysis attack
Malicious node adware	Traffic analysis damage	Malicious script	Man-in-the-middle attack
RF interference	RFID spoofing	Denial of service (DoS)	
Sleep deprivation attack	Denial of service (DoS)	Spyware and malicious node adware	
Node jamming	Sybil attack	Distributed denial of service (DDoS)	
Social engineering	Man-in-the-middle attack		
Malicious node attack injection on the node	Sinkhole attack		
Power wastage, e.g., battery depletion	RFID unauthorized attack		
Electromagnetic interference	RFID cloning		
	Replay		

nature, target, scope, capacity, and impact. Moreover, their skills and available tools motivate attackers to achieve their aim and goals.

Nature	Target	Scope	Capacity	Impact
Internal: e.g., rogue employees may collaborate with external attackers	One or more patients of interest	Small scale	Rigorous background checks on all employees. Regular training against social engineering	Depends on the network and the importance of the targets
External: malicious hackers	Large-scale target. May steal patients' data for sale to malicious third parties	Large scale	Encryption	Massive
Passive: attacker remains hidden. May collaborate with internal and external attackers	Intercept data and gather and exploit for more sophisticated cyberattack	Large scale	Firewall, AI-enabled IDS,	Massive
Active:	Intercept communication between source and destination aggressively	Small scale	AI-enabled IDS, multi-factor authentication, and authorization	Massive

8.5 TARGETED ARTIFICIAL INTELLIGENCE-ENABLED INTERNET OF MEDICAL THINGS (AIOMTS) SECURITY ASPECTS

The three main criteria for system security control are confidentiality, integrity, and availability principles. Confidentiality is a criterion in which information is not disclosed to processes and devices unless authorization exists. Integrity is the principle in which an unauthorized entity has not tampered with or destroyed the information. Finally, availability is the principle by which the information is accessible. These principles are taken into cognizance when looking at the targeted artificial intelligence-enabled Internet of medical things (AIoMTs) security aspects.

With the ubiquity of AIoMT, devices' security vulnerabilities and privacy are major concerns. The activities of malicious actors can compromise the medical data of the patient. These activities may lead to cyberattacks incapacitating the devices, blackmail, and false insurance claims among other vices. To address these issues, it becomes imperative to address these security vulnerabilities on four layers of security. The four layers include application security, connectivity security, device security, and cloud security.

8.5.1 APPLICATION SECURITY

The focus here is the protection of the integrity of data and code. Also, threats intelligence and vulnerability analysis are engaged to review known threats as well as third-party vulnerabilities. Management and analysis of big data amassed for artificial intelligence-enabled Internet of medical things (AIoMT) are challenging for healthcare organizations using conventional computing paradigms. Also, artificial intelligence-enabled Internet of medical things (AIoMT) devices have limited capabilities that rule out their use for computational-intensive tasks. Furthermore, artificial intelligence-enabled Internet of medical things (AIoMT) wireless communications are prone to confidentiality attacks. These include eavesdropping, packet capturing, data interception, dumpster diving, traffic analysis, and brute force attacks.

Ghubaish et al. [1] describe IoMT threats to patients' data at the following stages: collection, transit, and storage. The sensor layer is the first point of collection of patients' data; attacks at this stage could be software or hardware, hence efforts must be geared toward the protection of patients' data and lives at this stage. The Internet of medical things (IoMT) system is characterized by the transmission of data from one layer to another. Attackers can intercept data and destroy the integrity of the data or block the data from being transmitted. These informed the need to secure the IOMT system on the four layers. Ultimately patient data are stored in the cloud layer. Attacks on the cloud could be stealing account credentials for DOS and DDOS attacks. At these points, there is the need to protect the data from being accessed by malicious hackers at both the cloud layer and the visualization layer.

In the work of [8], the processing of data using edge technology was suggested. Adopting fog computing, cloudlet, and mobile edge computing approaches will reduce latency, increase availability, and reduce vulnerabilities in cloud computing. Developing security strategies for edge servers is less cumbersome than for the cloud itself. Bringing the analysis of data to edge devices allows decision-makers to gain actionable insights faster than the use of conventional paradigms.

8.5.2   CONNECTIVITY SECURITY

Artificial intelligence-enabled Internet of medical things (AIoMT) devices are connecting devices that are highly vulnerable to attacks. Therefore, interface security between connecting devices and APIs is equally essential. There is the need to ensure that API connections are secure. Unauthorized actors can exploit the vulnerabilities in APIs when proper security measures are not put in place.

Penetration testing could be performed, and wireless security systems analysis should be undertaken.

8.5.3   DEVICE SECURITY

Emphases are placed on side-channel analysis to prevent attempts at extracting secrets from devices as well as microcode tampering. In addition, periodic intrusion protection reviews are undertaken.

8.6   EXISTING SECURITY MEASURES IN THE MEDICAL DOMAIN

Due to the large volume of data generated by artificial intelligence-enabled Internet of medical things (AIoMT) systems, the collection and storage of healthcare over cloud storage are susceptible to various cyberattacks within the EHR system. The EHR is an electronic health records system that helps manage, collect, and control healthcare and information. In addition, other issues within the IoMT system are security and privacy issues that occur during the transmission of data from one network device to another or over the internet [37].

To achieve the potential of artificial intelligence-enabled Internet of medical things (AIoMT), there is a need for addressing these privacy and security concerns.

Different jurisdictions address these concerns by putting in place regulations to protect privacy and address security concerns. The European Union (EU) came up with the General Data Protection Regulation (GDPR) for its citizens [32]. The United States has the Health Insurance Portability and Accountability Act (HIPAA) and the Health Information Technology for Economic and Clinical Health (HITECH) Act [33].

In other words, the data protection policies stress the importance of transparency of AI-enabled systems as well as patients' consent while utilizing this artificial intelligence-enabled Internet of medical things (AIoMT) technologies [35].

Furthermore, data security in healthcare is important to protect medical information from unauthorized access and human error, while privacy requires that data is managed safely and effectively. It also involve, obtaining users' permission, adhering to regulatory policies, and providing notifications.

Aside from the aforementioned regulatory actions, other security measures can be taken to ensure the safety and security of artificial intelligence-enabled Internet of medical things (AIoMT) devices in the medical domain. These include encryption, access control, device authentication, software updates, network segmentation, penetration testing, data backup, and security training, among others.

8.6.1 ENCRYPTION

To ensure the security of information, various encryption algorithms exist. Medical information is sensitive, and there is a need to have a mechanism in place to protect the data of patients in AIoMT. Two-factor authentication and password protection are some ways in which data confidentiality and integrity are preserved.

Data in AIoMT devices are protected by encryption to guide again access if the devices are stolen or lost. Also, transport layer security helps to secure communication between devices over the Internet. Finally, end-to-end encryption helps protect the interaction between two AIoMT devices.

8.6.2 ACCESS CONTROL

AIoMT involves the transmission and storage of sensitive medical data, hence it is instinctive to prevent access to unauthorized individuals. Therefore, access control is key in the regulation of any entity (persons or systems) with permission to access AIoMT resources. Access control can be undertaken in several ways, including the following:

Role-based: This is concerned with the assignment of different levels of access based on job title. A hospital record attendant has less access than a nurse.

User authentication: This is concerned with the identity of a person before allowing access to a device or data. This can be carried out through passwords, two-factor authentication, tokens or biometrics, etc.

Restriction-based: This is concerned with restricting access to specific resources only based on the permission of the user. For instance, access could be read-only.

8.6.3 DEVICE AUTHENTICATION

To allow only authorized users to be able to connect to a network and access or transmit transit data, it is expedient to verify the identity of a device in AIoMT. Device authentication can be achieved by password-based authentication, which involves using a unique password for each device before a user can access it.

Also, biometric authentication delves into the use of unique anatomical characteristics of the user to verify their identity. Digital certificate involves the issue of digital certificates to each device. A trusted third party may issue the certificate. It could contain the serial number and the firmware of the manufacturer.

8.6.4 SOFTWARE UPDATES

Regular software updates are essential in enhancing the security of AIoMT. This evolution also involves the improvement in the functionalities of the software. This process allows for patches to remedy security vulnerabilities encountered in the case of the use of the software. Regular updates that address these vulnerabilities will help frustrate hackers from infiltrating the system.

Updates also involve improvements in user experience and the addition of new features to enhance the performance of the system. The organization must have policies that will ensure timely updates to help improve the overall performance, stability, and security of the AIoMT.

8.6.5 NETWORK SEGMENTATION

Network segmentation seeks to decompose a network into smaller subnetworks to enhance security. This is implemented by the use of firewalls intrusion detection and prevention systems, and access controls to deter unauthorized access to patients' data. Network segmentation deters a hacker from moving laterally and compromising nodes within a network.

Segmentation in AIoMT also ensures the confidentiality, integrity, and availability of devices in a network. By segmenting the network and prioritizing, separate secure areas for storing and accessing patients' information are created to enhance security controls and further protect against hackers [43].

8.6.6 PENETRATION TESTING

Penetration testing is an authorized simulated attack on a computer system to access its vulnerabilities using similar tools as criminal hackers. Penetration testing is categorized into, internal, external, and network testing. Internal testing is done with the perspective of insider work done by a rogue employee with access to the system. External testing is carried out with the perspective of an external attack on the system by criminal elements. Network testing involves testing the vulnerabilities inherent in the interactions between nodes in a network.

Penetration testing is necessary to discover vulnerabilities in the system and ensure the mitigation of these vulnerabilities before either rogue employees or external hackers exploit them.

8.6.7   DATA BACKUP

Data backup is periodically creating copies of data to protect against data loss due to software bugs, human error, cyberattacks, and other unforeseen events. In AIoMT, data backup is a key mechanism that will help ensure the availability and integrity of patients' records. There are several approaches to data backup. These include onsite backup, which involves creating copies of data and storing them on secondary storage devices (hard disk, flash drive, etc.) within the organization's premises. Also, cloud backup involves creating copies of data and storing them on a remote server, which a cloud service provider could provide. Finally, hybrid backups involve the use of onsite and cloud backup to enjoy the benefits of both approaches.

However, irrespective of the approach used, it is crucial to ensure that backups are in top shape in an emergency that could lead to data loss. A robust disaster recovery mechanism should be put in place to prevent disruptions in operations.

8.6.8   SECURITY TRAINING

Security training deals with educating employees, external collaborators, and other persons on how to recognize and prevent cyberattacks, as well as detecting unauthorized access to sensitive data and systems. In AIoMT, security training is key to ensuring the overall security of the system. Security training can be carried out using the following approaches: in-house training, online training, and simulation training.

First, in-house training delves into training sessions on various topics in cyberattacks, best practices to deter attacks, and emergency response procedures. Second, online training delves into providing employees with various online media like webinars, and targeted online courses, to enable them to study at their own pace. Third, simulation training involves the simulation of actual attacks and determining the best response to deter attacks when they happen.

Finally, whichever approach is used, the bottom line is that the confidentiality, integrity, and availability of patient data in AIoMT must be maintained and guarded properly through constant training and awareness of employees of various organizations in the healthcare sector.

8.7   A CONCEPTUAL FRAMEWORK FOR AIoMT SECURITY

The central idea behind exploring the targeted AIoMTs' security aspects is to provide a holistic approach to security AIoMTs. Hence, the security of the four layers is well fortified. Starting from the devices in the sensors layer, the size of the AIoMT system follows a pyramidal structure with the AIoMT data collection devices making the base of the pyramid. This layer could be made up of millions of devices and are essentially devices owned by patients (smartphones, smart watches, etc.). These devices are not within the purview of system providers.

It is a truism that attacks on wireless devices are much easier than those on wired devices. Hence, we drew inspiration from the work of Hassan [8] with the incorporation of edge technology in our proposed framework.

Cloudlets, a form of edge computing, are deployed as shown in Figure 8.2, to take care of latency-sensitive and computationally intensive tasks that otherwise cannot be implemented at the sensors layer. The cloudlets serve as the edge gateway to the cloud. AI-driven complex cryptographic algorithms can be resident on the cloudlets.

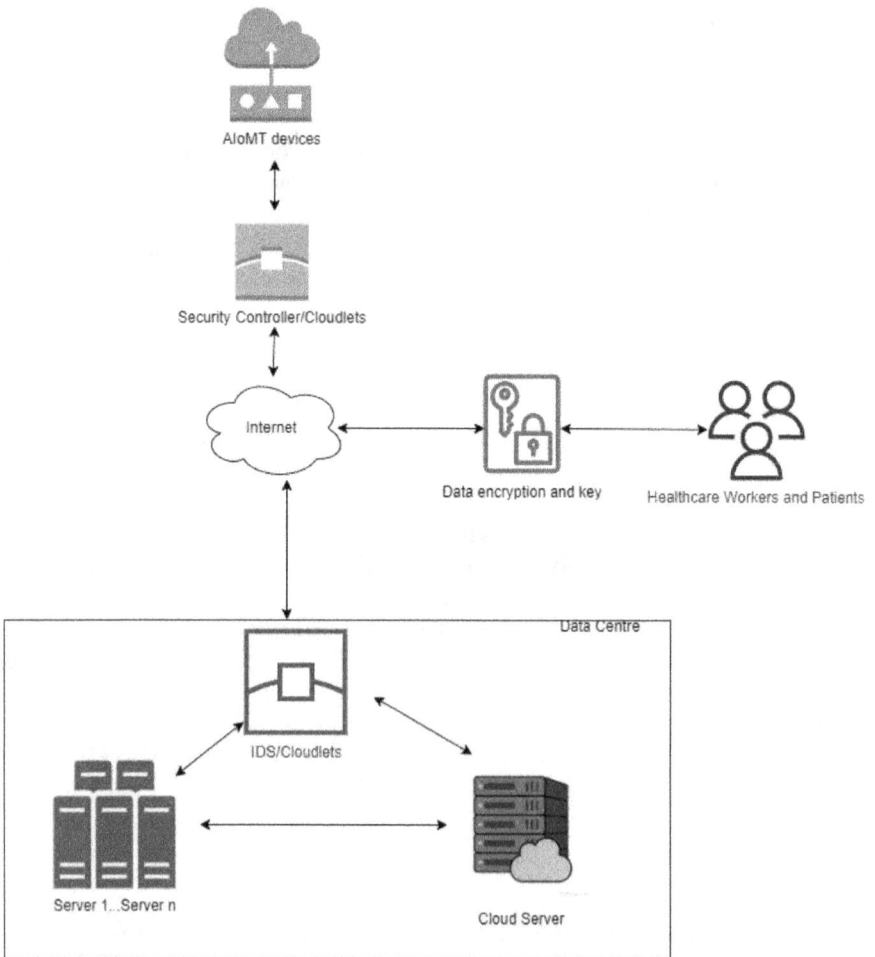

FIGURE 8.2   A proposed conceptual framework for AIoMT's security.

To enhance connectivity security, we proposed the incorporation of software-defined networking (SDN), which will be able to programmatically manage and control network resources such as switches and routers [9].

In Figure 8.2, healthcare workers and patients can access the system using a hybrid of AES and RSA encryption as suggested by [19]. At the visualization layer, multi-factor authentication will guide against bot attacks. The cloud layer is characterized by the presence of cloudlets that serve as instruction detection systems that mitigate DOS and DDOS attacks on the farm of servers and cloud servers. The servers in the data center are dedicated to different operations. Separate servers are reserved for authentication, AI-driven cryptography, and blockchain operations. The number of servers deployed depends on the size of the artificial intelligence-enabled Internet of medical things (AIoMT) system. Using multiple servers will ensure low latency in taking critical healthcare decisions [44].

The framework is geared toward the achievement of the CIANA principle that is elaborated upon in the introduction of the study.

In further work, we intend to develop a robust instruction detection algorithm using deep learning to mitigate against the various attacks discussed.

8.8 METHODOLOGY

This study uses machine learning to predict malware attacks using the WUSTL-EHMS-2020 dataset [36] (obtained from www.cse.wustl.edu/~jain/ehms/index.html) for Internet of Medical Things to simulate real-life attacks on the IDS/Cloudlets of our proposed framework. We proceed with the simulation thus:

First, collecting and labeling a dataset of network activity data. The dataset should contain both normal and malicious activity. Second, the data is preprocessed by cleaning the data, transforming categorical variables, scaling numerical values, and extracting only important features. Third, the data is split into training and testing sets, in which the model will be trained on the training set, while the model will be evaluated on the testing set. Fourth, an appropriate machine learning algorithm and hyperparameters are chosen at this stage. Fifth, the model is trained on the training set. Sixth, the model is evaluated on the testing set, and the hyperparameters are tuned if required.

Finally, the model is deployed in the network, and its performance is monitored. Eventually, the model can be used to classify new network activity data as normal or attack types. This process is represented in Figure 8.3.

8.8.1 DATA COLLECTION

Enhanced Healthcare Monitoring System (EHMS) dataset was used. The data is made up of network flow metrics and the patients' biometrics. The patients' data are collected from sensors attached to the patient's bodies. The data is sent to the edge server. An attacker interrupts this data before it arrives at the server. The man-in-the-middle attacks include spoofing and data injection. The dataset is made up of 44 features and 16,318 data points, of which 35 features are flow metrics for the network, 8 patients' biometrics, and the last feature for the label. The data points with the attack are labeled as 1, while the benign or normal situations are labeled as 0.

```
                          ┌─────────┐
                         (   Start   )
                          └─────────┘
                               │
                               ▼
                    ╱─────────────────────╱
                   ╱   Collection of data  ╱
                  ╱─────────────────────╱
                               │
                               ▼
                    ┌──────────────────┐
                    │ Data preprocessing│
                    └──────────────────┘
                               │
                               ▼
                    ┌──────────────────┐
                    │ Train/Test Data Split│
                    └──────────────────┘
                               │
                               ▼
                    ┌──────────────────┐
                    │ Choose Machine    │◄──────┐
                    │ Learning model and│       │
                    │ Hyperparameters   │       │
                    └──────────────────┘       │
                               │                │
                               ▼                │
                    ┌──────────────────┐       │
                    │  Train  model on  │       │
                    │   training set    │       │
                    └──────────────────┘       │
                               │                │
                               ▼                │
                    ┌──────────────────┐       │
                    │ Evaluate model on │       │
                    │   testing set     │       │
                    └──────────────────┘       │
                               │                │
                               ▼                │
                         ╱──────────╲           │
                        ╱ Are the      ╲   No    │
                       ⟨ hyperparameters ⟩───────┘
                        ╲ well-tuned ? ╱
                         ╲──────────╱
                               │
                              Yes
                               ▼
                    ┌──────────────────┐
                    │   Deploy model    │
                    └──────────────────┘
                               │
                               ▼
                          ┌─────────┐
                         (   Stop    )
                          └─────────┘
```

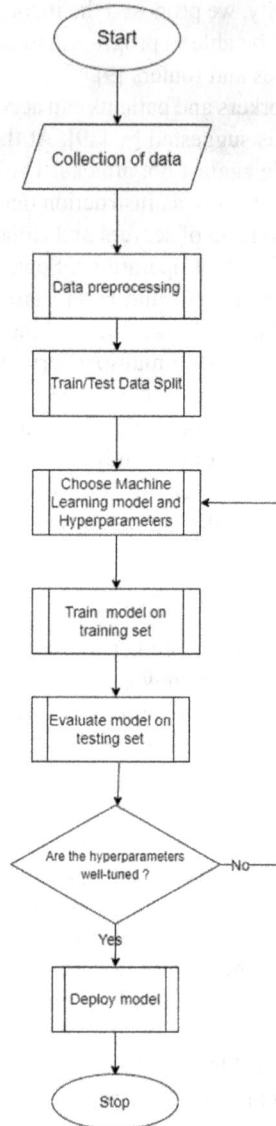

FIGURE 8.3   The flowchart of the machine learning process.

8.8.2   DATA PREPROCESSING

In machine learning experiments, there is the need to preprocess the data before use. The first need is to check for the features that will be relevant to the ML model at hand. Feature reduction has been a subject of research over the years. Techniques like principal component analysis (PCA) and singular value decomposition (SVD) have been used for many experiments. In this work, we checked the types of features and discovered eight of the features are of type objects. Hence, the following features were dropped to pave the way for features with type numerical types (float and int): Dir, Flgs, SrcAddr, DsrAddr, Sport, SrcMac, and DstMac.

The data was subsequently split into train and test datasets in the ratio 2:1 (10933: 5385).

Since attacks in the dataset are in the minority (12%), it informs the need to come up with a mechanism that will make the model predict accurately. We use synthetic minority over-sampling techniques (SMOTE) to balance the imbalanced data at the training stage.

8.8.2.1 Experimental Procedure

We performed the simulation of the intrusion detection system using a machine with the following specifications: HP Envy x 360 notebook with processor: Intel® Core i7 10th Gen with a capacity of 1.8 GHz with installed RAM: 12 GB, Windows 11 64-bit OS. Furthermore, software packages used include Python libraries such as Numpy, Sklearn, Pandas, and Imblearn. Matplotlib is used for data visualization, pandas is used for creating dataframes, imblearn is used for oversampling imbalanced data, and sklearn is used for the implementation of machine learning.

We used seven machine learning models for training and testing the systems against attacks. The ML models are k-nearest neighbor (kNN), naïve Bayes (NB), Logistic Regression (LR), support vector machines (SVM), decision tree (DT), random forest (RF), and extreme gradient boosting (XGBoost). Extensive details on these models can be found in the literature.

8.8.2.2 Standard Performance Metrics

The following metrics can measure the performance of machine learning models:

1. $accuracy = \dfrac{TP + TN}{TP + TN + FP + FN}$ 　　　　　　　　　　　　　　(8.1)

2. $precision = \dfrac{TP}{TP + FP}$ 　　　　　　　　　　　　　　　　　　　(8.2)

3. $sensitivity\,(TPR) = \dfrac{TP}{TP + FN}$ 　　　　　　　　　　　　　　　(8.3)

4. $specificity = \dfrac{TN}{TN + FP}$ 　　　　　　　　　　　　　　　　　　(8.4)

5. $F1\,score = 2 * \dfrac{precision * sensitivity}{precision + sensitivity}$ 　　　　　　　　　(8.5)

where TP = True Positives, TN = True Negatives, FP = False Positives, FN = False Negatives.

Other metrics are ROC and AUC.

The accuracy metric is a measure of the correct predictions made by the model concerning the total number of predictions made.

Sensitivity is a measure of the proportion of true positives that the model correctly predicts, while specificity is the measure of the proportion of true negatives correctly predicted by the model.

The F1 score is the harmonic mean of the precision and sensitivity score. F1 score is an evaluation metric that assesses the class-wise performance rather than the overall performance offered by the accuracy score.

Receiver over characteristics (ROC) measures the trade-off between sensitivity and specificity. AUC (area under the ROC curve) metric is used to validate the accuracy metric. It is used to evaluate how well the model can predict the classes accurately. The higher the value of these metrics, the better the models.

8.9   RESULTS AND DISCUSSIONS

The performance of the seven machine learning models was evaluated using the following metrics: accuracy, precision, sensitivity, specificity, F1 score, and AUC.

The results of the experiment in Table 8.4, show the extreme gradient boosting (XGBoost) model outperforming the other models in three metrics: accuracy (95.02%), F1 score (78.66%), and AUC (86.44%). The logistic regression model trumps other models in precision (93.03%) and specificity (99.51%). Finally, the decision tree model outperforms other models in sensitivity (89.51%). The bold figures are the highest for each metric. The higher the metrics, the better the performance of the algorithms.

The performance of the machine learning models using the following metrics: accuracy, precision, sensitivity, specificity, F1 score, and area under the roc curve (AUC). In Figure 8.4, XGBoost outperformed the other models with an accuracy score of 95.02%, logistic regression (LR) 93.05%, support vector machines (SVM) 90.68%, naïve Bayes (NB) 89.19%, random forest (RF) 78.40, k-nearest neighbor 77.25%, and decision tree (DT) 58.31%. The accuracy measure is germane because it gauges how the model can forecast future outcomes.

TABLE 8.4
The Performance Metrics in Percentage

ML Model	Accuracy	Precision	Sensitivity	Specificity	F1 Score	AUC
kNN	77.25	29.44	61.70	79.42	39.86	70.56
NB	89.19	56.91	47.57	94.99	51.82	71.28
LR	93.05	**93.03**	46.66	**99.51**	62.15	73.08
SVM	90.68	66.67	47.42	94.97	55.42	72.06
DT	58.31	21.30	**89.51**	53.97	34.41	71.74
RF	78.40	32.88	72.64	80.35	45.48	76.38
XGBoost	**95.02**	82.61	75.08	97.80	**78.66**	**86.44**

Note: The bold figures are the highest for each metric. The higher the metrics, the better the performance of the algorithms.

Accuracy

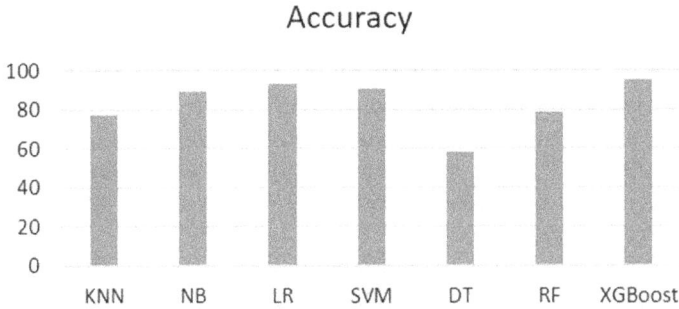

FIGURE 8.4   The accuracy graph with the XGBoost outperforming other models.

Precision

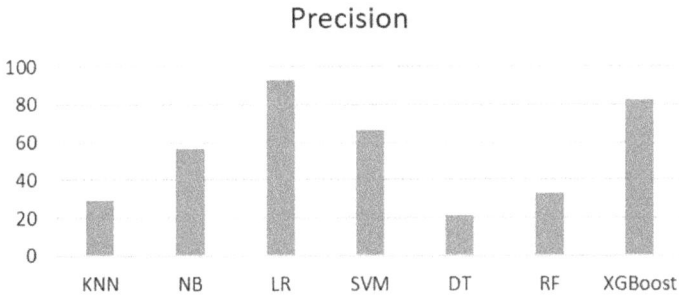

FIGURE 8.5   The precision graph with the logistic regression outperforming other models.

Sensitivity

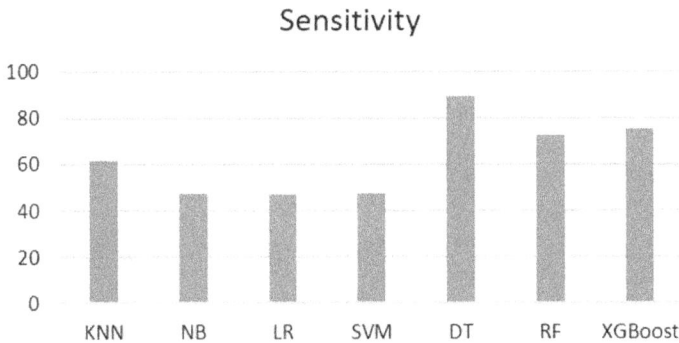

FIGURE 8.6   The sensitivity graph with the decision tree outperforming other models.

In Figure 8.5, the logistic regression outperforms other models with a precision score of 93.03%, XGBoost 82.61%, support vector machines (SVM) 66.67%, naïve Bayes (NB) 56.91%, random forest 32.88%, k-nearest neighbor 29.44%, and decision tree 21.30%. The precision seeks to determine the proportion of positive identification was correct.

In Figure 8.6, the decision tree outperforms other models with sensitivity scores of 89.51%, XGBoost 75.08%, random forest (RF) 72.64, kNN 61.70%, naïve Bayes (NB) 47.57%, support vector machines (SVM) 47.42%, and logistic regression (LR) 46.66%. The sensitivity score is a measure of how well the model can detect positive instances.

In Figure 8.7, logistic regression trumps other models with a specificity score of 99.51%, XGBoost 97.80%, naïve Bayes (NB) 94.99%, support vector machines (SVM) 94.97, random forest (RF) 80.35%, kNN 79.42%, and DT 53.97%. Specificity is the true negative rate.

In Figure 8.8, XGBoost surpasses other models with an F1 score of 78.66%, LR 62.15%, SVM 55.47%, naïve Bayes (NB) 51.82%, random forest (RF) 45.48%, kNN 39.86%, and DT 34.41%. The F1 score is the harmonic mean of the precision and sensitivity metrics.

In Figure 8.9, XGBoost outperforms other models with an AUC score of 0.8644, random forest 0.7638, logistic regression 0.7308, SVM 0.7206, DT 0.7174, NB 0.7128,

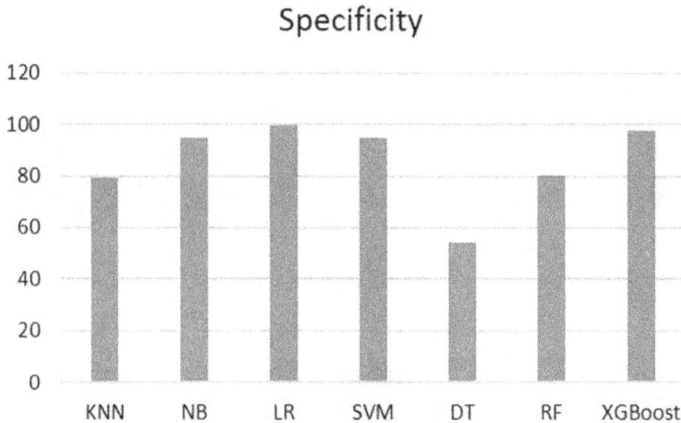

FIGURE 8.7   The specificity graph with the logistic regression outperforming other models.

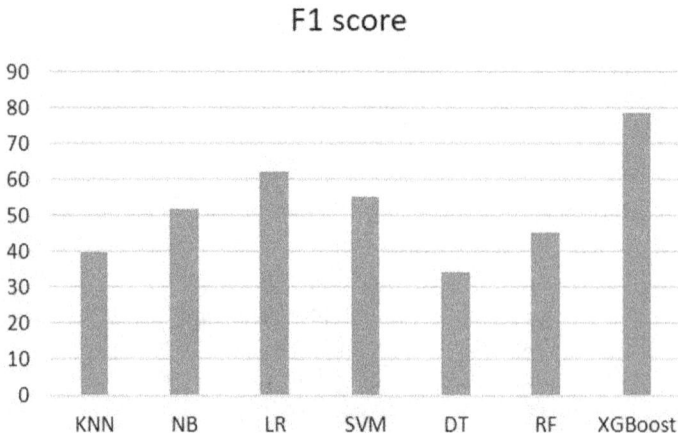

FIGURE 8.8   The F1 score graph with the XGBoost outperforming other models.

AUC

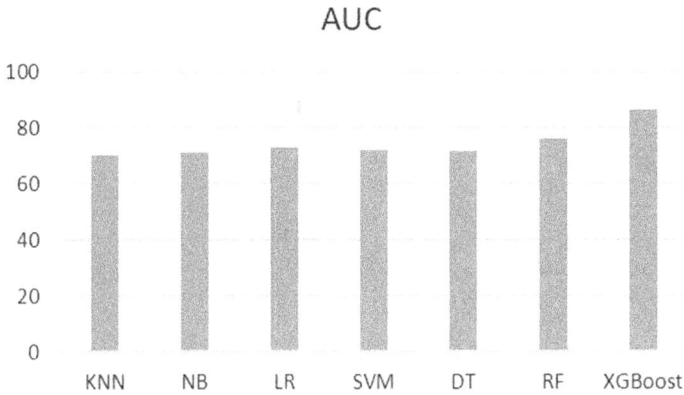

FIGURE 8.9   The AUC graph with the XGBoost outperforming other models.

and kNN 0.7056. AUC is a measure of the ability of a classifier to distinguish between classes. AUC values range from 0.0 to 1.0. The higher the AUC score, the better the model at distinguishing between classes. All the models have values close to 1, hence we can deduce that the models can distinguish between classes considerably.

Overall, XGBoost model surpasses other models in the following metrics: accuracy with 95.02%, F1 score 78.66%, and AUC 0.8644. The logistic regression outperforms other models in the following metrics: precision 93.03% and specificity 99.51%. Decision tree trumps other models only in sensitivity at 89.51%.

8.10   CONCLUSIONS AND FUTURE SCOPE

In this study, we investigated, highlighted, and reported recent advances and countermeasures on cyberattacks against artificial intelligence-enabled internet of medical things. Artificial intelligence-enabled Internet of medical things (AIoMT)'s architecture was tweaked to incorporate software-defined networking (SDN) to enable the development of an AI-based instruction detection system at the edge of the cloud using edge technology. Consideration was also given to categorizing and classifying the nature and types of cyberattacks prevalent in AIoMTs. It is worthy of note that the artificial intelligence-enabled Internet of medical things (AIoMT) comprises four pyramidal layers with the data collection devices, i.e., the sensors layer is the base. We simulated the IDS/Cloudnet of the framework with the flow metrics of the network and the biometrics of the patient using a testbed dataset. More work is required on the other parts of the framework and the implementation of a software-defined network.

Having considered the targeted AIoMTs aspects with the security of application, devices, cloud, and connectivity, we proposed a conceptual framework that gives a holistic coverage of the security and privacy concerns inherent in artificial intelligence-enabled Internet of medical things (AIoMT). Furthermore, the framework incorporated cloudlets—an edge technology—for low-latency and computationally intensive requirements in artificial intelligence-enabled Internet of medical things (AIoMT) systems. For example, cloudlets can be used as an instruction detection system, and it can be used to stem DoS and DDoS attacks.

Further works include using deep learning algorithms to provide a robust intrusion detection/prediction system using the advantage of edge technology and SDN technology.

ACKNOWLEDGMENT

The work of Agbotiname Lucky Imoize is supported in part by the Nigerian Petroleum Technology Development Fund (PTDF) and, in part, by the German Academic Exchange Service (DAAD) through the Nigerian-German Postgraduate Program under grant 57473408.

REFERENCES

[1]   A. Ghubaish, T. Salman, M. Zolanvari, and A. Al-Ali, "Recent Advances in the Internet-of-Medical Things (IoMT) Systems Security," *IEEE Internet of Things Journal*, vol. 8, no. 11, 2021

[2]   T. Belkhouja, S. Sorour, and M. S. Hefeida, "Role-Based Hierarchical Medical Data Encryption for Implantable Medical Devices," in *Proceedings of IEEE Global Communications Conference (GLOBECOM)*, Waikoloa, HI, 2019. doi: 10.1109/GLOBECOM38437.2019.9014192.

[3]   Y. Lu and L. D. Xu, "Internet of Things (IoT) Cybersecurity Research: A Review of Current Research Topics," *IEEE Internet of Things Journal*, vol. 6, pp. 2103–2115, 2019.

[4]   M. Shamila, K. Vinuthna, and A. K. Tyagi, "A Review on Several Critical Issues and Challenges in IoT Based E-Healthcare System," in *International Conference on Intelligent Computing and Control Systems (ICCS)* (pp. 1036–1043). IEEE, 2019.

[5]   J. B. Awotunde, R. G. Jimoh, S. O. Folorunso, E. A. Adeniyi, K. M. Abiodun, and O. O. Banjo, "Privacy and Security Concerns in IoT-Based Healthcare Systems," in *The Fusion of Internet of Things, Artificial Intelligence, and Cloud Computing in Health Care* (pp. 105–134). Springer, 2021.

[6]   E. Bout, V. Loscri, and A. Gallais, "How Machine Learning Changes the Nature of Cyberattacks on IoT Networks," *IEEE Communications Surveys & Tutorials*, vol. 24, no. 1, pp. 248–279, 2021.

[7]   T. Bhatia, A. K. Verma, and G. Sharma, "Toward a Secure Incremental Proxy Re-Encryption for E-Healthcare Data Sharing in Mobile Cloud Computing," *Concurrency and Computation Practice and Experience*, vol. 32, no. 5, p. e5520, 2019.

[8]   N. Hassan, S. Gillani, E. Ahmed, I. Yaqoob, and M. Imran, "The Role of Edge Computing in Internet of Things," *IEEE Communication Magazine*, 2018, https://doi.org/10.1109/MCON.2018.1700906.

[9]   S. Hyun, J. Kim, H. Kim, J. Jeong, S. Hares, L. Dunbar, and A. Farrel, "Interface to Network Security Functions for Cloud-Based Security Services," *IEEE Communications Magazine*, pp. 171–178, 2018, https://doi.org/10.1109/MCOM.2018.1700662.

[10] Y. Sun and B. Lo, "An Artificial Neural Network Framework for Gait-Based Biometrics," *IEEE Journal of Biomedical and Health Informatics*, vol. 23, no. 3, pp. 987–998, 2018, https://doi.org/10.1109/JBHI. 2018.2860780.

[11] G. Hatzivasilis, O. Soultatos, S. Ioannidis, C. Verikoukis, G. Demetriou, and C. I. Tsatsoulis, "Review of Security and Privacy for the Internet of Medical Things (IoMT)," in *15th International Conference on Distributed Computing in Sensor Systems (DCOSS)*, Santorini, Greece, 2019. doi: 10.1109/DCOSS.2019.00091.

[12] H. N. Dai, Z. Zheng, and Y. Zhang, "Blockchain for Internet of Things," *IEEE Internet of Things Journal*, vol. 6, no. 5, pp. 8076–8094, 2019.

[13] J. Sengupta, S. Ruj, and S. D. Bit, "A Comprehensive Survey on Attacks, Security Issues and Blockchain Solutions for IoT and IIoT," *Journal of Network and Computer Applications*, 2019, https://doi.org/10.1016/j.jnca.2019.102481.

[14] J. A. Yaacoub, M. Noura, H. N. Hassan, O. Salman, E. Yaacoub, R. Couturier, and A. Chehab, "Securing the Internet of Medical Things Systems: Limitations, Issues, and Recommendations," *Future Generation Systems*, vol. 105, pp. 581–606, 2020.

[15] Yanquig Yang, K. Zheng, C. Wu, X. Niu, and YixianYang, "Buliding an Effective Intrusion Detection System," *Applied Sciences, MDPI*, vol. 9, no. 238, 2019, https://doi.org/10.3390/app9020238.

[16] B. A. Alzahrani, A. Irshad, A. Albeshri, and K. Alsubhi, "A Provably Secure and Lightweight Patient-Healthcare Authentication Protocol in Wireless Body Area Networks," *Wireless Personal Communications*, vol. 117, pp. 47–69, 2021. https://doi.org/10.1007/s11277-020-07237-x.

[17] Y. Sun and B. Lo, "An Artificial Neural Network Framework for Gait-Based Biometrics," *IEEE Journal of Biomedical and Health Informatics*, vol. 23, no. 3, 2019.

[18] S. M. Tahsien, H. Karimipour, and P. Spachos, "Machine Learning Based Solutions for the Security of Internet of Things (IoT)," *Journal of Network and Computer Applications*, vol. 161, pp. 1–18, 2020.

[19] B. A. Alennizi, M. Humayun, and N. Z. Jhanjhi, "Security and Privacy Issues in Cloud Computing," *Journal of Physics*, 2021. https://doi.org/10.1088/1742-6596/1979/1/012038.

[20] A. Avinashiappan and B. Mayilsamy (eds.), *Internet of Medical Things, Internet of Things*, D. J. Hemanth et al. (eds.). Springer Nature, 2021.

[21] V. Mothukuri, P. Khare, R. M. Parizi, S. Pouriyeh, A. Dehghantanha, and G. Srivastava, "Federated Learning-based Anomaly Detection for IoT Security Attacks," *IEEE Internet of Things Journal*, vol. 9, no. 4, pp. 2545–2554, 2021.

[22] A. A. Süzen, B. Duman, D. J. Hermanth et al. (eds.), *Internet of Medical Things, Internet of Things*, Springer Nature, 2021.

[23] U. Inayat, M. F. Zia, S. Mahmood, H. M. Khalid, and M. Benbouzid, "Learning-Based Methods for Cyber Attacks Detection in IoT Systems: A Survey on Methods, Analysis, and Future Prospects," *Electronics MDPI*, vol. 11, no. 1502, 2022.

[24] P. Manickan, S. A. Mariappan, S. M. Murugesan, S. Hansda, A. Kaushik, R. Shinde, and S. P. Thipperudraswamy, "Artificial Intelligence (AI) and Internet of Medical Things (IoMT) Assisted Biomedical Systems for Intelligent Healthcare," *Biosensors*, vol. 12, p. 562, 2022. https://doi.org/10.3390/bios12080562.

[25] M. Maqsood, S. Yasmin, S. Gillani, F. Aadil, I. Mehmood, S. Rho, and S. Yeo, "An Autonomous Decision-Making Framework for Gait Recognition Systems Against Adversarial Attack Using Reinforcement Learning," *ISA Transactions*, vol. 132, pp. 80–93, 2022.

[26] S. Razdan and S. Sharma, "Internet of Medical Things (IoMT): Overview, Emerging Technologies, and Case Studies," *IEEE Technical Review*, vol. 39, no. 4, pp. 775–788, 2022.

[27] I. Andrea, C. Chrysostomou, and G. Hadjichristofi, "Internet of Things: Security Vulnerabilities and Challenges," in *IEEE Symposium on Computers and Communication (ISCC)* (pp. 180–187). IEEE, 2015.

[28] J. Deogirikar and A. Vidhate, "Security Attacks in IoT: A Survey," in *2017 International Conference on I-SMAC (IoT in Social, Mobile, Analytics and Cloud)(I-SMAC)* (pp. 32–37). IEEE, 2017.

[29] A. D. Wood and J. A. Stankovic, "Denial of Service in Sensor Networks," *Computer*, vol. 35, no. 10, pp. 54–62, 2002.

[30] G. Kaur and P. Gupta, "Detection of Distributed Denial of Service Attacks for IoT-based Healthcare Systems," *Computer Assisted Methods in Engineering and Science*, vol. 30, no. 2, pp. 167–186, 2022.

[31] A. I. Newaz, A. K. Sikder, L. Babun, and A. S. Uluagac, "Heka: A Novel Intrusion Detection System for Attacks to Personal Medical Devices," in *2020 IEEE Conference on Communications and Network Security (CNS)* (pp. 1–9). IEEE, 2022.

[32] [Online]: Chapter 3—Rights of the Data Subject—General Data Protection Regulation (GDPR), gdpr-info.eu, accessed December 9, 2022.

[33] A. Koren and R. Prasad, "IoT Health Data in Electronic Health Records (EHR): Security and Privacy Issues in Era of 6G," *Journal of ICT Standardization*, pp. 63–84, 2022.

[34] L. Sun, X. Jiang, H. Ren, and A. Yi Guo, "Edge-Cloud Computing and Artificial Intelligence in the Internet of Medical Things," *IEEE Access*, vol. 8, pp. 101079–101092, 2020.

[35] W. Moore and S. Frye, "Review of HIPAA, Part 1: History, Protected Health Information, and Privacy and Security Rules," *Journal of Nuclear Medicine Technology*, vol. 47, no. 4, pp. 269–272, 2019.

[36] A. A. Hady, A. Ghubaish, T. Salman, D. Unal, and R. Jain, "Intrusion Detection System for Healthcare Systems Using Medical and Network Data: A Comparison Study," *IEEE Access*, vol. 8, pp. 106576–106584, 2020, https://doi.org/10.1109/ACCESS.2020.3000421, https://ieeexplore.ieee.org/document/9109651

[37] A. T. Rufai, K. F. Dukor, O. M. Ageh, and A. L. Imoize, "XAI Robot-Assisted Surgeries in Future Medical Decision Support Systems," in *Explainable Artificial Intelligence in Medical Decision Support Systems*, 1st ed., A. L. Imoize, J. Hemanth, D.-T. Do, and S. N. Sur (eds.) (pp. 167–195). The Institution of Engineering and Technology, 2022.

[38] P. K. Sadhu, V. P. Yanambaka, A. Abdelgawad, and K. Yelamarthi, "Prospect of Internet of Medical Things: 'A Review on Security Requirements and Solutions'," *Sensors (Basel)*, vol. 22, no. 15, p. 5517, 2022, https://doi.org/10.3390/s22155517.

[39] A. Binbusayyis, H. Alaskar, T. Vaiyapuri, et al. "An Investigation and Comparison of Machine Learning Approaches for Intrusion Detection in IoMT Network," *The Journal of Supercomputing*, vol. 78, pp. 17403–17422, 2022, https://doi.org/10.1007/s11227-022-04568-3.

[40] J. Shahid, R. Ahmad, A. K. Kiani, T. Ahmad, S. Saeed, and A. M. Almuhaideb, "Data Protection and Privacy of the Internet of Healthcare Things (IoHTs)," *Applied Sciences*, vol. 12, no. 4, p. 1927, 2022, https://doi.org/10.3390/app12041927.

[41] R. Dwivedi, D. Mehrotra, and S. Chandra, "Potential of Internet of Medical Things (IoMT) Applications in Building a Smart Healthcare System: A Systematic Review," *Journal of Oral Biology and Craniofacial Research*, vol. 12, no. 2, pp. 302–318, 2022, ISSN 2212-4268, https://doi.org/10.1016/j.jobcr.2021.11.010.

[42] J. Nayak, S.K. Meher, A. Souri, et al., "Extreme Learning Machine and Bayesian Optimization-Driven Intelligent Framework for IoMT Cyber-Attack Detection," *The Journal of Supercomputing*, vol. 78, pp. 14866–14891, 2022, https://doi.org/10.1007/s11227-022-04453-z.

[43] R. Buenrostro-Mariscal, P. C. Santana-Mancilla, O. A. Montesinos-López, M. Vazquez-Briseno, and J. I. Nieto-Hipolito, "Prioritization-Driven Congestion Control in Networks for the Internet of Medical Things: A Cross-Layer Proposal," *Sensors*, vol. 23, no. 2, p. 923, 2023, https://doi.org/10.3390/s23020923.

[44] E. Yıldırım, M. Cicioğlu, and A. Çalhan, "Fog-Cloud Architecture-Driven Internet of Medical Things Framework for Healthcare Monitoring," *Medical & Biological Engineering & Computing*, pp. 1–15, 2023, https://doi.org/10.1007/s11517-023-02776-4.

9 Cyberattacks against AIoMT Architectures

Abasiama Godwin Akpan, Fergus Uchenna Onu, Flavious Bobuin Nkubli, Anayo Christian Okwor, and Geofery Luntsi

9.1 INTRODUCTION

AIoMT is an increasing technological advancement connecting diverse automated nodes to smart ecological network of things such as the *internet of medical things* [1]. Nevertheless, widespread and open location amplifies the possibility for cyber attackers to hack in order to exploit AIoMT terminals [2]. The nature of these terminals and their devices create unique opportunities for cybercriminals to target critical infrastructures leading to diverse attacks, such as distributed denial of service (DDoS), data injection, malware, botnet intrusion that breaches the privacy of information and its availability or even destroy the entire critical infrastructure [3]. Hence, AIoMT is vulnerable to several cyber threats, such as *identity theft, keylogging, phishing, malicious bot* [4]. The restriction of critical assets, scalability, allocation, mobility, and small latency are key issues that promote critical system attacks [5]. Information transmission is usually done with the assistance of a wireless infrastructure. Hence, it amplifies the possibilities of weaknesses due to the transmission of information via wireless medium. The hacker can simply snuffle information if no safety machinery is deployed [6]. Solitude and safety of patient's information are key factors in AIoMT and preserving them from loss becomes imperative [7]. Internet usage has increased over the years, paving way to the Internet of Things (IoT).

This has linked huge amount of information via linked nodes to the internet for communication [8]. This advancement assists in monitoring the health status of patients remotely combining several automated terminals accessible to the patient [9]. AIoMT is an emerging technology for improving healthcare services irrespective of time and location constraints. Nevertheless, AIoMT devices that make up the critical units of the network forming what is termed a Wireless Body Area Network are prone to several kinds of threats and attacks, causing major risk to patient's safety and privacy [10]. Safety and confidentiality are decisive factors for the thriving adaptation of AIoMT-enabled network technologies in healthcare. There is a necessity for novel safety methods to protect the safety and privacy of the AIoMT network since the present authentication methods to the Artificial Intelligence of Medical Things are complicated because of extremely dynamic and probably unprotected situations and a supply chain for the Internet of Things devices that are not trusted. Hence, understanding the exact requirement for an appropriate AIoMT

DOI: 10.1201/9781003370321-9

validation requires a total knowledge of the existing and potential threats to the AIoMT edge network [11]. The therapeutic information safety is experiencing an enormous threat as a result of the swift development in the Internet of Things utilization and mobile networks. The safety of clinical information is of huge significance in the AIoMT. Accessing clinical records of patients without permission can result in creating impairment, such as wrong prescription of drugs leading to the health risk of the patients or death. The proportion of internally generated safety threats to externally generated safety threats is alarming [12]. Hence, domestic safety threats are extremely critical and demanding to handle as compared to external safety threats. The AIoMT is a set of equipment linked to the networks of medical things to offer health-related services [13]. Essentially, AIoMT is a linked communication of clinical systems, for example, clinical equipment, applications, and routines. There is a clear indication that the linkage between clinical equipment and sensor-based terminals assists in managing medical processes in efficient ways regardless of the patient's location [14]. Connecting clinically related equipment will have a huge effect on patients and medical practitioners. AIoMT expertise is vital in advocating possible cure and rendering useless any extra attacks through remote monitoring by clinicians and self-monitoring [15, 16]. The key function of AIoMT is for detecting ailments in patients and having clinical insight into patients' health status [17, 18, 19]. Kandasamy et al. argued that AIoMT structures are in four (4) stages [20], namely:

i. *Devices that are wearable*: Typical examples are intelligent watches, sensors for measuring human body temperature, sensors for measuring human blood pressure, intelligent heart monitors, sensors for measuring human muscle activity, sensors for measuring human body glucose, and the biochemical processes of the body.
ii. *Devices that are implantable*: Camera capsule that can be swallowed for visualization of the gastrointestinal tract, embedded cardiac pacemakers, and implantable cardioverter-defibrillators.
iii. *Devices that are ambient*: Sensors for mobility of aging, sensors for unlocking automatic doors, sensors for vibration, etc.
iv. *Stationary devices*: Imaging modalities, such as Computerized Tomography (CT) and Magnetic Resonance Imaging (MRI) and some devices for surgery.

9.1.1 CONTRIBUTION OF THE CHAPTER

The significance of this chapter includes:

i. Identifying weaknesses based on the level of devices.
ii. Examining the nature, characteristics, and targeted AIoMT's security
iii. Classifying threats targeting AIoMT network
iv. Introduction of safety issues in AIoMT
v. Developing a link between threats and exploited weaknesses
vi. Examining of validation protocols and detecting methods for AIoMT networks

9.1.2 Chapter Organization

This chapter is presented in sections as follows: Section 9.1 explains the artificial intelligence of medical things (AIoMT). Section 9.2 presents the concept of cyber security. Section 9.3 presents a review of related works. Section 9.4 explains the concept of ML for cyber security tasks. Section 9.5 presents the functions of cyber security center. Section 9.6 discusses the AIoMT model. Section 9.7 discusses the nature of cyberattacks. Section 9.8 presents types of cyberattacks against AIoMT. Section 9.9 presents man-in-the-Middle attack mitigation in AIoMT. Section 9.10 presents Intrusion detection systems. Section 9.11 discusses cyberattacks on PACS. Section 9.12 presents the conclusion.

9.2 CONCEPT OF CYBER SECURITY

Cyberspace is a mutually dependent network that underpins several of our information technologies [21]. This constituent is a crucial entity of the world's economy critical infrastructure. Therefore, securing cyberspace is critical to the standard and the security of the world's economy [21]. Cyber security describes the standards and policy protection strategies espoused to restrain cyber criminality in the super highway [22]. Cyber security attempts to maintain critical infrastructures and national assets against risks. The technologies, procedures, and practices are designed to protect networks or unauthorized access. Abasiama et al. listed key objectives of cyber security to include [22]:

   i. Confidentiality
  ii. Integrity
 iii. Availability

Some of the key cyber security notions are elucidated herewith:

9.2.1 Cyber Threats

A cyber threat is an unauthorized access to manage devices via a network pathway. Threats to network nodes can emanate from different sources, such as unreceptive governments, radical groups, disgruntled staff, and cruel interlopers. Cyber threats with focus on *personality, brunt, source and perpetrator* can be classified as follows:

   i. *Intentional*: Sometimes referred to as *accidental threats,* they arise without deliberate intention. A typical example is a software failure or physical system malfunctions. Nevertheless, these threats result from premeditated acts against the security of a critical asset.
  ii. *Active:* This kind of threats is termed *Passive threats*, resulting from changes in the status of the system. A typical example is the *alteration of information, wiretapping, deep packet analysis, annihilation of physical devices, and eavesdropping.*
 iii. *Threat source*: This is regarded as a unit that needs to violate physical assets' security controls.

    iv. *Threat actor:* This is a unit that executes the attack or exploits the accident.
    v. *Vulnerability*: This is weakness in the system that includes lack of patch-
       ing software or configuration that is poor.

9.2.2 SECURITY RISK

This is the likelihood that a risk uses a weakness to break the safety of an asset.
However, efficient systems function with levels of exposure to risks, since total
removal of risk is high or unwanted.

9.2.3 COMPUTER EMERGENCY RESPONSE TEAM (CERT)

CERT is a professional group that is in charge of information security incidents.
CERT is the human equivalent of antivirus software. The main objectives of CERT
are listed here:

    i. Building capacity to speedily and efficiently manage interaction among
      professionals for safety measures
    ii. Creating consciousness about risk concerns across the network
    iii. Expanding the risk response plan
    iv. Recognizing and categorizing attack incidents
    v. Choosing devices, methods, and pathways for detecting and preventing
      attacks
    vi. Promoting awareness on cyber-security
    vii. Determining the extent of investigations once there is an attack

9.2.4 CYBER INCIDENT RESPONSE TEAM (CIRT)

The responsible of CIRT is to design plans for incident response and examination in
line with the incidence plan. The key objectives are listed as follows:

    i. Designing plans for cyber incident response
    ii. Recognizing and categorizing attack incident
    iii. Choosing devices, methods, and pathways for detecting and preventing attacks
    iv. Creating awareness on cyber-security
    v. Establishing extent for inquiry
    vi. Carry out inquiry on the occurrence of cyberattack

9.2.5 CYBER SECURITY STRATEGY

A cyber security threat is sophisticated because adversaries use new techniques like
cloud, mobile computing, big-data analytics, and artificial intelligence. There is no
enterprise that has the required potential to ease all cyber risks. Hence, collaboration
is significant and should include making inquiries, data, authority, and instruction.

International Telecommunication Union recognizes five important structures that support world cybersecurity programs. The structures include:

   i. Authorized procedures
  ii. Technological and routine procedures
 iii. Formation based on organization
  iv. Competence building
   v. Global cooperation

9.3   REVIEW OF RELATED WORKS

Ref.	Purpose	Findings
[21]	Painting a mounting scenario of a progression of new kind of war—the internet cybercrime.	Cybercrime is multifaceted. This act is carried out mainly from isolated locations.
[22]	Responding wisely in the age of uncertainty.	Cybercrime is aggressive and affect IT critical infrastructure.
[23]	Creating a platform for self-destruction of data.	Validating information security platform via files of diverse designs and a protected server making enhancement on the existing system.
[24]	Creating an intelligent reporting platform for crime using structured system analysis and design methodology. Implemented using Javascript, React, Firebase and Express web server.	Incorporation of attributes of a conventional reporting system with options for reporting crime.
[25]	Leveraging on cyber security for digital economy.	Unraveling different types of emerging cyber threats and new attack patterns.
[26]	Militating against cyber security threats and attacks.	Investigation of category of cyber threats and attacks; clarifying countermeasures to minimize existential security risk.
[27]	Creating a platform for software use in crime mapping.	Law enforcers adopting crime mapping software for detecting crime.
[28]	Statistical testing using differential privacy for MDSS.	Demonstration of findings from statistical analysis to reveal individual attribute values.
[29]	Developing a secure pandemic information handling using Blockchain technology.	Results revealed core structures with resilience for data handling.
[30]	Developing AI-IoMT for management of pandemic records.	Perceptive privacy-aware energy via AIoMT for COVID-19 pandemic information usage.
[31]	Reviewing different platforms for IoT, AI, and blockchain technology.	Unraveling trends among related technologies.
[32]	Integrating XNN in the prediction of diabetes mellitus.	Results revealed the effect of each variable on the overall model. XNN Model was assessed based on accuracy, sensitivity, specificity, recall, and F1.

(Continued)

(Continued)

Ref.	Purpose	Findings
[33]	Analytical approach to concerns of IoTs in healthcare.	Discovery mechanism was proposed as a means to secure AIoMT.
[34]	Highlighting cyberattacks on AIoMT.	Several means to detect different attacks were presented.
[35]	Designing security for medical cyber-physical systems.	The design of a threat model and proposing prospective attack techniques for medical imaging devices.
[36]	Reviewing threat challenges in PACS and medical imaging.	Integration of the clinical enterprise incorporation report and testing devices in PACS.
[37]	Developing a framework on one-pixel attacks against medical imaging.	Describing a theoretical structure of one-pixel attack and applying it to clinical tasks.
[38]	Reviewing cybersecurity in the internet of medical things.	Introduction of regulatory guidance documents emphasizing on device identification, legacy device management, enhanced physical security, and breach detection.
[39]	Modeling threats for IoMT using Markov chain and common vulnerability Scoring System.	Identification of any weaknesses in AIoMT set of connections.
[40]	Protecting medical records in heterogeneous IoTs.	Implementation of authorization in combination with permissions and roles.
[41]	Building secured IoTs.	A tamper-proof digital ledger implementation for nontrusted nodes.
[42]	Outlining cyber threats and mitigation in healthcare.	Security measures and cryptographic countermeasures to mitigate threats in e-healthcare environment.
[43]	Designing IDS for IoTS.	Experimental results showing detection of anomalies in network flow and patient's biometric readings.
[44]	Mitigating against MitM Attack in IoTs.	Proposed framework to prevent a MitM from disrupting the operations and prohibiting the raise of alarms by the remote healthcare monitoring system.
[45]	Creating privacy management in IoMT.	Classifying techniques and to characterize them in order to benefit from their positive aspects.
[46]	Developing a secure medical image-sharing system based on zero trust.	Result recommended blockchain technology for data integrity.
[47]	Securing picture archiving and communication system.	Implementing controls to safeguard medical images from cybersecurity and privacy threats.
[48]	Harnessing healthcare critical systems.	Safety measures among providers of healthcare devices.
[49]	A systematic literature review of blockchain cyber security.	Finding a means to assemble structures and to divide them into lesser units.
[50]	Analyzing PUF machines existing in the *Thing layer.*	Machines display a critical role in the validation of AIoMT machines.

9.4   ML FOR CYBER SECURITY TASKS

Recently, the improvement in artificial intelligent and machine learning as commanded recommendations; integrating machine learning techniques for privacy control have been in practice. Until lately, this practice fell nearly into the detective level of cyber security, where concentration is on *detecting spam*, *detecting intrusion*, and *detecting malware*. These methods are usually divided into *supervised learning* and *unsupervised learning* [51]. Supervised learning tagged datasets in order to use for training a replica to categorize new inputs. Unsupervised learning untagged datasets in order to examine or identify fundamental model within the data. Whichever methods can be helpful in detecting malicious traffic. To show how conventional ML methods are used cyber security, look at a few illustrations.

   i. *Detecting spam*: ML has been a key component of spam-detecting mechanism since early 2000s, and ML methods are in full usage up till today.
   ii. *Intrusion detecting*: Intrusion-detecting systems tries to determine the occurrence of unlawful processes within the networks, focusing on performance profiles and looking for malicious signs. These systems are grouped as *misuse-based* or *anomaly-based*.
   iii. *Malware detection*: Malware detecting systems scrutinize specific *files* to establish if files are cruel.

9.4.1   AI APPLICATIONS FOR THREATS PREVENTION

The initial phase of cyber security replica is prevention. Table 9.1 shows the AI application for threat prevention.

9.4.2   AI APPLICATIONS FOR THREAT DETECTION

Detecting threats is the least method where DL and ML techniques are regarded as a possible transformative strength [51]. Table 9.2 shows the AI application for threat detection.

TABLE 9.1
AI Application for Threat Prevention.

Cyber Security Functions	AI Applications	Importance of Function	AI Capability
Fuzzing	DL	Towering	Average Towering
Pentesting	RL	Towering	Average Towering
Bug Triage and categorization	NLP, ML	Average	Average
Susceptibility Strictness Assessment	NLP, ML	Average	Average Low

9.4.3   AI APPLICATIONS FOR THREAT RESPONSE AND RECOVERY

Response and recovery is an active and uninterrupted practice that is not broken into separate components [52]. Table 9.3 shows AI application for threat response and recovery.

9.4.4   AI APPLICATIONS FOR ACTIVE DEFENSE

Any organizations with safety needs must take practical measures to strengthen their cyber security policies in response to new threats [53, 54]. Table 9.4 shows AI application for active defense.

TABLE 9.2
AI Application for Threat Detection

Cyber Security Functions	AI Application	Importance of Function	AI capability
Precise Recognition	DL	Towering	Low
Alert Priority	DL	Average Towering	Average
Hardening of Detecting Systems	GANs	Average Towering	Average Low

TABLE 9.3
AI Application for Threat Response and Recovery

Cyber Security Functions	AI Application	Importance of Function	AI Capability
Adversary rendezvous	RL	Towering	Average Low
Target protection	RL	Towering	Average Low

TABLE 9.4
AI Application for Active Defense

Cyber Security Functions	AI Application	Importance of Function	AI capability
Deceptive document generation	NLP, GANs	Average Low	Towering
Honey potting	RL	Average	Average Towering
Phishing response	NLP, RL	Low	Average Towering
Dark web attack	NLP	Average	Average
Attack clusters	NLP, ML	Average Low	Average
Deanonymization of code	NLP	Low	Average Low

9.5   FUNCTIONS OF CYBER SECURITY CENTER

Preferably, a center for cyber security strives to make sure a secure and flexible cyber communications infrastructure supports national security. To achieve this, the center should:

i. Focus on organizing the avoidance and lessening of cyber threats that pose the greatest risk
ii. Follow operational incorporation via increasing and deepening commitment with its partners via data sharing to deal with threats, weaknesses, and occurrences
iii. Classify the barriers that hamper mutual data swap, situational responsiveness, and perceptive of threats and their effect
iv. Sustain willingness to react straight away and efficiently to any cyber occurrence on critical asset
v. Serve as a point for cyber safety concerns
vi. Defend the privacy of the citizens

9.6   AIOMT MODEL

AIoMT structural design assists in understanding the components of diverse layers of AIoMT. Several structural designs are proposed in various researches. The major structural design layers are:

i. Application
ii. Network
iii. Physical

i. Application Layer

This offers modified services based on user pertinent requirements [43]. The major function is connecting users and the applications. The implementation of the application layer is done via a dedicated application at the server end [23].

ii. Network Layer

This layer is charged with the tasks of forwarding data from source to destination via internet addressing points. It sends out and route information received from nodes, and creates connections among intelligent systems, such as servers and networking devices [55–59]. The standard for the transmission can be cabled or cableless [55].

iii. Perception Layer

A key function of this layer is information gathering and transferring of information to the network layer. It consists of nodes for detecting and collecting data concerning

TABLE 9.5
Internetworking Technologies for AIoMT

Network	Connectivity
Ethernet	Cabled
Wireless	Cableless
3G	Cableless
LAN	Cabled/Cableless
Bluetooth	Cableless
RFID	Cableless
ZigBee	Cableless

TABLE 9.6
Representation of Perception Layer Devices in AIoMT

AIoMT Device	Functions
Activity Monitor	Gyroscope sensors are used for monitoring patients' medical status.
Electronic Cardiogram	Ensuring safety for the heart.
Temperatures Measurement	Body temperature measurement.
Biometric Sensor	Identification of patients.
Locator	Location tracer for patients.
Biochemical Sensors	Detecting harmful substances.
Blood Pressure	Measuring blood pressure of patients.
Respiratory Rate	Breathing rate measurement for patients.
Pulse Oximeters	Pulse rate measurement for patients.
Heart Monitoring	Heartbeats measurement using electrocardiography.

the immediate environment. Table 9.7 shows the representation of the perception layer devices in AIoMT.

9.7 NATURE OF CYBERATTACKS

Primarily, cyberattacks are on data, network, and access [22]. Militating against these kinds of attacks will stop any effort to deteriorate the performance of an intelligent system or effort to trail clinical activities without permission [21, 22, 26]. Abasiama et al. discussed diverse kinds of rising threats and attack patterns on critical systems, such as AIoMT [26, 30]. The authors listed emerging cyber threats to include:

    i.   *Deepfakes*: Deepfakes occur whenever AI-based technology creates fake images and sounds in any critical physical systems that appear real. To reduce the threat, verification measures should be imposed.

    ii.   *Synthetic identities*: These are associated with identity scheme where a criminal uses genuine and conjured ID to creating a fake notion of

TABLE 9.7
AIoMT Attacks

Attacks	Typical Methods	Mitigating Channels
Self-directed AI	Devices that are closed-loop can maliciously distort information in patients' records	• Execute device audit • Replication of high-risk situation
Reduce Bluetooth power	Attacking Bluetooth stack rules in paired machines	• Cryptographic keys • Update OS regularly • Turn off Bluetooth at idle state
Convergent cloud	Attacks on the weak safety measures in cloud	• Update cloud security • Critical assets auditing • Integration of IDS • Data encryption • Backup critical data • Isolate critical networking infrastructures
Edging processes	Interfacing edging processes to cloud pose a risk	• Point-to-point connections should be afforded • Authenticate direct connections • Dedicated links should be deployed for critical systems
AIoMT diversity	State of dissimilar elements encourages novel hacking	• Extrapolation threats scene during modeling • Monitoring and managing critical infrastructures • End user's agreement implementation
OtS elements	Usage of off-the-shelf modules in AIoMT triggers maximal target for hackers	• Required standards for OTS should be implemented • Safety assessment of critical components should be done promptly
Physical landscape	hackers exploit nodes via stealing of concealed AIoMT	• Build AIoMT with unparalleled identification and trackers • AIoMT critical assets should be made accountable
Retrofitting	Security weaknesses in obsolete devices can be a point for compromising the entire system	• Enacting laws on duration of critical infrastructures usage • Risk analysis should be carried out on legacy systems to reduce device structures
Quantum computing	Computational requirements would turn some cryptographic devices not useful	• Encrypted algorithm to increase crypto-key parameters • Migrating critical infrastructures to quantum-safe encrypted level • Develop integrated quantum encrypted methods as safety means

an actual person. To reduce the risk, safekeeping of personal information and destruction of documents containing personal information is paramount.

  iii. *AI-powered cyberattacks:* Using AI, hackers create programs that replicate acknowledged human characters and use them to trick people. To reduce the risk, ML method deploys to train chronological datasets and detect anomalies.

  iv. *Poisoning attacks:* Hackers inject dreadful information into AI programs. This information can cause malfunctioning of the AI system. To reduce the risk, the latest patches on all software should be installed.

   v. *Ransomware attacks*: The hacker injects a victim's system with a malicious code that contains all of their data. The victim is requested to pay a ransom or lose critical information. To reduce the risk, perimeter security, such as firewalls should be installed to avert intruders from uploading to your systems.

  vi. *Denial-of-service (DOS) and attacks:* In this method of attack, critical systems resources are being overpowered, thereby preventing the system from responding to service requests. To reduce the risk, strong access control and policies should be established.

 vii. *Distributed denial-of-service (DDoS) attacks:* This attack is initiated from various host nodes polluted by software that are with malicious codes controlled by the hacker. To reduce the risk, blacklist IP addresses.

viii. *Man-in-the-middle (MitM) attack:* In this attack, the hacker introduces themselves between the *client* and a *server.* To reduce the risk, establish VPNs to protect links.

  ix. *SQL injection attack:* This attack occurs when an intruder performs an SQL query to the database via the input data. To reduce the risk, validating the input, querying parameters, procedure storing, and firewall should be applied.

   x. *Eavesdropping attack:* This is the interception of the traffic in the system where hackers get confidential information across the network. To reduce the risk, firewall and updating the antivirus software should be applied.

  xi. *Cross-site scripting (XSS) attack:* In this attack, a third party is used to script web browser application of the victim. To reduce the risk, use appropriate filters and encoding techniques.

9.8   TYPES OF CYBERATTACKS AGAINST AIOMT

Cyberattacks may create an impact on the privacy, reliability, or accessibility. Some threats on linked AIoMT are:

   i. *Eavesdropping attack*
  ii. *Brute force*
 iii. *Ransomware attacks*
 iv. *Replay*

    v. *Cross-site request forgery*
   vi. *Hijacking of session*
  vii. *XSS attack*
 viii. *SQL injection*
   ix. *Side channel*
    x. *Account hijacking*
   xi. *Tag cloning*
  xii. *Tampering devices*
 xiii. *Rogue access*

9.8.1 ONE-PIXEL ATTACKS

One pixel is an adversarial attack on critical AIoMT, such as medical imaging systems where one pixel of an image is distorted, resulting in false classification of the AI model. There are numerous attacks on DNNs that analyze images with the aim of image classification. There are illustrations of images and patches that generate redundant outcomes as soon as AI classifier is in use [61]. One-pixel attacks are known techniques of deceiving NN models. Altering a single pixel in an object makes the classification of the object as another class. One-pixel attack alters a single pixel in the image to deceive the AI model. This is a typical kind of threat against smart examination and analysis in clinical practice, particularly when the pixel is evidently well-known.

9.8.2 ATTACKS IN AIoMT

AIoMT attack, typical method, and mitigating channels are listed in Table 9.7.

9.8.3 CYBERATTACKS ON AIoMT

Trending adversarial attacks, defense techniques, causes, and possible threats are listed in Table 9.8.

9.8.4 SECURITY CHALLENGES IN HEALTHCARE SYSTEMS

Wael and Nidal posited that cyberattacks on healthcare critical systems cannot be less [62]. Nevertheless, security concerns weakening AIoMT connectivity as argued by researchers are listed by Owida et al. [63]. The list includes:

    i. *Exploitation of information*—the hacker modifies or deletes information on patients' records which can intimidate patient life.
   ii. Records of patients accessed by personnel can be a source for blackmail.
  iii. Noncompliance to standards by providers of health devices might ease hijacking process of patients' information.
  iv. Adoption of internet via public access in healthcare services exposes the entire healthcare network to intruders.

TABLE 9.8
Cyberattacks on AIoMT

Adversarial attacks	Defense techniques	Causes	Possible threats
Ransomware	Antimalicious code, knowledge-based approach through awareness and avoidance of private data	Usage of weak means of authentication, extortion from ransomware	Privacy, reliability, validation, and accessibility
Spyware	Updating of system applications, such as OS and updated antivirus	A definite host required	Privacy, reliability, validation, and accessibility
Trojan horse	Updating physical system components regularly, deploying intrusive detecting system	Indiscriminate software downloads and hidden software updating internally	Privacy, reliability, validation, and accessibility
Viruses	Antivirus solutions, Penetration tester-based approach	Breach/failure of defense network	Privacy, reliability, validation, and accessibility
Botnet	Penetration tester-based approach, intrusive detecting system, and anti-malicious code	Exploitation of AIoMT logical weaknesses	Privacy, reliability, validation, and accessibility
Rootkit	Effective configuration of system, managing system authentication, intrusive detecting system, and patch update	Operating system kernel exploitation and root attributes	Validation
Worm	Intrusive detecting system and anti-malicious code and antivirus solutions	Breach/failure of defense network	Privacy, reliability, validation, and accessibility

    v. Most AIoMT sensors are integrated with wireless network, hence exposed to wireless safety issues.

    vi. Lack of standard safety measures among providers of healthcare devices.

    vii. AIoMT devices are constrained by resources. Hence, applications of encryption keys are not appropriate.

    viii. DOS and DDoS attackers over flood healthcare servers with large amount of traffic.

9.8.5 AIoMT SECURITY TREPIDATION

In ensuring the safety of AIoMT set of connections arrangement, it is tremendously imperative to remove several possible risks to facilitate safety measures against any form of attack and violation of the safety of clinical information. AIoMT know-how is known to be a famous demanding expertise across emerging clinical processes. Safeguarding several levels of safety AIoMT platforms is demanding, since cyberattacks damage incorporated systems. Alteration inserted into any clinical records, by means of leaking may well intimidate the patient's safety. AIoMT critical infrastructural attacks include:

    i. *Spying:* This type of attack on set of connections within AIoMT is termed *eavesdropping.* Generally, this is achieved whenever critical information is stolen from any proprietary system in clinical sittings. The involvement of this type of attack is basically as a result of weaker AIoMT connections within the participatory units, such as client-server connections. Strategy used includes pickup equipment, passwords that are weak, networks that are open and transmitting links.

    ii. *Interception of data:* Hackers interrupt clinical records and forward patients' records to unknown destination at any point in time; allowing unauthorized persons to sniff into the protocol resolution address files that permit connectivity within the AIoMTs. Once entry is illegally made into the ARP, the hackers penetrate clinical records without permission and acquire encrypted keys.

    iii. *Attack through flooding:* This is an overcrowding of the AIoMT network traffic in order to bring down critical clinical infrastructures with the view to lessen system assets through flooding and infusing means through deceitful records and falsification of calls.

    iv. *Attacks through birthday:* Relying on fragile *hashes* especially in password utilization possibly will create a means for exploiting system vulnerability, making it easier to access healthcare records with no permission. The most excellent resolution to guard the AIoMTs would be to apply secure hash algorithm methods.

    v. *Attacks by worms:* This is the most hazardous and disparaging form of malicious code experience within AIoMTs. Self-reproductive in nature devoid of individual interference through linked machines, taking opportunity of loopholes in machine capabilities. Virtually all terminals on the network are affected leading to information loss and possible harm on the patient's health. It combines other threats such as botnets/ransomware activating its spreading capabilities across networks of AIoMT.

vi. *Attacks by dictionary:* Prevalent of any cyber threats through this form is by having access to clinical records devoid of permission. This is a typical case of less or no rigorous defense countermeasures on AIoMT.

vii. *Attacks by replay:* In this attack, a typical hacker signals AIoMT components by way of altering or modifying communication to forward false request to other AIoMT devices. Also, capturing and pilfering broadcasting clinical data is possible via a means of redirecting information to unknown destination. At the end, a severe material harm may be experienced by connected AIoMT terminals.

viii. *Attack by black-nursing:* Internet control message protocol threats are on central processing unit of computers and firewalls prompted by the denial of service threats averting clinical experts and clients from conveying network congestion across the LAN.

ix. *Attack through brute force:* This kind of threat typically involves guessing system security login information, encrypted keys, or hidden application sites. Hackers crack likely keywords to penetrate AIoMT networks for unauthorized functions by acquiring clinical records or patient identification. This threat involves nearly all beleaguered AIoMT apparatus. Also, brute forcing attacks are not restricted to remote clinical sensing of patients.

x. *Attacks by malicious scripting injection:* Incorrect scripting on scheme may provide a phony updating of records, where criminally minded elements may choose to imitate a genuine backup server within the system. The outcome is that the intruder can have accessible right into the AIoMT machines without permission.

9.9   MAN-IN-THE-MIDDLE ATTACK MITIGATION IN AIOMT

The attacker pretends to be a legitimate user and connects to the router. The attacker gets the data first before it travels to the monitoring systems. The artificial intelligence internet of medical things (AIoMT) is a set of medical sensors used to collect physiological data from the body of a remotely monitored patient [44].

9.10   INTRUSIVE DETECTING SYSTEMS

Intrusive Detecting System (IDS) is a platform deployed to screen linking system for cruel activities. The objectives are information spying, stealing, and infecting network protocols. It defends and detects diverse devices. Akpan et al. [21] summarily classified IDS thus:

i. *Host-based IDSs*
   * Receive auditing information from host auditing trials.
   * Perceive a lone host attack.

ii. *Distributed IDSs*
  - Collect auditing information from many hosts and the set of connections that links the hosts.
  - Perceive a multiple hosts attack.
iii. *Network-based IDSs*
  - Deploy set of connections traffic as auditing information source.
  - Perceive host's attack.
iv. *Misuse detection*
  - Get intrusions from the attributes of a recognized attack.
v. *Anomaly detection*
  - Perceive actions that change from the normal characteristics.

Figure 9.1 shows Intrusion Prevention System (IPS) disconnecting attackers automatically.

The functions of IDS, as enumerated by [60] are as follows:

  i. Intrusion classification
 ii. Providing intruder location
iii. Viewing of network activities
 iv. Preventing malicious activities
  v. Reporting suspicious actions to the host admin
 vi. Providing intrusion information

9.11   CYBERATTACKS ON PACS

Eichelberg et al. [36] described five attack incidents affecting PACS and therapeutic imaging connections to include the following:

  i. Importing of patient information from storage space including malware
 ii. Compromising the set of connections in the hospital
iii. Integration of malware in digital imaging
 iv. Interactions in medical images and reports
  v. Exploitation of a cruel imaging and a system permeation

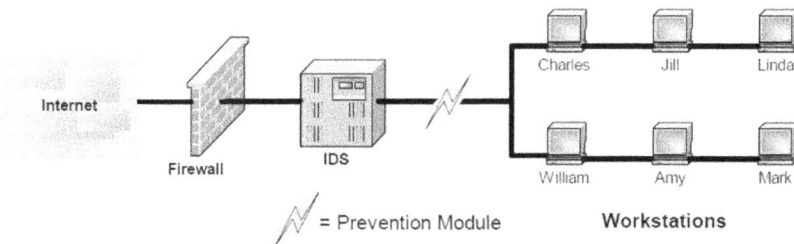

FIGURE 9.1   Intrusion Prevention System (IPS) disconnects attackers automatically [21].

9.11.1 Scenario 1: Importing of Patient Information from Storage Space Including Malware

Incidence is a contamination as a result of importing patient's information from storage space including malware. Figure 9.2 involves a malware infection of the computerized system through patient's compact disk creation.

Practical procedures to avoid this kind of attack are the usage of antivirus during medium creation. This will prevent the formation and circulation of infected storage space [36].

9.11.2 Attack 2: Compromising the Set of Connections in the Clinic

This incident is directed at the hacker who penetrates clinical network (local area network). Figure 9.3 depict the stages of the attack.

Depth defense is the practical procedure to curb the penetration attack.

9.11.3 Attack 3: Integration of Malware in Digital Imaging

The incident commences with importing of medical images or reporting from a medium presented by a patient or from an HER, as shown in Figure 9.4.

Thorough testing of vendor's applications is one key technical procedure to curb the attack.

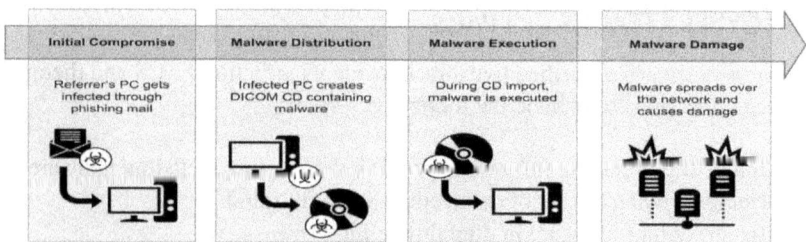

FIGURE 9.2 Malware infection of the computerized system through patient's compact disk creation [36].

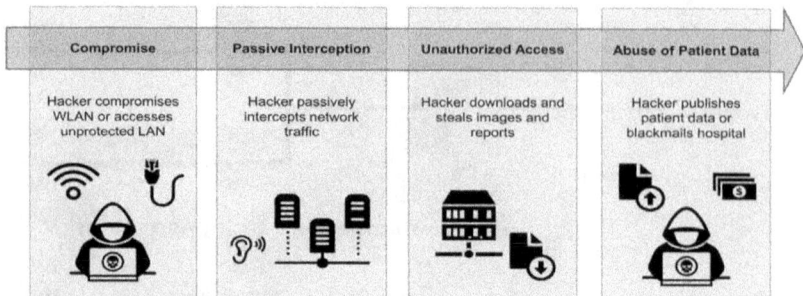

FIGURE 9.3 Hacker penetrates clinical network [36].

9.11.4   ATTACK 4: INTERACTIONS IN MEDICAL IMAGES AND REPORTS

The phase of a cyberattack is as a result of cruel exploitation of clinical images, as depicted in Figure 9.5.

Technical procedure to curb the attack is by using nontrivial PIN codes.

9.11.5   ATTACK 5: EXPLOITATION OF A CRUEL CLINICAL IMAGES AND A SYSTEM PERMEATION OF CRUEL HEALTH LEVEL INFORMATION

Practical procedures against this attack are protecting the information exchange with TLS using bidirectional certificate exchange.

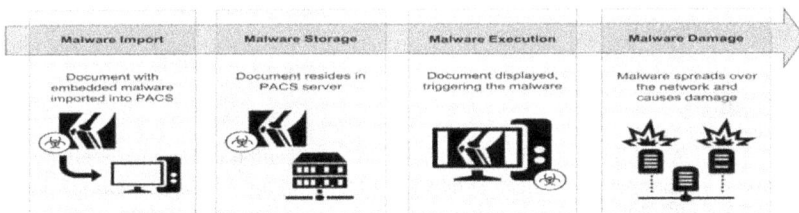

FIGURE 9.4   Virus fixed in medical images or reports [36].

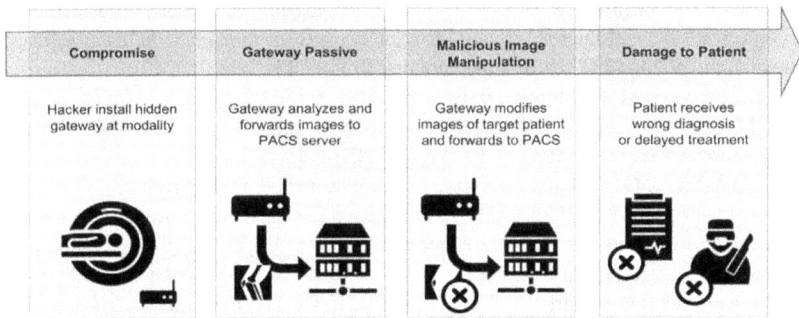

FIGURE 9.5   Malicious manipulation of medical images [36].

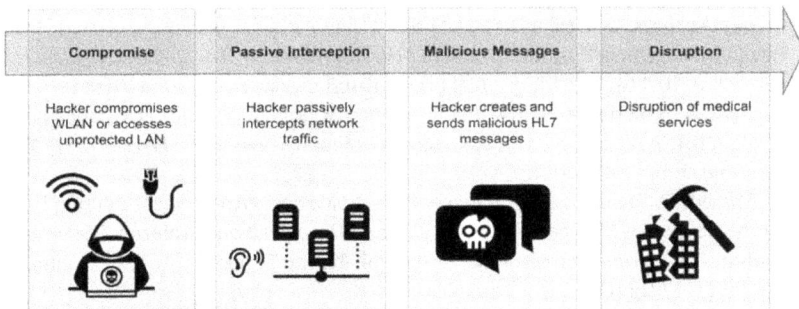

FIGURE 9.6   Connection infiltration by malicious code [36].

9.12   CONCLUSION

In this chapter, we provided an overview related of Artificial Intelligence of Medical Things (AIoMT) and presented AIoMT architecture. The most essential aspect of AIoMT is the connectivity it offers as systems are linked based on the network, and it is used in monitoring the patient with the help of remote sensors, assembling data, and forwarding patient's data to concerned parties. With all the advantages of AIoMT infrastructures in the healthcare ecosystem, its weaknesses call for concern. The safety aspect is extremely weak to violations; for this reason, this chapter focused on a number of cyberattacks on AIoMT, such as attack on PACS, accuracy and trust on DICOMS, and one-pixel attack. This chapter has identified and has technically addressed these issues by discussing and comparing various cyberattacks and the mitigations in AIoMTs. In the future, we hope to expand cyber-attack strategies for safety of AIoMT.

REFERENCES

[1]   T. Liaqat, A. Akhunzada, F. Shaikh, "SDN Orchestration to Combat Evolving Cyber Threats in Internet of Medical Things (IoMT)," *Computer Communications*, vol. 160, no. 7, pp. 697–705, 2020, https://doi.org/10.1016/j.comcom.2020.07.006.

[2]   I. Makhdoom, I. Abolhasan, J. Lipman, "Anatomy of Threats to the Internet of Things," *IEEE Communications Surveys and Tutorials*, vol. 21, no. 2, pp. 1636–1675, 2019, https://doi.org/10.1109/COMST.2018.2874978.

[3]   E. Sisinni, S. Saifullah, S. Han, U. Jennehag, "Industrial Internet of Things: Challenges, Opportunities, and Directions," *IEEE Transactions on Industrial Informatics*, vol. 14, no. 11, pp. 4724–4734, 2018, https://doi.org/10.1109/TII.2018.2852491.

[4]   P. K. P. Prajoy, M. R. Mondal, S. Bharati, "Review on the Security Threats of Internet of Things," *International Journal of Computers and Applications*, vol. 176, no. 41, pp. 37–45, 2020, https://doi.org/10.5120/ijca2020920548.

[5]   R. Chaudhary, G. S. Aujla, S. Garg, N. Kumar, J. J. P. C. Rodrigues, "SDN-Enabled Multi—Attribute-Based Secure Communication for Smart Grid in IIoT Environment," *IEEE Transactions on Industrial Informatics*, vol. 14, no. 6, pp. 2629–2640, 2018, https://doi.org/10.1109/TII.2018.2789442.

[6]   S. A. Butt, J. L. Diaz-Martinez, T. Jamal, A. Ali, E. De-La-Hoz-Franco, "IoT Sma[rt] Health Security Threats," *Proceeding of 19th International Conference on Computational Science Its Applications ICCSA*, vol. 2019, pp. 26–31, 2019, https://doi.org/10.1109/ICCSA.2019.000-8.

[7]   M. Amoon, M. Altameem, T. Altameem, "Internet of Things Sensor Assisted Security and Quality Analysis for Health Care Data Sets Using Artificial Intelligence Based Heuristic Health Management System," *Journal of the International Measurement Confederation*, vol. 161, p. 107861, 2020, https://doi.org/10.1016/j.measurement.2020.107861.

[8]   K. Fizza, A. Banerjee, K. Mitra, P. P. Jayaraman, R. Ranjan, P. Patel, D. Georgakopoulos, "QoE in IoT: A Vision, Survey, and Future Directions," *Discover the Internet of Things*, vol. 1, no. 1, pp. 1–14, 2021.

[9]   G. Ahmed, D. Mehmood, K. Shahzad, R. A. S. Malick, "An Efficient Routing Protocol for the Internet of Medical Things Focusing on Hot Spot Node Problems," *International Journal of Distributed Sensor Networks*, vol. 17, no. 2, pp. 115–163, 2021. https://doi.org/1550147721991706.

[10] M. Allouzi, J. I. Khan, "Identifying and Modeling Security threats for IoMT Edge Network Using Markov Chain and Common Vulnerability Scoring System," *Transactions on Emerging Telecommunications Technologies*, vol. 3, no. 5, pp. 23–27, 2021.

[11] M. Mushtaq, M. A. Shah, A. Ghafoor, "The Internet of Medical Things (IoMT): Security Threats and Issues Affecting Digital Economy," *COMSATS Institute of Information Technology*, pp. 1–6, 2021.

[12] R. Kishalaj, "AI Enabled Internet of Medical Things," *International Journal of Creative Research Thoughts (IJCRT)*, vol. 9, no. 12, pp. 579–602, 2021.

[13] M. Papaioannou, M. Karageorgou, G. Mantas, V. Sucasas, I. Essop, J. Rodriguez, D. Lymberopoulos, "A Survey on Security Threats and Countermeasures in Internet of Medical Things (IoMT)," *Transactions on Emerging Telecommunications Technologies*, vol. 7, no. 3, pp. 1–15, 2020.

[14] M. A. Habib, C. M. Nadeem Faisal, S. Sarwar, M. A. Latif, F. Aadil, M. Ahmad, R. Ashraf, M. Maqsood, "Privacy-Based Medical Data Protection Against Internal Security Threats in Heterogeneous Internet of Medical Things," *International Journal of Distributed Sensor Networks*, vol. 15, no. 9, pp. 1–12, 2019. https://doi.org/10.1177/1550147719875653

[15] R. Kishalaj, "AI Enabled Internet of Medical Things," *International Journal of Creative Research Thoughts (IJCRT)*, vol. 9, no. 12, pp. 579–602, 2021.

[16] A. S. Adly, M. S. Adly, "Approaches Based on Artificial Intelligence and the Internet of Intelligent Things to Prevent the Spread of COVID-19: Scoping Review," *Journal of Medical Internet Research*, vol. 22, no. 8, pp. 191–204, 2022.

[17] A. F. Alrefaei, Y. M. Hawsawi, D. Almaleki, T. Alafif, F. A. Alzahrani, M. A. Bakhrebah, "Genetic Data Sharing and Artificial Intelligence in the Era of Personalized Medicine Based on a Cross-sectional Analysis of the Saudi Human Genome Program," *Scientific Reports*, vol. 12, no. 1, pp. 1–10, 2022.

[18] C. Guo, J. Zhang, Y. Liu, Y. Xie, Z. Han, J. Yu, "Recursion Enhanced Random Forest with an Improved Linear Model (RERF-ILM) for Heart Disease Detection on the Internet of Medical Things Platform," *IEEE Access*, vol. 8, no. 5, pp. 9247–9256, 2022.

[19] P. Harvey, O. Toutsop, K. Kornegay, E. Alale, D. Reaves, "Security and Privacy of Medical Internet of Things Devices for Smart Homes," in *2020 7th International Conference on Internet of Things: Systems, Management and Security (IOTSMS)*, pp. 1–6. IEEE, 2020.

[20] K. Kandasamy, S. Srinivas, K. Achuthan, V. P. Rangan, "IoT Cyber Risk: A Holistic Analysis of Cyber Risk Assessment Frameworks, Risk Vectors, and Risk Ranking Process," *EURASIP Journal on Information Security*, vol. 20, no. 1, p. 8, 2020. https://jiseurasipjournals.springeropen.com/articles/10.1186/s13635-020-00111-0

[21] A. G. Akpan, S. Mmeah, B. Barida, "Cybercrime and Cyber Security: A Painted Scenario of a New Type of War," *Journal of Scientific and Engineering Research*, vol. 5, no. 10, pp. 185–197, 2018.

[22] A. G. Akpan, S. E. Eneji, "Cybercrime: Responding Sensibly in the Age of Uncertainty," *International Journals of Advanced Research in Computer Science and Software Engineering*, vol. 9, no. 4, pp. 17–28, 2019.

[23] A. G. Akpan, C. V. Umeakuka, "Self Destructive Data Security System: Towards an Improved Platform for Data Protection," *International Journals of Advanced Research in Computer Science and Software Engineering*, vol. 9, no. 4, pp. 9–16, 2019.

[24] A. G. Akpan, J. O. Ugah, V. N. Ezeano, "An Intelligent Crime Reporting System: A Proactive Method for Crime Prevention," *Journal of Scientific and Engineering Research*, vol. 9, no. 8, pp. 78–93, 2022.

[25] A. G. Akpan, J. O. Ugah, V. N. Ezeano, "Leveraging on Cyber Security for Digital Economy: Analysis of Emerging Cyber Security Threats and Attacks," *International Journal of Scientific & Engineering Research*, vol. 13, no. 7, pp. 663–674, 2022.

[26] J. J. Tom, A. G. Akpan, "Cyberspace: Mitigating Against Cyber Security Threats and Attacks," *International Journal of Engineering Research & Technology (IJERT)*, vol. 11, no. 11, pp. 327–332, 2022. https://doi.org/IJERTV11IS110028.

[27] A. G. Akpan, F. U. Onu, "Crime Mapping Software: A Tool for Effective Crime Detection and Control in Nigeria," *International Journal of Research*, vol. 6, no. 10, pp. 1269–1279, 2019.

[28] Y. Sei, A. Ohsuga, A. L. Imoize, "Statistical Test with Differential Privacy for Medical Decision Support Systems," in *Explainable Artificial Intelligence in Medical Decision Support Systems*, 1st ed., A. L. Imoize, J. Hemanth, D. T. Do, S. N. Sur, Eds. The Institution of Engineering and Technology, 2022, pp. 401–433.

[29] A. L. Imoize, D. O. Irabor, P. A. Gbadega, C. Chakraborty, "Blockchain Technology for Secure COVID-19 Pandemic Data Handling," in *Smart Health Technologies for the COVID-19 Pandemic: Internet of Medical Things Perspectives*, 1st ed., C. Chakraborty and J. J. P. C. Rodrigues, Eds. The Institution of Engineering and Technology, 2022, pp. 141–179.

[30] A. L. Imoize, P. A. Gbadega, H. I. Obakhena, D. O. Irabor, K. V. N. Kavitha, C. Chakrab, "Artificial Intelligence—Enabled Internet of Medical Things for COVID-19 Pandemic Data Management," in *Explainable Artificial Intelligence in Medical Decision Support Systems*, 1st ed., A. L. Imoize, J. Hemanth, D. T. Do, S. N. Sur, Eds. The Institution of Engineering and Technology, 2022, pp. 357–380.

[31] R. L. Kumar, Y. Wang, T. Poongodi, A. L. Imoize, *Internet of Things, Artificial Intelligence and Blockchain Technology*, 1st ed. Springer Nature, 2021.

[32] S. C. Nwaneri, C. Yinka-Banjo, U. C. Uregbulam, O. O. Odukoya, A. L. Imoize, "Explainable Neural Networks in Diabetes Mellitus Prediction," in *Explainable Artificial Intelligence in Medical Decision Support Systems*, 1st ed., A. L. Imoize, J. Hemanth, D. T. Do, S. N. Sur, Eds. The Institution of Engineering and Technology, 2022, pp. 313–334.

[33] P. Pandey, S. C. Pandey, U. Kumar, "Security Issues of Internet of Things in Health—Care Sector: An Analytical Approach," in *Advancement of Machine Intelligence in Interactive Medical Image Analysis, Algorithms for Intelligent Systems*, 1st ed., O. P. Verma et al., Eds. Springer Nature, 2020, pp. 307–329.

[34] S. Ghada, H. Ghada, K. Reham, "Modern Study on Internet of Medical Things (IOMT) Security," *IJCSNS International Journal of Computer Science and Network Security*, vol. 21, no. 8, pp. 254–266, 2021.

[35] Z. Wang, P. Ma, X. Zou, T. Yang, "Security of Medical Cyber—Physical Systems: An Empirical Study on Imaging Devices," *Beijing Electronic Science and Technology Institute*, vol. 5, no. 3, pp. 1–7, 2020. arXiv: 1904.00224v2.

[36] M. Eichelberg, K. Kleber, M. Kammerer, "Cybersecurity Challenges for PACS and Medical Imaging", *Special Report, The Association of University Radiologists*, vol. 27, no. 8, pp. 1126–1139, 2020. http://doi.org/10.1016/j.acra.2020.03.026.

[37] T. Sipola, T. Kokkonen, "One—Pixel Attacks Against Medical Imaging: A Conceptual Framework," in *Trends and Applications in Information Systems and Technologies (WorldCIST 2021)*, Alvaro Rocha, Hojjat Adeli, Gintautas Dzemyda, Fernando Moreira, and Ana Maria Ramalho Correria, Eds., vol. 1365, Advances in Intelligent Systems and Computing, Switzerland, Springer, 2021, pp. 197–203. https://doi.org/10.1007/978-3-030-72657-7_19.

[38] N. M. Thomasian, E. Y. Adashi. "Cybersecurity in the Internet of Medical Things," *Health Policy and Technology*, vol. 10, no. 2, pp. 1–9, 2021

[39] M. Allouzi, J. Khan, "Identifying and Modeling Security Threats for IoMT Edge Network using Markov Chain and Common Vulnerability Scoring System," *Computer Science Department*, Kent State University, USA. Unpublished, 2021.

[40] M. A. Habib, C. M. N. Faisal, S. Sarwar, M. A. Latif, F. Aadil, M. Ahmad, R. Ashraf, M. Maqsood, "Privacy-Based Medical Data Protection Against Internal Security Threats in Heterogeneous Internet of Medical Things," *International Journal of Distributed Sensor Networks*, vol. 15, no. 9, pp. 1–12, 2019. https://doi.org/10.1177/1550147719875653.

[41] N. Dilawar, M. Rizwan, F. Ahmad, S. Akram, "Blockchain: Securing Internet of Medical Things," *International Journal of Advanced Computer Science and Applications*, vol. 10, no. 1, pp. 227–232, 2019.

[42] D. G., *Cybersecurity Threats and Mitigations in the Healthcare Sector*. AIA—IE 3022, Sri Lanka Institute of Information Technology, Sri Lanka, Unpublished.

[43] D. Oladimeji, "An Intrusion Detection System for Internet of Medical Things," M.Sc. Dissertation in Computer Science, Dalhousie University, Halifax, Nova Scotia, 2021.

[44] O. Salem, K. Alsubhi, A. Shaafi, M. Gheryani, A. Mehaoua, R. Boutaba, "Man-in-the-Middle Attack Mitigation in Internet of Medical Things," *IEEE Transactions on Industrial Informatics*, vol. 18, no. 3, pp. 2053–2062, 2022.

[45] R. Hireche, H. Mansouri, A.-S.K. Pathan, "Security and Privacy Management in Internet of Medical Things (IoMT): A Synthesis," *Journal of Cybersecurity and Privacy*, vol. 2, no. 1, pp. 640–661, 2022. https://doi.org/10.3390/jcp2030033.

[46] M. Sultana, A. Hossain, F. Laila, K. A. Taher, M. N. Islam, "Towards Developing a Secure Medical Image Sharing System Based on Zero Trust Principles and Blockchain Technology," *BMC Medical Informatics and Decision Making*, 20, p. 256, 2020. https://doi.org/10.1186/s12911-020-01275-y.

[47] B. Hodges, J. Kuruvilla, K. Littlefield, B. Niemeyer, C. Peloquin, S. Wang, R. Williams, K. Zheng, "Securing Picture Archiving and Communication System (PACS): Cybersecurity for the Healthcare Sector," *NIST Special Publication 1800 –24, National Institute of Standards and Technology*, pp. 1–255, 2020. https://doi.org/10.6028/NIST.SP.1800-24.

[48] T. Wael, T. Nidal, "A Survey on Security Threats in the Internet of Medical Things (IoMT)," *Journal of Theoretical and Applied Information Technology*, vol. 100, no. 10, pp. 3361–3371, 2022.

[49] P. J. Taylor, T. Dargahi, A. Dehghantanha, R. M. Parizi, K. K. Raymond Choo, "A Systematic Literature Review of Blockchain Cyber Security," *Digital Communications and Networks*, vol. 6, no. 2, pp. 147–156, 2020.

[50] P. Harvey, O. Toutsop, K. Kornegay, E. Alale, D. Reaves, "Security and Privacy of Medical Internet of Things Devices for Smart Homes," *2020 7th International Conference on Internet of Things: Systems, Management and Security (IOTSMS)*, Paris, France, vol. 7, pp. 1–6, 2020.

[51] J. Jacobs, "Improving Vulnerability Remediation through Better Exploit Prediction," *Journal of Cybersecurity*, vol. 6, no. 1, pp. 156–162, 2020. https://doi.org/10.1093/cybsec/tyaa015.

[52] M. Pereira, S. Christiansen, "Identifying Security Bug Reports Based Solely on Report Titles and Noisy Data," *Microsoft*, March 6, 2020. https://docs.microsoft.com/en-us/security/engineering/identifying-security-bug-reports.

[53] B. Buchanan, J. Bansemer, D. Cary, J. Lucas, M. Musser, "Automating Cyber Attacks," *Center for Security and Emerging Technology*, 2020. https://doi.org/10.51593/2020CA002.

[54] M. Musser, A. Garriott, "Machine Learning and Cyber Security: Hype and Reality," *Emerging Technology*, 2021. https://doi.org/10.51593/2020CA004.

[55] S. Rizvi, A. Kurtz, J. Pfeffer, M. Rizvi, "Securing the Internet of Things (IoT): A Security Taxonomy for IoT," in *Proceedings—17th IEEE International Conference on Trust, Security a^{nd} Privacy in Computing and Communications and 12th IEEE International Conference on Big Data Science and Engineering, Trustcom/BigDataSE*, vol. 17. Institute of Electrical and Electronics Engineers, Inc., pp. 163–168, 2018.

[56] F. R. Labs, "Connected Medical Device Security: A Deep Dive into Healthcare Networks," *Techrep Report*. https://www.forescout.com/resources/connected-medical-device-security-a-deep-dive-into-healthcare-networks/

[57] "Introduction to HL7 Standards | HL7 International," Accessed 2021-04-13 [Online]. Available: www.hl7.org/implement/standards/index.cfm?ref= Nav

[58] "DICOM," Accessed 13-04-2021 [Online]. Available: www.dicomstandard.org/

[59] "Point-of-Care Testing Standards Documents—CLSI Shop," Accessed 2021-04-13 [Online]. Available: https://clsi.org/standards/products/point-ofcare-testing/documents/

[60] M. Wazid, A. K. Das, J. J. Rodrigues, S. Shetty, Y. Park, "IoMT Malware Detection Approaches: Analysis and Research Challenges," *IEEE Access*, vol. 7, no. 5, pp. 182–459, 2019.

[61] T. Sipola, S. Puuska, T. Kokkonen, "Model Fooling Attacks Against Medical Imaging: A Short Survey," *Information & Security: An International Journal*, vol. 46, no. 2, pp. 215–224, 2020. https://doi.org/10.11610/isij.4615

[62] T. Wael, T. Nidal, "A Survey on Security Threats in the Internet of Medical Things (IoMT)," *Journal of Theoretical and Applied Information Technology*, vol. 100, no. 10, pp. 3361–3371, 2022.

[63] H. A. Owida, J. I. Al-Nabulsi, N. M. Turab, F. Alnaimat, H. Rababah, M. Y. Shakour, "Autocharging Techniques for Implantable Medical Applications," *International Journal of Biomaterials*, vol. 10, no. 8, pp. 20–21, 2021.

10 Local Differential Privacy for Artificial Intelligence of Medical Things

Yuichi Sei, Akihiko Ohsuga, J. Andrew Onesimu, and Agbotiname Lucky Imoize

10.1 INTRODUCTION

The collection of personal health data and medical data can assist in the creation of machine learning (ML) models that have tangible benefits for private companies and public entities, such as hospitals and pharmaceutical companies [1–3]. However, key considerations when developing and using ML models that depend on personal data are those of privacy and fairness [4, 5].

This study assumes a scenario in which there already exists a relatively small sample of data, such as data from fewer than 10,000 individuals, which has been obtained through the use of local differential privacy (LDP) [6]. This privacy notion is used in many studies [7, 8] (Figure 10.1). Each individual in Figure 10.1 transfers her/his attribute values (e.g., location and health status) to a server, and all data values are protected using LDP techniques. Due to this, it is impossible for the server to learn the true attribute value. The server trains a model of ML using the stored DP data.

LDP is an extension of differential privacy (DP), particularly for collecting data from each individual. Various organizations, including technology companies such as Google and Apple, have leveraged LDP to protect privacy [9]. A general method for implementing LDP involves adding Laplace noise to numerical data [10]. Each individual sends perturbed data to a central aggregator, which is only able to view the perturbed data.

In this study, a decision tree algorithm is taken as the focal point. Despite the rise of the deep learning era, decision tree algorithms are still ubiquitous in practical applications, as well as academic research [12–16]. The accuracy of decision trees is lower than deep learning algorithms in general, but their nonparametric design, high human interpretability, and other characteristics represent significant advantages [17–19]. In particular, when ML is used for medical or pharmaceutical purposes, humans need to be able to understand the ML output. Therefore, it is sometimes desirable to use decision trees.

In recent years, DP decision tree generation algorithms have been proposed widely [19–22]. In the available studies, raw (non-privatized) data are used for DP

DOI: 10.1201/9781003370321-10

Health and medical data collection
under differential privacy in the past.

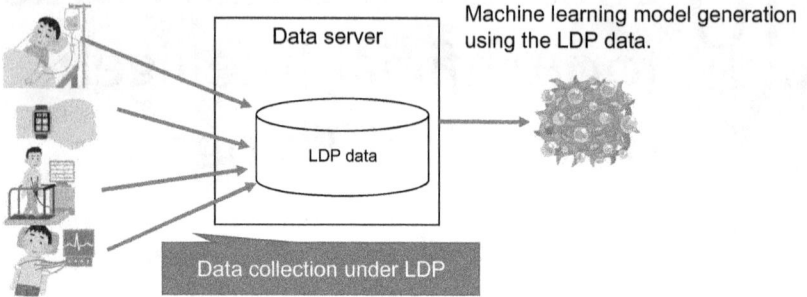

FIGURE 10.1   Research scenario: a data server, which stores LDP data, uses the data to generate an accurate ML model.

decision tree generation. By contrast, this study seeks to create decision trees from locally stored LDP data.

We adopted the copula used in financial studies [23] in this research. The original copula algorithm does not take LDP into account. While LDP can protect individual privacy, a lot of noise is added. As a result, the copula's accuracy deteriorates. We propose a new preprocessing algorithm to generate synthetic datasets using copulas while removing the effects of noise added by LDP. The proposed algorithm includes three steps: generation of covariance matrix from LDP numerical data, generation of discrete cumulative distribution function (CDF) from LDP numerical data, and generation of numerical samples by copula. The generated dataset is used for training an ML model.

Although this research focuses on decision trees, we also simulate deep neural networks (DNN), k-nearest neighbors (kNN), and support vector machines (SVM). The proposed algorithm improves the model accuracy for kNN and DNN, but not for SVM.

There are four contributions of this research. First, we introduced the relationship between the covariance/variance of the LDP numerical data and the covariance/variance of the raw data. Second, we introduce the algorithm that estimates variances and covariances, and creates a copula model. Third, in copula space, we present an algorithm to convert discrete CDF to continuous CDF and generate effective ML models. The final contribution is that this study used simulation results of real and synthetic data for performance evaluation. The proposed algorithm is expected to increase the number of patients who will be granted permission to use the algorithm for data analysis. This will allow for rapid and highly accurate machine learning, such as countermeasures to COVID-19. An earlier version of the chapter appeared in [11].

This chapter is structured as follows: the assumptions in this research are described in Section 10.2; a discussion of LDP and decision trees are presented in Section 10.3; the impact of LDP on decision trees is analyzed in Section 10.4; Section

10.5 introduces the proposed algorithm; the performance evaluation and its results are shown in Sections 10.6 and Section 10.7, respectively; and Section 10.8 provides concluding remarks.

10.2 ASSUMPTION

10.2.1 TARGET SCENARIO

The entity that generates the ML model is referred to as the *data server*. The available techniques fall into three categories, which are discussed in the next paragraphs. In the first category, it is assumed that the data server—in this case, a trusted entity—stores the raw personal data, which is not yet privatized; the generated LDP machine learning models are published to third parties. Various studies that have investigated LDP decision trees have utilized this category of techniques [19–22].

In this study, the assumption is made that the data server is a semi-honest entity. As a result, it is not permitted direct access to the raw data. This assumption is also employed in model generation techniques of the second and third categories. The distinguishing feature between the second and third categories relates to the variable of whether the data server can indirectly access the raw data when generating ML models.

The second category of LDP ML model generation technology consists of technologies that utilize accumulated LDP data without accessing the raw data. This research is conducted on this premise. There exist a variety of reasons why such data would be stored by the data server, including:

- *To use in the future*: Some organizations collect and store privacy-preserving data for future use [24–26]. The accumulated data is used when it comes to generating ML models.
- *To generate efficient ML modes*: Training data are critical for model debugging and the performance analysis of trained models [27, 28].
- *To facilitate fairness auditing*: The challenge of ML models' biased output for personal attributes such as gender and race is broadly acknowledged as a fairness problem in ML. It is necessary to analyze training data [29–31] to audit fairness or develop fair ML models. Furthermore, the question of how bias is defined is dependent on individuals' attitudes, and such assessments are subject to future change, which represents another use case for storage.

The third category assumes the data server accesses to the LDP information of the raw data stored in third parties. In this category of technology, data servers work with multiple personal data holders to train ML models. Each personal data holder submits data to train ML models without violating privacy. This approach has many advantages, but when the data server trains the ML model, it must access the information necessary to update ML parameters from third parties that have the raw data. However, the access to data cannot be guaranteed in the future. Federated learning techniques belong to this category, and although there are several in deep neural networks, there are a limited number of them in decision trees. Techniques of this kind have been extensively studied, but for the reasons given earlier, our research in this chapter focuses on the second category.

In recent years, smartphones and smartwatches have generated people's medical data on a daily basis. Such data can be collected by smartphone application providers for statistical analysis using LDP techniques.

10.2.2 TARGET ML MODEL

Despite advances in deep neural networks and extensive research in this field over the previous decade, the human-interpretability of these models is low, which means their outputs are challenging to understand. While techniques exist to aid interpretability, numerous challenges persist [32].

The decision tree algorithm is among the widest-used ML algorithms. It has a high level of human interpretability. The principal limitation of the decision tree algorithm is the tendency it has to overfit the data, as well as its lack of stability when minor changes happen within the data. Nevertheless, tree depth can be limited to lessen this limitation, along with utilizing ensembles rather than individual trees and pruning leaf nodes that are unreliable [19]. While the proposed algorithm is applicable to any ML algorithm, its effectiveness is greatest for the decision trees. This is due to the substantial noise that characterizes all LDP data, where decision trees overfit this noise. In Section 10.6, however, the adaptable nature of the proposed algorithm to various ML algorithms is demonstrated, by applying it to SVM, kNN, and DNN.

10.2.3 TARGET DATA TYPE

In this research, we focus on Internet of Medical Things (IoMT) data. Such data includes the body temperature, heart rate of patients, and so on [33–35]. Given the ease with which one can convert numerical data into categorical data, and thus the higher utility of numerical data, numerical data are utilized in this study.

Such medical data is highly sensitive data. Therefore, collecting and analyzing the raw data in its raw form risks compromising the privacy of the patient. Of course, if the data is directly necessary for the patient's treatment, the server's collection of the patient's raw data does not pose a problem because of the patient's consent. However, when data is utilized not for treatment but for statistical analysis, consideration of patient privacy is necessary.

Encrypting data prevents a third party from intercepting the data, but the entity performing the statistical analysis can see the patient's data as it is. On the other hand, secret computation techniques that perform statistical processing while encrypting the data have been studied. By using secret computation techniques, statistical processing can be performed without anyone being able to check the raw data. However, the problem is that the computational complexity is very large. Recently, secret computation techniques with reduced computational complexity have been proposed, but it is difficult to construct complex machine learning models in a short time.

The differential privacy technique used in this study disturbs data at the patient's hand. Therefore, the computational cost is small. Moreover, even if risks to conventional encryption arise in the future, such as the development of quantum computation technology, it will be impossible to recover individual data from the disrupted data. With such advantages in mind, this study assumes a scenario in which numerical data is protected by differential privacy and then collected.

10.3 RELATED WORK

10.3.1 LOCAL DIFFERENTIAL PRIVACY (LDP)

Differential privacy (DP) is regarded as the principal metric for privacy [36]. The topic of DP of ML models has been intensively researched over the previous decade [10, 19]. A central model rather than a local model is assumed for DP, which means that the anonymizer is the holder of all raw data (see Section 10.2 for an introduction to the first category). By contrast, the local model is assumed in LDP, wherein each individual obfuscates the values of their personal data attributes locally.

The symbols X and Z represent a set of raw data and a set of privatized data, respectively.

Definition 1 (ε -LDP): *A satisfies ε-LDP if, for every $x_1, x_2 \in X$ and $z \in Z$,*

$$P(A(x_1)=z) \le e^\varepsilon \, Pr(A(x_2)=z) \tag{10.1}$$

The Laplace mechanism is used for numerical attributes in a large number of LDP methods [10]. In this case, X represents numerical values. The difference between the minimum value of X and the maximum value of X is represented by Δ. A noise that is drawn from a Laplace distribution is added to the raw value. The mean and the scale of the Laplace distribution are zero and Δ/ε, respectively.

A significant proportion of the literature on LDP, including [37–39], is principally focused on the generation of multi-dimensional contingency table of the collected values. If the resulting multi-dimensional contingency table has sufficient accuracy, it is able to estimate a target value from the other values like the ML model.

In recent years, researchers have proposed several other mechanisms for numerical attributes. Wang et al. developed a piecewise mechanism that estimates the mean value with high accuracy [40]. This mechanism was extended by Li et al., in which the authors proposed a square-wave mechanism [41]. The mechanism outputs $\tilde{v} \in [v-b, v+b]$ for an input domain $[0,1]$, an output domain $[-b, 1+b]$, and a true value v, with a probability of $2be^\varepsilon/(2be^\varepsilon +1)$. For other values, the probability is $1/(2be^\varepsilon +1)$.

A mechanism for estimating value distributions is needed in this study due to the fact that they are necessary to generate training samples for ML models. We assume the employment of the Laplace mechanisms for realizing LDP, given that these mechanisms are characterized by their status as the most fundamental mechanisms, and they focus on our proposed approach. It is also assumed in this study that the data server stores LDP data. If the data were privatized using another mechanism, the corresponding method could be used to estimate the numerical distributions. For this reason, it is possible to improve on the method through the application of other extended mechanisms to the method.

10.3.2 LDP ML MODEL GENERATION FROM RAW DATA

The data server's possession of raw data is an assumption that many researchers posit, on the basis of which they have developed methods that create LDP ML models [42–48]. This study draws the assumption that the data server is not trustworthy, which necessitates the use of other approaches.

10.3.3 ML MODEL GENERATION FROM LDP DATA

This approach is the category into which the proposed algorithm fits. In the current research, generating an ML model following the collection of LDP data is regarded as a baseline method [49]. This is due to the fact that it is complex to improve the accuracy of a model after LDP data are collected. DNN models are generated using a collection of LDP data, and there is no objective to develop enhanced algorithms. Scenarios exist in which the data server has a set of LDP data but lacks the ability to access the raw data in a direct or indirect way. As a result, proposing an algorithm with the ability to generate high-performance ML models using locally stored LDP data is a worthwhile task.

10.3.4 ML MODEL GENERATION WITH INDIRECT LDP ACCESS TO RAW DATA

Over the previous decade, substantial research activity has been dedicated to federated learning techniques [50–52], particularly for DNNs. In federated learning, the data owners are distributed, and an ML model is generated by the data server with only indirect access to the data. It is possible to offer some level of privacy protection for all the data because the data server lacks direct access to the personal data. Rather than sending the raw data, each data owner sends other information, such as the model gradient information, to the data server. In recent literature, it has been pointed out that the risk of privacy leakage exists in the model gradient information [53], which prompted the development of LDP federated learning algorithms [54–60]. The value of such techniques is their ability to safeguard privacy and promote high utility at the same time.

The shuffle model for LDP has been the target of growing research attention in recent years [61]. This model has the capability to mitigate noise added through LDP, under the assumption that there exists a perfectly secure primitive [62]. In addition, it is not possible for the data server under this scenario to store LDP data.

10.3.5 LDP SYNTHETIC DATA GENERATION

A range of models exist that can be used to generate an LDP dataset using samples of raw data [63–66]. An assumption drawn in these models is that raw data samples are held in the server, where the objective is to create a synthetic dataset that has a high level of similarity compared to the data samples. By contrast, in this study, the assumption is drawn that raw data samples are not held in the server; the aim is to facilitate ML model generation using LDP data samples.

Table 10.1 summarizes the perspectives of the various types of generated ML model described in the literature with LDP and LDP synthetic data generation. The

TABLE 10.1
Perspectives in Related Literature

Category	Data	Owner of data
LDP ML Model Generation from Raw Data	Raw data	Data server
ML Model Generation from LDP Data	LDP data	Data server
ML Model Generation with Indirect LDP Access to Raw Data	Raw data's partial information necessary for updating ML model	Third parties
LDP synthetic data generation	Raw data	Data server

focus of this study is the second category, which is characterized by the data server lacking raw data but owning LDP data.

10.3.6 Copula

The covariance matrix Σ of each pair of attributes and the cumulative distribution function (CDF) F_j of each attribute are necessary for creating the copula model. The created copula model can generate an arbitrary number of samples that maintain the characteristics of the data. Let $s_{i,j}$ denote individual i's jth attribute value, and let n be the number of individuals. Each data of individual i is represented by $s_i = \{s_{i,1}, \ldots, s_{i,g}\}$. The collected data is represented by $\{s_1, \ldots, s_n\}$. Let σ_j represent jth attribute's standard deviation. First, the standardization is conducted, that is,

$$s_{i,j} \leftarrow s_{i,j} / \sigma_j. \tag{10.2}$$

For each value of the samples, the values of the CDF of $N(0,1)$ were calculated:

$$t_{i,j} = \frac{1}{2}\left[1 + \mathrm{erf}\left(\frac{s_{i,j}}{\sqrt{2}}\right)\right]. \tag{10.3}$$

Following this, we attain the associated value from $t_{i,j}$. In particular, the following is calculated:

$$u_{i,j} = F_j^{-1}\left(t_{i,j}\right) \tag{10.4}$$

where F_j^{-1} is an inverse function of F_j.

The resulting $u_i = \{u_{i,1}, \ldots, u_{i,g}\}$ is a generated sample.

Rocher et al. [67] developed a copula approach for predicting the number of individuals in a population with a specific set of attribute values. However, LDP and other privacy measures were not employed (i.e., the assumption was made that they have raw data). Researchers have examined data generation based on a copula technique, which has potential usage in the training of ML models [68–70]. Nevertheless, LDP data are not considered. In recent literature, researchers have generated copula models on the basis of LDP data [71, 72], but numerical data have not been focused on.

Furthermore, the objectives of previous researchers have not been centered around ML model training, and instead, researchers have sought to re-identify individuals using partial datasets and facilitate multi-dimensional contingency table generation.

10.4　DECISION TREE WITH LDP DATA

10.4.1　CATEGORICAL DATA

The purpose of a decision tree is to assist in the analysis of data using a tree-like model, where internal nodes represent rules for data splitting. A range of tree generation algorithms exist, including [73–75].

The concept of information gain is used in most algorithms. The information gain is calculated as the impurity of a node minus the sum of the weighted impurity of its child nodes. In many cases, the impurity is calculated as an entropy or Gini impurity.

Let f represent the number of categories and p_j represent the ratio of samples with category j. The Gini impurity is calculated as

$$H(jini)=1-\sum_{j=1}^{f}\left(p_j\right)^2,\tag{10.5}$$

and the entropy is calculated by

$$H(entropy)=-\sum_{j=1}^{f}p_j\log_2\left(p_j\right).\tag{10.6}$$

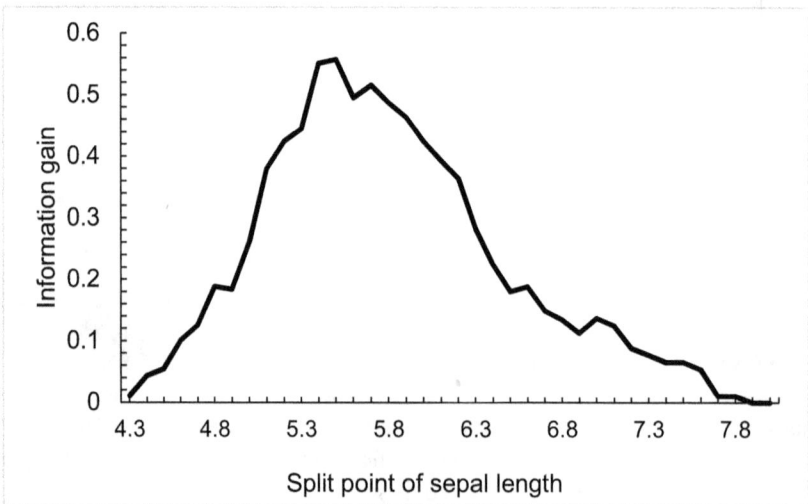

FIGURE 10.2　Relationship between the split point and information gain (entropy is used as impurity).

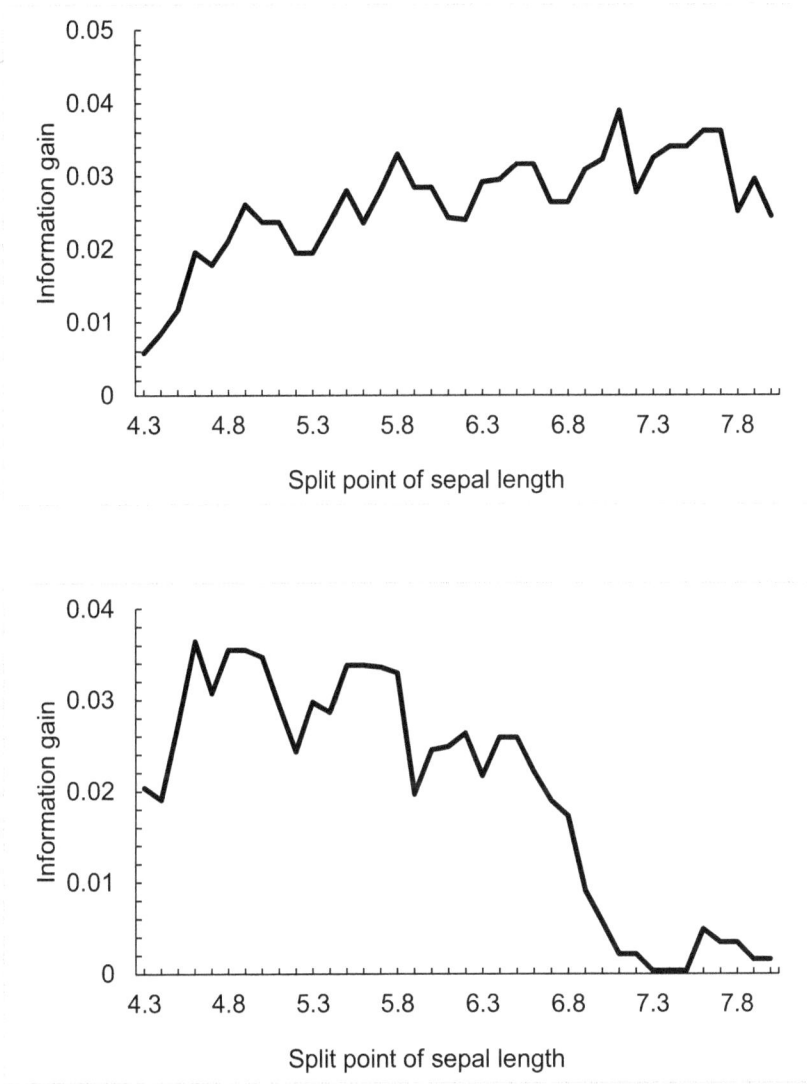

FIGURE 10.2 (Continued)

Because a random noise generated based on Laplace distribution is added to each data, finding the optimal split point is difficult. Figure 10.2 shows poor partitioning examples. Here we used the famous iris dataset [76]. This dataset consists of five attributes and class labels (Setosa, Versicolour, Virginica). It has a mountain shape, and the information gain is maximized when the dividing point is 5.5. Figures 10.2b and 10.2c are when each data was collected under LDP. The value of ε is 1. In Figure 10.2b, the amount of information is maximized when the division point is 7.1, and in Figure 10.2c, the amount of information is maximized when the division point is

4.6. Because of this stochastic amount of noise in LDP, different results are obtained. Also, regardless of the division point, the value of the overall information gain is much smaller than the value of the information gain in Figure 10.2a.

10.4.2 Numerical Data

The mean squared error (MSE) measure is applied to identify each attribute's optimal splitting point for regression trees treating numerical data. The objective is to identify the attribute and its splitting point that minimizes the weighted average of the MSE (WAMSE) of the child nodes, ensuring it reaches the lowest value.

Decision tree algorithms find it challenging to split the tree effectively when each value contains Laplace noise. This arises given that it is not possible to calculate the WAMSE correctly due to the noise. An example in which the split does not work is provided in Figures 10.3a–10.3c. In this example, a Boston dataset [77, 78] with 13 feature attributes was used, where the feature attributes included each town's crime rate, along with a target attribute (housing prices). Figure 10.3a shows the association between the split point of the town's crime rate and the corresponding WAMSE. There is a convex downward shape, and when the split point is 7, the minimization of the WAMSE occurs. Figures 10.3b and 10.3c present scenarios where LDP is applied for the collection of the data samples, and ε is set to 5. In Figure 10.3b, the minimization of the WAMSE occurs when the split point is set to 37, and in Figure 10.3c, when the split point is 59. Every run produces differing results, given the stochastic production of noise in LDP, as the figures indicate. Additionally, all values of the

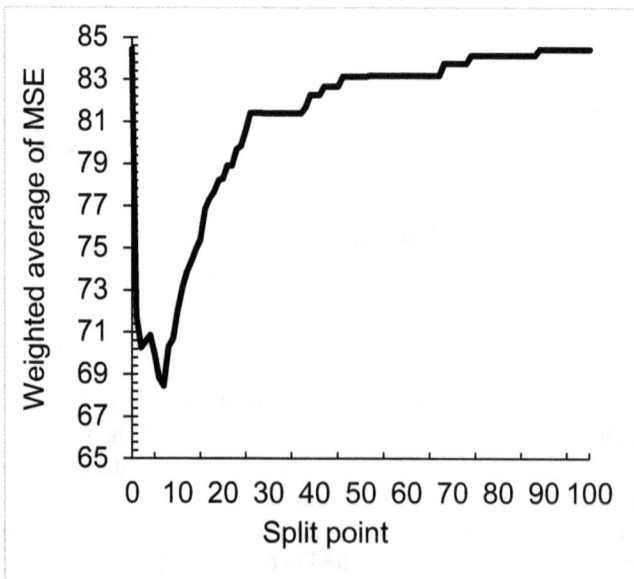

FIGURE 10.3 The average of MSE and split point in decision trees.

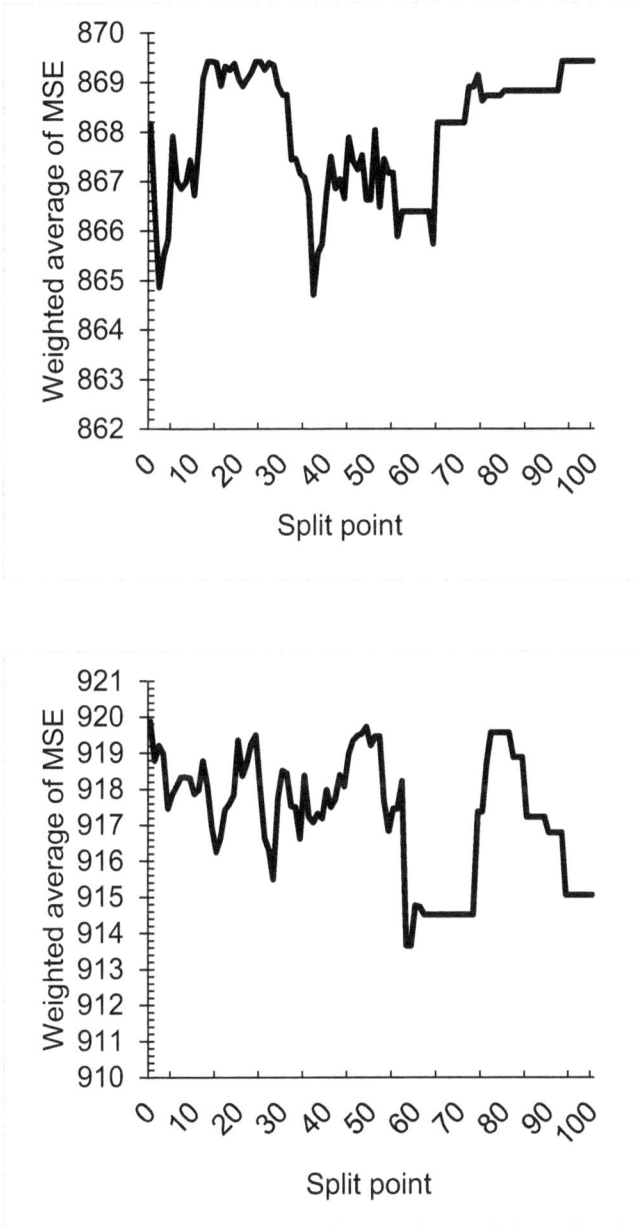

FIGURE 10.3 (Continued)

WAMSE significantly exceed that of the raw value in Figure 10.3a. For this reason, determining the split point is a significant challenge in cases where the noise of LDP is added to all data samples. Due to this, the generation of an accurate decision tree model faces complexities under LDP.

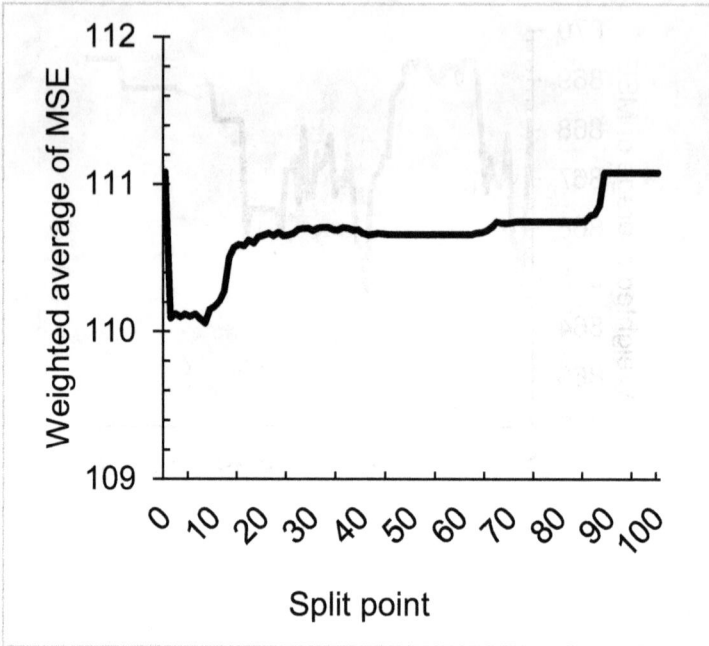

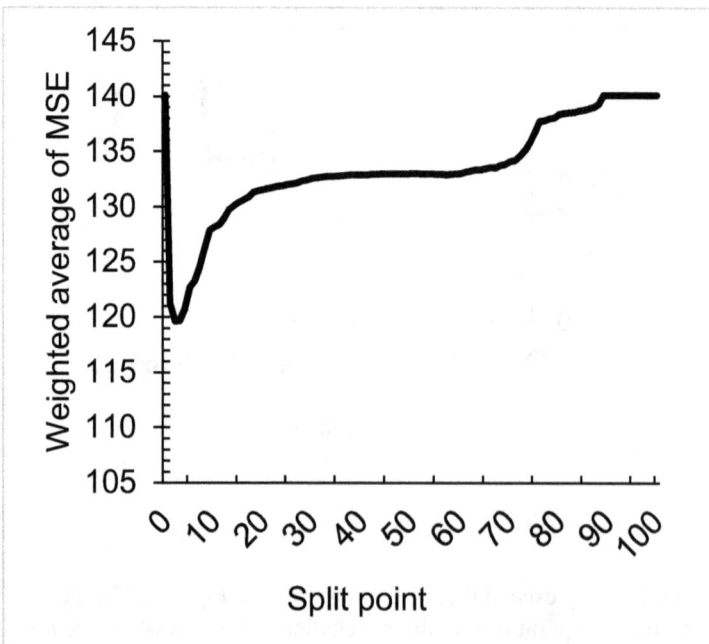

FIGURE 10.3   (Continued)

By contrast, the results for the pseudodata generated using the proposed algorithm are presented in Figures 10.3d and 10.3e. Due to the generation of pseudodata in the proposed algorithm that preserves each attribute's statistical trend, the shapes in Figures 10.3d and 10.3e—the splitting points for which are 8 and 3, respectively—resemble the raw shape in Figure 10.3a. Both splitting points are near the splitting point of 7, which is the optimal splitting point.

It is also noteworthy that under LDP data, the relationships between information attributes are eliminated. For this reason, if a node is deeper when generating a decision tree from LDP data, the significance of the effect of the error increases. Dissimilarly, the correlation information of attributes is reconstructed by the pseudo dataset based on the proposed algorithm. As a result, it is possible to suppress the declining accuracy of the decision tree even in situations when the nodes are deeper.

10.5 PROPOSED ALGORITHM

The Laplace function with mean μ, scale s, and a random variable $x \in X$ is represented by $L(x;\mu,s)$. $L(x;s)$ is used for the same meaning as $L(x;0,s)$ for simplicity.

10.5.1 OUTLINE

Researchers have investigated copula-based data synthesis for the production of perturbed data and the incorporation of fine-grained statistical information. The protocol presented in this study consists of the following steps: generating a covariance matrix from the LDP numerical data (Section 10.5.2), generating a discrete CDF (Section 10.5.3), and generating copula samples (Section 10.5.4). The copula samples resulting from the final step are utilized for ML model training. A summary of the proposed algorithm is presented in Figure 10.4, and the algorithms used in each step were designed as part of this research.

10.5.2 COVARIANCE MATRIX GENERATION FROM LDP DATA

The variance and covariance of the raw values based on observing LDP values are calculated. The random variable of the ith attribute of data is represented by H_i. The random variable of Laplace noise is represented by L_i. $H_b i$ is defined as

$$\hat{H}_i = H_i + L_i. \tag{10.7}$$

Based on the linearity of expectation property, it follows that

$$E\left[\hat{H}_i\right] = E\left[H_i + L_i\right] = E\left[H_i\right] + E\left[L_i\right] = E\left[H_i\right], \tag{10.8}$$

because the mean of Z is zero.

Let σ_{Hi}^2 denote the variance of H_i. The following equation can be used to calculate $\sigma^2 Hi$:

$$\sigma_{\hat{H}_i}^2 = E\left[\left(\hat{H}_i - E\left[\hat{H}_i\right]\right)^2\right] = E\left[\left(H_i + L_i - E\left[H_i\right]\right)^2\right]$$

$$= E\left[\left(H_i - E\left[H_i\right]\right)^2\right] + 2E\left[H_i L_i\right] - 2E\left[H_i\right]E\left[L_i\right] + E\left[L_i^2\right] \qquad (10.9)$$

$$= \sigma_{H_i}^2 + 2E\left[H_i L_i\right] - 2E\left[H_i\right]E\left[L_i\right] + E\left[L_i^2\right]$$

In addition, we have $E[H_i L_i] = E[L_i] = 0$ and

$$E\left[L_i^2\right] = \int_{x=-\infty}^{\infty} x^2 \mathcal{L}\left(x; 1/\varepsilon_i\right) dx = \frac{2}{\varepsilon_i^2} \qquad (10.10)$$

Therefore,

$$\sigma_{H_i}^2 = \max\left(\sigma_{\hat{H}}^2 - \frac{2}{\varepsilon_i^2}, 0\right) \qquad (10.11)$$

where it is ensured that the variance is greater than or equal to zero.

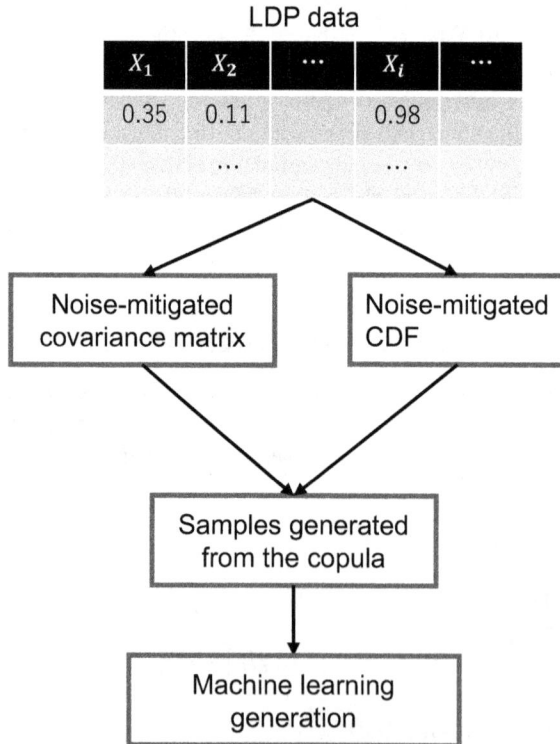

FIGURE 10.4 Structure of the algorithm.

Let $\sigma_{Hi, Hj}$ denote the covariance of H_i and H_j. The covariance of $\sigma_H b_{i,H} c_j$ is denoted by the following equation:

$$
\begin{aligned}
\sigma_{\hat{H}_i,\hat{H}_j} &= E\left[\left(\hat{H}_i - E\left[\hat{H}_i\right]\right)\left(\widehat{H}_j - E\left[\widehat{H}_j\right]\right)\right], \\
&= E\left[\left(H_i + L_i - E\left[H_i\right]\right)\left(H/ + L_j - E\left[H_j\right]\right)\right] \\
&= E\left[\left(H_i - E\left[H_i\right]\right)\left(H_j - E\left[H_j\right]\right)\right] + E\left[L_i L_j\right] \\
&+ E\left[\left(H_j - E\left[H_j\right]\right)L_i\right] + E\left[\left(H_i - E\left[H_i\right]\right)L_j\right].
\end{aligned}
\tag{10.12}
$$

The following equation is attained as L_i and L_j are independent, and $E[L_i]=E[L_j]= 0$.

$$
\sigma_{H_i, H_j} = \sigma_{\hat{H}_i, \widehat{H}_j}.
\tag{10.13}
$$

A covariance matrix is represented by Σ, which is calculated from Equations 10.12 and 10.13. The matrix may not be positive definite due to the Laplace noise. Therefore, we should repair it. Let λ_i and q_i represent the ith eigenvectors and eigenvalues, respectively, of matrix Σ. Based on order of magnitude, sort q_i and its corresponding λ_i; in turn, two matrices are generated as follows:

$$
D = \begin{pmatrix}
q_1 & 0 & \cdots & 0 \\
0 & q_2 & \cdots & 0 \\
0 & \cdots & \cdots & 0 \\
0 & \cdots & \cdots & q_g
\end{pmatrix},
\tag{10.14}
$$

and

$$
\Lambda = \left(\lambda_1, \lambda_2, \ldots, \lambda_g\right),
\tag{10.15}
$$

where g represents the number of attributes. We have the following equation:

$$
\Sigma = D \Lambda D^{-1}.
\tag{10.16}
$$

The PDM version can be obtained in the following way:

$$
\Sigma' = D \Lambda' D^{-1}
\tag{10.17}
$$

where Λ' represents the matrix that replaces the negative values of Λ with small positive values.

10.5.3   CDF GENERATION FROM LDP DATA

It is assumed in this study that the data server already has LDP data. Let $\tilde{v}_i$ denote the LDP value of the raw value v_i of individual i. In this research, the following hyperparameters are used: b, denoting the number of separations in X for constructing a CDF, and r, which determines the range of Z. These values have no impact on privacy, but they influence ML model accuracy. Theoretically, the output domain can be $[-\infty, \infty]$ because we assume that a Laplace mechanism is used to realize LDP. Nevertheless, the accuracy declines when the output domain is set too wide. The maximum and minimum raw values are represented by M and m, respectively. The maximum and minimum output values are represented by M^{pri} and m^{pri}, respectively.

We have

$$\int_{x=-\infty}^{m^{pri}} L\left(x; \frac{M-m}{\epsilon}\right) dx = 1-r. \tag{10.18}$$

Through solving Equation (10.18), we have

$$m^{pri} = m + \frac{(M-m)\log 2(1-r)}{\epsilon}. \tag{10.19}$$

Similarly, we have

$$M^{pri} = M + \frac{(M-m)\log 2r}{\epsilon}. \tag{10.20}$$

Let w denote each bin's width, namely,

$$w = \frac{M-m}{b}. \tag{10.21}$$

Let b^{pri} represent the number of separations of r. This value is calculated by

$$b^{pri} = \frac{M^{pri} - m^{pri}}{w}. \tag{10.22}$$

Let $L(x; \mu, s)$ denote the CDF of the Laplace distribution, where the mean and scale are μ and s, respectively. Equation 10.23 calculates the probability that a true value in b_i is privatized to b^{pri}_j:

$$P_{i,j} = \begin{cases} S_{|i-j|+1} & \left(j \neq 1, j \neq b^{pri}\right) \\ H_0 + S_1 & (i=1, j=1) \\ H_0 - \sum_{k=2}^{i} P_{i,k} & (i \neq 1, j=1) \\ 1 - \sum_{k=1}^{b^{pri}-1} P_{i,k} & \left(j = b^{pri}\right) \end{cases} \tag{10.23}$$

where for arbitrary m, it follows that

$$H_0 = \int_{t=m}^{m+w} \frac{\mathcal{L}(m;t,s)dt}{w} = \frac{s - e^{-w/s}s}{2w} \qquad (10.24)$$

and for arbitrary m and $i \in \{1,\ldots,b^{pri}\}$, it follows that

$$S_i = \int_{t=m}^{m+i*w} \frac{\mathcal{L}(m;t,s)dt}{w} - \int_{t=m}^{m+(i-1)*w} \frac{\mathcal{L}(m;t,s)dt}{w}$$

$$\qquad (10.25)$$

$$= \begin{cases} \dfrac{e^{-i*w/s}\left(-1+e^{w/s}\right)^2 s}{2w} & (i \geq 2) \\[3mm] 1 + \dfrac{-1+e^{-w/s}s}{w} & (i = 1) \end{cases}$$

Expectation-maximization-based algorithms such as [9] can be used for estimating a CDF of the true values based on Equation 10.23 and LDP values.

10.5.4 COPULA SAMPLE GENERATION

Suppose that $F_j(k)$ is the probability that k is greater than or equal to the random variable of the jth attribute. For all i and j, the values of $t_{i,j}$ are calculated using Equation 10.3. Let m_k denote the minimum value of k, which satisfies $F_j(k) \geq t_{i,j}$. In turn, the following is calculated:

$$\begin{cases} u'_{i,j} = \dfrac{t_{i,j}}{F_j(0) \times b} & (m_k = 0) \\[3mm] u'_{i,j} = \dfrac{m_k - F_j(m_k - 1) + t_{i,j}}{\left(F_j(m_k) - F_j(m_k - 1)\right)b} & \text{(otherwise.)} \end{cases} \qquad (10.26)$$

Figure 10.5 shows an example of calculating Equation 10.26, representing the case where $b = 4$.

10.6 EVALUATION

Focusing on the decision tree, we conducted a comparative analysis of the case where the decision tree was created as it is and the case where the decision tree was created using the learning data created by the proposed algorithm. We also conducted a comparative analysis of methods for generating training data using normal copulas [67] and constructing decision trees. In addition, we compared our algorithm with

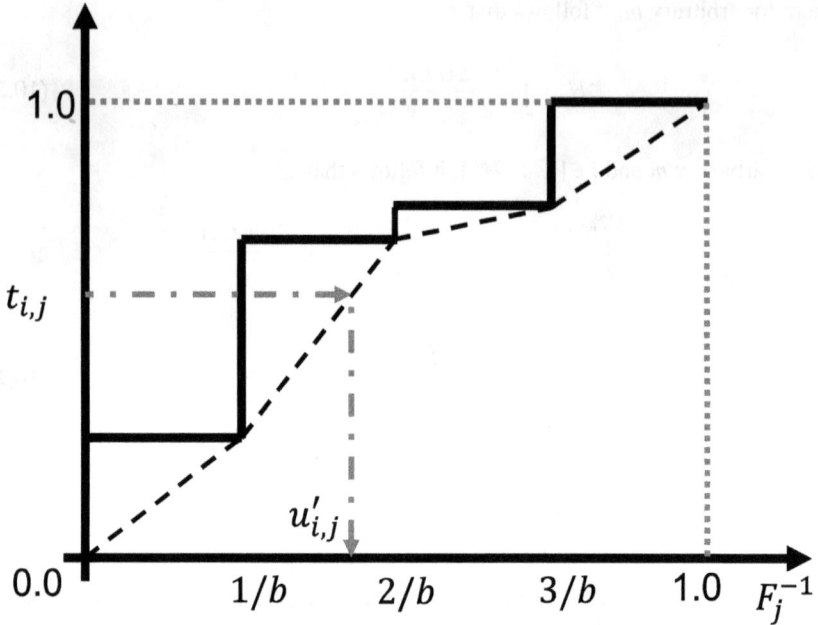

FIGURE 10.5   Calculation $u'_{i,j}$ in $b = 4$ case.

data augmentation methods, which are often used in practice to increase the size of the training data sample.

Generating multi-dimensional contingency tables from LDP data can be achieved using a range of techniques. This study presents the results of [37] for the purposes of comparison. The authors proposed IDUE on the basis of RAPPOR [79], along with IDUE based on OUE [80]. We refer to these methods as IR and IO.

Among the methods under comparison, the hyperparameters of each ML algorithm are common. Ten simulations were performed, and their average was calculated, where each simulation was undertaken with identical settings.

10.6.1   SYNTHETIC DATASETS

In this study, three probability distributions, multivariate normal distribution (MND), multivariate t-distribution (MTD), and negative multinomial distribution (NMD), were used to generate synthetic datasets. The number of attributes (g) and the number of people (n) were used as parameters for dataset generation.

The simulation results are shown in Figure 10.6, where n is assigned a static value of 1,000 and ε varies over the range 0.01–10 for each attribute. The value g was set to 30. When ε is smaller, the value of MSE is greater. Virtually no difference exists in outcome between data augmentation (Aug.+DT), using decision tree as is (DT), and the copula method [67] (Copula+DT). In view of this, it is clear that accuracy does not improve through the simple addition of the copula model to LDP.

The method proposed in this study (Proposal+DT) attained greater accuracy (the reader will note that high accuracy is reflected by a low MSE value). The estimation accuracy of IR and IO is relatively low. In addition, it is important to note that these methods are able to construct a multi-dimensional contingency table of all combinations of attribute values (i.e., the primary aim of these methods is not to predict one attribute value).

Following this, ε was set to 1.0, and the experiment was performed by varying n over the range 1,000–10,000. Figure 10.7 shows the results. The proposed algorithm's accuracy increased with an increase in the value of n. This can be accounted for by referencing the fact that when n is greater, the accuracy of the estimated covariance matrix improves, along with the reconstruction accuracy of the CDF. An improvement also occurs in the accuracy of IR and IO when n increases. Generally, methods that generate multi-dimensional contingency tables using LDP data necessitate the presence of substantial volumes of data. The expectation is that the accuracy of these methods improves with the availability of large datasets. Contrastingly, the degree to which the other methods were accurate did not improve with an increase in n. It is not expected that the ML models' accuracy will improve, due to the considerable impact of noise in LDP.

10.6.2 Experiment with Real Datasets

For the purposes of the evaluation, two real datasets were used in this study. Descriptions of these datasets are provided next.

The number of attributes in the real datasets was 11 for diabetes and 6 for AReM. These datasets are publicly accessible. Given that this study focuses on the intersection between privacy and ML technologies, well-known datasets relating to these fields were selected. For diabetes, this dataset is part of the scikit-learn framework

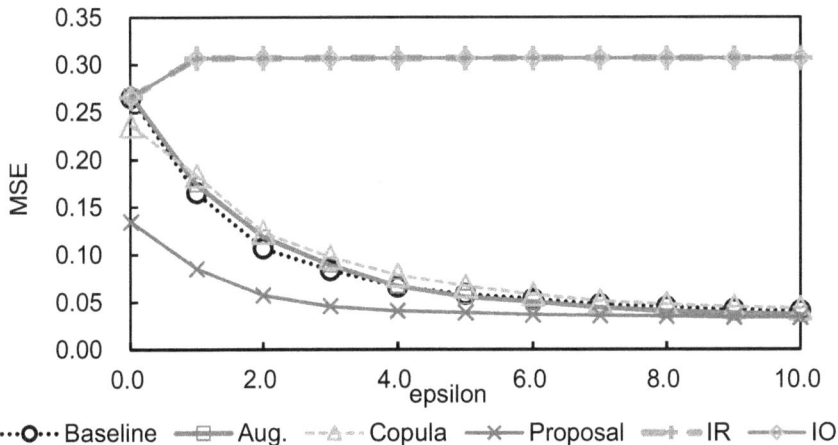

FIGURE 10.6   MSE values of ($g = 30$, $n = 1,000$).

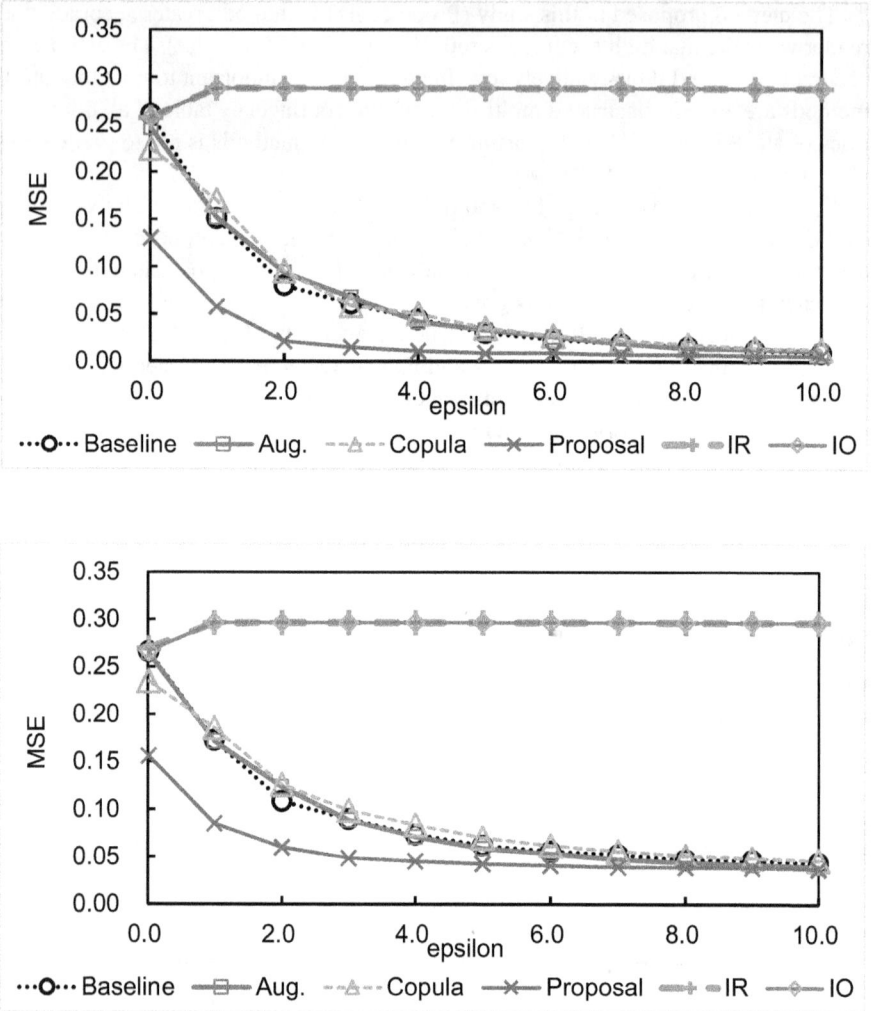

FIGURE 10.6   (Continued)

and so is well-known in the ML community, given scikit-learn's status as the primary ML framework today. For AReM, this dataset is a benchmark in the field of behavior recognition applications. An overview of each dataset is given as follows:

- *Diabetes*
  - The diabetes dataset [81] is part of scikit-learn. A reason for designing the dataset was to assist in the prediction of diabetes progression after 12 months, utilizing the test results of diabetic individuals. Four hundred and forty-two records are contained in the dataset with 11 attributes in total. A considerable number of studies have employed the diabetes dataset for the evaluation of techniques in the domain of data mining [82, 83].

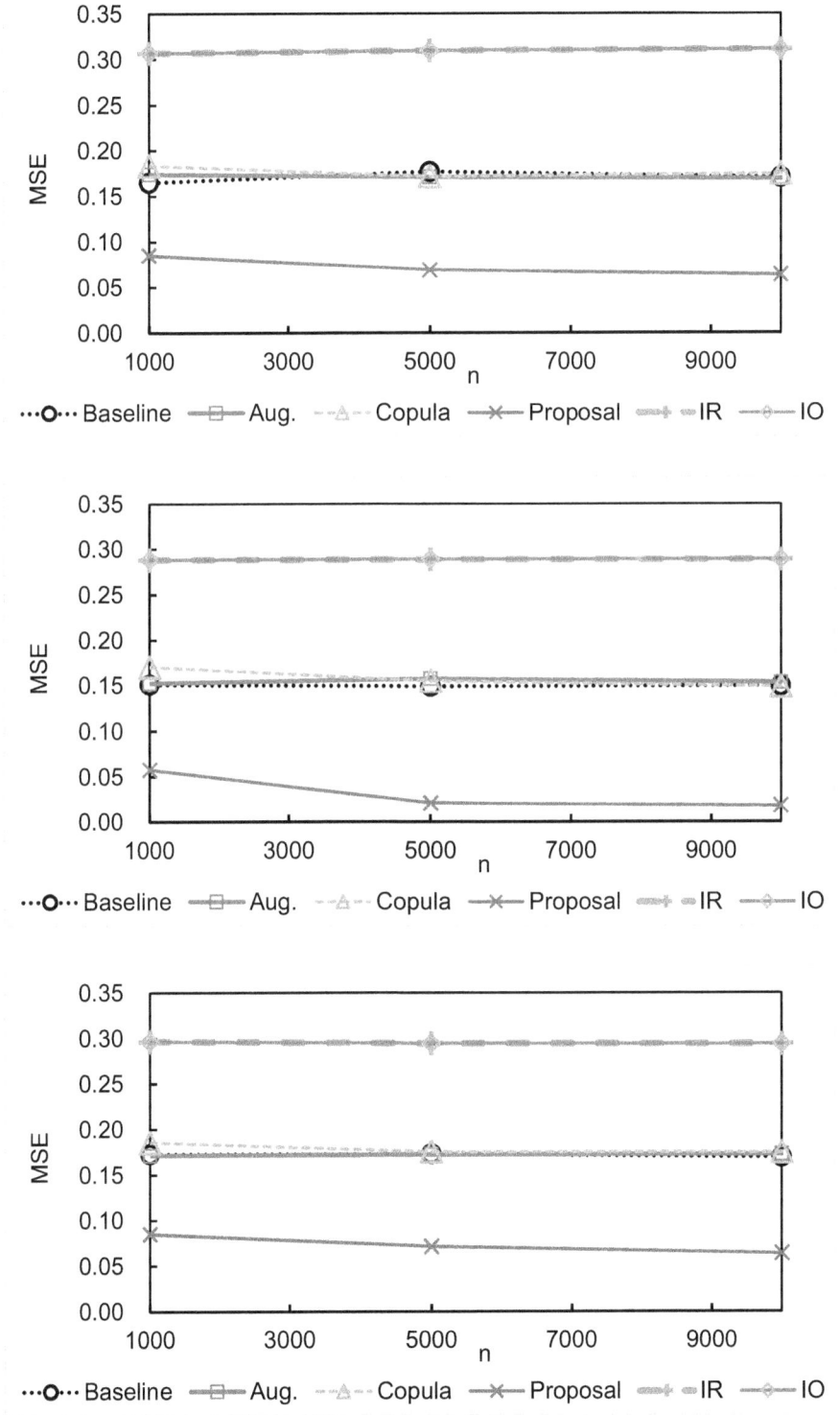

FIGURE 10.7 MSE values ($g = 30$, $\varepsilon = 1.0$).

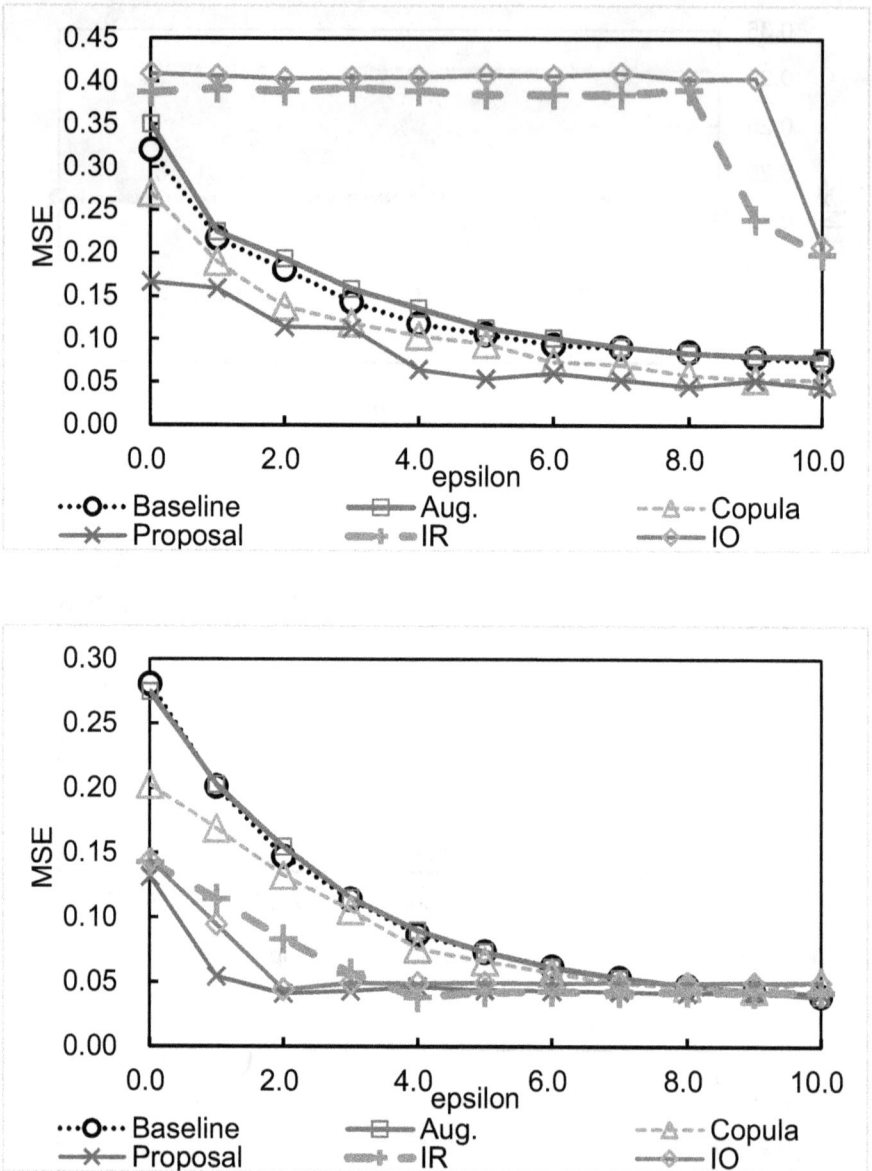

FIGURE 10.8 MSE values.

- *AReM*
  - This data set can be used as a task to infer user activity based on infor-
    mation from inertial sensors embedded in the smartphone carried by
    the user and information obtained from wireless sensors installed in the
    environment or on the user himself.

Figure 10.8 shows the results. We know from the figure that the accuracy of the proposed algorithm is overwhelming.

Lastly, experiments were conducted on DNN, SVM, and kNN to ascertain the feasibility of applying the proposed algorithm to ML algorithms. Figure 10.9 shows the results. The increased ratio shows how much the proposed algorithm reduces the MSE. When the increase ratio is less than zero, it means that the proposed algorithm could reduce the MSE. For DNN, kNN, and DT, the effectiveness of the proposed algorithm is evident. The results indicate that the proposed algorithm is not effective for SVM.

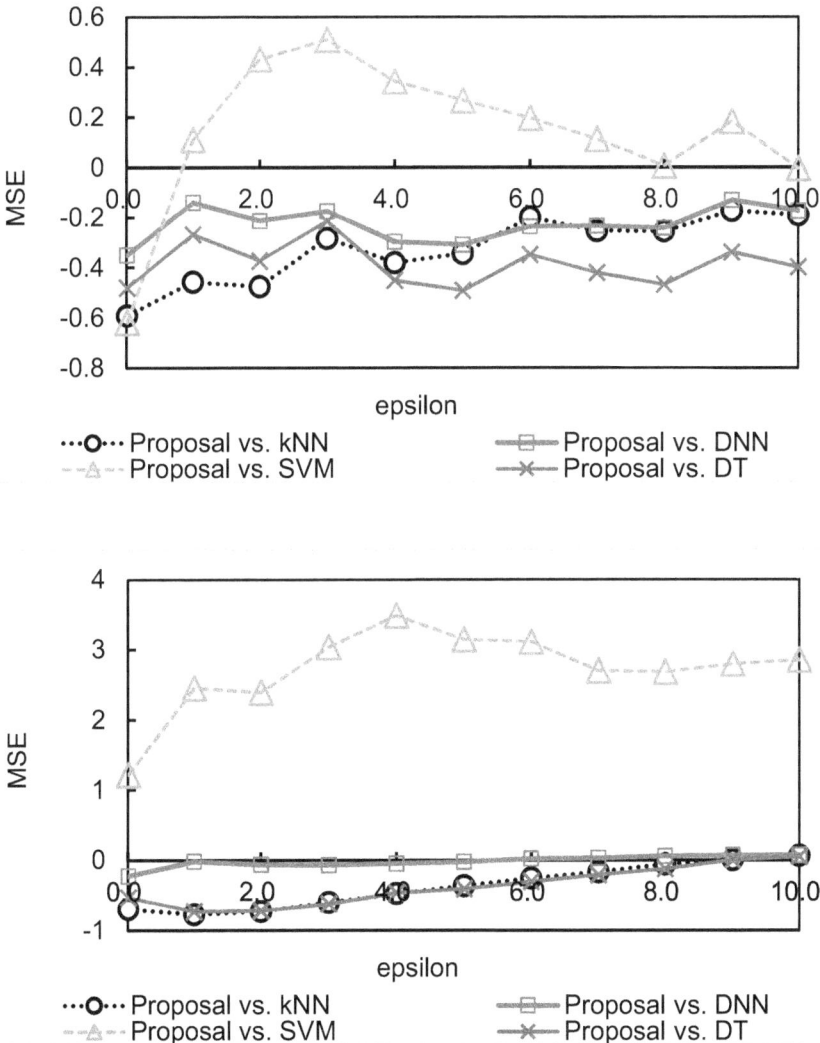

FIGURE 10.9 Increased ratio of MSE.

10.7 DISCUSSION

10.7.1 ADVANTAGES AND LIMITATIONS

The previous section presented a comparative assessment of data augmentation, the copula method, and multi-dimensional contingency table generation methods (IR and IO). The experimental results indicate that the computational complexity exceeds the copula method. In the case of data augmentation, the method's computational complexity is low, but it suffers from low accuracy.

10.7.2 COMPARISON OF ML ALGORITHMS

Section 10.4 provides an overview of the reason why the proposed algorithm works effectively for decision trees. Given that LDP data are characterized by high noise, this reduces the accuracy of the ML models that are trained on such data. Noteworthily, a range of ML algorithms are characterized by high robustness to data of this kind.

In general, DNN is considered to be robust to noise [84]. However, the ability to cancel noise is limited. In this research, we obtained the result that the accuracy of DNN is improved when the proposed algorithm is adopted.

A feature of SVM for regression is the use of an e-insensitive loss function, which penalizes predicted values that are more than the value of e away from the intended output, making the e-insensitive region less sensitive to noisy inputs [85]. This SVM characteristic may have had a positive effect on LDP data characterized by noise. Making the SVM verification process more detailed is for further study.

On the other hand, the high sensitivity of kNN to noisy data is well established in the literature [86]. Therefore, the results of the proposed algorithm using kNN are also satisfactory as shown by the experimental results.

10.7.3 HANDLING HIGH-DIMENSIONAL DATA

Given the suitability of a copula model for data characterized by low dimensionality, it is challenging to handle high-dimensional data. A range of research projects have demonstrated that dimensionality reduction improves ML model accuracy [87, 88]. To perform PCA with LDP data, it is possible to use the algorithm proposed by Wang and Xu [89].

In the case of DNN, a range of models utilize data with high dimensionality. Despite this, a collection of studies have generated DNN models with high accuracy using PCA and other dimensionality reduction techniques, including [90]. The focal point of this study is data with a limited number of attributes, and so the effectiveness of the method is not yet confirmed for high-dimensional data without dimensionality reduction. In view of this, investigating the degree to which the proposed algorithm works effectively in both the presence and absence of dimensionality reduction is an area for future research.

The high level of human interpretability of decision trees is an important rationale for having focused on them in this study. At the same time, however, multiple research projects have sought to interpret the behavior and outputs of DNNs. Nascita et al. developed an algorithm to generate global DNN interpretations [91].

Interpreting model behavior in the process of constructing DNN models using the method proposed in this study is another consideration for future research.

10.7.4 Preprocessing Techniques

A range of general preprocessing techniques have been developed, including data cleaning and dimensionality reduction [92]. These techniques do not consider LDP numerical data, which are characterized by high levels of noise, but where the noise's probability distribution follows the Laplace distribution. The method proposed in this study facilitates the generation of synthetic data that leads to the reduction of the noise arising from LDP. One of the other preprocessing techniques utilized for growing the size of training data is data augmentation. Additionally, LDP data are not considered in this technique, which means that it has a negligible impact on elevating ML accuracy. The experimental results in this chapter indicate that the proposed algorithm performed more effectively.

10.8 CONCLUSION

In this study, a scenario in which data is collected while protecting privacy using LDP was envisioned for medical data. The objective of this study is to construct a highly accurate machine-learning model from differential privacy data. Data collection is happening at an accelerating rate in the era of IoT, but such data are often noisy due to the widespread use of LDP. This study developed a novel method for generating high-accuracy ML models, focusing in particular on decision tree models, on the basis of datasets with LDP noise. Through experiments on real and synthetic datasets, we showed that the proposed algorithm led to an improvement in ML model accuracy. The proposed algorithm is expected to increase the number of patients who will be granted permission to use the algorithm for data analysis. This will allow for rapid and highly accurate machine learning, such as countermeasures to COVID-19.

We aim to extend the proposed algorithm in future research to other types of datasets for which LDP is applicable. This includes time-series data, data containing graph structures, and image data. In particular, we plan to apply the proposed algorithm to medical-specific images, such as CT images; CT images are among the most important medical data, and research to construct them with high accuracy is still active [93]. Several methods have been proposed for applying differential privacy techniques to image data [94]. We believe that the proposed algorithm should be integrated with the results of such research.

ACKNOWLEDGMENT

The work of Agbotiname Lucky Imoize is supported in part by the Nigerian Petroleum Technology Development Fund (PTDF) and, in part, by the German Academic Exchange Service (DAAD) through the Nigerian-German Postgraduate Program under grant 57473408.

REFERENCES

[1] Xiong J, Xiong Z, Chen K, et al. Graph neural networks for automated de novo drug design. *Drug Discovery Today.* 2021;26(6):1382–1393.

[2] Lakhan A, Mastoi QUA, Elhoseny M, et al. Deep neural network-based application partitioning and scheduling for hospitals and medical enterprises using IoT assisted mobile fog cloud. *Enterprise Information Systems.* 2022;16(7):1883122. Available from: www.tandfonline.com/doi/abs/10.1080/17517575.2021.1883122.

[3] Keidar D, Yaron D, Goldstein E, et al. COVID-19 classification of X-ray images using deep neural networks. *European Radiology.* 2021;31(12):9654–9663. Available from: https://link.springer.com/article/10.1007/s00330-021-08050-1.

[4] Shokri R, Shmatikov V. Privacy-preserving deep learning. In: *Proc. ACM CCS*; 2015, pp. 1310–1321. Available from: https://dl.acm.org/doi/abs/10.1145/2810103.2813687.

[5] Toreini E, Aitken M, Coopamootoo K, et al. The relationship between trust in AI and trustworthy machine learning technologies. In: *Proc. ACM FAccT*; 2020. Available from: https://dl.acm.org/doi/abs/10.1145/3351095.3372834.

[6] Duchi JC, Jordan MI, Wainwright MJ. Local privacy and statistical minimax rates. In: *Proc. IEEE FOCS*; 2013, pp. 429–438. Available from: https://ieeexplore.ieee.org/document/6686179.

[7] Murakami T, Takahashi K. Toward evaluating re-identification risks in the local privacy model. *arXiv:2010.08238.* 2020.

[8] Hassan MU, Rehmani MH, Chen J. Differential privacy techniques for cyber physical systems: A survey. *IEEE Communications Surveys & Tutorials.* 2020;22(1):746–789.

[9] Murakami T, Kawamoto Y. Utility-optimized local differential privacy mechanisms for distribution estimation. *Proc USENIX Security Symposium.* 2019:1877–1894.

[10] Zhu T, Ye D, Wang W, et al. More than privacy: Applying differential privacy in key areas of artificial intelligence. *IEEE Transactions on Knowledge and Data Engineering.* 2020;1:1–20.

[11] Sei Y, Onesimu JA, Ohsuga A. Machine learning model generation with copula-based synthetic dataset for local differentially private numerical data. *IEEE Access.* 2022;10: 101656–101671.

[12] Yoo SH, Geng H, Chiu TL, et al. Deep learning-based decision-tree classifier for COVID-19 diagnosis from chest X-ray imaging. *Frontiers in Medicine.* 2020;7:1–8.

[13] Toraih EA, Elshazli RM, Hussein MH, et al. Association of cardiac biomarkers and comorbidities with increased mortality, severity, and cardiac injury in COVID-19 patients: A meta-regression and decision tree analysis. *Journal of Medical Virology.* 2020;92(11):2473–2488.

[14] Jiang J, Zhu X, Han G, et al. A dynamic trust evaluation and update mechanism based on C4.5 decision tree in underwater wireless sensor networks. *IEEE Transactions on Vehicular Technology.* 2020;69(8):9031–9040.

[15] Hou Q, Zhang N, Kirschen DS, et al. Sparse oblique decision tree for power system security rules extraction and embedding. *IEEE Transactions on Power Systems.* 2021;36(2):1605–1615.

[16] Lu H, Ma X. Hybrid decision tree-based machine learning models for short-term water quality prediction. *Chemosphere.* 2020;249:126169.

[17] Huysmans J, Dejaeger K, Mues C, et al. An empirical evaluation of the comprehensibility of decision table, tree and rule based predictive models. *Decision Support Systems.* 2011;51(1).

[18] Murphy KP. *Machine Learning: A Probabilistic Perspective.* The MIT Press; 2012.

[19] Fletcher S, Islam MZ. Decision tree classification with differential privacy: A survey. *ACM Computing Surveys.* 2019;52(4):83:1–83:33.

[20] Zhao L, Ni L, Hu S, et al. In private digging: Enabling tree-based distributed data mining with differential privacy. In: *Proc. IEEE INFOCOM*; 2018, pp. 2087–2095. Available from: https://ieeexplore.ieee.org/document/8486352.

[21] Sun Z, Wang Y, Shu M, et al. Differential privacy for data and model publishing of medical data. *IEEE Access.* 2019;7(Mi):152103–152114.

[22] Wang S, Chang JM. Privacy-preserving boosting in the local setting. *IEEE Transactions on Information Forensics and Security.* 2021;99:1–15.

[23] Patton AJ. A review of copula models for economic time series. *Journal of Multivariate Analysis.* 2012;110:4–18.

[24] Khan NA, Habib MA, Jamal S. Effects of smartphone application usage on mobility choices. *Transportation Research Part A: Policy and Practice.* 2020;132(January):932–947.

[25] Krieter P, Breiter A. Analyzing mobile application usage: Generating log files from mobile screen recordings. *Proc MobileHCI*; 2018, pp. 1–10. Available from: https://dl.acm.org/doi/10.1145/3229434.3229450.

[26] Peköz ÜG. Product usage data collection and challenges of data anonymization. In: *Lecture Notes on Data Engineering and Communications Technologies.* Springer; 2018, pp. 117–136.

[27] Breck E, Cai S, Nielsen E, et al. The ML test score: A rubric for ML production readiness and technical debt reduction. *Proc IEEE BigData*; 2017, pp. 1123–1132. Available from: https://ieeexplore.ieee.org/document/8258038.

[28] Simard PY, Amershi S, Chickering DM, et al. Machine teaching: A new paradigm for building machine learning systems. 2017. Available from: https://arxiv.org/abs/1707.06742.

[29] Holstein K, Wortman Vaughan J, Daume H, et al. Improving fairness in machine learning systems: What do industry practitioners need? In: *Proc. ACM CHI*; 2019, pp. 600:1–600:16. Available from: https://dl.acm.org/doi/10.1145/3290605.3300830.

[30] Saleiro P, Kuester B, Hinkson L, et al. Aequitas: A bias and fairness audit toolkit. *arXiv.* 2018. Available from: http://arxiv.org/abs/1811.05577.

[31] Tramer F, Atlidakis V, Geambasu R, et al. FairTest: Discovering unwarranted associations in data-driven applications. In: *Proc. IEEE European S&P*; 2017, pp. 401–416. Available from: https://arxiv.org/abs/1510.02377.

[32] Liang Y, Li S, Yan C, et al. Explaining the black-box model: A survey of local interpretation methods for deep neural networks. *Neurocomputing.* 2021;419:168–182.

[33] Gupta D, Bhatia MPS, Kumar A. Resolving data overload and latency issues in multivariate time-series IoMT data for mental health monitoring. *IEEE Sensors Journal.* 2021;21(22):25421–25428.

[34] Haque RU, Hasan ASMT. Privacy-preserving multivariant regression analysis over blockchain-based encrypted IoMT data. In: *Artificial Intelligence and Blockchain for Future Cybersecurity Applications.* 2021, pp. 45–59. Available from: https://link.springer.com/chapter/10.1007/978-3-030-74575-2_3.

[35] Gao Y, Lin H, Chen Y, et al. Blockchain and SGX-enabled edge-computing-empowered secure IoMT data analysis. *IEEE Internet of Things Journal.* 2021;8(21):15785–15795.

[36] Wang T, Zhang X, Feng J, et al. A comprehensive survey on local differential privacy toward data statistics and analysis. *Sensors.* 2020;20(24):1–48.

[37] Gu X, Li M, Xiong L, et al. Providing input-discriminative protection for local differential privacy. *Proc ICDE*; 2020, pp. 505–516. Available from: https://doi.ieeecomputersociety.org/10.1109/ICDE48307.2020.00050.

[38] Murakami T, Hino H, Sakuma J. Toward distribution estimation under local differential privacy with small samples. *Proceedings on Privacy Enhancing Technologies.* 2018;2018(3):84–104.

[39] Sei Y, Ohsuga A. Differentially private mobile crowd sensing considering sensing errors. *Sensors.* 2020;20(10):2785:1–2785:25.

[40] Wang N, Xiao X, Yang Y, et al. Collecting and analyzing multidimensional data with local differential privacy. In: *Proc. IEEE ICDE*; 2019, pp. 638–649. Available from: https://doi.ieeecomputersociety.org/10.1109/ICDE.2019.00063.

[41] Li Z, Wang T, Lopuhaa-Zwakenberg M, et al. Estimating numerical distributions under local differential privacy. In: *Proc. ACM SIGMOD*; 2020, pp. 621–635. Available from: https://dl.acm.org/doi/abs/10.1145/3318464.3389700.

[42] Chaudhuri K, Monteleoni C, Sarwate AD. Differentially private empirical risk minimization. *Journal of Machine Learning Research.* 2011;12(29):1069–1109.

[43] Fang X, Yu F, Yang G, et al. Regression analysis with differential privacy preserving. *IEEE Access.* 2019;7:129353–129361.

[44] Smith MT, Alvarez MA, Zwiessele M, et al. Differentially private regression with gaussian processes. In: *Proc. AIStat*; 2018, pp. 1195–1203. Available from: https://proceedings.mlr.press/v84/smith18a.html.

[45] Barrientos AF, Reiter JP, Machanavajjhala A, et al. Differentially private significance tests for regression coefficients. *Journal of Computational and Graphical Statistics.* 2019;28(2):440–453.

[46] Abadi M, Chu A, Goodfellow I, et al. Deep learning with differential privacy. In: *Proc. ACM CCS*; 2016, pp. 308–318. Available from: https://dl.acm.org/doi/10.1145/2976749.2978318.

[47] Lin Y, Bao LY, Li ZM, et al. Differential privacy protection over deep learning: An investigation of its impacted factors. *Computers and Security.* 2020;99:102061.

[48] Bu Z, Dong J, Long Q, et al. Deep learning with gaussian differential privacy. *Harvard Data Science Review.* 2020;2(3):1–31. Available from: https://hdsr.mitpress.mit.edu/pub/u24wj42y.

[49] Sei Y, Okumura H, Ohsuga A. Privacy-preserving publication of deep neural networks. In: *Proc. IEEE DSS*; 2017, pp. 1418–1425. Available from: https://ieeexplore.ieee.org/document/7828543.

[50] Mothukuri V, Parizi RM, Pouriyeh S, et al. A survey on security and privacy of federated learning. *Future Generation Computer Systems.* 2021;115(October):619–640.

[51] Hao M, Li H, Luo X, et al. Efficient and privacy-enhanced federated learning for industrial artificial intelligence. *IEEE Transactions on Industrial Informatics.* 2020; 16(10):6532–6542.

[52] Yang Q, Liu Y, Cheng Y, et al. Federated learning-challenges, methods, and future directions. *Synthesis Lectures on Artificial Intelligence and Machine Learning.* 2020;13(3):1–207.

[53] Song M, Wang Z, Zhang Z, et al. Analyzing user-level privacy attack against federated learning. *IEEE Journal on Selected Areas in Communications.* 2020;38(10):2430–2444.

[54] Xu J, Glicksberg BS, Su C, et al. Federated learning for healthcare informatics. *Journal of Healthcare Informatics Research.* 2021;5(1):1–19.

[55] Wei K, Li J, Ding M, et al. Federated learning with differential privacy: Algorithms and performance analysis. *IEEE Transactions on Information Forensics and Security.* 2020;15:3454–3469.

[56] Truex S, Liu L, Chow KH, et al. LDP-fed: Federated learning with local differential privacy. In: *Proc. ACM EdgeSys*; 2020, pp. 61–66. Available from: https://dl.acm.org/doi/abs/10.1145/3378679.3394533.

[57] Wu N, Farokhi F, Smith D, et al. The value of collaboration in convex machine learning with differential privacy. In: *Proc. IEEE S&P*; 2020, pp. 304–317. Available from: https://doi.org/10.1109/SP40000.2020.00025.

[58] Chuanxin Z, Yi S, Degang W. Federated learning with gaussian differential privacy. In: *Proc. RICAI*; 2020, pp. 296–301. Available from: https://dl.acm.org/doi/10.1145/3438872.3439097.

[59] Wang D, Xu J. On sparse linear regression in the local differential privacy model. In: *Proc. ICML*; 2019, pp. 6628–6637. Available from: https://proceedings.mlr.press/v97/wang19m.html.

[60] Mahawaga Arachchige PC, Bertok P, Khalil I, et al. Local differential privacy for deep learning. *IEEE Internet of Things Journal*. 2020;7(7):5827–5842. Available from: https://ieeexplore.ieee.org/document/8894030.

[61] Erlingsson U, Feldman V, Mironov I, et al. Amplification by shuffling: From local to central differential privacy via anonymity. *Proc. Annual ACM-SIAM Symposium on Discrete Algorithms*. 2019, pp. 2468–2479. Available from: https://dl.acm.org/doi/10.5555/3310435.3310586.

[62] Balle B, Bell J, Gascon A, et al. The privacy blanket of the shuffle model. *Lecture Notes in Computer Science*. 2019;11693 LNCS(1565387):638–667.

[63] Zhang Z, Wang T, Li N, et al. PrivSyn: Differentially private data synthesis. In: *30th USENIX Security Symposium*; 2021. Available from: https://www.usenix.org/system/files/sec21fall-zhang-zhikun.pdf.

[64] Vietri G, Tian G, Bun M, et al. New oracle-efficient algorithms for private synthetic data release. In: *Proc. ICML*; 2020, pp. 9707–9716. Available from: https://proceedings.mlr.press/v119/vietri20b.html.

[65] Harder F, Adamczewski K, Park M. DP-MERF: Differentially private mean embeddings with random features for practical privacy-preserving data generation. In: *Proc. AISTAT*, vol. 130; 2021; pp. 1819–1827. Available from: http://proceedings.mlr.press/v130/harder21a/harder21a.pdf.

[66] Cai K, Lei X, Wei J, et al. Data synthesis via differentially private Markov random fields. *Proc VLDB*. 2021;14(11):2190–2202.

[67] Rocher L, Hendrickx JM, de Montjoye YA. Estimating the success of reidentifications in incomplete datasets using generative models. *Nature Communications*. 2019;10(1):1–9.

[68] Chen Y. A copula-based supervised learning classification for continuous and discrete data. *Journal of Data Science*. 2016;14(4):769–790.

[69] Gonçalves AR, Zuben FJV, Banerjee A, et al. Multi-task sparse structure learning with gaussian copula models. *Journal of Machine Learning Research*. 2016;17(33):1–30.

[70] Carrillo JA, Nieto M, Velez JF, et al. A new machine learning forecasting algorithm based on bivariate copula functions. *Forecasting*. 2021;3(2):355–376.

[71] Sei Y, Onesimu JA, Okumura H, et al. Privacy-preserving collaborative data collection and analysis with many missing values. *IEEE Transactions on Dependable and Secure Computing*. 2022;20(3): 2158–2173. Available from: https://ieeexplore.ieee.org/document/9774940.

[72] Sei Y, Okumura H, Ohsuga A. Re-identification in differentially private incomplete datasets. *IEEE Open Journal of the Computer Society*. 2022;3:62–72.

[73] Breiman L, Friedman JH, Olshen RA, et al. *Classification and Regression Trees*. Routledge; 1984.

[74] Quinlan JR. Induction of decision trees. *Machine Learning*. 1986;1(1).

[75] Quinlan JR. *C4.5: Programs for Machine Learning*. Morgan Kaufmann; 1993.

[76] Dua D, Graff C. *UCI Machine Learning Repository*; 2019. Available from: http://archive.ics.uci.edu/ml.

[77] Chen JM. An introduction to machine learning for panel data. *International Advances in Economic Research.* 2021;27(1).

[78] Breiman L. Bagging predictors. *Machine Learning.* 1996;24(2).

[79] Erlingsson U, Pihur V, Korolova A. RAPPOR: Randomized aggregatable privacy-preserving ordinal response. In: *Proc. ACM CCS*; 2014, pp. 1054–1067. Available from: https://dl.acm.org/doi/10.1145/2660267.2660348.

[80] Wang T, Blocki J, Li N, et al. Locally differentially private protocols for frequency estimation. In: *Proc. USENIX Security Symposium*; 2017, pp. 729–745. Available from: https://www.usenix.org/conference/usenixsecurity17/technical-sessions/presentation/wang-tianhao.

[81] Efron B, Hastie T, Johnstone I, et al. Least angle regression. *The Annals of Statistics.* 2004;32(2).

[82] Zhao L. Privacy-preserving distributed analytics in fog-enabled IoT systems. *Sensors.* 2020;20(21):1–23.

[83] Kwon S, Kim Y, Choi H. Sparse bridge estimation with a diverging number of parameters. *Statistics and its Interface.* 2013;6(2):231–242.

[84] Rolnick D, Veit A, Belongie S, et al. Deep learning is robust to massive label noise. *arXiv.* 2017:1–10. Available from: https://arxiv.org/abs/1705.10694v3.

[85] Awad M, Khanna R. Support vector regression. In: *Efficient Learning Machines.* Apress; 2015, pp. 67–80.

[86] Saez JA, Luengo J, Herrera F. Predicting noise filtering efficacy with data complexity measures for nearest neighbor classification. *Pattern Recognition.* 2013;46(1):355–364.

[87] Suleiman A, Tight MR, Quinn AD. Hybrid neural networks and boosted regression tree models for predicting roadside particulate matter. *Environmental Modeling and Assessment.* 2016;21(6):731–750.

[88] Caggiano A, Angelone R, Napolitano F, et al. Dimensionality reduction of sensorial features by principal component analysis for ANN machine learning in tool condition monitoring of CFRP drilling. *Procedia CIRP.* 2018;78:307–312.

[89] Wang D, Xu J. Principal component analysis in the local differential privacy model. *Theoretical Computer Science.* 2020;809:296–312.

[90] Gadekallu TR, Khare N, Bhattacharya S, et al. Deep neural networks to predict diabetic retinopathy. *Journal of Ambient Intelligence and Humanized Computing.* 2020;1:1–14.

[91] Nascita A, Montieri A, Aceto G, et al. XAI meets mobile traffic classification: Understanding and improving multimodal deep learning architectures. *IEEE Transactions on Network and Service Management.* 2021;18(4):4225–4246.

[92] Benhar H, Idri A, L Fernandez-Alemán J. Data preprocessing for heart disease classification: A systematic literature review. *Computer Methods and Programs in Biomedicine.* 2020;195:1–30.

[93] Mizusawa S, Sei Y, Orihara R, et al. Computed tomography image reconstruction using stacked U-Net. *Computerized Medical Imaging and Graphics.* 2021;90(101920).

[94] Fan L. Image pixelization with differential privacy. In: *Proc. IFIP Annual Conference on Data and Applications Security and Privacy (DBSec)*; 2018, pp. 148–162. Available from: https://link.springer.com/chapter/10.1007/978-3-319-95729-6_10.

11 Artificial Intelligence of Internet of Medical Things (AIoMT) in Smart Cities
A Review of Cybersecurity for Smart Healthcare

Kassim Kalinaki, Mugigayi Fahadi,
Adam A. Alli, Wasswa Shafik,
Magombe Yasin, and Nambobi Mutwalibi

11.1 INTRODUCTION

In the twenty-first century, we have seen a plethora of technological advancements that have changed the way we live. One such breakthrough is the Internet of Things (IoT), which is capable of transforming various aspects of our lives by connecting every digital object to the Internet and enabling Machine-to-Machine communication between devices. The IoT has far-reaching implications for various fields, such as surveillance, agriculture, military, manufacturing, energy generation, healthcare, and more, all of which hold immense potential for shaping the human race for the better [1, 2]. In this regard, healthcare can be considered as one such major domain this IoT is being served. This use of IoT in healthcare is also known as the Internet of Medical Things or IoMT [3]. Most of the IoMT applications and services in healthcare possess the capabilities for providing quality and comprehensive patient care within less time and are applicable in numerous clinical contexts that include nursing homes, hospitals, communities, and individual homes among others [4].

Within the context of smart healthcare as a major component of smart cities, AI is highly used in line with IoMT for inferring the meaning of gathered pathological data and taking timely and precise decisions on underlying pathological conditions. This collation is known as AIoMT [5] and is playing a significant role in ameliorating the well-being and health of billions of people, all around the world. In various aspects of healthcare, especially in disease diagnosis, patient condition monitoring, clinical environment monitoring, surgical procedures, and pandemic situation management/surveillance, these AIoMT technologies are highly used owing to their ubiquitous nature and yield benefits such as aiding in taking timely and precise decisions [5]. This has also given rise to many healthcare applications, such as applications for elderly care, remote health monitoring, chronic disease management, and fitness programs to mention but a few [6, 7].

In recent years, this AIoMT has attracted so much attention from academia, industry, and researchers as a result of the many benefits it has, among which include minimizing the massive burden in healthcare brought about by a shortage of medical staff, the rise of global pandemics such as SARS, and the still prevalent COVID-19 deadly pandemic, the upsurge of aging population, and rise of chronic diseases [8, 9]. As the AIoMT ecosystem itself is often involving and dealing with highly sensitive patient data, owing to the ever-changing attack vectors in the modern threat landscape, this AIoMT is becoming a critical and frequent target, that various cyber attackers are paying higher attention to [10, 11]. If the intruders can penetrate such AIoMT devices, they will be able to access personal and medical information stored on the devices along with gaining control over the devices which eventually leads to major health issues and potential loss of lives. Nevertheless, they could have also access to the underlying highly sensitive patient information and could have sold this information for higher prices on the dark web's black market, which eventually tarnishes the reputation of medical organizations [3]. As for that, higher attention must be paid to the security of the entire AIoMT ecosystem otherwise that will endanger the lives of patients and tarnish the reputation of medical organizations.

11.1.1　Chapter Contributions

The integration of AI in the healthcare industry is poised to revolutionize the way we deliver and manage healthcare services in smart cities. This chapter explores the various ways in which AI is shaping the health sector in smart cities, highlighting the following contributions:

1. Overview of AI's impact on healthcare in smart cities and its applications in smart healthcare
2. Overview of the cybersecurity aspect of AIoMT in smart cities
3. Proposal for a secure framework for AI-enabled Medical Technologies in smart cities
4. Analysis of potential risks and vulnerabilities of AIoMT, particularly concerning cyberattacks and patient data security
5. Discussion of measures to protect against cyberattacks and other security and privacy breaches in AIoMT
6. Exploration of future developments and advancements in AIoMT in the healthcare industry

11.1.2　Chapter Organization

Following the introduction in Section 11.1, the rest of this article is organized as follows: Section 11.2 describes the different applications of AI in smart healthcare.

Section 11.3 highlights the cybersecurity aspect of AIoMT in a smart city. Section 11.4 proposes a secure AIoMT framework for smart healthcare in smart cities based on edge technologies. Threats and cyberattacks targeting the IoMT as well as proposed countermeasures are discussed in Section 11.5. Lessons learned are highlighted in Section 11.6. Anticipated future directions are elaborated on in Section 11.7 and the conclusion is depicted in Section 11.8.

11.2 APPLICATIONS OF AI IN SMART HEALTHCARE

The application of AI in the health sector has the potential to progressively revolutionize the landscape of the health sector in a more advanced way in what is now referred to as AI-enabled healthcare (smart health or e-health). This AI-enabled healthcare constitutes a broad technological perspective of independent machines that entails reinforcement learning, supervised, and non-supervised learning coupled with deep learning. Figure 11.1 illustrates AI sub-domains in healthcare in a smart way both supervised and non-supervised machine learning (ML) arrangements. Smart healthcare offers countless opportunities to use AI for more accurate and effective patient care due to the availability of a plethora of medical data [12].

This subsection, therefore, affords AI applications in the smart health setup even though the level of acceptance and influence of the technologies has been discussed in a more detailed way in several technological and medical pieces of literature.

11.2.1 SURGICAL ROBOTS

Feasibly, the utmost famous robots in use nowadays are those used in surgery in the medical industry. Medical centers are increasingly using robotic surgery to establish

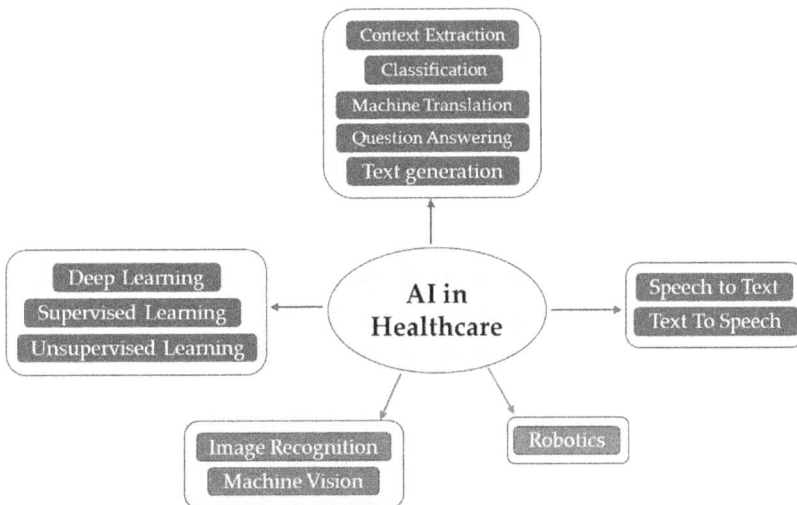

FIGURE 11.1 Artificial intelligence sub-domains in healthcare, as adapted from [13].

themselves as industry pioneers in cutting-edge medicine [14]. There are still concerns regarding the efficiency and overall cost-benefit of surgery helped by a robot. A demonstrated example of such concerns includes undermining the integrity of surgery as a result of a bug within an algorithm [15]. The technological problem is to figure out how to let the AI-enabled machine make up for human error while also letting the human operator keep control in the event of an AI machine's failure [16].

11.2.2   Exoskeletons

Lower human exoskeletons with robotics, such as the Ekso, are being utilized to help individuals with spinal cord injuries and strokes regain their walking. The Ekso's algorithms and AI hardware interact magically [17], enabling persons with physical disabilities to move independently, increasing self-reliance, boosting muscular growth, and decreasing the physical toll on therapists for human recovery. The "ReWalk" has successfully fulfilled the stringent safety requisites, akin to the prevalent utilization of canes, crutches, and electric wheelchairs, hinting at a future where artificial intelligence becomes ubiquitously embraced [18].

11.2.3   Prosthetics

This is now a common AI application for patients that have body amputations, and it has seen considerable technological advancements in the earlier decades. For instance, intelligent robotic prosthetics like the DEKA Arm for amputees' controllable system using MG signals for muscle growth has been unveiled [19].

11.2.4   Artificial Organs

The use of the gadget by the patient is very strictly controlled by the conditions of an end-user licensing contract (EULA). Illustrated examples of such organs include artificial joints, lungs, hearts, kidneys, skins, bones, cochlear, and retina implants, among others, which are available for human usage [20]. Subsequently, producers can adopt the contentious business strategies employed in mass marketing consumer products with vendor lock-in and deliberate obsolescence. The EULAs require software upgrades frequently or creating new gear that isn't compatible with previous or future models. It was also discovered that the risk of major injustice is allowed by EULAs [21].

11.2.5   Healthcare Automation Robots

Healthcare facilities and pharmaceuticals are also transforming as a result of AI evolution. In this attempt, hospitals are now adopting strategies from the manufacturing industry to reduce expenses via AI applications to boost productivity. AI that can make deliveries on its own is utilized to bring supplies, meals, linens, and medications within hospitals, allowing nurses and support workers to focus on other duties. Delivery intelligent bots, for example, RoboCourier [22] and HOSPI are exploring the hospital halls while avoiding hazards [23].

11.2.6 Autonomous Identification of Diseases

The effectiveness of AI is demonstrated in the diagnosis of skin cancer [24], breast cancer [25, 26], and eye illnesses [27] when natural language processing, machine vision, and data mining techniques are applied. Additionally, one application where AI techniques have been successfully used is in the prediction of glucose levels [28, 29]. AI techniques can be employed for psychosis prediction and TB diagnosis [30]. These researched AI technologies could be implemented via an artificial intelligence distribution platform to give clients and end users direct access to them. In light of the current pandemic, Iskander et al. [31] deployed deep transfer learning-based algorithms to analyze, classify, and predict COVID-19 infections using X-ray images, which were essential in real-time communication and diagnosis helping prevent the spread of the virus

11.2.7 Personalized Medicine

Tailoring treatment to the individual characteristics of a patient is referred to as personalized medicine. The approach is rooted in understanding an individual's specific molecular and genetic makeup and how it predisposes them to certain diseases. To apply treatments more successfully, personalized medicine also emphasizes early disease detection [32]. AI-enable machines can track patient diagnoses together with data, depending on information supplied on already trained AI techniques, AI-enable machines could recommend the best courses of action and/or medications to the patient.

11.2.8 Medication Errors

AI techniques are employed in smart health care to increase medication nonadherence and detect medication mistakes. An AI-powered screening system can be developed to find potential drug flaws and produce alerts for clinical systems [33]. Medication adherence has been improved by using AI techniques for instance neural networks to track patient access to drugs. Healthcare service providers can be able to access these techniques through AI-distribution platforms as a service.

11.2.9 Candidate Identification Meant for Clinical Trials

Finding attendees in clinical trials is crucial for producing more thorough trials at a cheaper cost. AI can help with medical trial design and discover a massive data set model to find suitable patients earlier to start medical testing. During clinical studies, AI can be employed for better, more precise patient follow-up. AI techniques have been shown to boost clinical trial enrolment [34]. Additionally, the application of AI techniques improves patient identification who are qualified for medical trials among other identifiable benefits like epidemic outbreak predictions and management [8] and diagnostics of medical images [35].

11.2.10 Cybersecurity

As the reliance on data continues to increase, protecting sensitive information and preventing cyberattacks becomes increasingly challenging. AI has emerged as a powerful solution to this problem, and many companies are investing in AI to protect their data. The healthcare sector, in particular, has been hardest hit by cyberattacks, and these attacks are rising at an alarming rate [36]. Healthcare organizations are recognizing the benefits of AI in identifying and neutralizing threats, maintaining compliance, and minimizing human error. AI-powered programs can analyze large volumes of data, uncovering new insights about unfamiliar patterns and suspicious activity by cyber criminals and system vulnerabilities [37]. However, no technology can be entirely secure, and there will always be a risk of hackers breaching AI systems.

11.2.11 HEALTHCARE MONITORING AND WEARABLES

As individuals become increasingly invested in their health and wellness, the demand for health monitoring and wearable devices is skyrocketing. These wearables are designed to track various physical parameters such as strain, pressure, temperature, heartbeat, and other biological variations within the body [12]. Furthermore, AI-powered devices equipped with smart sensors have the potential to aid in early diagnosis, remote patient monitoring, and managing chronic conditions, as well as assist in emergency health situations. The integration of state-of-the-art technologies that include but are not limited to IoT, Big Data, and 5G is expected to improve the performance and versatility of health monitoring through wearable devices [8, 15].

11.2.12 AI IN HEALTH FRAUD DETECTION

According to [38], fraud, waste, and abuse (FWA) accounts for a significant portion of healthcare claims in the United States, costing insurance providers and other stakeholders billions of dollars. Health fraud originates from a myriad of sources, such as insurance carriers, subscribers, and service providers. As noted in [15], the healthcare industry generates a large amount of data over an extended period, making detecting fraudulent activity a complex and labor-intensive task. However, automation of the process can be achieved by using data mining and ML techniques, resulting in quicker detection, and saving organizations millions of dollars in FWA-related costs. Regardless of the promising advantages, the adoption of AI for fraud detection and control will vary across industries, companies, and countries.

Overall, as technology continues to advance, the use of AI in healthcare is expected to become even more prevalent, providing several benefits to patients, healthcare providers, and the healthcare industry as a whole. The diagram in Figure 11.2 summarizes the aforementioned AI applications in healthcare.

A summary of the AI algorithms applied in healthcare including neural networks, Naive Bayes, k-nearest neighbor, decision tree, logistic regression, random forest, and support vector machine is depicted in Table 11.1.

11.3 CYBERSECURITY ASPECTS OF AIOMT IN SMART CITIES

The challenge for most IoMT systems is to ensure the security of medical endpoint devices (MePD), which generate a large amount of data from connected devices. This is because devices in such networks capture sensitive data about patients,

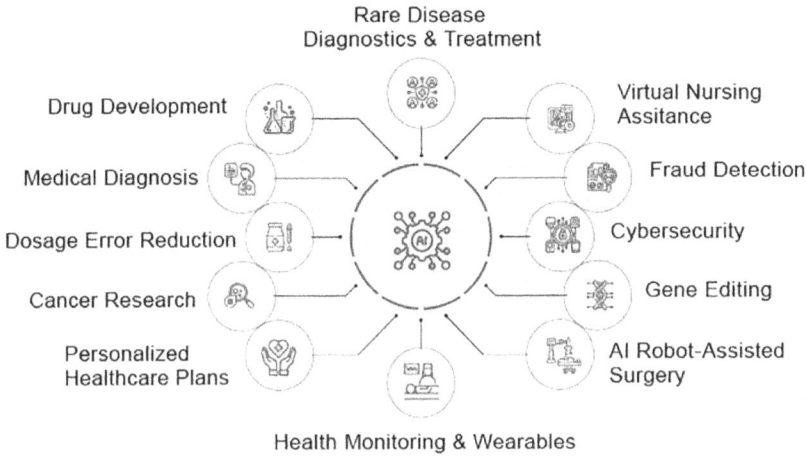

FIGURE 11.2 Artificial intelligence applications in healthcare [38].

TABLE 11.1
Summary of AI Algorithms and Their Applications in AI-Enabled Healthcare

AI Algorithms	Applications in Healthcare	References
Logistic regression (LR)	Healthcare-monitoring System	[39]
	Pandemic resource management	[40]
	Glucose monitoring for diabetes	[41]
Random Forest (RF)	Heart-disease prediction	[42]
	Healthcare nursing	[25]
	Disease(s) predictions	[43]
Decision Tree (DT)	Surgery	[44]
	Medical diagnosis	[45]
	Glucose monitoring for diabetes	[41]
k-nearest neighbor (kNN)	Heart-disease prediction	[46]
	Healthcare monitoring	[39]
	Computer-aided diagnosis	[47]
	Disease prediction	[48]
Naïve Bayes (NB)	Medical diagnosis	[49]
	Disease prediction	[50]
Neural Network (NN)	Diabetes prediction	[51]
	Image-based cardiac monitoring	[52]
	Cancer diagnosis	[53]
	COVID-19 prediction	[31]
	Surgery	[54]
Support Vector Machine (SVM)	Predicting surgical site infection	[55]
	Cancer diagnosis	[56]
	Psychiatric disorders	[57]

compatibility, and complex issues that are often private. Security and privacy issues at the MePD are difficult to resource due to the heterogeneous nature of MePD. Mawgoud et al. [58] noted that most security vulnerabilities and breaches occur during medical emergencies when medical personnel are in a rush to use IoMT solutions without considering the security aspect. During this period, security and issues relating to Confidentiality, Integrity, and Availability (CIA) are ignored. The security concerns raised included controlling, monitoring, and operating the MePD.

The confidentiality aspect concerns safeguarding data from unauthorized access, raising questions about how to maintain confidentiality at both the MePD and individual levels while ensuring proper data management through proper authorization of both MePD and individuals on the network. Integrity ensures the authenticity of the data being transmitted and stored on the system so that no creation or modification of data occurs without proper authorization. Availability ensures that data on the system is accessible at any time as needed by authorized personnel. Authentication ensures that all MePDs verify each other's identity thus ensuring that information is accessed by permitted devices and personnel and only limited to that information on which they have access permissions [59, 60].

Moreover, the IoMT system enforces privacy regulations in the IoMT environment, granting access to the personal details of various users. These rules are crafted to prevent unauthorized disclosure of patient information and must adhere to legal and ethical laws of privacy, such as the Health Insurance Portability and Accountability Act (HIPAA) and the General Data Protection Regulation (GDPR) [61, 62]. Finally, the non-repudiation aspect ensures that the communicating parties within an IoMT environment cannot deny participation in the exchange of information [63].

11.4   SECURE AIOMT FRAMEWORK FOR SMART HEALTHCARE IN SMART CITIES

The framework in this article is deployable for personal area and home area-oriented remote medical surveillance based on edge technologies. The framework captures, transmits, analyses, and stores health data from multiple sources. The source of data could be sensors, smart watches, wristbands, smartphones, or any other medical data acquisition systems [37]. Despite the numerous potentials envisioned by the framework, the immediate challenge to be addressed is to access the information without compromising privacy [64]. The privacy concern is about who accesses what information, and the authentication and authorization of different actors like doctors, patients, guardians, nurses, and hospital administration.

All the data captured from the patient is sent from the MePDs to the medical midpoint Devices (MiPD) (fog/mist/edge) for processing using AI systems. In some situations, the data could be complex requiring more advanced AI methods that may not fit the processing power of MiPD. In such scenarios, the data is sent for processing in the cloud system for medical applications. At each of these levels, AI-enabled processing is used to derive meaning and relationships underlying datasets being collected in real time from MePD [65].

This framework is modeled with security components at each level to secure both data and related insights by detecting suspicious activities in an attempt to breach the system [64]. The services provided by this framework enable doctors, nurses, and other hospital staff to gain controlled access to the information to be used in clinical situations to diagnose, treat, and predict future ailment trends of the patient.

The framework in Figure 11.3 is proposed to deter challenges that MePD face; these include limited system resources (memory, energy, processing power, interoperability, etc.). The diverse heterogenous nature of MePD limits the scalability and performance of the whole AIoMT systems [66].

In this framework, processing large data is forwarded to MiPD, whereas big processes are pushed to the Cloud AIoMT. The MiPD runs the AI algorithms, given that they have better resources and provide real-time processing of the unstructured, structured, and complex data that are ever growing in size, produced at high velocity let alone being very diverse [67, 68]. Earlier studies have noted the importance of ensuring the safekeeping of medical and healthcare information from the security and privacy context in which the cloud and fog application in IoMT introduced non-compliance and other risk factors in a medical environment [69].

MePD devices capture data about the patients and the environment through sensor actuators, smart wristbands, and other medical data acquisition systems, which provide continuous monitoring that generates massive medical data (big medical data) upon which health workers can make rational decisions about medical events [37]. The information processing can be used for medical transactions that happen daily, weekly, monthly, and quarterly. Further processes support decisions at the hierarchies of the health system starting from the transactional level to the executive level, which requires knowledge and experiences of doctors and/or consultants. This knowledge extraction and analysis follows a complex process that needs to be

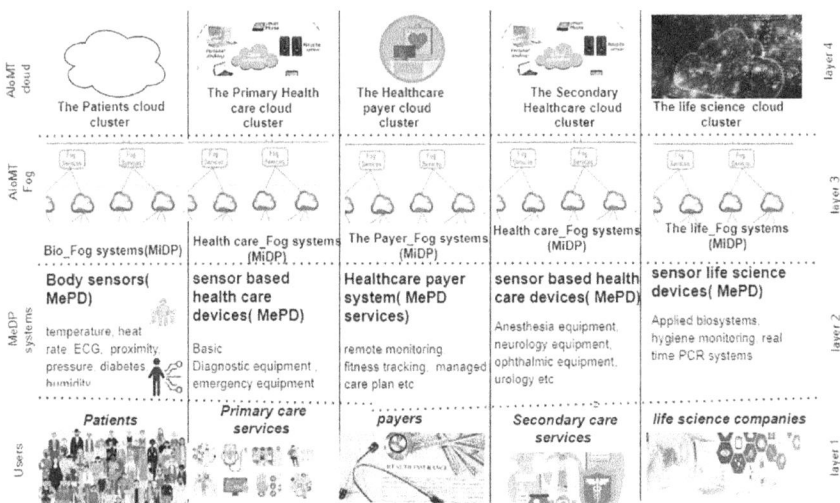

FIGURE 11.3 Secure AIoMT ecosystem.

secured [70] to ensure that no third parties have access to the data and that authorized access is limited to the data that is needed.

Due to the resource limitations of MePD, the generated data is sent to MiPD (Edge/Fog device) through a secure gateway [70], which ensures the security of data and performs analysis, exploration, and filtering of the collected information. Whilst in the fog, AI models are applied to the data for classification and non-private data to be transmitted securely to the cloud, where health professional personnel can securely access the information to provide quality diagnosis, decisions, and treatment based on the cleaned information [65, 71]. The AI Models significantly diminish the burden on health personnel, and expenses along with eliminating other health hazards such as radiation exposure in traditional imaging systems while recognizing patterns that otherwise would be missed by the human eye [65, 72].

11.5   IOMT ATTACKS, THREATS, AND COUNTERMEASURES FOR SMART HEALTHCARE

With many IoMT being connected in smart cities, they face countless threats and attacks that can lead to patient data leaks, which may result in patients being publicly harassed and traumatized along with tarnishing the reputation of medical organizations. A simple search in scholarly repositories shows that there is no size-fits-all security solution for IoMT systems to safeguard against security and privacy breaches [73]. This section briefly discusses the attacks and threats against IoMT together with their proposed countermeasures.

Multi-vector attacks on IoMT devices in smart cities such as Distributed Denial of services (DDoS) have the potential to disrupt the end-user experience in the IoMT environment by denying legitimate users (patients and medical personnel) from access to MePD or systems [74]. Such an attack affects the system and medical device availability and ultimately prevents access to medical records by medical personnel, and the patients will be denied access to their prescribed medication and care.

Malware attacks are other forms of attacks to which IoMT environments are prone. These malware include spyware, worms, trojans, viruses, ransomware, and many more that can exploit security loopholes and spread very fast across the network thereby threatening the integrity and confidentiality of the IoMT network and devices [75–77]. Their ability to have unauthorized access to medical records can lead to modification, loss, and leaks of patient records. Therefore, combating malware attacks on medical systems becomes so crucial to mitigate the fallout from loss and unauthorized access to patient and medical-related data within the IoMT environment.

Attacks such as eavesdropping have been reported, which have the means to listen and collect information from medical sensors [36]. Salem et al. [78] identified the man-in-the-middle (Mitm) attack as a common attack on IoMT systems and proposed its countermeasure. Such an attack has the means to identify healthcare emergencies of patients being monitored and retransmit the unmodified physiological data to prevent the healthcare system from activating an alarm. A system that prohibits a MitM from disrupting performance and preventing alarms from going off by the remote healthcare monitoring system was proposed.

Yaacoub et al. [74] have reported that IoMT devices are susceptible to botnets or 'zombies' attacks, which can cause physical harm to patients. As described in their modus operandi, these botnets can logically exploit a drug dose that when prescribed to a patient, can kill or result in life-threatening complications. Additionally, IoMT devices can be remotely hijacked and used for targeted assassinations by terrorists [79].

Other reported attacks in the IoMT environment include brute force, jamming attacks, packet analysis attacks, flooding attacks, resource depletion attacks (such as buffer overflow, sleep deprivation, and battery drain), false data injection, hardware trojans, and social engineering [80]. Table 11.2 summarizes them along with the impacts they have on the AIoMT system.

TABLE 11.2
Summary of AIoMT Attacks, Their Impacts, and Countermeasures

Attack	Impact	Countermeasures	References
DDoS	All	DDoS protection services, firewalls, content delivery networks (CDNs), etc.	[74]
Malware attack	Integrity, availability	Anti-virus and anti-malware software, two-factor authentication	[75–77]
Eavesdropping/ wiretapping or snooping attack	Confidentiality, non-repudiation, privacy	Use secure protocols (IPsec, SSL), use firewalls, virtual private networks (VPNs), intrusion detection systems (IDS), and intrusion prevention systems (IPS)	[36]
MITM attack	Confidentiality, integrity	Use secure protocols (IPsec, SSL), VPNs, digital signatures, public key infrastructure (PKI), firewalls, etc.	[77]
Botnets	Availability, confidentiality	Using anti-virus and anti-malware software, network-based IDS, host-based IDS, implement honeypots	[74]
Brute force attack	Confidentiality, integrity	Use strong passwords, two-factor authentication, limit password attempts, use password manager, deploy CAPTCHA, monitor suspicious activity, etc.	[79, 81]
Jamming attack	Availability	Use encryption, use a dedicated jamming detection system, etc.	[82]
Packet analysis/ sniffing attacks	Packet analysis attacks integrity, confidentiality, non-repudiation, privacy	Use VPNs, IDS/IPS, firewalls and network segmentation, etc.	[83]
Flooding attack	Availability	Use rate limiting, CDNs, Firewalls, IDS/IPS, etc.	[74]
Resource depletion attacks (such as buffer overflow, sleep deprivation, and battery drain)	Availability	Monitor suspicious activity, use firewalls, use CDNs, traffic shaping, and management, etc.	[74, 84]

(Continued)

TABLE 11.2 (*Continued*)
Summary of AIoMT Attacks, Their Impacts, and Countermeasures

Attack	Impact	Countermeasures	References
False data Injection	Confidentiality, integrity, privacy non-repudiation	Use authentication and access control, data validation, data integrity techniques, IDPS, etc.	[63]
Hardware Trojan	All	Use secure supply chain techniques, use hardware-assisted security, use run-time monitoring and detection, use physical security, etc.	[80]
Social Engineering (Reverse Engineering, Shoulder-surfing)	All	Educate employees on its dangers, implement security policies and procedures, use anti-phishing software, etc.	[74, 80]

Khan and Adnan [85] put forth a novel hybrid deep learning-powered intelligent software-defined network (SDN)-based malware detection framework for swift and efficient detection of advanced malware attacks in the IoMT environment. This framework is designed to harness the potential of resource-constrained IoMT devices without overwhelming them. Also, Lorenzo et al. [86] presented an innovative, intelligent, and dynamic system that aims to effectively combat the spread of ransomware in integrated health environments. This system utilizes advanced ML methods to precisely identify and categorize the different stages of ransomware spreading within integrated health environments.

Threats can be attributed not only to the technical skills of the hackers when targeting IoMT systems but to the unskilled end-users as well. Authors in [87] have indicated that issues such as stakeholders' unfamiliarity with security and privacy solutions together with overlooking the inbuilt features of medical devices can create attack opportunities. Such threats can lead to serious breaches in the IoMT environment from unsuspecting individuals, thereby resulting in the loss of patient data. As a countermeasure, the authors proposed an ontology-based security recommendation framework consisting of context-aware protocols for the IoMT that empowers stakeholders to make well-informed decisions. The overall mechanism of this framework ensures the classification of security threats in the IoMT environment and provides automatic recommendations for the required security controls to be applied for each threat [87].

Mohan [88] identified the low battery power limitation on MePDs that posed threats to the comprehensive cybersecurity of the IoMT environment in terms of confidentiality, integrity and availability. To negate such risks, he proposed transferring software details to the cloud-based platforms of service providers and deploying lightweight cryptographic keys to safeguard patient data. Additionally, Varshney et al. [60] proposed attributes to the cybersecurity solutions in the IoMT environment such as having lightweight MePDs with low power consumption rates, policies that regulate and ensure data on the IoMT network are protected at all levels from the collection, transmission, and storage, as well as having lightweight key management mechanisms, since MePDs have to communicate in a secure way amongst themselves. Lu and Cheng [89] subsequently suggested a system for secured data-sharing that ensures the safeguarding of information, allowing access to mutual information as well as prevention of transmission of incorrect computations from customers through integrity verification tests.

The heterogeneity and ubiquitous nature of IoMT devices further create a problem of ensuring holistic secure communication among them due to the uniqueness of security measures inherent in them from their manufacturers. Such differences provide countless opportunities for hackers to take advantage of weak and obscure security measures, which may result in compromising the security of the entire network. As one of the countermeasures, Allouzi and Khan [90] deployed a Multiparty Trust Negotiation (MTN) system using the SOTER framework that secures communication among MePDs and healthcare personnel. This was achievable through the gradual exchange of established digital credentials, which are based purely on personalized Access Control Policies.

To protect data confidentiality and ensure the integrity of transmitted data in resource-restricted IoMT devices and IoMT edge network environment, data encryption has been implemented [91]. Additionally, authors in [69] devised a cloud-based security and privacy solution for IoMT that used the asymmetric encryption standard (AES), where keys were generated using the attribute-based encryption (ABE) protocol. Such cryptographic methods maintained the integrity of IoMT-generated patient data.

A BIoMT, a four-component framework based on blockchain technology, was proposed for security and privacy preservation in smart healthcare systems that use IoMT by Seliem and Elgazzar [92]. These components included the smart medical devices, medical facility, network cluster, and cloud server, which provided a non-significant overhead capable of meeting most of the IoMT security and privacy requirements. Another blockchain-based secure e-health records storage management prototype known as MedRrec was proposed by Azaria et al. [93]. This prototype addressed patient privacy issues, improved the secure presence of medical research data, and prevented modification of patient records using cryptographic-based hashes [94].

Saheed and Arowolo [95] highlighted the results of merging a deep recurrent neural network (DRNN) with ML models such as RF, kNN, DT, and ridge classifiers to effectively detect and predict advanced cyber threats. When features from a bio-inspired particle swarm algorithm where optimized, the proposed model outshined existing models in terms of performance.

An AUDIT system for detecting inaccurate measurements of physiological data from sensors in real-time was proposed by [96] to distinguish erroneous and faulty data in health events. This system has the potential to save lives as medical personnel is becoming constantly reliant on MePDs to make health-related decisions.

Finally, Karmakar et al. [97] put forth an IoMT security architecture that leverages virtual network functions, which are developed and implemented as components and services. The security and privacy-preserving mechanism of the architecture lies in its ability to allow only authenticated and trusted MePDs in the IoMT environment to serve patients through an encryption-based communication protocol. With the help of an application, the security services provided by this architecture can be used on demand.

Overall, as the healthcare industry continues to integrate AI, it is imperative to prioritize security and privacy to ensure the safe and responsible use of these technologies, especially in emerging smart cities. The future of AIoMT in healthcare is promising, but it is crucial to address these security challenges to guarantee the accountable deployment of AI in healthcare and the protection of patient data. To fully harness the potential of AIoMT for society, further research and collaboration between AI and healthcare experts are essential to design and implement security measures for AIoMT.

11.6 LESSONS

This chapter has provided a comprehensive examination of the impact of AI on the healthcare sector in smart cities. Through an overview of the current state of AI in healthcare, the chapter has highlighted the potential benefits of AI such as improved efficiency, cost-effectiveness, and better patient outcomes. However, it also emphasized the importance of addressing the potential challenges that arise from the integration of AI in healthcare, specifically in terms of ensuring the security of AIoMT against cyberattacks and safeguarding patient data. To mitigate these challenges, the chapter proposed a secure framework for AIoMT in smart cities and discussed countermeasures to protect against cyberattacks. Furthermore, the chapter also presented an in-depth analysis of the potential risks and vulnerabilities of AIoMT.

11.7 FUTURE DIRECTIONS

Around the world, healthcare systems are undergoing a lot of pressure as a result of an increase in population, an increase in the number of disaster incidences as a result of global climatic changes, let alone the appearance of new strains of diseases that don't have treatment available [8]. In addition, the lifestyle we have adopted as a people over the years have made communicable illness become rampant. The overall population of the world is expected to hit close to 9 billion by 2050 [98] and yet the number of health professionals is likely to be 5.73 per 1,000 persons; this by itself makes health care expensive and exclusive thereby requiring the adoption of healthcare technology. Adoption of health technologies helps care providers in increasing capacity in engaging more patients and achieving better outcomes hence achieving one step ahead of their counterparts.

AIoMT is expected to uplift the precision of wearable devices in collecting data about patients' conditions. This will enable doctors to engage with their patients using telemedicine to gain better healthcare services. The new ways of getting healthcare services will considerably lower the healthcare cost for all groups of patients. Second, as a base technology beneath virtual reality and augmented reality [99], AIoMT will provide a tool for doctors to acquire data and experience of the patients in real-time allowing for precise prescription of medicine and other related healthcare procedures. Further, AIoMT forms the foundation of chatbot technologies (voice assistants) that provide clear information about clinical processes, and measurements from patients' activities as well as health care support, especially during health emergencies/pandemics. Voice assistants such as Apple Siri, Google Assistant, and Amazon Alexa have been very useful along with WhatsApp text-based chatbots, which were able to respond to COVID-19-related public questions [100]. These trends are seen to transform healthcare systems as a whole in the future as they become fully embraced.

The adoption of intelligent things and medical big data analytics as applied in AIoMT technologies will trend health care through digitized health care cutting across digital health records that may be useful in remote diagnosis, medical communication, and body and bio-hacking [37]. This could involve numerous trends in gene editing and advancements in prosthetics along with increasing the lifespan of the human body [101].

Another visible trend is seen in robots and nanobots finding their way into a healthcare setting as effective devices that can perform surgery and AI-based exoskeletons for disabled persons that enable them for example walk [102]. In addition to that, nanobots may also be injected into the human body at a specific and targeted place in the body for specialized medication. Generally, the trends cited here form a very lucrative place for the IoMT, which is estimated to be more than $158 billion market worth in the near future [103].

11.8   CONCLUSION

As smart cities continue to integrate more IoT devices and the convergence of AI and IoMT in smart healthcare gains momentum, this review delves into how AI is transforming the healthcare sector. By examining the ecosystem of AIoMT based on edge technologies, discussing the cybersecurity concerns in smart healthcare, identifying potential threats, proposing countermeasures, and exploring future developments, this review serves as a comprehensive guide for understanding the current state and future direction of AIoMT in healthcare.

One of the major strengths of this review is its ability to provide readers with a comprehensive understanding of how AI is revolutionizing healthcare, as well as the potential risks and vulnerabilities that internet-facing medical devices in the IoMT environment may face, and their corresponding solutions. Additionally, the future trends discussed in the review are yet to be fully realized as the adoption of smart healthcare is still in its early stages.

In conclusion, as different cities continue to explore the opportunities brought by the increased application of AI in smart healthcare, it is crucial to also consider the potential cyber threats and attacks that may compromise patient data, damage the reputation of medical providers, and potentially lead to loss of lives. Medical device manufacturers, software developers, and security architects must implement measures to mitigate the fallout from any cyberattacks on the IoMT environment. This review will serve as a valuable resource for researchers, students, and other stakeholders with an interest in this field.

REFERENCES

[1]   A. Alabdulatif, N. N. Thilakarathne and K. Kalinaki, "A Novel Cloud Enabled Access Control Model for Preserving the Security and Privacy of Medical Big Data," Electronics, vol. 12, no. 12, pp. 2646, 2023, doi: 10.3390/electronics12122646.

[2] W. D. de Mattos and P. R. L. Gondim, "M-Health Solutions Using 5G Networks and M2M Communications," *IT Prof*, vol. 18, no. 3, pp. 24–29, 2016, doi:10.1109/MITP. 2016.52.

[3] G. J. Joyia, R. M. Liaqat, A. Farooq, and S. Rehman, "Internet of Medical Things (IOMT): Applications, Benefits and Future Challenges in Healthcare Domain," *J Commun*, 2017, doi:10.12720/jcm.12.4.240-247.

[4] A. A. Alli and M. M. Alam, "The Fog Cloud of Things: A Survey on Concepts, Architecture, Standards, Tools, and Applications," *IoT*, vol. 9, p. 100177, 2020, doi:10.1016/ j.iot.2020.100177.

[5] T. Davenport and R. Kalakota, "The Potential for Artificial Intelligence in Healthcare," *Future Healthc J*, vol. 6, no. 2, pp. 94–98, 2019, doi:10.7861/futurehosp. 6-2-94.

[6] H. Kaur, Mohd. Atif, and R. Chauhan, "An Internet of Healthcare Things (IoHT)-Based Healthcare Monitoring System," in *Advances in Intelligent Computing and Communication*, 2020, pp. 475–482, doi:10.1007/978-981-15-2774-6_56.

[7] F. Alshehri and G. Muhammad, "A Comprehensive Survey of the Internet of Things (IoT) and AI-Based Smart Healthcare," *IEEE Access*, vol. 9, pp. 3660–3678, 2021, doi:10.1109/ACCESS.2020.3047960.

[8] N. L. Bragazzi, H. Dai, G. Damiani, M. Behzadifar, M. Martini, and J. Wu, "How Big Data and Artificial Intelligence Can Help Better Manage the COVID-19 Pandemic," *Int J Environ Res Public Health*, vol. 17, no. 9, p. 3176, 2020, doi:10.3390/ijerph17093176.

[9] A. L. Imoize, D. O. Irabor, P. A. Gbadega, and C. Chakraborty, "Blockchain Technology for Secure COVID-19 Pandemic Data Handling," in *Smart Health Technologies for the COVID-19 Pandemic: Internet of Medical Things Perspectives*, 2022, pp. 141–179, doi:10.1049/PBHE042E_CH6.

[10] H. Habibzadeh, B. H. Nussbaum, F. Anjomshoa, B. Kantarci, and T. Soyata, "A Survey on Cybersecurity, Data Privacy, and Policy Issues in Cyber-Physical System Deployments in Smart Cities," *Sustain Cities Soc*, vol. 50, p. 101660, 2019, doi:10.1016/j.scs.2019. 101660.

[11] S. M. Ahmed and A. Rajput, "Threats to Patients' Privacy in Smart Healthcare Environment," in *Innovation in Health Informatics*, Elsevier, 2020, pp. 375–393, doi:10.1016/B978-0-12-819043-2.00016-2.

[12] L. Syed, S. Jabeen, M. S., and A. Alsaeedi, "Smart Healthcare Framework for Ambient Assisted Living Using IoMT and Big Data Analytics Techniques," *Future Gener Comp Syst*, vol. 101, pp. 136–151, 2019, doi:10.1016/j.future.2019.06.004.

[13] A. Panesar, "Machine Learning Algorithms," in *Machine Learning and AI for Healthcare*, Berkeley, CA: Apress, 2021, pp. 85–144, doi:10.1007/978-1-4842-6537-6_4.

[14] "Robotic Surgery Symptoms, Risk Factors, Diagnosis and Treatment I Narayana Health." www.narayanahealth.org/robotic-surgery (accessed Jan. 20, 2023).

[15] J. Andreu-Perez, C. C. Y. Poon, R. D. Merrifield, S. T. C. Wong, and G.-Z. Yang, "Big Data for Health," *IEEE J Biomed Health Inform*, vol. 19, no. 4, pp. 1193–1208, 2015, doi:10.1109/JBHI.2015.2450362.

[16] A. L. Imoize, J. Hemanth, D.-T. Do, and S. N. Sur, Eds., "*Explainable Artificial Intelligence in Medical Decision Support Systems*; 2022, doi:10.1049/PBHE050E.

[17] "What is a Robotic Exoskeleton?—Levitate Tech—The AIRFRAME™," www.levita-tetech.com/2017/10/19/what-is-a-robotic-exoskeleton/ (accessed Jan. 20, 2023).

[18] Z. Kappassov, J.-A. Corrales, and V. Perdereau, "Tactile Sensing in Dexterous Robot Hands—Review," *Rob Auton Syst*, vol. 74, pp. 195–220, 2015, doi:10.1016/j.robot. 2015.07.015.

[19] "FDA Approves the Deka Arm, the First Commercial Mind-Controlled Prosthetic Arm—ExtremeTech," www.extremetech.com/extreme/182202-fda-approves-the-deka-arm-the-first-commercial-mind-controlled-prosthetic-arm (accessed Jan. 21, 2023).

[20] "Artificial Organs: Let us Welcome an Era Where Transplants Are Obsolete," https:// iheartintelligence.com/artificial-organs-transplants/ (accessed Jan. 20, 2023).

[21] E. Fleck, S. Staley, K. Ryszka, and J. A. Potkay, "BIO16: Toward a Blood-Compatible, 3D Printing Resin for Microfluidic Artificial Organs," *ASAIO J*, vol. 68, no. Supplement 2, pp. 18–18, 2022, doi:10.1097/01.mat.0000840800.55807.ab.

[22] "Healthcare Automation—RPA in Healthcare | UiPath," www.uipath.com/solutions/ industry/healthcare-automation (accessed Jan. 20, 2023).

[23] T. Kruse, A. K. Pandey, R. Alami, and A. Kirsch, "Human-aware Robot Navigation: A Survey," *Rob Auton Syst*, vol. 61, no. 12, pp. 1726–1743, 2013, doi:10.1016/j.robot. 2013.05.007.

[24] S. MacDonald, K. Steven, and M. Trzaskowski, "Interpretable AI in Healthcare: Enhancing Fairness, Safety, and Trust," in *Artificial Intelligence in Medicine*, Singapore: Springer Nature Singapore, 2022, pp. 241–258, doi:10.1007/978-981-19-1223-8_11.

[25] T. A. Patel et al., "Correlating Mammographic and Pathologic Findings in Clinical Decision Support Using Natural Language Processing and Data Mining Methods," *Cancer*, vol. 123, no. 1, pp. 114–121, 2017, doi:10.1002/cncr.30245.

[26] S. M. McKinney et al., "International Evaluation of an AI System for Breast Cancer Screening," *Nature*, vol. 577, no. 7788, pp. 89–94, 2020, doi:10.1038/s41586-019-1799-6.

[27] J. de Fauw et al., "Clinically Applicable Deep Learning for Diagnosis and Referral in Retinal Disease," *Nat Med*, vol. 24, no. 9, pp. 1342–1350, 2018, doi:10.1038/s41591- 018-0107-6.

[28] ClinicalTrials.gov, "Adult Accuracy Study of the Elite 3 Glucose Censor (E3)," www. clinicaltrials.gov/ct2/show/study/NCT02246582?term=NCT02246582&rank=1&sec t=X0123456/ (accessed Oct. 17, 2022).

[29] S. C. Nwaneri, C. Yinka-Banjo, U. C. Uregbulam, O. O. Odukoya, and A. L. Imoize, "Explainable Neural Networks in Diabetes Mellitus Prediction," in *Explainable Artificial Intelligence in Medical Decision Support Systems*, pp. 313–334, 2022, doi:10.1049/PBHE050E_CH11.

[30] X. Liu et al., "A Comparison of Deep Learning Performance Against Health-Care Professionals in Detecting Diseases from Medical Imaging: A Systematic Review and Meta-Analysis," *Lancet Digit Health*, vol. 1, no. 6, pp. e271–e297, 2019, doi:10.1016/ S2589-7500(19)30123-2.

[31] A. I. Iskanderani et al., "Artificial Intelligence and Medical Internet of Things Framework for Diagnosis of Coronavirus Suspected Cases," *J Healthc Eng*, vol. 2021, pp. 1–7, 2021, doi:10.1155/2021/3277988.

[32] S. Erikainen and S. Chan, "Contested Futures: Envisioning 'Personalized,' 'Stratified,' and 'Precision' Medicine," *New Genet Soc*, vol. 38, no. 3, pp. 308–330, 2019, doi:10.10 80/14636778.2019.1637720.

[33] G. D. Schiff et al., "Screening for Medication Errors Using an Outlier Detection System," *J Am Med Inform Assoc*, vol. 24, no. 2, pp. 281–287, 2017, doi:10.1093/jamia/ ocw171.

[34] D. Calaprice-Whitty, K. Galil, W. Salloum, A. Zariv, and B. Jimenez, "Improving Clinical Trial Participant Prescreening with Artificial Intelligence (AI): A Comparison of the Results of AI-Assisted vs Standard Methods in 3 Oncology Trials," *Ther Innov Regul Sci*, vol. 54, no. 1, pp. 69–74, 2020, doi:10.1007/s43441-019-00030-4.

[35] A. Chellasamy and A. Nagarathinam, "An Overview of Augmenting AI Application in Healthcare," in *Computer Networks, Big Data and IoT*, 2022, pp. 397–407, doi:10. 1007/978-981-19-0898-9_31.

[36] J. Beavers and S. Pournouri, "Recent Cyber Attacks and Vulnerabilities in Medical Devices and Healthcare Institutions," in *Blockchain and Clinical Trial*, 2019, pp. 249– 267, doi:10.1007/978-3-030-11289-9_11.

[37] S. Oniani, G. Marques, S. Barnovi, I. M. Pires, and A. K. Bhoi, "Artificial Intelligence for Internet of Things and Enhanced Medical Systems," in *Bio-inspired Neurocomputing*, 2021, pp. 43–59, doi:10.1007/978-981-15-5495-7_3.

[38] "Artificial Intelligence in Healthcare I AI Healthcare Tools and Applications," www.delveinsight.com/blog/top-applications-of-artificial-intelligence-in-healthcare (accessed Jan. 22, 2023).

[39] S. N. Alaziz, B. Albayati, A. A. El-Bagoury, and W. Shafik, "Clustering of COVID-19 Multi-Time Series-Based K-Means and PCA With Forecasting," International Journal of Data Warehousing and Mining (IJDWM), 2023, vol. 19, no. 3, pp. 1–25, doi: 10.4018/IJDWM.317374.

[40] M. Goswami and N. J. Sebastian, "Performance Analysis of Logistic Regression, KNN, SVM, Naïve Bayes Classifier for Healthcare Application During COVID-19," in *Innovative Data Communication Technologies and Application*, 2022, pp. 645–658, doi:10.1007/978-981-16-7167-8_47.

[41] M. Shokrekhodaei, D. P. Cistola, R. C. Roberts, and S. Quinones, "Non-Invasive Glucose Monitoring Using Optical Sensor and Machine Learning Techniques for Diabetes Applications," *IEEE Access*, vol. 9, pp. 73029–73045, 2021, doi:10.1109/ACCESS.2021.3079182.

[42] C. Martin-Isla et al., "Image-Based Cardiac Diagnosis with Machine Learning: A Review," *Front Cardiovasc Med*, vol. 7, 2020, doi:10.3389/fcvm.2020.00001.

[43] M. Khalilia, S. Chakraborty, and M. Popescu, "Predicting Disease Risks from Highly Imbalanced Data Using Random Forest," *BMC Med Inform Decis Mak*, vol. 11, no. 1, p. 51, 2011, doi:10.1186/1472-6947-11-51.

[44] F. Galbusera, G. Casaroli, and T. Bassani, "Artificial Intelligence and Machine Learning in Spine Research," *JOR Spine*, vol. 2, no. 1, p. e1044, 2019, doi:10.1002/jsp2.1044.

[45] N. A. Fauziyyah, S. Abdullah, and S. Nurrohmah, "Reviewing the Consistency of the Naïve Bayes Classifier's Performance in Medical Diagnosis and Prognosis Problems," in *Proceedings of the 5th International Symposium on Current Progress in Mathematics and Sciences (ISCPMS2019)*, 2020, p. 030019, doi:10.1063/5.0007885.

[46] D. Rahmat, A. A. Putra, Hamrin, and A. W. Setiawan, "Heart Disease Prediction Using K-Nearest Neighbor," in *2021 International Conference on Electrical Engineering and Informatics (ICEEI)*, 2021, pp. 1–6, doi:10.1109/ICEEI52609.2021.9611110.

[47] C. Li et al., "Using the K-Nearest Neighbor Algorithm for the Classification of Lymph Node Metastasis in Gastric Cancer," *Comput Math Methods Med*, vol. 2012, pp. 1–11, 2012, doi:10.1155/2012/876545.

[48] S. Uddin, I. Haque, H. Lu, M. A. Moni, and E. Gide, "Comparative Performance Analysis of K-Nearest Neighbour (KNN) Algorithm and its Different Variants for Disease Prediction," *Sci Rep*, vol. 12, no. 1, p. 6256, 2022, doi:10.1038/s41598-022-10358-x.

[49] Y. Shen, Y. Li, H.-T. Zheng, B. Tang, and M. Yang, "Enhancing Ontology-Driven Diagnostic Reasoning with a Symptom-Dependency-Aware Naïve Bayes Classifier," *BMC Bioinform*, vol. 20, no. 1, p. 330, 2019, doi:10.1186/s12859-019-2924-0.

[50] M. Langarizadeh and F. Moghbeli, "Applying Naive Bayesian Networks to Disease Prediction: A Systematic Review," *Acta Inform Med*, vol. 24, no. 5, p. 364, 2016, doi:10.5455/aim.2016.24.364-369.

[51] Y.-T. Kwon, H. Kim, M. Mahmood, Y.-S. Kim, C. Demolder, and W.-H. Yeo, "Printed, Wireless, Soft Bioelectronics and Deep Learning Algorithm for Smart Human-Machine Interfaces," *ACS Appl Mater Interfaces*, vol. 12, no. 44, pp. 49398–49406, 2020, doi:10.1021/acsami.0c14193.

[52]   W. Shafik, S. M. Matinkhah, and M. Ghasemzadeh, "Theoretical Understanding of Deep Learning in UAV Biomedical Engineering Technologies Analysis," *SN Comput Sci*, vol. 1, no. 6, p. 307, 2020, doi:10.1007/s42979-020-00323-8.

[53]   E. Svoboda, "Artificial Intelligence is Improving the Detection of Lung Cancer," *Nature*, vol. 587, no. 7834, pp. S20–S22, 2020, doi:10.1038/d41586-020-03157-9.

[54]   M. Chang, J. A. Canseco, K. J. Nicholson, N. Patel, and A. R. Vaccaro, "The Role of Machine Learning in Spine Surgery: The Future is Now," *Front Surg*, vol. 7, 2020, doi:10.3389/fsurg.2020.00054.

[55]   C. Soguero-Ruiz et al., "Data-driven Temporal Prediction of Surgical Site Infection," *AMIA Annu Symp Proc*, vol. 2015, pp. 1164–1173, 2015.

[56]   N. H. Sweilam, A. A. Tharwat, and N. K. Abdel Moniem, "Support Vector Machine for Diagnosis Cancer Disease: A Comparative Study," *Egypt Inform J*, vol. 11, no. 2, pp. 81–92, 2010, doi:10.1016/j.eij.2010.10.005.

[57]   G. Orrù, W. Pettersson-Yeo, A. F. Marquand, G. Sartori, and A. Mechelli, "Using Support Vector Machine to Identify Imaging Biomarkers of Neurological and Psychiatric Disease: A Critical Review," *Neurosci Biobehav Rev*, vol. 36, no. 4, pp. 1140–1152, 2012, doi:10.1016/j.neubiorev.2012.01.004.

[58]   A. A. Mawgoud, A. I. Karadawy, and B. S. Tawfik, "A Secure Authentication Technique in Internet of Medical Things through Machine Learning," *arXiv:1912.12143*, 2019, doi:10.6084/m9.figshare.13311479.v2.

[59]   A. A. Alli, M. Fahad, and A. Cherotwo, "Chapter Four Blockchain and Fog Computing: Fog-Blockchain Concept, Opportunities, and Challenges," in *Blockchain in Data Analytics*, 2020, pp. 75–101. Cambridge Scholars Publishing, Lady Stephenson Library, Newcastle upon Tyne, NE6 2PA, United Kingdom.

[60]   T. Varshney, N. Sharma, I. Kaushik, and B. Bhushan, "Architectural Model of Security Threats & Their Countermeasures in IoT," in *2019 International Conference on Computing, Communication, and Intelligent Systems (ICCCIS)*, 2019, pp. 424–429, doi:10.1109/ICCCIS48478.2019.8974544.

[61]   A. Mosenia and N. K. Jha, "A Comprehensive Study of Security of Internet-of-Things," *IEEE Trans Emerg Top Comput*, vol. 5, no. 4, pp. 586–602, 2017, doi:10.1109/TETC.2016.2606384.

[62]   M. Shuaib, S. Alam, M. Shabbir Alam, and M. Shahnawaz Nasir, "Compliance with HIPAA and GDPR in Blockchain-Based Electronic Health Record," *Mater Today Proc*, 2021, doi:10.1016/j.matpr.2021.03.059.

[63]   A. I. Newaz, A. K. Sikder, M. A. Rahman, and A. S. Uluagac, "A Survey on Security and Privacy Issues in Modern Healthcare Systems: Attacks and Defenses," ACM Transactions on Computing for Healthcare, vol. 3, no. 3, pp 1–44, 2020, doi: 10.1145/3453176.

[64]   P. Podder, M. R. H. Mondal, S. Bharati, and P. K. Paul, "Review on the Security Threats of Internet of Things," *Int J Comput Appl*, vol. 176, no. 41, pp. 37–45, 2020, doi:10.5120/ijca2020920548.

[65]   Y.-K. Chan, Y.-F. Chen, T. Pham, W. Chang, and M.-Y. Hsieh, "Artificial Intelligence in Medical Applications," *J Healthc Eng*, vol. 2018, pp. 1–2, 2018, doi:10.1155/2018/4827875.

[66]   A. A. Alli and M. M. Alam, "SecOFF-FCIoT: Machine Learning Based Secure Offloading in Fog-Cloud of Things for Smart City Applications," *IoT*, vol. 7, p. 100070, 2019, doi:10.1016/j.iot.2019.100070.

[67]   V. Tsoutsouras, D. Azariadi, K. Koliogewrgi, S. Xydis, and D. Soudris, "Software Design and Optimization of ECG Signal Analysis and Diagnosis for Embedded IoT

Devices," in *Components and Services for IoT Platforms*, Cham: Springer International Publishing, 2017, pp. 299–322, doi:10.1007/978-3-319-42304-3_15.

[68]   S. Ge, S.-M. Chun, H.-S. Kim, and J.-T. Park, "Design and Implementation of Interoperable IoT Healthcare System Based on International Standards," in *2016 13th IEEE Annual Consumer Communications & Networking Conference (CCNC)*, 2016, pp. 119–124, doi:10.1109/CCNC.2016.7444743.

[69]   R. M. P. H. K. Rathnayake, M. S. Karunarathne, N. S. Nafi, and M. A. Gregory, "Cloud Enabled Solution for Privacy Concerns in Internet of Medical Things," in *2018 28th International Telecommunication Networks and Applications Conference (ITNAC)*, 2018, pp. 1–4, doi:10.1109/ATNAC.2018.8615361.

[70]   P. K. Binu, K. Thomas, and N. P. Varghese, "Highly Secure and Efficient Architectural Model for IoT Based Health Care Systems," in *2017 International Conference on Advances in Computing, Communications and Informatics (ICACCI)*, 2017, pp. 487–493, doi:10.1109/ICACCI.2017.8125887.

[71]   A. I. Iskanderani et al., "Artificial Intelligence and Medical Internet of Things Framework for Diagnosis of Coronavirus Suspected Cases," *J Healthc Eng*, vol. 2021, pp. 1–7, 2021, doi:10.1155/2021/3277988.

[72]   S. Vishnu, S. R. J. Ramson, and R. Jegan, "Internet of Medical Things (IoMT)—An Overview," in *2020 5th International Conference on Devices, Circuits and Systems (ICDCS)*, 2020, pp. 101–104, doi:10.1109/ICDCS48716.2020.243558.

[73]   A. A. Alli, K. Kassim, N. Mutwalibi, H. Hamid, and L. Ibrahim, "Secure Fog-Cloud of Things: Architectures, Opportunities and Challenges," in *Secure Edge Computing*, 1st ed., M. Ahmed and P. Haskell-Dowland, Eds. Cleveland, Ohio, CRC Press, 2021, pp. 3–20.

[74]   J.-P. A. Yaacoub et al., "Securing Internet of Medical Things Systems: Limitations, Issues and Recommendations," *Future Gener Comp Syst*, vol. 105, pp. 581–606, 2020, doi:10.1016/j.future.2019.12.028.

[75]   M. K. Hasan et al., "A Review on Security Threats, Vulnerabilities, and Counter Measures of 5G Enabled Internet-of-Medical-Things," *IET Comm*, vol. 16, no. 5, pp. 421–432, 2022, doi:10.1049/cmu2.12301.

[76]   M. Wazid, A. K. Das, J. J. P. C. Rodrigues, S. Shetty, and Y. Park, "IoMT Malware Detection Approaches: Analysis and Research Challenges," *IEEE Access*, vol. 7, pp. 182459–182476, 2019, doi:10.1109/ACCESS.2019.2960412.

[77]   K. Kalinaki, N. N. Thilakarathne, H. R. Mubarak, O. A. Malik, and M. Abdullatif, "Cybersafe Capabilities and Utilities for Smart Cities", in *Cybersecurity for Smart Cities, Springer, Cham*, 2023, pp. 71–86, doi: 10.1007/978-3-031-24946-4_6.

[78]   O. Salem, K. Alsubhi, A. Shaafi, M. Gheryani, A. Mehaoua, and R. Boutaba, "Man-in-the-Middle Attack Mitigation in Internet of Medical Things," *IEEE Trans Industr Inform*, vol. 18, no. 3, pp. 2053–2062, 2022, doi:10.1109/TII.2021.3089462.

[79]   G. W. Clark, M. V. Doran, and T. R. Andel, "Cybersecurity Issues in Robotics," in *2017 IEEE Conference on Cognitive and Computational Aspects of Situation Management (CogSIMA)*, 2017, pp. 1–5, doi:10.1109/COGSIMA.2017.7929597.

[80]   S. S. Hameed, W. H. Hassan, L. Abdul Latiff, and F. Ghabban, "A Systematic Review of Security and Privacy Issues in the Internet of Medical Things; The Role of Machine Learning Approaches.," *PeerJ Comput Sci*, vol. 7, p. e414, 2021, doi:10.7717/peerj-cs.414.

[81]   D. Stiawan, M. Y. Idris, R. F. Malik, S. Nurmaini, N. Alsharif, and R. Budiarto, "Investigating Brute Force Attack Patterns in IoT Network," *J Electr Comp Eng*, vol. 2019, 2019, doi:10.1155/2019/4568368.

[82]   Y. Sun, F. P.-W. Lo, and B. Lo, "Security and Privacy for the Internet of Medical Things
       Enabled Healthcare Systems: A Survey," *IEEE Access*, vol. 7, pp. 183339–183355, 2019,
       doi:10.1109/ACCESS.2019.2960617.
[83]   T. W. Tseng, C. T. Wu, and F. Lai, "Threat Analysis for Wearable Health Devices and
       Environment Monitoring Internet of Things Integration System," *IEEE Access*, vol. 7,
       pp. 144983–144994, 2019, doi:10.1109/ACCESS.2019.2946081.
[84]   M. Shafiq, Z. Tian, A. K. Bashir, X. Du, and M. Guizani, "IoT Malicious Traffic
       Identification Using Wrapper-Based Feature Selection Mechanisms," *Comput Secur*,
       vol. 94, p. 101863, 2020, doi:10.1016/j.cose.2020.101863.
[85]   S. Khan and A. Akhunzada, "A Hybrid DL-Driven Intelligent SDN-Enabled Malware
       Detection Framework for Internet of Medical Things (IoMT)," *Comput Commun*, vol.
       170, pp. 209–216, 2021, doi:10.1016/j.comcom.2021.01.013.
[86]   L. Fernández Maimó, A. Huertas Celdrán, Á. Perales Gómez, F. García Clemente,
       J. Weimer, and I. Lee, "Intelligent and Dynamic Ransomware Spread Detection and
       Mitigation in Integrated Clinical Environments," *Sensors*, vol. 19, no. 5, p. 1114, 2019,
       doi:10.3390/s19051114.
[87]   F. Alsubaei, A. Abuhussein, and S. Shiva, "Ontology-Based Security Recommendation
       for the Internet of Medical Things," *IEEE Access*, vol. 7, pp. 48948–48960, 2019,
       doi:10.1109/ACCESS.2019.2910087.
[88]   A. Mohan, "Cyber Security for Personal Medical Devices Internet of Things," in *2014
       IEEE International Conference on Distributed Computing in Sensor Systems*, 2014,
       pp. 372–374, doi:10.1109/DCOSS.2014.49.
[89]   X. Lu and X. Cheng, "A Secure and Lightweight Data Sharing Scheme for Internet
       of Medical Things," *IEEE Access*, vol. 8, pp. 5022–5030, 2020, doi:10.1109/
       ACCESS.2019.2962729.
[90]   M. A. Allouzi and J. I. Khan, "Soter: Trust Discovery Framework for Internet of
       Medical Things (IoMT)," in *2019 IEEE 20th International Symposium on "A World of
       Wireless, Mobile and Multimedia Networks" (WoWMoM)*, 2019, pp. 1–9, doi:10.1109/
       WoWMoM.2019.8792971.
[91]   M. Papaioannou et al., "A Survey on Security Threats and Countermeasures in Internet
       of Medical Things (IoMT)," *Trans Emerg Telecommun Technol*, vol. 33, no. 6, 2022,
       doi:10.1002/ett.4049.
[92]   M. Seliem and K. Elgazzar, "BIoMT: Blockchain for the Internet of Medical Things," in
       *2019 IEEE International Black Sea Conference on Communications and Networking
       (BlackSeaCom)*, 2019, pp. 1–4, doi:10.1109/BlackSeaCom.2019.8812784.
[93]   A. Azaria, A. Ekblaw, T. Vieira, and A. Lippman, "MedRec: Using Blockchain
       for Medical Data Access and Permission Management," in *2016 2nd International
       Conference on Open and Big Data (OBD)*, 2016, pp. 25–30, doi:10.1109/OBD.2016.11.
[94]   "Internet of Things, Artificial Intelligence and Blockchain Technology," in *Internet of
       Things, Artificial Intelligence and Blockchain Technology*, 2021, doi:10.1007/978-3-
       030-74150-1.
[95]   Y. K. Saheed and M. O. Arowolo, "Efficient Cyber Attack Detection on the Internet
       of Medical Things-Smart Environment Based on Deep Recurrent Neural Network
       and Machine Learning Algorithms," *IEEE Access*, vol. 9, pp. 161546–161554, 2021,
       doi:10.1109/ACCESS.2021.3128837.
[96]   L. Ben Amor, I. Lahyani, and M. Jmaiel, "AUDIT: AnomaloUs Data Detection and
       Isolation Approach for Mobile Healthcare Systems," *Expert Syst*, vol. 37, no. 1, 2020,
       doi:10.1111/exsy.12390.

[97]   K. K. Karmakar, V. Varadharajan, U. Tupakula, S. Nepal, and C. Thapa, "Towards a Security Enhanced Virtualised Network Infrastructure for Internet of Medical Things (IoMT)," in *2020 6th IEEE Conference on Network Softwarization (NetSoft)*, 2020, pp. 257–261, doi:10.1109/NetSoft48620.2020.9165387.

[98]   UN, "World Population Projected to Reach 9.8 Billion in 2050," www.un.org/en/desa/world-population-projected-reach-98-billion-2050-and-112-billion-2100 (accessed Nov. 4, 2022).

[99]   R. Dwivedi, D. Mehrotra, and S. Chandra, "Potential of Internet of Medical Things (IoMT) Applications in Building a Smart Healthcare System: A Systematic Review," *J Oral Biol Craniofac Res*, vol. 12, no. 2, pp. 302–318, 2022, doi:10.1016/j.jobcr.2021.11.010.

[100] E. Sezgin, Y. Huang, U. Ramtekkar, and S. Lin, "Readiness for Voice Assistants to Support Healthcare Delivery During a Health Crisis and Pandemic," *NPJ Digit Med*, vol. 3, no. 1, p. 122, 2020, doi:10.1038/s41746-020-00332-0.

[101] P. Manickam et al., "Artificial Intelligence (AI) and Internet of Medical Things (IoMT) Assisted Biomedical Systems for Intelligent Healthcare," *Biosensors (Basel)*, vol. 12, no. 8, p. 562, 2022, doi:10.3390/bios12080562.

[102] P. Simoens, M. Dragone, and A. Saffiotti, "The Internet of Robotic Things," *Int J Adv Robot Syst*, vol. 15, no. 1, p. 172988141875942, 2018, doi:10.1177/1729881418759424.

[103] "Medtech and the Internet of Medical Things | Deloitte US," www2.deloitte.com/us/en/pages/life-sciences-and-health-care/articles/medtech-internet-of-medical-things.html (accessed Jan. 20, 2023).

12 Digital Twins in the AIoMT

Qian Qu and Yu Chen

12.1 INTRODUCTION

The unprecedented proliferation of the smart Internet of Things (IoT) and edge-fog-cloud computing paradigm makes the concept of Smart Cities realistic [1], which consists of intelligent services covering variant aspects of human society, like smart transportation [2], smart grid [3], smart public safety surveillance [4], and smart healthcare service [5]. Among the fast-growing smart city applications, digital healthcare is recognized as one of the most investigated areas [6]. Research is investigated from different sectors in both health and digitalization technologies. The global Internet of Medical Things (IoMT) market size will expand to USD 188.2 billion by 2025, compared to USD 72.5 billion in 2020 [7]. Digital Twin (DT) technology is considered to play an essential role that allows business operations to be managed remotely and product/system development processes to be accelerated [8]. In a report by Gartner, one of the leading research organizations in the world, it is stated that the subject of "Digital Twins in Healthcare" is on the rise and the interest in technology is gradually increasing [9]. DT technology is expected to increase both the number and diversity of healthcare activities and offers promising revolutionary solutions.

As an emerging concept of the interconnects between physical and virtual entities, DT virtually represents both the structural elements and dynamics of a physical entity (e.g., a patent) throughout its lifetime. With the help of smart sensors, physical models, and statistical techniques, DT provides reflection, simulation, and prediction of a certain system. As shown in Figure 12.1, a DT consists of three major components: physical object (PO), logical object (LO), and data. With the successful applications in industrial manufacturing, integrating DT with IoMT and data-driven methods (e.g., machine learning) is promising to provide efficient and accurate personalized, digital healthcare services (DHS). DT-based healthcare systems not only allow for continuous monitoring, fast diagnosing, and accurately predicting aspects of the health of individuals, but it also reduces uncertainty related to the effectiveness and progression of medical treatments by healthcare professionals.

The current application of DT in AIoMT can be categorized into three major areas [7]:

- *Medical resource optimization.* With the help of DT technology, medical institutes can provide optimized resource allocation including beds in hospitals,

DOI: 10.1201/9781003370321-12

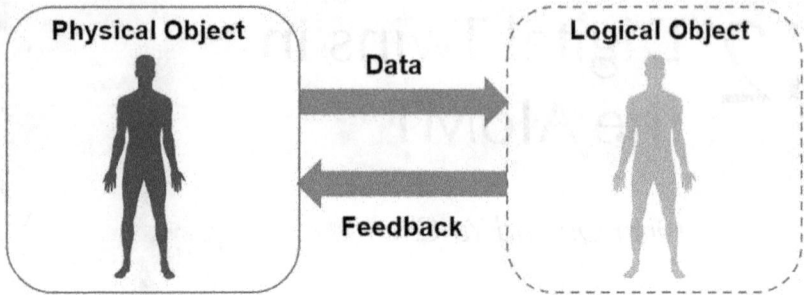

FIGURE 12.1 Digital twin model.

ventilators, MRI, CT, etc. This technique can help countries short of medical resources during the COVID-19 pandemic.

- *Digital organs.* Based on the collected data, DT can create digital models for the patients. For example, Siemens created digital organ models for the simulation of medical treatments, including definitive diagnosis and therapy trials.
- *Digital patient.* Using modern wearable devices, we can create DT for individuals who require real-time body information, body status prediction, and continuous monitoring. By examining the collected data and simulation results, the authorized doctor can monitor the situation after the treatment and provide real-time adjustments accordingly.

12.1.1 KEY CONTRIBUTIONS OF THE CHAPTER

The following are the key contributions of this chapter:

1. An overview of applications of DT technology in IoMT and AIoMT areas and current state-of-the-art research.
2. A detailed SafeTwins architecture that integrates DT and AIoMT for health services.
3. As a case study, the application of SafeTwins architecture for senior safety monitoring is highlighted through an experimental study.

12.1.2 CHAPTER ORGANIZATION

Section 12.2 overviews the current application of DT technology in IoMT and AIoMT. Section 12.3 presents SafeTwins, a DT-AIoMT framework, and the design rationales and key function blocks are illustrated. Taking senior safety monitoring as a case study, Section 12.4 presents the experimental investigation of SafeTwins-based virtual health service to protect seniors living alone. Section 12.5 discusses existing challenges, opportunities, and other problems in Digital Twins-based AIoMT.

12.2 DIGITAL TWINS IN AIOMT: AN OVERVIEW

12.2.1 An Introduction to Digital Twins

Digital Twins (DT) was conceptually introduced in the area of manufacturing and was first presented in 2003 [10]. This new term drew great attention from both industrial and academic. At first, the digital twin models were introduced to various manufacturing scenarios [11]. As the definition of the PO is extended, the application of DT soon attracts interest from different domains, including areas of the IoT and IoMT.

12.2.1.1 Industrial Manufacturing

The early usage of DT originates from the manufacturing process of an industrial artifact [12]. Different procedures in the lifecycle of a product can benefit from the usage of DT models, such as design, production, testing, and disposal. Using various types of sensors, multiple parameters are collected from the product (PO) and LOs are created in virtual space. By observing the LOs in a virtual space, the manufacturer can monitor, predict, and modify the lifecycle of the product. The typical lifecycle of a product and the role DT plays can be illustrated as follows [8]:

- *Design*: The design phase of a product is where the key characteristics are defined. Characteristics like various parameters are expected to be limited in a certain interval. However, unpredicted situations or design mistakes can lead to anomaly values or outliers. DT models assisting the design procedure help to identify these characteristics in the early stage by simulating the behavior of the product in a virtual space. Thus, some design failures can be avoided even before the product is produced and industrial resources can be saved.
- *Production*: The production phase is where the product is manufactured according to the designed prototype. The main function of DT is to help measure whether the key characteristics are properly produced and whether the behavior of the product is normal. During this phase, some simulations are operated.
- *Testing*: Unlike the simulations in the production phase, the DT model would use more tools to test the possible behaviors of the product in different circumstances. For example, certain stress tests are quite necessary for some products before they are sold to customers. In this case, the DT would create some extreme environments such as extreme temperature, high/low pressure, or other critical situations. This phase may use some platforms or AI tools to get better prediction or simulation results.
- *Disposal*: In this phase, the product passes the production and testing phases, and the lifecycle is ended. DT models help to collect the data of the products and assist the future storage process.

12.2.1.2 Internet of Things

As the definition of DT became more general, its applications quickly expanded to variant areas of IoT [13]. The capability of DT in predicting the behavior and optimizing the performance of an object combined with AI/ML technology shows great potential. There have been numerous research works in this direction, here we highlight two top concerned areas: Smart Grid [14] and Smart Driving [15].

- *Smart Grid*: The applications of DTs in power systems leverage their capability of supporting simulation, prediction, and optimization. Relevant research includes the areas of power system simulation, online analysis, and real-time optimization. Using dynamic DT models, the power system can be updated or adjusted according to the real-time results of the simulation. With the help of ML/AI technologies, the power grid can achieve self-intelligence together with other additional functions. Online analysis of the power grid can also benefit from the introduction of DT techniques. For example, combining traditional Supervisory Control and Data Acquisition (SCADA) systems with DTs is already a widely investigated topic in the community [16]. By introducing a new data path and ML methods, the hybrid system achieves fast dynamic security assessment (DSA), whose response speed is in seconds compared to traditional minutes count. Real-time optimization is another important aspect of Smart Grid. Different situations can lead to various needs for power. For example, the operation of a certain wind farm can be affected by numerous factors, such as the weather forecast, the status of birds nearby, and the real-time exchange rates in the market [17]. In addition, recent studies introduce AR techniques for users to visit certain wind farms [18]. The AR-enabled DT platform provides visualization of current weather conditions, geographical information, and the process of the construction of wind energy converters (WEC). Thus, managers of wind farms can carry out different tasks like daily maintenance, emergency exams, or online optimizations accordingly.
- *Smart Driving*: One of the most popular topics of Smart Driving is autonomous driving. This technology domain involves multiple subjects, including mechanical engineering, electrical engineering, and AI. DTs are more suitable compared to traditional simulation methods, and the application of DT models enables more intelligent driving systems, including better path planning [15]. Moreover, other aspects of Smart Driving take advantage of DT's capability of prediction and optimization. For example, DT-enabled platforms may record the driving styles of different users and help to save extra energy and provide a more pleasant driving experience. Using DT models, some systems can predict certain characteristics of the motor like torque to deal with different driving environments and save more energy. Combining DT and ML methods can also help to reduce the risks of accidents [19].

12.2.2 APPLICATIONS OF DT IN IoMT

Early applications of DTs in IoMT are dated back to the case of medical equipment [20]. DTs help to build models for the maintenance of prediction and optimization. As mentioned in the first section, current applications in IoMT/AIoMT can be classified into three major domains:

1. **Medical resource optimization**

   The applications of DTs in optimizing medical resources are widely adopted by large healthcare enterprises. For example, DT-enabled platforms are built for hospital management, including functions for predicting resource consumption and optimizing allocation [21]. These approaches have more significance during the COVID-19 pandemic as the hospitals have limited capacity compared to the booming demand for medical resources in certain regions [22]. By establishing DT systems, some hospitals improve the quality of service (QoS) using combined technology of AI and simulation tools [20]. The prediction results help the medical professionals to better understand the real demand of the patients and adjust the resource accordingly, including equipment, beds, and medicine. Some hospitals may face similar challenges like the shortage of beds, various patent needs, aging medical equipment, and increasing appointment amounts. Leveraging suitable AI methods and DT systems, these urgent issues can be solved in an efficient way.

2. **Digital organs**

   Digital organs have been an attractive field for applying DT in IoMT. By creating a digital replicant of the human organ in the virtual space, doctors can set different scenarios for the digital organs to test the corresponding outcomes of the patient. This hypothetical procedure highly improves the accuracy of diagnosis and reduces the risk. However, unlike traditional DT modeling in industrial manufacturing, it is impossible to place all kinds of sensors on the organs (PO). Most of the data on the organs including medical parameters are collected during medical examinations [20]. That is to say, the real-time twining process is not guaranteed in most Digital Organs systems. Therefore, the applications of DTs in this domain highly rely on the completeness of the database. A comprehensive, massive data set helps the ML/AI process to generate training models with high quality and to provide more accurate predictions and diagnoses.

3. **Digital Patient**

   Digital Patient refers to creating a virtual replica of a patient using historical data and/or a real-time data stream, which is collected by various sensors [8]. Combining the currently collected data and historical reports, a complete medical record can provide reliable information about the patient for further medical services including regular medical examination, diagnosis, etc.

With the fast development of IoMT devices like smartwatches and smart rings, low-cost medical sensors have entered our daily life and made the concept of Digital Patients more realistic [21]. Therefore, a patient does not require hospitalization when continuous medical monitoring is in service. It is no longer mandatory that a patient has to live in a single room in a nursing house or alone at home. The availability of different sensors, the growing computation power of edge devices, and the fast evolution of communication techniques make Digital Patient a promising solution for modern medical services. Digital Patient provides medical professionals with a more efficient way to monitor the behaviors of a patient in real time. The collected data such as physiological status, actions, environmental data, and other parameters will be processed with AI technology to both improve the patient's treatment and reduce potential risks [22, 23].

The high-quality data collected from the users is essential for Digital Patients [24]. The data source can be not only the patients but also the environment they live in. The sensors may include medical sensors attached to the patient's body, which are responsible for collecting real-time parameters such as body temperature, blood pressure, heart rate, glycemia level, etc. Moreover, a complete Digital Patient system may contain extra devices like smart cameras, motion detectors, and other sensors, which collect environmental data. Smart cameras give patients more options to enjoy medical services with high quality as well as have their private information protected. Combining state-of-the-art AI technology [25] and smart cameras, the Digital Patient system can mask or obscure the collected image or video frame to protect the sensitive information of the patients. For example, by leveraging machine learning and a smart camera, the output of the data stream can be turned into a body skeleton frame that only shows points and lines [26]. Thus, the system can run simulations or predictions according to the coordinates of these points and report alarms when an emergency happens (e.g., the patient falls on the floor). Figure 12.2 shows an example of a corresponding skeleton image where the 20 points represent the key skeletal joints that can describe the movement of the target patient [26].

Apart from the data directly collected from sensors, Digital Patient can also leverage indirect information to improve the QoS. Under the permission and authorization of the users, the DT can collect information from the patient's daily life like laughter

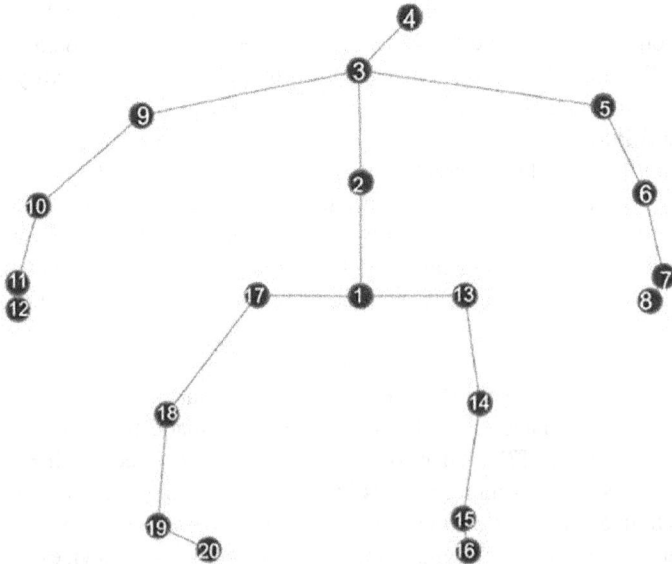

FIGURE 12.2 Skeleton image [26].

to evaluate certain psychological statuses [27]. Moreover, data from other anonymized patients with similar characteristics can help the DT to give certain medical advice about food intake, daily habits, and other behaviors. It is worth noting that all these activities of the system should have the patients' permission and be under the supervision of medical professionals.

Digital Patient is established on the foundation of the patient's medical data. This necessitates a high standard for the protection of personal information, in terms of both security and privacy. However, security and privacy issues are beyond the scope of this chapter; interested readers may find more from some high-quality survey papers on this important topic [28, 29].

12.3   INTEGRATING DIGITAL TWIN TECHNOLOGY AND AIOMT

As mentioned in the previous section, Digital Patients can satisfy different demands of patients in various scenarios. Considering this technology is highly associated with AI for simulation, prediction, and evaluation, this section introduces a system called SafeTwins that integrates DT, blockchain, NFT, and IoMT technologies under the context of Digital Patient.

12.3.1   System Architecture

The main system architecture of the SafeTwin framework is shown in Figure 12.3. This conceptual architecture utilized the DT technology to build a three-layer virtual healthcare system aiming to provide continuous monitoring of the patients as well as medical services.

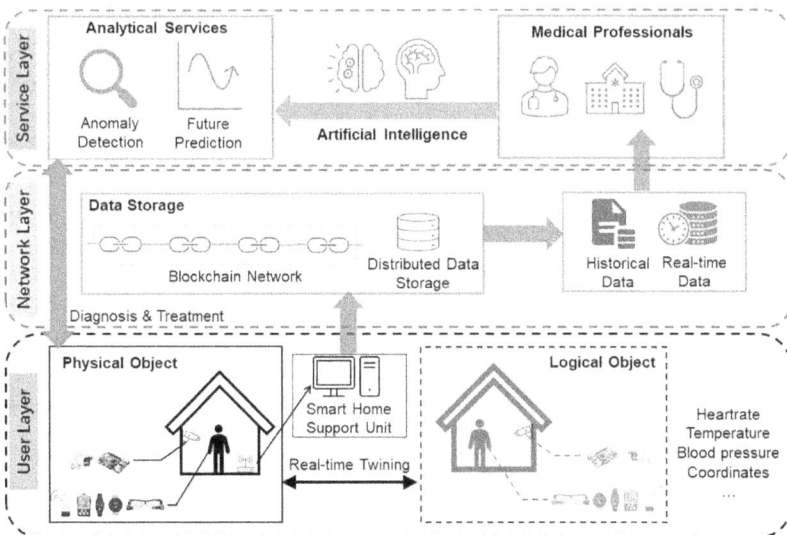

FIGURE 12.3   SafeTwins system architecture.

1. *User layer*: The user layer is the infrastructure layer consisting of multiple personal domain networks. Each domain contains a smart home environment such as a single room in a nursing house or an apartment for a patient who lives alone. This scenario contains a trust support unit that is deployed on a personal computer (PC) or an edge server and other registered IoMT devices within the network. The support unit works as a gateway that aggregates data streams from IoMT devices, and it also plays the role of data processing, senior patients' virtual space maintenance, and primary intelligent decision-making operations, like ML-based abnormal event detection and on-site emergency alarms. The PO essentially is the senior who lives in the house with a smart camera providing continuous monitoring and wearable devices carrying various on-body sensing functions. Since the collected data from POs may be transmitted in various communication protocols, it is required to make them uniform before using DT technology to create corresponding LOs in the virtual space. DT allows the link of POs in a smart home and LOs of the virtual space, and DT models for senior patients can be constructed by the support unit.

2. *Network layer*: The network layer enables efficient and secure data stored in either a central or a distributed network environment. According to the demand of patients, the data can be stored in a cloud server or in a distributed network (e.g., on a blockchain). The medical data may contain various information such as electrocardiograms (ECGs). To avoid directly storing the data with a large volume on the Blockchain, we bring Distributed Data Storage (DDS) into the network layer as off-chain storage. Inter Planetary File System (IPFS) is one practical solution to store data in a resilient system of file storage and sharing.

3. *Service layer*: The service layer can be viewed as a *system brain*, which provides intelligent healthcare applications by combining ML and Big Data technologies. The DT model of a senior patient contains abundant information, including personal body status, environment data, and location coordinates. Using these real-time along with historical records, analytical services like anomaly detection and future activity prediction can be provided with the help of statistical algorithms and ML methods. In addition, the DTH model can set required privacy policies for emergencies according to the demands and situations of the patients. For instance, the smart camera could generate the body skeleton image of the physical person to protect users' privacy and a smartwatch can be used to test the heart rate [21]. Furthermore, all collected personal data by support units and historical medical records managed by medical service providers can be shared with different professionals for further diagnosis and governmental institutions for medical resource allocations.

12.3.2 Major Function Blocks

1. *Physical object*: The PO in SafeTwins is the patient (user) together with the smart home environment. According to the demand of the patient, various

sensors are deployed on the patient's personal network and in the environment. For example, body sensors may contain smart watches, smart glasses, and portable glucose monitoring devices. Smart cameras, motion detectors, and thermometers may be mounted inside the house to detect the daily behavior of the patients as well as the environmental parameters according to users.

2. *Logical object*: The LO is established and maintained in the virtual space using the data collected by the sensors from the PO. The data is transmitted and unified for the DT model. As shown in Figure 12.3, the parameters may contain medical information about the patient like heart rate, body temperature in different areas, blood pressure and glycemia level, etc. In addition, smart cameras may capture the behaviors of the patient at different privacy levels. The information may only contain coordinates of the body skeleton for emergency alarm or contain a clear frame of the patient to judge whether they are in pain or at risk. The LO may also include certain information about the environment like the season, time, room temperature, and humidity. These parameters can also help to train prediction models for the AI processes.

3. *Data storage*: As mentioned, medical data can be classified as historical data and real-time data. Most of the real-time data is the live feed from the sensors in a lightweight format. However, some of the historical data like medical records may contain images like ECGs or even short videos. Although privacy and security issues are beyond the scope of this chapter, the SafeTwins framework adopts Blockchain technology for data storage security. To avoid storing a large volume of data on the blockchain network, an off-chain storage approach is adopted by SafeTwins to mitigate this challenge.

4. *Medical professionals*: The medical professionals in this system mainly refer to authorized doctors, hospitals, or other medical institutions. They are responsible for the daily examination of the patient's status, online follow-up treatment, and emergency diagnosis.

5. *Analytical services*: Analytical services depend on mathematical methods and AI technology. Using massive data from the patients or even historical record data set, this function domain may create different intelligent models for various purposes such as emergency alerts and future predictions.

12.4   CASE STUDY: DT-AIOMT ENABLED SENIOR SAFETY MONITORING

In this section, using senior safety monitoring as a case study, an experimental evaluation of the SafeTwins framework is presented. A simple hybrid model using singular spectrum analysis (SSA) and long short-term memory (LSTM) network is integrated to test the feasibility and performance of the SafeTwins system.

12.4.1   HYBRID SSA-LSTM DETECTION AND PREDICTION MODEL

The SSA algorithm is one of the sequential change-point detection approaches for time series problems [30]. The essential of the SSA algorithm is to extract different components from the target series including periodical parts, long-term trends, and noises. As a non-parametric method, SSA does not require any pre-consumption of the series and can deal with time series with relatively small sizes. These characteristics make SSA suitable for edge-fog scenarios, especially in the context of AIoMT [31].

The LSTM is a special kind of Recurrent Neural Network (RNN) that was first introduced in 1997 [32]. Instead of having a simple repeating module structure, LSTM has four neural network layers. Each memory cell contains three gates: input gate, forget gate, and output gate. While the function of input and output gates is receiving and outputting parameters, the forget gate determines the forgotten degree of the information from previous neurons. This specific characteristic makes the LSTM neural network a promising way to process and analyze sequence information problems like time series data.

However, using a single forecasting model may have deficiencies or bring inaccuracy due to essential characteristics of the parameters. To improve the accuracy of prediction, many researchers combine ML with other statistical analysis methods such as SSA [33, 34]. These hybrid models focus on prediction in areas such as load demand in power systems and financial data in the stock market. In this chapter, we adopt the SSA-LSTM model in the context of future prediction in the SafeTwins system.

12.4.2 EXPERIMENTAL STUDY

The analytical service scheme in the SafeTwin framework combines SSA and LSTM to achieve efficient predictions for anomaly events in DTH systems. Figure 12.4 illustrates the hybrid SSA-LSTM prediction framework used in analytic service, which consists of multiple parallel SSA-enabled data processors and an LSTM network. The details of the SSA-LSTM framework are described as follows.

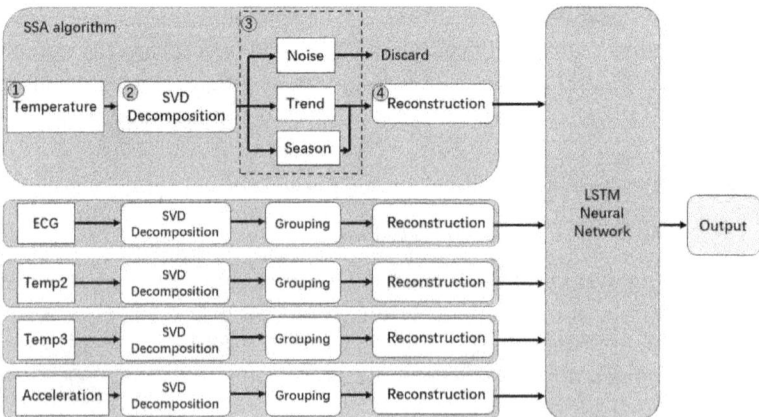

FIGURE 12.4 Hybrid SSA-LSTM prediction framework in analytic service.

In the scenario of seniors' safety monitoring, five parameters are used for this case study, and they are three-lead ECG, distal phalanx (first segment) PPG sensor temperature, proximal phalanx (base segment) PPG sensor temperature, InvenSenseMPU-9250 IMU temperature, and acceleration in the x-direction(g). All the parameters are collected simultaneously and unified into time series with the same sample rate. The time series of a wearable sensor on a patient's body is handled by an SSA processor that aims to extract features and remove noise from raw data. We use the body temperature parameter as an example to explain the workflow of an SSA processor, which can be divided into four steps:

1. *Embedding*: We can first turn the body temperature collected from the patient into a one-dimensional time series $x = \left[x_1, \ldots, x_N \right]$, and we denote the length as N. Then we define a certain window size L ($L < N$) and rewrite X into multiple vectors $\vec{X_i}$. At last, we can define a new trajectory matrix $X = \left[\vec{X_1}, \vec{X_2}, \ldots, \vec{X_M} \right]$, where $M = N - L + 1$.

2. *Decomposition*: To extract the eigenvalues of the new matrix X, we adopt SVD (Singular Value Decomposition). The results including eigenvalues and eigenvectors will be listed in descending order.

3. *Categorizing*: Using the eigenvalues from step 2, we can easily turn matrices $\vec{X_i}$ into certain groups and categorize them into different signals such as trends, seasons, and noises. Here we define a subset $I = i_1, i_2, \ldots, i_l$ where $l < L$ and the corresponding matrix would be $X_I = X_{i_1} + X_{i_2} + X_{i_j}$.

4. *Reconstruction*: In this section, we aim to extract the essential component of the time series and to ignore the noise. So we choose $I = i_1$. Then the reconstructed series is one of the features that would be fed into the LSTM.

Finally, all features of parameters are extracted from different sensors by the SSA processors, then they are fed into the LSTM neural network for training. In this experiment, we chose to use mean square error (MSE) as the loss function, Adam optimizer for optimization training, and set the Epochs as 10. Then, we use the trained model to generate a prediction value to compare with the real value from body sensors. The results of predicting the temperature from the distal phalanx (first segment) with LSTM alone are shown in Figure 12.5, and Figure 12.6 shows the results of using a hybrid SSA-LSTM model. The introduction of the SSA algorithm as a pretreatment of the raw data collected from the sensors benefits the prediction process of LSTM. By discarding the noise, the SSA-LSTM method improves the accuracy of the prediction. Meanwhile, as a lightweight algorithm, SSA will not have much impact on the workload of the on-site smart home support unit.

12.5   CONCLUSIONS AND OPEN CHALLENGES

This chapter introduces the current landscape of the application of Digital Twins technology in the AIoMT domains. Considering the growing need for digital health

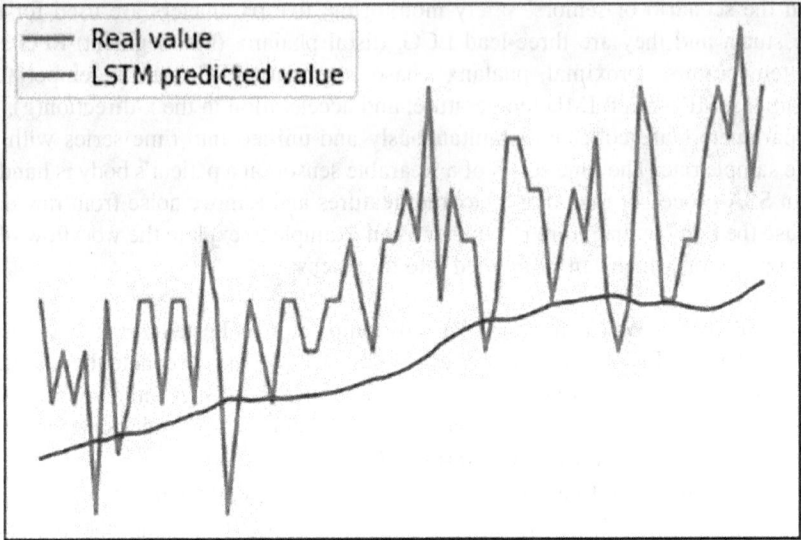

FIGURE 12.5 Prediction result of single LSTM.

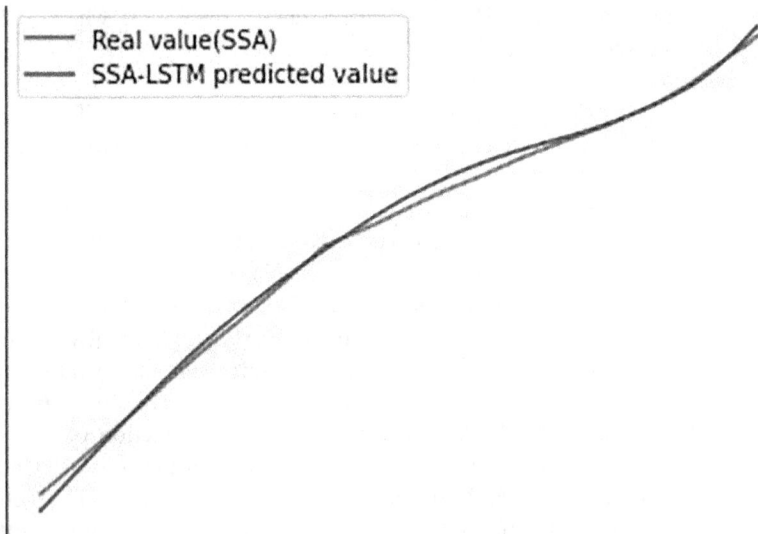

FIGURE 12.6 Prediction result of SSA-LSTM.

services in continuous monitoring in the background of the aging society and the ongoing COVID-19 pandemic, DT-enabled AIoMT systems are a promising approach to providing healthcare services with better qualities.

However, there are still many open questions yet to be thoroughly investigated before DT technology can be widely applied in digital healthcare applications

[35–37]. At the end of this chapter, the following most compelling issues are listed in the hope more novel ideas will be inspired in the community.

- *Data security and privacy*: The sensitivity of medical data asks for robust protection in terms of information security and privacy preservation. Consequently, it is mandatory to focus on new technical approaches for preserving the private information of the patients and other different security issues, including various potential attacks. In addition, the application of DTs in healthcare should not violate governmental rules and policies. The process of data collection should be carefully supervised.
- *Highly heterogenous application contexts* and *standardization*: While it is widely recognized that a well-defined standard will accelerate the design, implementation, and deployment of a DT-based e-healthcare system, the requirements for healthcare services are highly disease or individual-dependent. It is an open challenge for the community of digital healthcare to settle down a balance between standardization and compatibility.
- *Efficient architectures for healthcare*: In recent years, there are multiple architectures proposed to leverage the DTs in variant healthcare systems. However, most of them are still general DT frameworks instead of customized to meet specific requirements in the healthcare domains. It is nontrivial to find an optimal DT design and DT deployment strategy within a certain context.
- *Technical education for healthcare workers*: We have witnessed a lot of cases in which first-line healthcare workers are reluctant to adopt new equipment or devices built on top of cutting-edge technologies. The lack of knowledge is the top reason. Insufficient communication and/or education is a critical factor, which often leads to a design that is not user-friendly at all. There is a compelling need for technical education programs and materials for healthcare workers.

REFERENCES

[1] Kirimtat, Ayca, Ondrej Krejcar, Attila Kertesz, and M. Fatih Tasgetiren. "Future trends and current state of smart city concepts: A survey." *IEEE Access* 8 (2020): 86448–86467.

[2] Zantalis, Fotios, Grigorios Koulouras, Sotiris Karabetsos, and Dionisis Kandris. "A review of machine learning and IoT in smart transportation." *Future Internet* 11, no. 4 (2019): 94.

[3] Dileep, G. "A survey on smart grid technologies and applications." *Renewable Energy* 146 (2020): 2589–2625.

[4] Chen, Ning, Yu Chen, Xinyue Ye, Haibin Ling, Sejun Song, and Chin-Tser Huang. "Smart city surveillance in fog computing." In *Advances in mobile cloud computing and big data in the 5G era*. Cham: Springer, 2017, pp. 203–226.

[5] Jin, Zhanpeng, and Yu Chen. "Telemedicine in the cloud era: Prospects and challenges." *IEEE Pervasive Computing* 14, no. 1 (2015): 54–61.

[6] Siriwardhana, Yushan, Gürkan Gür, Mika Ylianttila, and Madhusanka Liyanage. "The role of 5G for digital healthcare against COVID-19 pandemic: Opportunities and challenges." *ICT Express* 7, no. 2 (2021): 244–252.

[7]   Erol, Tolga, Arif Furkan Mendi, and Dilara Doğan. "The digital twin revolution in healthcare." In *2020 4th International Symposium on Multidisciplinary Studies and Innovative Technologies (ISMSIT)*. Istanbul: IEEE, 2020, pp. 22–24.

[8]   Minerva, Roberto, Gyu Myoung Lee, and Noel Crespi. "Digital twin in the IoT context: A survey on technical features, scenarios, and architectural models." *Proceedings of the IEEE* 108, no. 10 (2020): 1785–1824.

[9]   Craft, Laura, and Mike Jones. "Hype Cycle for Healthcare Providers, 2020," *Gartner*, Aug. 05, 2020. www.gartner.com/en/documents/3988462 (accessed Sep. 23, 2020).

[10]   Grieves, M., "Digital twin: Manufacturing excellence through virtual factory replication," *White Paper*, Jan. 2015. https://www.3ds.com/fileadmin/PRODUCTS-SERVICES/ DELMIA/PDF/Whitepaper/DELMIA-APRISO-Digital-Twin-Whitepaper.pdf.

[11]   Van Schalkwyk, P. *The Ultimate Guide to Digital Twins.* https://xmpro.com/ digital-twins-the-ultimate-guide//2019

[12]   E. Glaessgen and D. Stargel, "The digital twin paradigm for future NASA and U.S. air force vehicles," in *Proceeding of 53rd AIAA/ASME/ASCE/AHS/ASC Structures, Structural Dynamics and Materials Conference, 20th AIAA/ASME/AHS Adaptive Structures Conference 14th AIAA*, Honolulu, HI, 2012, p. 114, https://doi.org/10.2514/6.2012-1818.

[13]   Jones, David, Chris Snider, Aydin Nassehi, Jason Yon, and Ben Hicks. "Characterising the digital twin: A systematic literature review." *CIRP Journal of Manufacturing Science and Technology* 29 (2020): 36–52.

[14]   Pan, Huaming, Zhenlan Dou, Yanxing Cai, Wenzhu Li, Xing Lei, and Dong Han. "Digital twin and its application in power system." In *2020 5th International Conference on Power and Renewable Energy (ICPRE)*. Shanghai: IEEE, Sept. 12–14, 2020, pp. 21–26.

[15]   Damjanovic-Behrendt, Violeta. "A digital twin-based privacy enhancement mechanism for the automotive industry." In *2018 International Conference on Intelligent Systems (IS)*. Funchal: IEEE, Sept. 25–27, 2018, pp. 272–279.

[16]   Zhou, Mike, Jianfeng Yan, and Donghao Feng. "Digital twin framework and its application to power grid online analysis." *CSEE Journal of Power and Energy Systems* 5, no. 3 (2019): 391–398.

[17]   Sivalingam, Krishnamoorthi, Marco Sepulveda, Mark Spring, and Peter Davies. "A review and methodology development for remaining useful life prediction of offshore fixed and floating wind turbine power converter with digital twin technology perspective." In *2018 2nd International Conference on Green Energy and Applications (ICGEA)*. Singapore: IEEE, March 24–26, 2018, pp. 197–204.

[18]   Pargmann, Hergen, Dörthe Euhausen, and Robin Faber. "Intelligent big data processing for wind farm monitoring and analysis based on cloud-technologies and digital twins: A quantitative approach." *2018 IEEE 3rd International Conference on Cloud Computing and Big Data Analysis (ICCCBDA)*. Chengdu: IEEE, April 20–22, 2018.

[19]   Bhatti, Ghanishtha, Harshit Mohan, and R. Raja Singh. "Towards the future of smart electric vehicles: Digital twin technology." *Renewable and Sustainable Energy Reviews* 141 (2021): 110801.

[20]   Barricelli, Barbara Rita, Elena Casiraghi, and Daniela Fogli. "A survey on digital twin: Definitions, characteristics, applications, and design implications." *IEEE Access* 7 (2019): 167653–167671.

[21]   Liu, Ying, Lin Zhang, Yuan Yang, Longfei Zhou, Lei Ren, Fei Wang, Rong Liu, Zhibo Pang, and M. Jamal Deen. "A novel cloud-based framework for the elderly healthcare services using digital twin." *IEEE Access* 7 (2019): 49088–49101.

[22] Imoize, A. L., P. A. Gbadega, H. I. Obakhena, D. O. Irabor, K. V. N. Kavitha, and C. Chakraborty, "Artificial intelligence-enabled internet of medical things for COVID-19 pandemic data management," in *Explainable Artificial Intelligence in Medical Decision Support Systems*, 1st ed., A. L. Imoize, J. Hemanth, D.-T. Do, and S. N. Sur, Eds. London: The Institution of Engineering and Technology, 2022, pp. 357–380.

[23] Kumar, R. L., Y. Wang, T. Poongodi, and A. L. Imoize, Eds., *Internet of Things, Artificial Intelligence and Blockchain Technology*, 1st ed. Switzerland, AG: Springer Nature, 2021.

[24] Rivera, Luis F., Miguel Jiménez, Prashanti Angara, Norha M. Villegas, Gabriel Tamura, and Hausi A. Müller. "Towards continuous monitoring in personalized healthcare through digital twins." In *Proceedings of the 29th Annual International Conference on Computer Science and Software Engineering*, Toronto, Canada, Nov. 4–6, 2019, pp. 329–335.

[25] Ayoade, O. B. et al., "Explainable artificial intelligence (XAI) in medical decision systems (MDSSs): Healthcare systems perspective," in *Explainable Artificial Intelligence in Medical Decision Support Systems*, 1st ed., A. L. Imoize, J. Hemanth, D.-T. Do, and S. N. Sur, Eds. London: The Institution of Engineering and Technology, 2022, pp. 1–43.

[26] Sun, Han, and Yu Chen. "Real-time elderly monitoring for senior safety by lightweight human action recognition." In *2022 IEEE 16th International Symposium on Medical Information and Communication Technology (ISMICT)*. Lincoln, NE: IEEE, May 2–4, 2022.

[27] Bisogni, Carmen, Aniello Castiglione, Sanoar Hossain, Fabio Narducci, and Saiyed Umer. "Impact of deep learning approaches on facial expression recognition in healthcare industries." *IEEE Transactions on Industrial Informatics* 18, no. 8 (2022): 5619–5627.

[28] Chacko, Anil, and Thaier Hayajneh. "Security and privacy issues with IoT in healthcare." *EAI Endorsed Transactions on Pervasive Health and Technology* 4, no. 14 (2018): e2.

[29] Rieke, Nicola, Jonny Hancox, Wenqi Li, Fausto Milletari, Holger R. Roth, Shadi Albarqouni, Spyridon Bakas et al. "The future of digital health with federated learning." *NPJ Digital Medicine* 3, no. 1 (2020): 1–7.

[30] Polunchenko, Aleksey S., Grigory Sokolov, and Wenyu Du. "Quickest change-point detection: A bird's eye view." *arXiv preprint arXiv:1310.3285* (2013).

[31] Yang, Zekun, et al. "A novel PMU fog based early anomaly detection for an efficient wide area PMU network." In *2018 IEEE 2nd International Conference on Fog and Edge Computing (ICFEC)*. Washington, DC: IEEE, May 1–3, 2018.

[32] Hochreiter, Sepp, and Jürgen Schmidhuber. "Long short-term memory." *Neural Computation* 9, no. 8 (1997): 1735–1780.

[33] Pham, Manh-Hai, Minh-Ngoc Nguyen, and Yuan-Kang Wu. "A novel short-term load forecasting method by combining the deep learning with singular spectrum analysis." *IEEE Access* 9 (2021): 73736–73746.

[34] Tang, Qi, et al. "Prediction of financial time series based on LSTM using wavelet transform and singular spectrum analysis." *Mathematical Problems in Engineering* 2021 (2021).

[35] Alazab, Mamoun, Latif U. Khan, Srinivas Koppu, Swarna Priya Ramu, et al. "Digital twins for healthcare 4.0-recent advances, architecture, and open challenges." *IEEE Consumer Electronics Magazine* (2022), IEEE, Sept. 2022.

[36] Bruynseels, Koen, Filippo Santoni de Sio, and Jeroen Van den Hoven. "Digital twins in health care: Ethical implications of an emerging engineering paradigm." *Frontiers in Genetics* (2018): 31.

[37] Popa, Eugen Octav, Mireille van Hilten, Elsje Oosterkamp, and Marc-Jeroen Bogaardt. "The use of digital twins in healthcare: Socio-ethical benefits and socio-ethical risks." *Life Sciences, Society and Policy* 17, no. 1 (2021): 1–25.

13 Artificial Intelligence-Assisted Internet of Medical Things Enabling Medical Image Processing

Ajimah Nnabueze Edmund, Christopher Akinyemi Alabi, Oluwaseun Olayinka Tooki, Agbotiname Lucky Imoizeand, and Tanko Daniel Salka

13.1 INTRODUCTION

Medical imaging is the process of creating images of a person's internal organs and tissues for use in clinical research, medical diagnosis, and therapeutic intervention [1]. Medical imaging aims to reveal internal structures concealed by the skin and bones while also diagnosing and treating diseases and illnesses. Through medical imaging, organized collections of normal anatomy and physiology are created, making the abnormal easier to identify. The set of techniques or procedures adopted for the non-invasive image generation of a body's internal parts is referred to as medical imaging. While it is possible to obtain images of organs and tissues that have been removed from the body, such procedures are considered under pathology rather than medical imaging. Medical imaging is analogous to the inverse problem in mathematics; the cause of a disease can be deduced from its observable (through medical images) impact on the part of interest.

Medical imaging instruments operate using various basic principles. The ultrasound scanning machine, for instance, uses ultrasonic pressure waves and echoes that travel inside the tissue to reveal internal structure. Radiations are absorbed differently by various types of body tissues, such as the muscular, bony, or fatty parts [2]. Ionizing and non-ionizing radioactivity can be used to expose the intrinsic body structure on an image receptor by showcasing these differences through absorption, or in the case of X-rays, the absorption of X-ray photons by the higher density materials. Radiographic anatomy is a practice that entails the study of anatomy using radiographic images. Radiographers typically acquire medical radiography, while radiologists typically perform image analysis. Medical radiography encompasses a variety of modalities that generate numerous image types, each with a distinct clinical application.

Scientific development in AI and IoMT have continued to push traditional methods of medical data acquisition, transmission, and processing to the edges. Today, devices or sensors such as the ingestible camera can be used to collect and transmit medical data, including images, to designated cloud based destination for analysis. Due to the complexity and peculiarity of medical images, AI is employed for medical data processing to facilitate diagnostic procedures and enhance quality decision-making [3].

13.1.1   KEY CONTRIBUTIONS

This chapter offers the following significant contributions:

i. The chapter provides a comprehensive guide to understanding medical image processing, from image acquisition techniques to image enhancement, segmentation, feature extraction, and image visualization.
ii. An objective review of Artificial Intelligent techniques and methods used in medical image processing was presented.
iii. An AI-based COVID-19 diagnostic experiment was carried out using a convolution neural network (CNN).

13.1.2   CHAPTER ORGANIZATION

Section 13.2 presents fundamental concepts of medical images and their acquisition techniques. Section 13.3 discusses the key tasks involved in medical image processing: image enhancement, segmentation, feature extraction, and image visualization. In Section 13.4, related works on artificial intelligence-based Medical Image Processing were reviewed. Section 13.5 presents an experimental diagnosis of COVID-19 disease using CNN trained model. The section provides students and researchers with useful guide on implementing AI based methods for medical diagnosis. Section 13.6 highlights how AI in health care affects the Radiologist as a professional. Section 13.7 presents and overview of research trends and gaps in AI based medical image processing. Section 13.8 summarizes the chapter and presents future direction on the subject matter.

13.2   MEDICAL IMAGES AND THEIR ACQUISITION TECHNIQUES

An image is simply a representation of a real object. The image is said to be digital if the visual data is represented using binary. It is a multi-dimensional pictorial signal representation of an object that has been sampled in space and/or time and quantized in amplitude. Digital images can be classified as either vector images or raster images [4]. While most digital images acquired through medical imaging tools are raster images with a large number of pixels, vector images are more desirable for numerical analysis. Some standard digital image formats include JPEG, PNG, SVG, GIF, TIFF, etc. Every image is made up of elemental components. The pixel is the element that makes up a two-dimensional image, while voxels are the elemental components of three-dimensional image elements. For four-dimensional images and higher, the elements are called hypervoxels. In order to sufficiently represent certain anatomical and topological complexities, such as the brain's white matter connection, the use of hypervoxel based framework is preferable as it provides much more details than the 3D voxel grids [5].

Digital images are interpreted as 2D or 3D matrices by the computer, and each pixel value in the matrix represents the amplitude or intensity of the pixel. Typically, we deal with eight-bit images, with amplitude values ranging from 0 to 255. Thus, digital images are seen as either two-variable (binary/grayscale images) or three-variable (RGB images) functions of the pixel coordinates.

Diagnostic radiography refers to the technical aspects of medical imaging, particularly image acquisition [2]. Radiographers are usually in charge of obtaining medical diagnostic images. The different techniques used in acquiring medical images are called medical imaging modalities. While there are several techniques or modalities for medical image acquisition, the common ones include the X-ray, Computed Tomography (CT), ultrasound, and Magnetic Resonance Imaging (MRI). A comprehensive description of the various medical image acquisition techniques is presented in this section:

13.2.1 RADIOGRAPHY (X-RAY)

To view an object's internal structure, radiography uses X-rays, gamma rays, or other types of radiation—ionizing or non-ionizing. Two key areas of radiography application are the medical and industrial fields. In conventional radiography, an image is produced when X-ray is beamed toward the target body. The amount of radiation absorbed by the body depends on its density and design features. An X-ray detecting material such as a photographic film or a digital detector is placed behind the object, which picks up the X-rays that travel through. This technique produces flat two-dimensional images as shown in Figure 13.1, and is known as projectional radiography.

13.2.2 COMPUTERIZED TOMOGRAPHY (CT)

In computerized tomography, a conical X-ray beam is created, and the subject is passed through the rotating X-ray source and its related detectors. Each point on the subject's body is traversed by a variety of beams from different angles. The beam or radiation's absorption or attenuation information is gathered and analyzed to generate two-dimensional images in three planes [6, 7]. Although a CT scan has many uses, it's particularly helpful for immediately assessing patients who might have internal injuries from automobile accidents or other similar accidents[1, 7–9]. Figure 13.2 provides a picture of a typical CT scanner.

13.2.3 MAGNETIC RESONANCE IMAGING (MRI)

Magnetic resonance imaging is a diagnostic method that uses magnetic field and computer-generated radio signals to produce detailed organ and tissue images. The

Projectional radiography

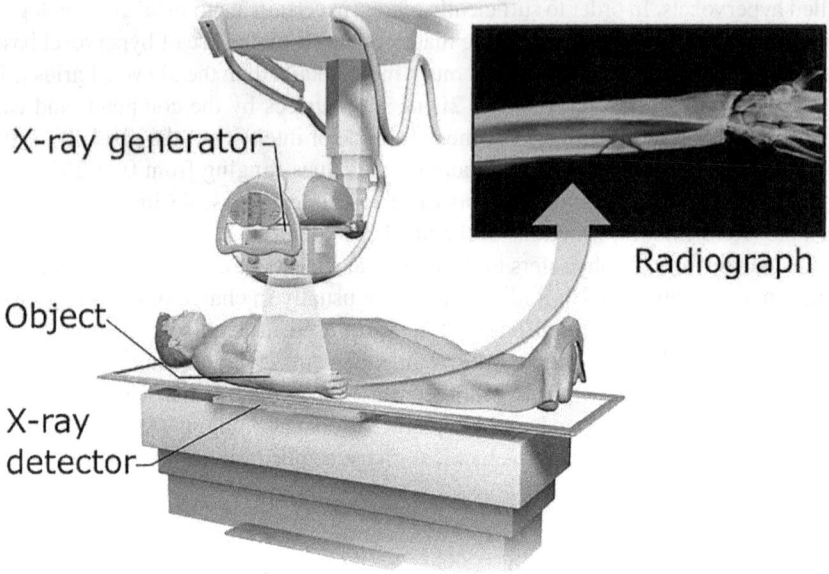

X-ray generator

Radiograph

Object

X-ray
detector

FIGURE 13.1 Typical set-up for radiography acquisition with X-ray.

Source: [6]

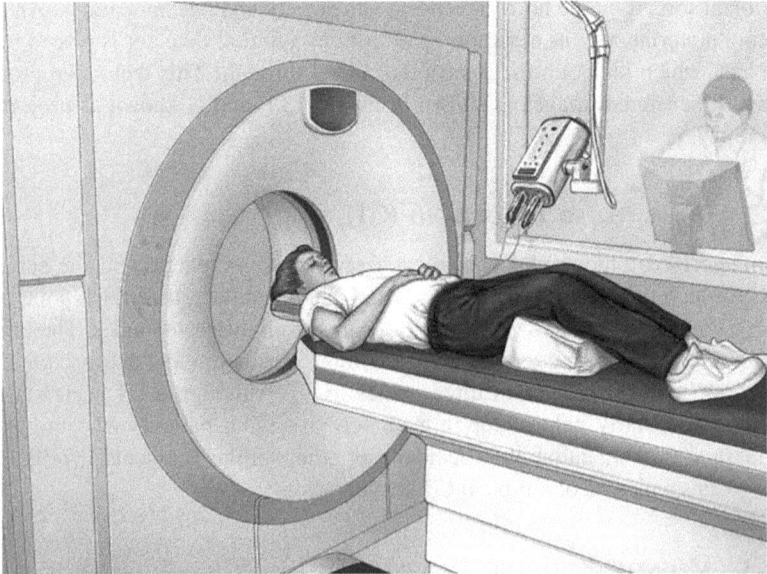

FIGURE 13.2 CT scanning machine.

Source: [6]

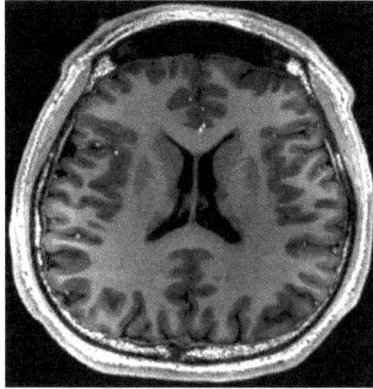

FIGURE 13.3   MRI image of the brain.

Source: [9]

water in a subject's body is temporarily re-adjusted by the magnetic field. The radio waves are released in bursts over the affected area, causing the tissue to resonate and give off weak signals that are used to create cross-sectional images, such as the one shown in Figure 13.3. The 3D images produced by the MRI machine aids viewing from different perspectives, helping the physician to investigate organs, tissues, and skeletal systems. MRI imaging is useful for the diagnosis of a variety of medical problems [9].

13.2.4   NUCLEAR MEDICINE IMAGING

Nuclear medicine is a branch of radiology that utilizes minute quantities of radioactive substances to evaluate organ structure and function [6]. This is essential because without the use of a contrast agent, it is difficult to see soft tissue such as the intestines, muscles, and blood arteries on X-rays.

During the procedure, a trace amount of a radioactive substance (known as a radionuclide) is introduced into the body and absorbed by the tissue under investigation to aid in the examination. Elements such as technetium, thallium, gallium, iodine, and xenon are used as radionuclides [8, 10]. The radionuclide used depends on nature of the study or the peculiarities of the body part being investigated.

Nuclear imaging can show organ and tissue structure as well as physiology. The functionality of a given organ or tissue is indicated by the extent to which it absorbs the radioactive material used. Hence, nuclear imaging is suitable for studying organs and tissues functionality [7, 8, 11].

13.2.5   ULTRASOUND

Diagnostic ultrasound, also known as sonography, is a medical imaging modality that uses sound waves to generate images of the body structures [12]. Although some scans require the introduction of a small device into the body, most ultrasound examinations are done using external ultrasound probe or scanner.

There are various medical applications of ultrasound. It is commonly used in monitoring the health of a developing baby and viewing the internal organs of the woman's body during pregnancy. It is also used in gallbladder disease identification and in blood flow examination. With the help of the ultrasound, a physician's needle can be guided to treat a tumor or perform biopsy; lumps can be identified in the breast; thyroid and prostate gland issues examined. Cases of joint inflammation and bone diseases can also be examined [8].

13.2.6 ELASTOGRAPHY

An elastography is a type of imaging test typically used to detect fibrosis in the liver. Fibrosis is a condition that causes a decrease in the blood flow to and within the liver. Scar tissue forms as a result of this. Elastography is a painless examination that employs low-frequency vibrations to assess the elasticity of your body's organs. Tissues that lack elasticity and are stiff may indicate disease, particularly in the liver [13].

Naturally, elastography finds application in organs and diseases where conventional palpation is already common. Breast, thyroid, and prostate cancers are detected and diagnosed using elastography. Some elastography techniques are also appropriate for musculoskeletal imaging, as they can assess the mechanical characteristics and condition of tendons and muscles [13].

13.2.7 PHOTOACOUSTIC IMAGING

Photoacoustic imaging is also called optoacoustic imaging. It is a medical imaging modality that makes use of the photoacoustic effect to create images. In this imaging technique, pulses of non-ionizing laser are fired into a target body part or tissue. Some of the energy transferred into the tissue is absorbed and converted to heat, causing momentary thermo-elastic expansion as a result of which a wideband ultrasonic emission is produced. The ultrasonic wave given off is detected and analyzed by ultrasonic transducers to produce images. There is a close correlation between a body's physiological features like hemoglobin level and oxygen saturation and its level of optical absorption. Hence, the physiological optical absorption contrast is revealed by the magnitude of ultrasonic emission. The targeted areas can then be represented as 2D or 3D images [12].

13.2.8 ECHOCARDIOGRAPHY

An echocardiogram or cardiac echo is a heart ultrasound. It is a kind of cardiac medical imaging that uses either regular or Doppler ultrasound [13]. It offers a wealth of useful information, including measurements of the size and shape of the heart, its capacity to pump blood, the location and severity of any tissue damage, and the evaluation of the heart's valves. An echocardiogram can also help medical experts to estimate other heart functions, such as cardiac output, ejection fraction, and diastolic

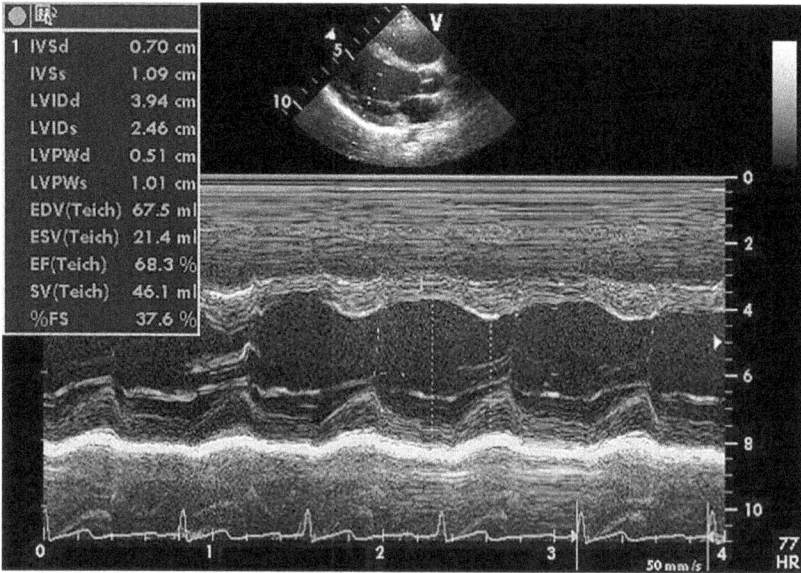

FIGURE 13.4   Parasternal view of heart ventricle echocardiogram.

Source: [14]

function. Echocardiography is a valuable tool for detecting abnormal motion in the cardiac wall of a patient [14].

The most significant benefit of echocardiography is its non-invasiveness (does not require surgical opening of the patient's body), and there are no identified adverse effects. An echocardiogram does not only produce ultrasound structural images of the heart, it also uses Doppler echocardiography, which provides an accurate evaluation of blood flow through the heart. Doppler echocardiography of tissues uses the Doppler technique to quantify tissue motion and velocity [15].

13.2.9   FUNCTIONAL NEAR-INFRARED SPECTROSCOPY

Functional near-infrared spectroscopy (fNIRS) is used for physiological neuroimaging. It's a medical imaging modality that employs near-infrared spectroscopy to optically monitor brain activity. To achieve this, the cortical hemodynamic activity that happens in response to neural activity is simulated with near-infrared light [15].

This optical imaging technique detects variations in hemoglobin's absorption of near-infrared light. From relatively straightforward blood-oxygen measurements to a sophisticated technique for capturing in-the-moment brain activity related to a variety of activities and cognitive tasks, fNIRS has advanced. Although fNIRS has less spatial resolution than fMRI, it has a big benefit over that technology in that it lets participants move around, talk, and engage with their surroundings while being scanned [16, 17].

13.2.10 Magnetic Particle Imaging

Super-paramagnetic nano particle tracers can be directly detected using the novel non-invasive tomographic approach known as magnetic particle imaging (MPI) [17]. The technology might be used in material science and diagnostic imaging. To pinpoint the three-dimensional position and concentration of nanoparticles, it is now employed in medical research. Imaging can produce a signal at any depth inside the body without using ionizing radiation. Super-paramagnetic iron oxide (SPIO) nanoparticles in MPI systems generate a signal by switching magnetic fields [17]. These fields are designed specifically to create a single region devoid of magnetic fields. Only in this region is a signal generated. An image is produced by moving this region across a specimen. A signal is only noticed when the tracer is injected because there is no organic SPIO in tissue. This produces background-free images. To determine the position of the tracer, MPI is usually used with anatomical imaging methods (such CT or MRI) [17].

From the highlight of the various medical image modalities in this subsection, it is obvious that they are complementary as each one provides a different view and insight into the same anatomy.

13.3 MEDICAL IMAGE PROCESSING

Medical image processing (MIP) involves the investigative analysis and use of three-dimensional image datasets of the human anatomy to diagnose pathologies and/or provide the basis for informed medical interventions. Medical image processing enables physicians and researchers to conduct thorough but non-invasive exploration of internal anatomy.

Medical Image processing is a vast and complex field in which numerous algorithms and techniques are used to achieve various outcomes.

The approach adopted in processing any medical image is determined primarily by the specific objective or problem at hand. Irrespective of the approach taken, the purpose is usually to achieve selective visualization for better diagnosis or treatment option determination. It may also be to prepare the medical data for further analysis. Images are processed or manipulated to achieve the following objectives:

i. Reduce noise and blur
ii. Identify structures within the image
iii. Extract useful information from the image
iv. Prepare the image for visualization

13.3.1 Basic Medical Image Processing Tasks

This section will go over some of the most common Medical Image processing tasks and how they are carried out.

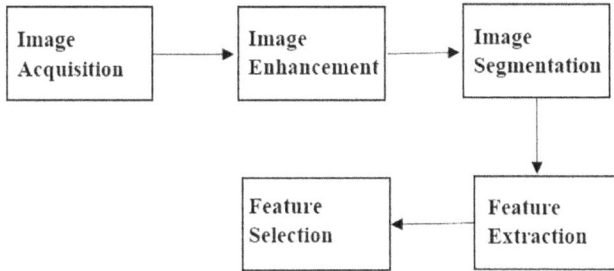

FIGURE 13.5   Block diagram showing basic medical image processing tasks.

13.3.1.1   Image Enhancement

Medical Image enhancement refers to efforts toward improving the quality of a Medical Image. Enhancement of medical images becomes necessary in the following scenarios:

   i. When image contrast is low and it is difficult to distinguish between tissues. This can be due to the unique features of the physiological system under investigation or the image capture procedure used.
   ii. When there is too much noise in the image due to interference from unwanted sources.
   iii. When image artifacts obscure the true picture of an image, making visualization difficult. An artifact is something seen in an image that in reality is not present.

The purpose of image enhancement is to make an image more useful for a certain activity, such as making it more aesthetically appealing for human sight. Ad hoc image-enhancing methods are widely used, although estimation of the real image deterioration process is rarely made. Some of the operations involved in image enhancement include an increase in image contrast, noise removal, emphasizing edges, and shape modification. A major concern is not to alter the information during the image enhancement process. The aim of enhancing the image is to increase the interpretability of information inside the image for feature extraction or human viewers and produce an image that is better than the initial image by changing of pixel intensity of the input image [18]. The contrast of a Medical Image is the difference in brightness between its brightest and darkest areas. The overall brightness of a Medical Image can be increased by increasing the contrast, making it easier to see. The brightness of a Medical Image refers to its overall lightness or darkness. A Medical Image can be made lighter by increasing the brightness, making it easier to see [10, 19, 20].

Due to the reduced pixel density per square inch, a medical image with ideal contrast and brightness may appear blurry when it is upscaled. Image Super-Resolution, a relatively new and significantly more sophisticated concept, is applied to this issue in order to create a high-resolution medical image from its low-resolution equivalent.

13.3.1.1.1   Medical Image Restoration

Medical Image quality may degrade for a variety of reasons, particularly photos taken before cloud storage was widely available. Medical Images scanned from hard copies taken with old instant cameras, for example, frequently acquire scratches. With Medical Image Restoration techniques damaged historical documents can be restored and large chunks of missing information from torn documents may be revealed. This is made possible by powerful Deep Learning-based Image restoration algorithms. For instance, a texture synthesis algorithm can be employed for image inpainting, where missing pixels in a medical image are generated [10].

13.3.1.1.2   Noise Reduction/Removal

During the image acquisition, coding, transmission, and processing steps, noise is always present. Noise is defined as an abrupt change in pixel values in an image. A number of noise-filtering methods are highlighted. The noise behavior can be used to select the appropriate filter.

Filters help remove noise from images while preserving the details. The filter to be used is determined by the filter's behavior and the type of data. When it comes to image filtering, the first thought that comes to mind is to replace the value of each pixel with the average of the pixels around it. The following are some other enhancement techniques for the improvement of medical images:

   i. Medical image brightening
  ii. Medical image sharpening
 iii. Deblurring of medical images
 iv. Contrasting of medical images
  v. Grayscale medical image histogram equalization

13.3.1.2   Image Feature Extraction

Feature extraction is aimed at reducing the number of features in a dataset by generating new and fewer features from the existing ones. This reduction in the dataset's dimension is to simplify data processing. The dimensionality of a dataset refers to the number of variables used to represent the dataset. These variables require a significant amount of computing power to process.

A classifier model may overfit the training set and fail to generalize to new data if it has too many variables, which requires a lot of memory and processing power. The phrase "feature extraction" refers to a large category of techniques for building correlations that get around these problems while still accurately describing the data [21]. The key to creating effective models, according to many machine learning experts, is feature extraction that has been properly optimized [7, 21, 22].

13.3.1.3   Image Feature Selection

Feature extraction and feature selection are the two ways to get a subset of features. By rating the features in some order of relevance and eliminating the less significant ones, feature selection aims to reduce the amount of features in an original dataset rather than adding new features from existing ones. While feature selection chooses a subset of the initial set of features, feature extraction extracts features with possible differentiating power. The primary goal of feature selection is to choose a subset of input parameters by eliminating characteristics that possess little to no predicting information while ensuring or improving classification accuracy. It is impossible to eliminate highly relevant set of features without incurring a decrease in classification accuracy. A feature may occasionally improve classification accuracy if it is weakly relevant [24–26]. In classification problems, choosing the most meaningful features is essential because (1) it takes time to identify all possible feature subsets obtainable from the original set, (2) every feature is important for at least some types of discrimination, and (3) the number of variations both within and between classes is not excessive. When additional features are added past a certain point, performance degrades rather than improves. Discriminating information that allows one object to be separated from others is a crucial component of a strong feature set. The feature coding must be as resilient as possible to ensure uniqueness of objects belonging to the same class. The set of features chosen should be small enough to efficiently discriminate between a variety of classes but are comparable for trends in the same class [26].

13.3.1.4   Image Segmentation

Medical image segmentation is the process of separating areas of interest (ROI) from 3D image data, such as that obtained from MRI or CT scans. It involves the separation of an image into various homogeneous regions or the separation of features of interest in an image from each other's backgrounds. Image Segmentation presents a labeling problem in machine learning. The primary goal of segmenting this data is to identify different anatomical regions needed for a specific study, such as simulating CAD-designed implants' physical characteristics or their virtual placement inside a patient. The segmentation of medical images can take some time, but recent advancements in AI software applications are making it simpler to achieve. One of the primary advantages of using medical image segmentation enables more accurate anatomical data analysis by isolating regions necessary only. Additionally, segmentation allows for the separation of various tissues, such as bone and soft tissues, and eliminates any extraneous information from a scan, such as air. When combined with other software processing options, clinicians and researchers could indeed create segmented masks in a series prepared for additional analysis [7]. Therefore, segmentation generally functions by creating a disguise using information from the backdrop picture data when working with scans such as MRI and CT. Depending on the assignment, users can modify their 2D or 3D scans. Different tools and techniques are available in segmentation software, including manual options to paint on the data or semi-automated processes like thresholding and region growth. There are also applications for cardiovascular image segmentation, with specific options for working with different applications seeking special remedies for treating various heart issues [11, 23, 24].

Many instances requiring medical information may involve the use of segmentation tools. As mentioned earlier, studying medical device placement can involve actions to segment areas of absorption in a bone, which is frequently possible by robots using scripts or related methods. However, some efforts, especially those that entail strange pathologies or complicated contusions, more time, and a larger selection of software features may be required to achieve the segmentation result that is needed [8–10, 15].

Segmentation finds applications in several medical diagnostic procedures and studies. These include coronary border detection in angiography, quantification of multiple sclerosis lesions, tumor identification and volume determination, surgical simulation and planning, functional mapping, automated classification of blood cells, cancer detection in mammograms, etc.

Image segmentation is an important step in image processing as it makes further analysis such as feature extraction and image measurement easier to accomplish. Hence, there exist several types or classes of segmentation techniques. The basis of classification differs from one classification scheme to the other. Table 13.1. presents a comprehensive classification of image segmentation techniques.

13.3.1.5   Medical Image Classification

Image classification is an image processing task that involves the prediction of the class to which an unknown data instance belongs using the training data membership as a basis. It is applicable to differentiate between regions depending on the kind of property used. Land-use data are frequently used during urban planning. Very high-resolution imagery can also be used to assess the effects and destruction of natural disasters like floods, volcanoes, and severe droughts. Image classification is a complicated procedure that depends on various components. Several of the proposed techniques, issues, and additional image order opportunities are discussed here. The focus will be on cutting-edge classification methods used to improve characterization precision. Furthermore, some critical issues about gathering execution are discussed in [16, 27]. Various techniques for image classification are highlighted in Table 13.2.

Considering the findings of the literature review, the table compares the performance of the fuzzy measure, decision tree, SVMs, and artificial neural network methods to that of recent studies on image classification [7, 28, 29].

13.3.2   Quantitative Measurement of Medical Imaging

Developed models need to be evaluated to confirm their reliabilities.

13.3.3   Image Data Visualization

The exploration, transformation, and viewing of data in the form of images to gain insight into the data are known as data visualization. Medical data, sourced from various points, are converted into visual content to aid medical experts as well as patients' understanding of the condition under investigation.

A huge amount of data is generated in the health sector today. Medical data sources include remote health monitoring and sensing devices or IoMTs, disease registers in health care centers, medical laboratories, hospital management information systems (HMISs). Given the growth of technology and the increased adoption of IoT

TABLE 13.1
Classification of Image Segmentation Techniques [25]

	Classification of Image Segmentation Techniques				
Category	Classical Image Segmentation Methods			Machine Learning-based Image Segmentation Methods	
Subcategory	Edge-based Techniques	Region-based Techniques	Threshold-based Techniques	Neural Network (NN) based Techniques	Other Machine Learning Model-based Techniques
Suitability of Technique	Suitable for images with well-defined edges	Suitable for noisy images with no distinct edges	Suitable for images with simple-intensity distribution	Suitable for a wide range of image types. It is robust toward noise	Suitable for a wide range of image types
Example of Techniques	Classified by operator [26] • Sobel • Robert Cross • Canny • Prewitt • Laplacian of Gaussian	Classified by algorithm [26] • Watershed • Region split and merge • Region growing	Classified by operator • Global • Local • Dynamic Other Classes: • Simple • Adaptive • Otsu's	• Convolution NN • Pulse Coupled NN • Kohonen NN • Deep NN • Spiking NN • Probabilistic NN • General Regression NN	• k-means clustering • c-means clustering • Support Vector Machine • Random Forest • Bayesian Classifier

TABLE 13.2
Image Classification Techniques

Classification techniques	Benefits	Assumptions and/or limitations
Neural network	• Suitable for classification • Capable of representing Boolean operations • Non-receptive to noisy inputs • Use of multiple outputs to categorize instances	• Complex in understanding the algorithm framework • Quite so many qualities can result in overfitting • Only experimenting can find the optimal network framework
Support vector machine	• Model types non-linear class boundary lines • Overfitting is unlikely • Model types of non-linear class boundary lines • Overfitting is unlikely • Computational burden reduced to a non-linear optimization problem • Decision rule complexity and error frequency are easily controllable	• Training is slower than Bayes and decision trees; • determining optimal process parameters is challenging when training data is not linearly separable; and • knowledge of the structure of a method is complicated.
Fuzzy logic	• Properties can be described using various stochastic connections	• Previous knowledge is essential for good results • Accurate solutions are not acquired if the judgment direction is unclear
Genetic algorithm	• Could be used in showcase classification and feature selection • Mainly used during optimization • Very often uncovers a "good" remedy • Could indeed handle big, complex, continuity and consistent, and multimodal spaces • Effective search technique for a complicated issue space	• Significant computation or progression of the scoring system • Possibly not the most effective technique of finding some optimum values, rather than global • Side effects in the interpretation of training/output data

in health care service delivery, that is IoMTs, the amount of medical data available is bound to grow astronomically. According to Statista, the amount of health data generated in 2013 was 153 exabytes, which had already grown to 2,314 exabytes by the end of 2020 [30].

TABLE 13.3
Performance Metrics for Medical Image Tasks

S/N	Tasks	Performance Metrics
1	Classification	- Accuracy
		- AUC-ROC
2	Segmentation	- Dice scores
		- Intersection over union
		- Pixel-wise accuracy
		- Jaccard index
		- Dice coefficient
		- Sensitivity
		- Specificity
3	Image Translation and Style Transfer	Microscopy Application
		- Structural Similarity Index
		- Peak Signal to Noise Ratio
		Structural Content Comparison Application
		- Pearson correlation coefficient

To draw useful inferences from a large amount of medical data available today, visualization is paramount. Data points can be aggregated and visually presented in the form of charts, tables, and scatter plots. This simplifies the work of the medical officials as it reduces result interpretation time, reveals trends and patterns in the medical data, and facilitates better health management decisions [31].

3D visualization and 3D printing have become very necessary in varieties of fields such as medical, education, and clinical practice. In medical image segmentation, complex computer tools are required for quantification and visualization. The recent technology development in AI technology, tumors can be swiftly identified and profiled using quality visual medical images [32].

Some examples of open-source visualization platforms for medical image exploration and analysis are thus [33]:

   i. QuIP—A quick image processing software
  ii. caMicroscope
 iii. QuPath
  iv. Pathology Image Informatics Platform
   v. Digital Slide Archive
  vi. Cytomine

13.4   RELATED WORKS ON AI-ENABLED
MEDICAL IMAGE PROCESSING

Information content existing in images is difficult to distinguish from human visual inspection. However, the use of artificial intelligence (AI)-based tools draws out solutions using trained associate image type A with image type B. In histopathology, deep learning (DL) technologies can be used to classify identified problems into four groups: classification, segmentation, image translation, and image style transfer.

Classification of images touches on the task of allocating a tag to an image. The most acceptable algorithms for the detection and classification of images for nucleated cells are convolutional neural networks (CNNs) [34, 35]. Researchers have developed different CNN architectures. However, some CNN architectures, such as ResNets, LeNet-5, Sanghvi nets, Inception nets, and shift-invariant neural networks are predominantly used owing to their effectiveness over a broad variety of tasks. Image segmentation or pixel-level classification applies to the process of allocating addresses to certain regions of an image. U-nets, the most commonly used DL architecture for image segmentation, can also perform the task of image enhancement.

Image translation is the transformation of an image from one form to another. It has been discovered that some DL model characteristics are advantageous for image analysis and image-based medical diagnosis. Image diagnosis entails finding abnormalities, evaluation of measurement, and detection of changes over a certain period [36]. Information processing and precise diagnosis, DL techniques offer the ability to provide cutting-edge, unbiased, automated interpretation of varieties of medical images. Generative adversarial networks (including their variants) are the well-known models used for translation images. Computational pathology uses style transfer, which is the process of applying the style of a reference image to the content of an input image, to create an output image [34].

The difficulty of interpretability and explain ability [37], which are critical in the medical industry, is a shortcoming in machine learning approaches. Deep learning models are like black boxes that accept inputs such as a medical image and come up with output based on the intelligence gained from training. When human actors such as medical personnel and radiologist do not clearly understand the procedure, criteria, and considerations used by an AI model, issues of trust and acceptability arise. While [38] conducted a review of various approaches in the literature to achieving AI interpretability, [39] reviewed explainable AI methods used for medical imaging.

The review by [35] highlighted recent development in the application of machine learning, artificial intelligence, and deep convolution neural network in medical image processing. The researchers reiterated the reason why the CNN model, among neural network techniques, is widely used for image analysis. Additionally, CNN can be used to detect blood cells in hyperspectral medical images [14]. In malaria diagnosis, researchers have also proposed 16-layer CNN to examine red blood cells with parasite infections in blood smears. Researchers are now applying AI algorithms to different facets of medical technologies such as diagnostic planning, microscopic image analysis, and tomographic image reconstruction since it offers hope in the area of better and prompt diagnosis and planning of treatment. Despite these benefits, the albatross of AI breakthrough is that millions of jobs are going to be lost [40, 41].

The work of [41] established the success of DL for medical imaging and proved its dependence on the massive, labeled data set. However, the researchers traced the challenges associated with the use of supervised DL for medical image segmentation to the inadequacy of labeled data sets. This was linked to the cost and time taken for the collection of labeled data. In the work, the researchers proposed a novel semi-supervised technique for medical imaging segmentation. The labeled inputs and both the labeled and unlabeled data, a weighted mixture of common supervised and regularization loss, were optimized. The drawback of work is the concept that data with and without labels come from the same distribution. An intelligent-based approach to classify medical images using a binary residual feature fusion (BARF), a fusion model with a module for uncertainty awareness, was presented in [36]. The BARF proposed is of two types: direct-based and cross-based. [42] presented a triple-clipped histogram model to enhance the features of medical images. The features considered were brightness, contrast, and preservation, which incorporate both the equalized image and the input image. In their work, the limitations of the spatial domain, one of the two categories of contrast enhancement technique, were highlighted. Instead, the researchers proposed a framework that uses the fusion method that combines the characteristics of the input image and the equalized image. Their choice of histogram equalization model was guided by its wide acceptability for image enhancement.

The outcome of image enhancement techniques by harnessing chest X-ray images on the detection of COVID-19 was probed [18]. The researchers proposed the use of radiography images, such as computed tomography (CT) or chest X-ray (CXR), a common technique for detecting lung-related diseases, in the diagnosis of coronavirus (COVID-19). The research assessed the suitability of CXR in the diagnosis of COVID-19 against the established Reverse Transcription Polymerase Chain Reaction (RT-PCR) diagnostic method. Since X-ray machines are portable, they provide faster, and more accurate COVID-19 diagnosis. CXRs are found to be a plausible alternative for detecting COVID-19 if incorporated with AI because it is less harmful to the human system, compared to CT.

The genetic algorithm-based adaptive histogram equalization (GAAHE) method, for better Magnetic Resonance Imaging (MRI) images, was proposed in [43]. This technique is also called the adaptive image enhancement technique. The technique was proven to be superior to other known enhancement techniques. Low-contrast medical images were improved visually using adaptive threshold values, and the procedure was made more adaptable using a genetic algorithm.

13.5   AI-BASED EXPERIMENT ON COVID-19 DETECTION

13.5.1   PROPOSED MODEL DESCRIPTION

This experiment is aimed at presenting the reader with the basic method of implementing AI techniques in medical applications. This study proposed a CNN-based model to detect COVID-19 infection using chest X-ray images as shown in Figure 13.6. A dataset of chest X-ray images from the Kaggle data base consisting of 5,860 images divided into two parts Normal and COVID-19 were used, as shown in Table 13.4.

13.5.2   METHODOLOGY

The image was converted from BGR (blue, green, red) color space to RGB (red, green, blue) color space three-channel image. This is to fine-tune the existing CNN models pre-trained on color (RGB) images. To do this, we applied a bilateral low-pass filter

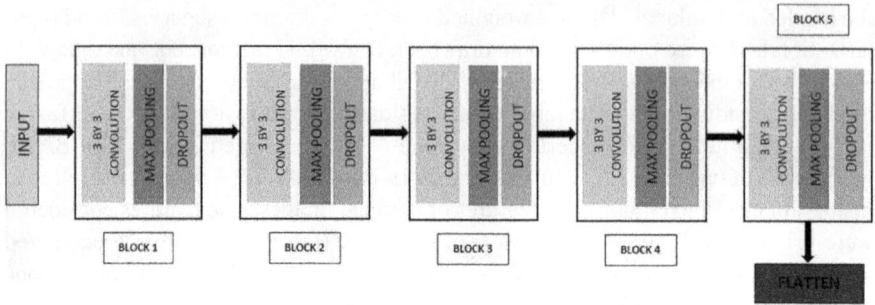

FIGURE 13.6   Architectural illustration of VGG16-based CNN model.

TABLE 13.4
Distribution of Cases in Two Subsets

S/N	Image Data Subset	Training	Testing	Validation
1	Normal case	1,341	234	9
2	COVID-19 case	3,875	390	9
3	Total number of cases	5,216	624	18

and an image noise-filtering procedure to remove the diaphragm area. The VGG16 CNN model was used in this work. The simplified architecture of the VGG16 CNN model is shown in Figure 13.6.

The original chest X-ray is 968 × 768 pixels. To fit into the VGG16 model, which was pre-trained with images of 512 × 512 pixels, each chest X-ray was down sampled to 512 × 512 pixels. Images for training and evaluation of the proposed VGG16-based transfer learning CNN model were then randomly selected from the entire image dataset of 5,860 cases and divided into three independent subgroups for training, validation, and testing. The test subgroup has been assigned of 624 cases; of the cases, 18 and 5,216 cases were allocated to the validation and training subsets, respectively.

There are various techniques available for handling imbalanced data. In this chapter, class-weighting procedure was adopted to reduce the possible outcomes of imbalanced data during training. The class weight method adjusts the weights inversely with the number of classes in the input data. The weights w_i for class i are computed using Equation 13.1. The model is fitted using the class weights. Higher values are given to instances of smaller classes in our loss function. The calculated loss is consequently a weighted average, and throughout the loss computation, the weight of each sample corresponding to each class is represented by w_i

$$w_i = \frac{Total\,number\,of\,cases}{(number\,of\,classes) \times (Number\,of\,cases\,in\,class)i} \tag{13.1}$$

Multiple iterations (Epochs) were implemented to train the CNN model based on VGG16. Using the data from the training subset, the model was initially trained before being verified. In order to minimize the overall performance between training and validation, the optimizer makes an effort to compel the architecture to learn extra information throughout training. In this work, we capped model training epochs at 128 to prevent overfitting and retain training effectiveness. Using the testing data, the trained model was saved and tested subset at the end of 128 epochs.

13.5.3 RESULT AND DISCUSSION

The diagram in Figure 13.7 presents trend curves of the VGG16-based CNN model's testing and training accuracy in two trials utilizing various training and testing of subsets. The two curves show that as the training iterations increase during training, the validation subset's ability to accurately anticipate changes significantly and then converges progressively to a greater level of accuracy. After epoch 64, the validation accuracy for both subsets follows the training accuracy, indicating that learning happens at several epochs. The trend graph additionally demonstrates that the suggested method does not significantly overfit or underfit our model.

Table 13.6. shows results of our model with an overall accuracy of 95%, and Table 13.7 shows a comparison of our proposed method and another method. Figure 13.8 and Figure 13.9 show the prediction of our model as positive for COVID-19 and normal for COVID-19, respectively.

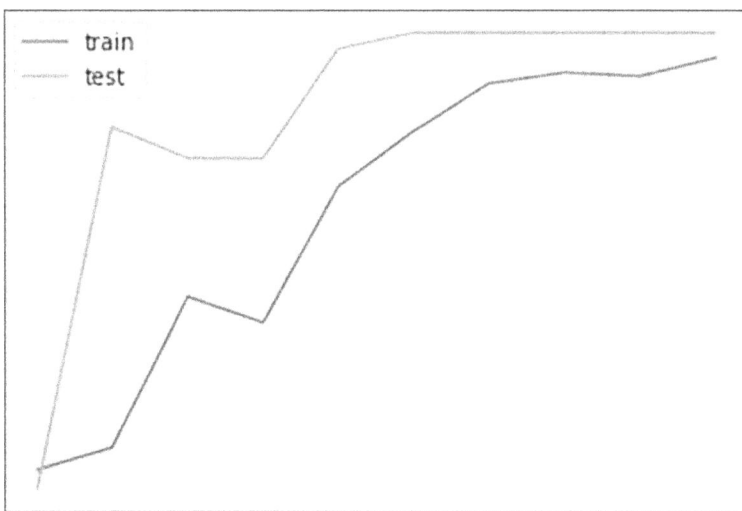

FIGURE 13.7(A)   Training accuracy for two-class classification.

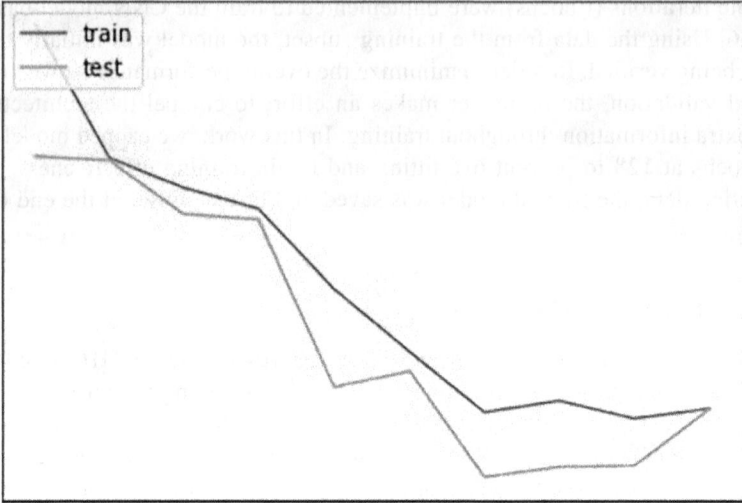

FIGURE 13.7 (B)   Training loss for two-class classification.

TABLE 13.6
Result of Our Proposed Method

Method	Accuracy (%)	Loss (%)	Val. Accuracy (%)	Val. Loss (%)
VGG16-based CNN model 2 class Classification	95	19	95	19

TABLE 13.7
Comparison of our Proposed Method and Other Methods

S/N	Method	Accuracy (%)
1	XGBoot (XGB) [48]	82
2	Random forest [48]	77
3	VGG16-based CNN model 2 class classification.	95

13.6   AIOMT AND THE RADIOLOGIST

The interpretation of medical images is typically performed by a radiologist or a physician who specializes in radiology; however, this can be performed by any healthcare professional who is trained and certified in radiological clinical evaluation.

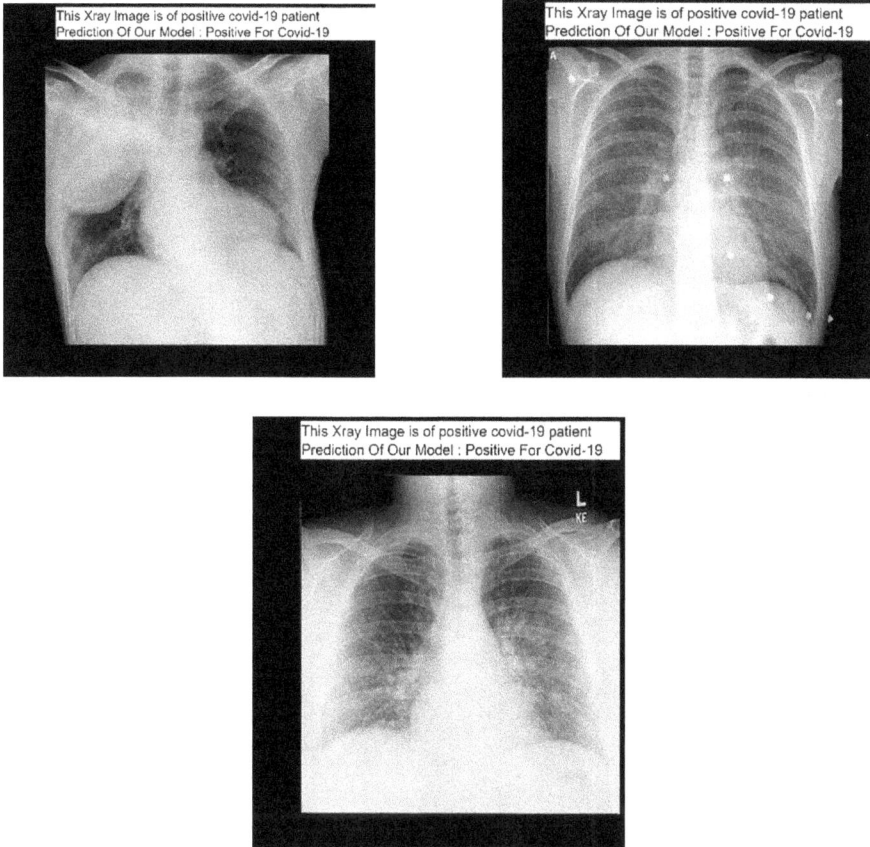

FIGURE 13.8 X-ray image of positive COVID-19 patient: prediction of our model: positive for COVID-19.

With the adoption of AI in health care, [40] classified the effect of computer-aided diagnostics systems on the work of radiologists. The classification is into three categories which are as follows:

i. AI-Replace (AI-R)
ii. AI-Assist (AI-A)
iii. AI-Extend (AI-X)

AI-replace (AI-R) suggests a scenario in which the radiologist's work of medical image interpretation is done by AI-enabled machines. AI-R finds application both in tertiary healthcare centers and in remote locations where radiologists are not readily available. For instance, the use of BoneXpert software to measure a child's bone age does not require the expertise of a radiologist.

Further, in AI-assist (AI-A), AI presents as a tool that helps the radiologist perform his normal tasks more efficiently. AI-A systems enhance the capability of a

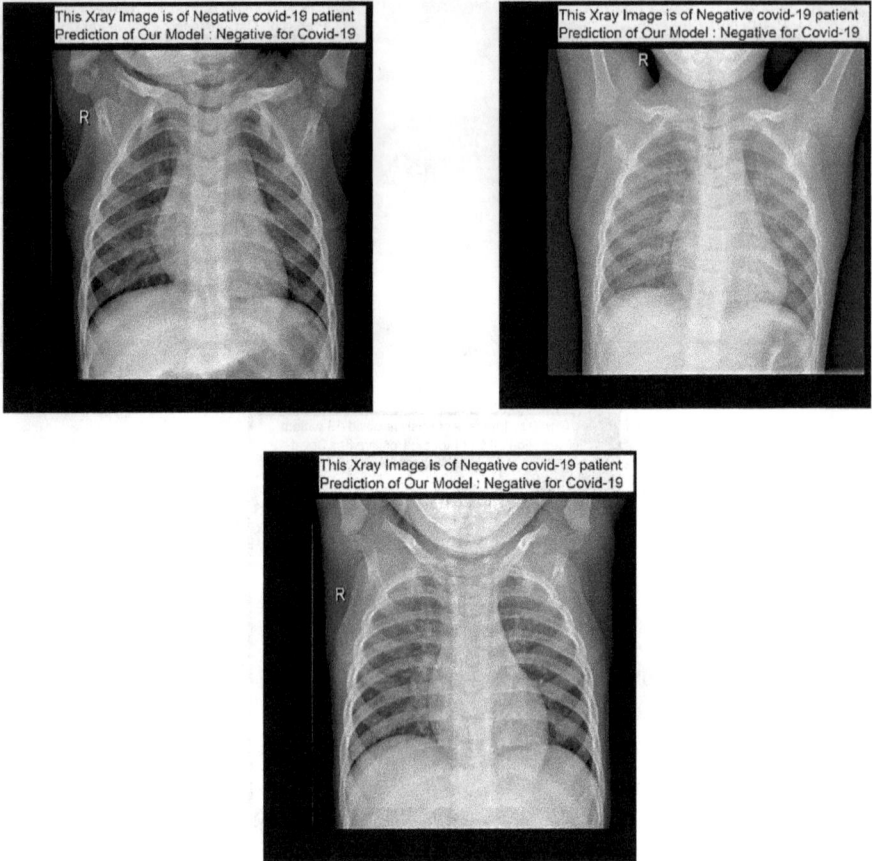

FIGURE 13.9 X-ray image of negative COVID-19 patient: prediction of our model: negative for COVID-19

radiologist, for instance, when used to check the veolity for lung cancer screening, it reduces the reading time by almost half. Lastly, AI-extend (AI-X) uses AI to execute completely new activities that were previously impossible. AI-X systems allow us to obtain more information from the captured data, thereby aiding the detection of ailments hitherto difficult to spot by trained radiologists.

13.7   RESEARCH ADVANCES AND GAPS IN AI-BASED MEDICAL IMAGE PROCESSING

Technological advances in the healthcare industry are leading to improved clinical decision-making. Medical experts are assisted in decision-making during image-aided diagnosis. The continued adoption of artificial intelligence in health care delivery is gradually turning conventional medical imaging into a fully automated diagnostic tool. Medical imaging techniques are now being used in the evaluation of several ailments and diseases, such as renal dysfunction or chronic kidney disease

[44]. Image fusion finds application in lesion detection, classification, and segmentation. Despite the benefit of image fusion, it is however prone to artifacts, distortion, and information loss [45].

Despite the volume of research into the adoption of AI for medical image processing, there remains a wide range of open issues to contend with. Some of these issues include the need for automated methods to accurately create a patient-specific anatomic model from images and an image-based simulation environment for medical procedure rehearsal and planning [46]. While several works have been done in the area of AI interpretability and transparency [38, 39], the issues of trust and acceptance for medical diagnostic applications remain open. More work is required to establish widely acceptable explainable and interpretable AI models for medical imaging applications. Deep learning AI techniques are known to perform well in image recognition applications; hence, they are widely used in medical image classification problems. However, they require massive amounts of data, which are rarely available in the required quantity. Therefore, researchers resort to transfer learning in which pre-trained networks are adapted for medical image applications [47].

13.8 CONCLUSION AND FUTURE DIRECTION

This chapter is a comprehensive guide to understanding AI-enabled medical image processing. It highlights the fundamentals and major goals of medical image processing and presents how they are enhanced with AI techniques and methods. VGG16-based CNN model was developed for the COVID-19 diagnostic experiment. X-ray images were subjected to the developed model to identify positive or normal patients. A prediction accuracy of 95% was achieved with the developed model. This is significantly higher than the accuracy obtained for other existing models in the literature. The developed model exemplifies the practical application of AI in medical image processing and disease diagnosis. In order to develop better models, more work is required in the area of data acquisition; raw data in the form of medical images, especially for newer diseases such as COVID-19, must be acquired for the training of neural networks from scratch.

ACKNOWLEDGMENTS

The work of Agbotiname Lucky Imoize is supported in part by the Nigerian Petroleum Technology Development Fund (PTDF) and in part by the German Academic Exchange Service (DAAD) through the Nigerian-German Postgraduate Program under Grant 57473408.

REFERENCES

[1] S. H. Hawkins et al., "Predicting Outcomes of Nonsmall Cell Lung Cancer Using CT Image Features," *IEEE Access*, vol. 2, pp. 1418–1426, 2014, doi:10.1109/ACCESS.2014. 2373335.

[2] E. P. Papageorgiou, B. E. Boser, and M. Anwar, "Chip-Scale Angle-Selective Imager for in Vivo Microscopic Cancer Detection," *IEEE Trans. Biomed. Circuits Syst.*, vol. 14, no. 1, pp. 91–103, 2020, doi:10.1109/TBCAS.2019.2959278.

[3]   A. Imoize, G. Peter, H. Obakhena, D. Irabor, K. V. N. Kavitha, and C. Chakraborty, "Artificial Intelligence-enabled Internet of Medical Things for COVID-19 Pandemic Data Management," in *Explainable Artificial Intelligence in Medical Decision Support Systems*, 2022, pp. 357–380, doi:10.1049/PBHE050E_ch13.

[4]   S. Roy, S. Bhattacharjee, B. K. Mandal, andM. Saha, "A Comparative Study on Different Techniques for Classification of Brain Waves from EEG Signals," *Am. J. Sci. Eng.*, vol. 2, no. 4, 2022, doi:10.15864/ajec.2401.

[5]   P. A. L. Laguna et al., "Hypervoxels: A Multidimensional Framework for the Representation and Analysis of Neuroimaging Data," *bioRxiv*, pp. 1–36, 2022, doi:10.1101/2022.04.11.485553.

[6]   S. Masoudi et al., "Deep Learning Based Staging of Bone Lesions from Computed Tomography Scans," *IEEE Access*, vol. 9, pp. 87531–87542, 2021, doi:10.1109/ACCESS.2021.3074051.

[7]   M. A. Alzubaidi, M. Otoom, and H. Jaradat, "Comprehensive and Comparative Global and Local Feature Extraction Framework for Lung Cancer Detection Using CT Scan Images," *IEEE Access*, vol. 9, pp. 158140–158154, 2021, doi:10.1109/ACCESS.2021.3129597.

[8]   A. Yang, X. Yang, W. Wu, H. Liu, and Y. Zhuansun, "Research on Feature Extraction of Tumor Image Based on Convolutional Neural Network," *IEEE Access*, vol. 7, pp. 24204–24213, 2019, doi:10.1109/ACCESS.2019.2897131.

[9]   S. Chen et al., "U-Net Plus: Deep Semantic Segmentation for Esophagus and Esophageal Cancer in Computed Tomography Images," *IEEE Access*, vol. 7, pp. 82867–82877, 2019, doi:10.1109/ACCESS.2019.2923760.

[10] A. Ahmed and S. J. Malebary, "Query Expansion Based on Top-Ranked Images for Content-Based Medical Image Retrieval," *IEEE Access*, vol. 8, pp. 194541–194550, 2020, doi:10.1109/ACCESS.2020.3033504.

[11] H. Gao, Z. Chen, and C. Li, "Sandwich Convolutional Neural Network for Hyperspectral Image Classification Using Spectral Feature Enhancement," *IEEE J. Sel. Top. Appl. Earth Obs. Remote Sens.*, vol. 14, pp. 3006–3015, 2021, doi:10.1109/JSTARS.2021.3062872.

[12] C. H. Leow et al., "3-D Microvascular Imaging Using High Frame Rate Ultrasound and ASAP Without Contrast Agents: Development and Initial in Vivo Evaluation on Nontumor and Tumor Models," *IEEE Trans. Ultrason. Ferroelectr. Freq. Control.*, vol. 66, no. 5, pp. 939–948, 2019, doi:10.1109/TUFFC.2019.2906434.

[13] S. Reis et al., "Automated Classification of Breast Cancer Stroma Maturity from Histological Images," *IEEE Trans. Biomed. Eng.*, vol. 64, no. 10, pp. 2344–2352, 2017, doi:10.1109/TBME.2017.2665602.

[14] Y. Li, C. P. Ho, M. Toulemonde, N. Chahal, R. Senior, and M. X. Tang, "Fully Automatic Myocardial Segmentation of Contrast Echocardiography Sequence Using Random Forests Guided by Shape Model," *IEEE Trans. Med. Imaging*, vol. 37, no. 5, pp. 1081–1091, 2018, doi:10.1109/TMI.2017.2747081.

[15] M. Toulemonde et al., "High-Frame-Rate Contrast Echocardiography Using Diverging Waves: Initial in Vitro and in Vivo Evaluation," *IEEE Trans. Ultrason. Ferroelectr. Freq. Control.*, vol. 65, no. 12, pp. 2212–2221, 2018, doi:10.1109/TUFFC.2018.2856756.

[16] Z. Wang, J. Zhang, Y. Xia, P. Chen, and B. Wang, "A General and Scalable Vision Framework for Functional Near-Infrared Spectroscopy Classification," *IEEE Trans. Neural Syst. Rehabil. Eng.*, vol. 30, pp. 1982–1991, 2022, doi:10.1109/TNSRE.2022.3190431.

[17] J. Choi et al., "Machine Learning Approach for Classifying College Scholastic Ability Test Levels with Unsupervised Features from Prefrontal Functional Near-Infrared Spectroscopy Signals," *IEEE Access*, vol. 10, pp. 50864–50877, 2022, doi:10.1109/ACCESS.2022.3173629.

[18] T. Rahman et al., "Exploring the Effect of Image Enhancement Techniques on COVID-19 Detection Using Chest X-ray Images," *Comput. Biol. Med.*, vol. 132, no. March, p. 104319, 2021, doi:10.1016/j.compbiomed.2021.104319.

[19] E. N. Ajimah, O. N. Iloanusi, M. C. Eze, and S. Olisa, "Adaptive Encryption Technique to Protect Biometric Template in Biometric Database using a Modified Gaussian Function," *IJSER* vol.8 no. 11 December, 2017.

[20] R. Mary Lourde and D. Khosla, "Fingerprint Identification in Biometric Security Systems," *Int. J. Electr. Comput. Eng.*, vol. 2, no. 5, pp. 5–8, 2010.

[21] C. Vimala and V. Radha, "Suitable Feature Extraction and Speech Recognition Technique for Isolated Tamil Spoken Words," *Int. J. Comput. Sci. Inf. Technol.*, vol. 5, no. 1, pp. 378–383, 2014.

[22] U. Rajanna, A. Erol, and G. Bebis, "A Comparative Study on Feature Extraction for Fingerprint Classification and Performance Improvements Using Rank-Level Fusion," *Pattern Anal. Appl.*, vol. 13, no. 3, pp. 263–272, 2010, doi:10.1007/s10044-009-0160-3.

[23] H. Kwon, Y. Kim, H. Yoon, and D. Choi, "Selective Audio Adversarial Example in Evasion Attack on Speech Recognition System," *IEEE Trans. Inf. Forensics Secur.*, vol. 15, p. 526–538, 2019, doi:10.1109/TIFS.2019.2925452.

[24] J. Stastny, M. Munk, and L. Juranek, "Automatic Bird Species Recognition Based on Birds Vocalization," *Eurasip J. Audio, Speech, Music Process.*, vol. 2018, no. 1, 2018, doi:10.1186/s13636-018-0143-7.

[25] M. Jena, S. P. Mishra, and D. Mishra, "A Survey on Applications of Machine Learning Techniques for Medical Image Segmentation," *Int. J. Eng. Technol.*, vol. 7, no. 4, pp. 4489–4495, 2018, doi:10.14419/ijet.v7i4.19005.

[26] S. Dubey, and Y.K. Gupta, "Computational Comparison of Various Existing Edge Detection Techniques for Medical Images," International Journal of Computing and Applications, vol. 16, no. 1, pp. 185–193, 2018, ISSN: 0973-5704

[27] M. Y. Kiang, "A Comparative Assessment of Classification Methods," *Decis. Support Syst.*, vol. 35, no. 4, pp. 441–454, 2003, doi:10.1016/S0167-9236(02)00110-0.

[28] M. Ismail et al., "Development of a Regional Voice Dataset and Speaker Classification Based on Machine Learning," *J. Big Data*, vol. 8, no. 1, 2021, doi:10.1186/s40537-021-00435-9.

[29] S. Uddin, A. Khan, M. E. Hossain, and M. A. Moni, "Comparing Different Supervised Machine Learning Algorithms for Disease Prediction," *BMC Med. Inform. Decis. Mak.*, vol. 19, no. 1, pp. 1–16, 2019, doi:10.1186/s12911-019-1004-8.

[30] "c2e2745029ce98f79133381dd72e5d712f75996f @ www.statista.com," www.statista.com/statistics/1037970/global-healthcare-data-volume/

[31] "Medical Healthcare Data Visualization Applications." https://lightningchart.com/blog/medical-healthcare-data-visualization/

[32] G. Jia et al., "Artificial Intelligence-Based Medical Image Segmentation for 3D Printing and Naked Eye 3D Visualization," *Intell. Med.*, vol. 2, no. 1, pp. 48–53, 2022, doi:10.1016/j.imed.2021.04.001.

[33] A. S. Panayides et al., "AI in Medical Imaging Informatics: Current Challenges and Future Directions," *IEEE J. Biomed. Heal. Inform.*, vol. 24, no. 7, pp. 1837–1857, 2020, doi:10.1109/JBHI.2020.2991043.

[34] T. Abraham, A. Todd, D. A. Orringer, and R. Levenson, "Applications of Artificial Intelligence for Image Enhancement in Pathology," in *Artificial Intelligence and Deep Learning in Pathology*. Elsevier Inc., 2021. doi:10.1016/b978-0-323-67538-3.00007-5.

[35] Z. Huang, Q. Li, J. Lu, J. Feng, J. Hu, and P. Chen, "Recent Advances in Medical Image Processing," *Acta Cytol.*, vol. 65, no. 4, pp. 310–323, 2021, doi:10.1159/000510992.

[36] M. Abdar et al., "BARF: A New Direct and Cross-Based Binary Residual Feature Fusion with Uncertainty-Aware Module for Medical Image Classification," *Inf. Sci. (Ny).*, vol. 577, pp. 353–378, 2021, doi:10.1016/j.ins.2021.07.024.

[37] J. B. Awotunde, E. A. Adeniyi, S. A. Ajagbe, A. L. Imoize, O. A. Oki, and S. Misra, "Explainable Artificial Intelligence (XAI) in Medical Decision Support Systems (MDSS): Applicability, Prospects, Legal Implications, and Challenges," in *Explainable Artificial Intelligence in Medical Decision Support Systems.* Institution of Engineering and Technology, 2022, pp. 45–90. doi:10.1049/PBHE050E_ch2.

[38] Z. Salahuddin, H. C. Woodruff, A. Chatterjee, and P. Lambin, "Transparency of Deep Neural Networks for Medical Image Analysis: A Review of Interpretability Methods," *Comput. Biol. Med.*, vol. 140, no. October 2021, p. 105111, 2022, doi:10.1016/j.compbiomed.2021.105111.

[39] B. H. M. van der Velden, H. J. Kuijf, K. G. A. Gilhuijs, and M. A. Viergever, "Explainable Artificial Intelligence (XAI) in Deep Learning-Based Medical Image Analysis," *Med. Image Anal.*, vol. 79, p. 102470, 2022, doi:10.1016/j.media.2022.102470.

[40] S. Mandal, A. B. Greenblatt, and J. An, "Imaging Intelligence: AI is Transforming Medical Imaging Across the Imaging Spectrum," *IEEE Pulse*, vol. 9, no. 5, pp. 16–24, 2018, doi:10.1109/MPUL.2018.2857226.

[41] X. Li, L. Yu, H. Chen, C. W. Fu, L. Xing, and P. A. Heng, "Transformation-Consistent Self-Ensembling Model for Semisupervised Medical Image Segmentation," *IEEE Trans. Neural Netw. Learn. Syst.*, vol. 32, no. 2, pp. 523–534, 2021, doi:10.1109/TNNLS.2020.2995319.

[42] S. Kumar, A. K. Bhandari, A. Raj, and K. Swaraj, "Triple Clipped Histogram-Based Medical Image Enhancement Using Spatial Frequency," *IEEE Trans. Nanobioscience*, vol. 20, no. 3, pp. 278–286, 2021, doi:10.1109/TNB.2021.3064077.

[43] U. K. Acharya and S. Kumar, "Genetic Algorithm Based Adaptive Histogram Equalization (GAAHE) Technique for Medical Image Enhancement," *Optik (Stuttg).*, vol. 230, no. January, p. 166273, 2021, doi:10.1016/j.ijleo.2021.166273.

[44] I. Alnazer et al., "Recent Advances in Medical Image Processing for the Evaluation of Chronic Kidney Disease," *Med. Image Anal.*, vol. 69, p. 101960, 2021, doi:10.1016/J.MEDIA.2021.101960.

[45] H. Hermessi, O. Mourali, and E. Zagrouba, "Multimodal Medical Image Fusion Review: Theoretical Background and Recent Advances," *Signal Process.*, vol. 183, 2021, doi:10.1016/j.sigpro.2021.108036.

[46] J. Suckling, "Medical Image Processing," *Webb's Phys. Med. Imaging, Second Ed.*, no. November, pp. 713–738, 2016, doi:10.1201/b12218-21.

[47] S. Laddha et al., "COVID-19 Diagnosis and Classification Using Radiological Imaging and Deep Learning Techniques: A Comparative Study COVID-19," *Diagnostics (Basel)*, vol. 12, no. 8, p. 1880, 2022.

[48] Moura, LuísVinícius de, et al. "Explainable Machine Learning for COVID-19 Pneumonia Classification with Texture-Based Features Extraction in Chest Radiography," *Front. Digit. Health*, vol.3, p. 662343,2022.

14 Application of AIoMT in Medical Robotics

Aishat Titilola Rufai, Adewole Usman
Rufai, and Agbotiname Lucky Imoize

14.1 INTRODUCTION

The Internet of Things (IoT) can be defined as the connection of physical devices and objects over a network or the internet [1], which implies that data transfer occurs between devices depending on domain-specific applications. In other words, IoT is a technology that connects a wide range of smart devices, sensors, frameworks, and intelligent devices over a network or the internet [2]. The concept of connecting devices over the internet has been in existence for over five decades—it was commonly referred to as "embedded internet" or "pervasive computing" [3]. However, Kevin Ashton introduced the term "Internet of Things" in 1999 and described it as uniquely identifiable connected objects with radio-frequency identification (RFID) [3]. IoT's inception did not garner much recognition until the past decade (the 2010s) when IoT has become an essential tool in all aspects of life. The advancement of the digital era, proliferation of mobile and computer technologies, novel technologies, and easy access to wireless networks have contributed significantly to the growth of IoT.

IoT technologies have recently been widely adopted in various healthcare sectors. This rapid adoption of IoT systems is due to technological advances such as artificial intelligence (AI) techniques, fast internet services, smartphones, and mobile technologies [4]. The application of IoT systems in the medical field is known as the Internet of Medical Things (IoMT). IoMT systems consist of wearable devices, ingestible capsules, and implantable medical devices. For example, AI-enabled IoMT (e.g., smart watches) can assist medical professionals in early predicting, detecting, and managing diseases and remote monitoring of patients, among others. The use of AI and IoMT systems was significantly impacted by the COVID-19 pandemic, where healthcare professionals utilized remote monitoring platforms and telemedicine systems for attending to patients. In other words, the COVID-19 pandemic highlighted the significance of an efficient medical decision support system (MDSS) [5, 6]. Thus, with the integration of AI and IoMT technologies in healthcare, the healthcare delivery system will continue to experience massive technological growth/transformation.

The COVID-19 pandemic and the increasing demands for healthcare practitioners have driven the growth of IoMT. These IoMT systems have contributed to the healthcare industry by assisting medical practitioners in improving their performance and accuracy in their routine activities. Furthermore, the applications of artificial intelligence and the internet of medical things (AIoMT) play a major role in medical decision support systems. Other applications of AIoMT include drug management, assistive technologies, surgical robots, etc. The growing number of AIoMT technologies generates a large volume of medical data. The data collected from these IoMT systems are analyzed using machine learning (ML) and artificial intelligence (AI) techniques. ML and AI technologies are used to extract useful information from the data. Despite the numerous advantages of these novel technologies, they present several limitations ranging from data storage, data quality, and data bias to making accurate decisions and/or predictions in the healthcare field. This is a major concern as the results of these AI/ML technologies could affect patients' outcomes.

In this chapter, we will focus on the applications of AIoMT in medical robotics. Hence, with the application of AIoMT in medical robotics, a new field emerges artificial intelligence of medical robotics things (AIoMRT). This field combines AIoMT technologies with other technologies for efficient and accurate healthcare systems. Although AIoMRT is still a relatively new field, medical practitioners are already benefiting from applying such technologies in the medical field. AIoMRT applications include robotic surgeries, assistive technologies, patient care, prosthetics, and remote monitoring of patients. This field has not been fully integrated into the medical domain due to various constraints of AIoMRT systems.

Furthermore, the increasing use of IoT systems has led to growing security and privacy concerns within these IoT devices [7, 8]. The transfer of information over the internet has made IoT systems susceptible to various security threats and attacks. These IoT threats or attacks are critical in the medical field since patients' lives depend on these IoMT technologies. For example, if an attacker gains access to these IoMT devices [8], such as robotic surgery, this can harm the patient and may lead to his/her death. Thus, most researchers agree that for the full implementation of the AIoMRT system, privacy, and security concerns must be addressed by all stakeholders to achieve a smart and robust healthcare system.

This chapter presents the IoMT applications, challenges, and opportunities. In addition, we will highlight the development of medical robotics, current trends in medical robotics, the application of AI in medical robotics, the research trends of AIoMRT, issues, benefits, and their applications.

14.1.1 KEY CONTRIBUTIONS OF THE CHAPTER

The following are the significant contributions of this chapter:

i. The chapter explores the integration of AI and IoT, for application in medical robotics.
ii. The chapter presents the challenges and prospects of AIoMT for medical robotics.
iii. This chapter reviews the current research trends of AIoMT in medical robotics.

14.1.2 Chapter Organization

Section 14.2 shows the related works on the application of AIoMT in the medical field. Section 14.3 presents the challenges of IoMT applications in medical systems, and Section 14.4 presents the experimental results and discussion. Section 14.5 explains the future research direction of AIoMT in medical robotics and the medical field at large, and finally, Section 14.6 concludes the chapter with future direction.

14.2 RELATED WORK

Due to recent technological advances, robots are designed to perform various tasks in the medical field [9]. With the aid of AI-enabled systems, there has been a wide increase in the development of robots, particularly for the healthcare system. Medical robots are designed to perform tasks that are difficult to perform by humans. Prior studies classify the application of medical robotics into three subfields: robot-assisted surgeries and assistive and rehabilitative systems [10, 11]. Thus, medical robotics are often known for their application in surgery, using robots and software to precisely handle surgical tools through minimally invasive incisions [9].

Guo et al. [10] outlined the medical and social factors for the rapid development of medical robotics. This study highlighted the technical, economic, and regulatory issues faced in medical robotics. However, this study focused on the challenges and opportunities of the development of medical robotics in China.

Trocazz et al. [11] presented robotic systems' recent trends and future perspectives in achieving a smaller, safer, more convenient, and more accessible use in clinical environments. Also, this study described the role computer vision, sensors, and robotics play in improving patient-specific treatment. The authors also highlighted the significance of surgical robotics systems for driving the growth of AI in the medical field. This is due to the information gathered during surgery. This information can be analyzed using AI techniques and can be used for real-time decision-making. In addition, AI in surgery can help detect real-time complications during, before, and after surgery. However, the AI models used for surgical interventions were not discussed.

One of the major challenges of medical robotics is the cost of implementation. This is because only a few organizations control the sector. Thus, Kim et al. [12] proposed developing a model for providing technology commercialization information to new businesses. Although few companies possess the technology, transferring this knowledge to new companies through technology commercialization is essential. Various approaches (such as machine learning (ML)) are used to obtain this technical knowledge. However, this knowledge transfer can be challenging when competitors utilize this technology commercialization technique.

Taylor et al. [13] also provided a general overview of medical robots as well as current trends and challenges of this robotics system. The authors presented an overview of medical robotics technology in remote surgery and robotics. This past decade has seen wide use of medical robotics. Medical robotics is used to perform both surgical and non-surgical tasks in healthcare.

Alessandri et al. [14] described the application of AI techniques to medical robotics, where AI techniques utilized a sequence of operations that is understandable by the robot's control system to carry out partially automated surgical tasks. The simulation was implemented in a virtual environment where the surgeon observes the robot's response to each sequence of tasks. This study allows surgical operations to be replicated effectively in a simulated environment. Since these simulations were carried out in a virtual environment, there is a need to perform these types of tasks in the real world to determine the effectiveness of AI techniques in robotic surgeries.

Future applications of surgical robotics are geared towards autonomous robotic systems where these robotic systems aim to perceive, decide, and act with little to no human interventions. The robot either learns how to perform surgeries by observing a surgeon's operation or videos of surgeons during surgeries or is taught by following instructions (through programming language). Ozmen et al. [15] emphasized the benefits of integrating autonomous robotic systems and AI models. These technologies can improve dexterity, and reduce surgery time and complication rates. Thus, AI for surgical robotics systems can improve patients' outcomes and reduce hospital stay.

Yogananda et al. [16] outlined AI and robots' retrospective and prospective applications for diseases during a pandemic. This study discussed the impact of AI and robots during the COVID-19 pandemic. This pandemic created huge opportunities for AI and automated robots to be used to perform different tasks to aid and support clinicians. This study highlighted the use of AI for patient monitoring, classifying different stages of diseases, and looking for critical cases that require immediate medical attention. Table 14.1 summarizes related works on medical robotics.

14.2.1 MEDICAL ROBOTICS SYSTEM AND APPLICATIONS

Medical robotics are robotic systems used for medical purposes. Robots are designed to carry out tasks for humans, specifically difficult tasks that require energy and fast-processing time. The initiation of robots in healthcare can be traced back to the 1960s. Medical robots were designed to perform surgeries and were fully implemented in 1985 using a PUMA 560 robot manipulator with a surgical arm mounted on its end effector [27]. Recently, the most common medical robot applications include robotic surgery, rehabilitation robots, wearable robots, assistive technologies, telemedicine diagnosis, drug delivery, magnetic actuation, capsule robots, minimally invasive surgery, and robotic laparoscopy, non-laparoscopic robots, soft robotics continuum robotics, and other applications [28, 29]. Also, robots can assist patients, carers, and clinicians by performing tasks such as food delivery and patient monitoring. According to [28], robotic laparoscopy is one of the most promising and oldest subfields of medical robots. In addition, medical robots can be used for prostheses that imitate human movements and can assist people with disability. For surgical applications, robots can be used to support surgeons in surgery and can be used to undergo difficult tasks [30]. For example, in orthopedic surgery, surgeons are prone to radiation as well as fatigue during surgery [30–32].

Surgeons can remotely control robotic surgeries, but they are yet to reach full autonomy due to safety concerns [29]. A study has classified medical robots into six autonomy levels, as described in Table 14.2.

TABLE 14.1
Summary of Application of Medical Robotics

Reference	Medical robotics application	Technologies used/ Discussed	Focus/Results	Limitations
[15]	Artificial intelligence for next-generation medical robotics	-AI/ML techniques -Computer vision -Natural language processing -Artificial neural networks	Discusses the benefits of AI/ML techniques in surgeries as well as recent trends and future advances of autonomous surgical robotics	-Data quality -AI inability to detect a causal relationship -Autonomous robots are yet to be fully implemented in real-world applications
[17]	Orthopedic robotic surgery	Convolutional Neural Network (CNN)	-Use of (AI) for MDSS for diagnosis and treatment for orthopedic surgery -Use of robotic surgery in surgical treatment	-AI and robots' helplessness during complications -AI and robots' non-liability -difficult to incorporate due to its complex technology
[18]	Machine learning in the optimization of robotics in the operative field—Robot-assisted urologic surgery		Highlights recent findings and applications of machine learning in robotic-assisted urologic surgery	-ML techniques not well-established in surgery -Security of high-volume surgical data
[11]	Frontiers of medical robotics	Computer vision Sensors	Outlines future outlook of robotic intervention Provides analysis of robotic interventions Investigates the notion of perception, decision, and action for improving patients' outcome	Bulky robots Robots not well integrated into clinical settings
[14]	Application of AI to medical robotics	AI techniques	Describes the application of AI techniques for a robotic surgical system	The simulation was conducted in a virtual environment but not in a clinical setting

(Continued)

TABLE 14.1 (Continued)
Summary of Application of Medical Robotics

Reference	Medical robotics application	Technologies used/ Discussed	Focus/Results	Limitations
[12]	Development of medical robotics technology commercialization model		Proposed a model for providing technology commercialization information for medical robotics to new companies	Fails during the market competition Technical barrier
[10]	Medical robotics opportunities in China		Outlines opportunities for various robotics applications in medicine	-Review limited on China -Economic, technical, and regulatory barriers
[16]	Retrospective and prospective application of robots and artificial intelligence in global pandemic and epidemic diseases		Discusses the impact of various AI and robotics applications in managing epidemic and pandemic diseases	
[19]	Review on artificial intelligence in robot-assisted surgery		Analyzes various works to identify challenges of the application of AI in robot-assisted surgery	-Data bias -Low-quality data -Lack of explainability -Data heterogeneity
[20]	Robots in healthcare—What do patients say?		Reviews patient perspective on the application of robots and AI in healthcare	-Ambivalent opinions from patients and/ or citizens
[21]	History of robotic surgery		Provides the evolution of robotic surgery over the years	
[22]	Robots in medicine: Past, present and future		Discusses the history of robots in the medical field as well as recent technological advancement, future opportunities, challenges, and applications in various medical domains	-For unskilled surgeons, robotic heart surgery could take longer than traditional surgery -No touch sensation for surgeons -High cost of setup and maintenance -Cell handling and DNA sequencing

Ref	Title	Method	Contribution	Features/Limitations
[23]	Artificial intelligence application in minimally invasive surgery		Analyzes the progress and barriers to the development of AI and medical robotics in minimally invasive surgery	-Poor ability to discern major factors for their result
[24]	Artificial intelligence and robots in healthcare		Developed framework for leading factors for a technology-based healthcare system	Implementation of real interactive procedures for healthcare delivery
[25]	Prediction of task-based, surgeon efficiency metrics during robotic-assisted minimally invasive surgery	Regression trees	Presented ML techniques for assessing surgeons' skills for future tasks based on the previous task	
[26]	Medical robots for infectious diseases: Lessons and challenges from the COVID-19 pandemic		Highlighted the unmet needs for technological advances in the medical field / Presented an overview of key research and barriers that need to be addressed to combat infectious diseases	
[13]	Medical robotics in computer-integrated surgery		Provides an overview of medical robotics. used in surgery and design issues of medical robotics	-Physical Human Robot Interaction (HRI) -Control -Sensing -Mobility -Actuation -Manipulation -Safety -Kinematics -Stiffness redundancy -Human-machine interface

TABLE 14.2
Levels of Robot Autonomy

Levels	Autonomy	Description
0	No autonomy	This system is handled manually by following the user's commands
1	Robot assistance	Robots assist while the user maintains control
2	Task autonomy	Robots perform certain tasks autonomously
3	Conditional autonomy	A task strategy can be generated. However, it is dependent on the user to choose and approve the strategy
4	Full autonomy	The robot is fully autonomous but requires human supervision
5	High autonomy	Robots perform tasks automatically without human expert

Currently, the highest automation level for robotics is conditional autonomy. Since the level of autonomy requires careful consideration, researchers are yet to develop a robotics system with human surgeons' technical know-how/competency. However, some scholars argue that autonomous systems should be fully implemented in the future. Nevertheless, due to patient safety and privacy concerns, researchers have yet to agree on the application of fully autonomous systems in surgeries.

In addition, medical robotics may be broadly divided into the following categories: intended operating environment, the motion of robotic systems (e.g., kinematics); level of autonomy, targeted anatomy, or technique [13].

Advantages of medical robotics include enhancing surgeon's performance, promoting surgical safety, consistent execution of tasks, etc. [13]. Furthermore, with the advancement of technology, AI can be applied to robotic surgery to improve surgical outcomes and enhance decision-making during surgeries. Thus, in the next subsection, we will discuss the various applications of medical robots.

14.2.2 CURRENT APPLICATION OF MEDICAL ROBOTS

Figure 14.1 shows the different applications of medical robotics.

Rehabilitation systems: These robots are used to assist patients with disability and elderly patients. They can be used for monitoring patients, checking patients' vital signs, and performing minor tasks that physicians, surgeons, or clinicians will do for patients. For example, robots can be used for mobility support. As discussed earlier, these rehabilitation systems employ various technologies such as IoMT, AI, and robotics.

Robotics systems employ IoT, AI, and other smart technologies for patient care and assistive technologies to monitor and care for patients with life-threatening conditions. In addition, these technologies assist in effectively managing diseases, thereby improving healthcare systems.

Robotic surgery: Robots are used to perform surgeries and assist surgeons during surgeries; thus, it has several advantages over conventional surgery. This includes flexibility—medical robots can be used in areas where it is difficult for human hands

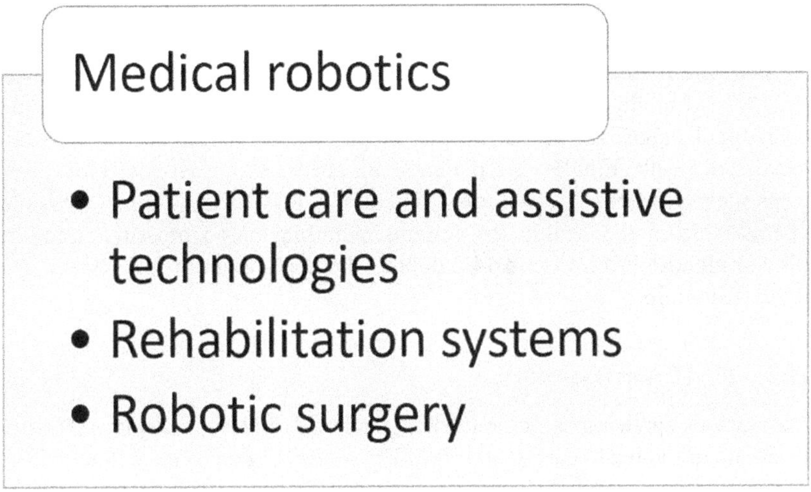

FIGURE 14.1 Application of medical robotics.

to perform surgery. In addition, it reduces the risk of infection for patients and provides computer-aided vision (3D vision) to surgeons [32]. However, the use of robotic surgery also has limitations, such as the cost of setup and difficulty in handling robotic arms [32]. Although medical robots have their benefits, it has yet to achieve their full potential due to limitations. Thus, AI aims to improve the implementation of robotic surgeries.

14.3 CONCEPT OF AIoMT IN MEDICAL ROBOTICS

Recently, IoT has become a significant aspect of the healthcare system. IoT aims to connect users (patients, medical practitioners, etc.) and/or objects to effectively monitor patients' biomedical signals and detect abnormalities within the collected data. The fundamental building block for IoT technology is the internet. Other technologies are used with IoT devices to attain a smart healthcare system. These technologies include AI/ML techniques, cloud computing, etc. IoT devices are used as the internet of medical things (IoMT) for medical purposes. In the subsequent subsection, we discuss how IoT technologies work, IoT architecture, technologies incorporated with IoT, and the applications of IoMT.

14.3.1 How IoMT Works

IoT combines different technologies such as sensors, network systems, and radio data processing and analytics [33]. IoT uses sensors or wearable devices to obtain patients' data or information from their environment (such as blood pressure and heart rate). The patient's electronic health records are transferred via the internet to a temporary or permanent storage unit. The process of transferring information from sensors to end-users requires communication protocols such as wireless networks, Bluetooth, wireless networks, and wireless local area networks (WLAN). After that, the data is analyzed with the aid of AI, ML, and/or big data techniques. ML/AI models obtain meaningful insights from the data. Then, the medical personnel makes recommendations or an efficient treatment plan based on the analyzed result. Finally, the patients can access this treatment plan through smartphones or mobile technologies. Therefore, IoT devices collect physiological parameters in the healthcare system, including blood pressure, heart rate, and blood glucose level. Figure 14.2 depicts the application of IoT systems in the healthcare domain.

14.3.2 IoMT APPLICATIONS

IoT has various applications in the medical field, and Table 14.1 displays the various applications in the healthcare sector. IoMT systems are emerging technologies that comprise sensors, network technologies, storage platforms, and processing platforms (AI and ML analysis tools) to assist clinicians in decision-making. Sensors are used to monitor patients' biomedical signals and vital information remotely. According to [34], IoT devices are used for remote monitoring of heart diseases, blood pressure, brain, and neurological diseases, monitoring fall detection for elderly patients, and tracking of ingestible sensors, among others. For tracking of ingestible sensors, these sensors are swallowed by the patient for early detection and monitoring of diseases such as cancer, and it makes use of smartphone technologies and other monitoring applications [35]. For extracting various patient information, sensors such as pulsometers, pedometers, and cameras, are used. Finally, network technologies such as mobile technologies (GSM), Bluetooth, and Wi-fi are utilized to transfer this information.

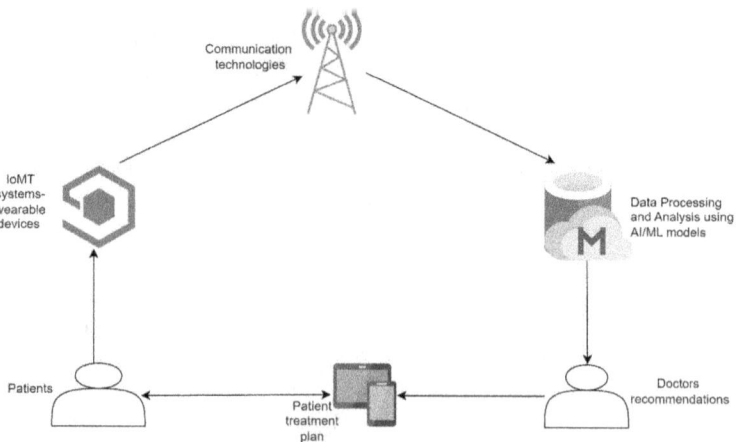

FIGURE 14.2 IoMT system.

Furthermore, sensors are used to track patients' movements—particularly elderly patients with the use of gyroscope sensors, accelerometer sensors, vibration sensors, wireless motes-based fall detection systems, and alarm systems for fall detection [36, 37]. However, the traditional remote monitoring platforms were uncomfortable for patients due to their size and the frequent need for charging these IoT devices [34]. However, IoMT systems address these issues by developing lightweight and low-power sensors [34].

Furthermore, IoT systems can be used to monitor a person's mood, some studies [38, 39] have highlighted IoT devices that detect different types of moods, such as anger, stress, terror, calm, excitement, and sadness. In addition, a real-time mood measurement system known as "Meezaj" has been developed [40]. Furthermore, machine learning algorithms are used to detect a person's mood. For example, a convolutional neural network (CNN) detects different moods, such as sadness, happiness, and stress. Some systems inform a person about their mood. Thus, mood detection can be used to discover the mood of patient's with mental health challenge.

Since most patients forget the time for medication, IoT-based systems are used to remind patients of the particular time to take their drugs. This will reduce the complication because of not taking drugs. For example, a platform for monitoring IVF patients since it has strict adherence to medications.

Furthermore, [41] described implementing an IoT-based medical nursing system (MNS) that uses smart technologies such as WSN, sensors, Wi-fi, and RFID for data transmissions. This MNS allows the easy and efficient supply of the drug.

Furthermore, the authors of [42–44] have stressed the importance of a secure and smart healthcare system. The work [42] designed an IoT-based tool known as mHealth. This m-health system tracks the patient's heart rate, which is extracted using a heart band. This extracted information is then transferred to the patient's family or friends. In addition, [43] provided an IoT-based plan and design for smart hospital systems. This smart hospital system hopes to manage healthcare data, allowing authorized users easy access to important healthcare information. [44] describes how medical practitioners can access patient data and how to maintain a secure and smart healthcare delivery system. Also, IoT systems can be used to assist clinicians with medical decision support systems, such as diagnosis and drug discovery. Furthermore, [45] described the connection of m-health with machine-to-machine and 5G technologies. [46] developed a concept that is used to train a bot using resources and information from medical books. This can educate nonprofessionals about different types of diseases. With the aid of IoT, this bot can be embedded with various sensors on smartphones and other smart/wearable devices, e.g., smartwatches. During the COVID-19 pandemic, IoMT systems were useful for the treatment of orthopedic patients. These treatments range from the bones, tendons, ligaments, joints, muscles [47]. The proposed IoMT systems for orthopedic patients make use of the following IoMT technologies: wearable devices, smart healthcare systems, internet-based services, and remote monitoring systems [47]. These healthcare solutions reduced the tasks of medical professionals by implementing the technologies mentioned previously—machine learning algorithms, and other smart technologies. These emerging technologies can be applied to different healthcare domains. Thus, several other applications of IoT-based systems in healthcare assist clinicians and patients in achieving reliable smart healthcare systems. The focus areas of IoMT and their gaps in healthcare are given in Table 14.3.

TABLE 14.3
Focus Areas of IoMT and Their Gaps in Healthcare

References	IoMT Applications	Focus	Gaps
[34]	Remote monitoring	*i.* Remote Monitoring for various diseases such as—heart diseases, diabetics, and brain and neurological diseases *ii.* Remote monitoring of fall detection for elderly patients *iii.* Tracking of ingestible sensors	Security and privacy concerns
[51]		*i.* Electrocardiogram (ECG) monitoring *ii.* Various disease monitoring such as asthma, glucose level, blood pressure, and oxygen saturation *iii.* Mood monitoring *iv.* Medication management *v.* Rehabilitation system *vi.* Wheelchair management	-Servicing and maintenance cost -Power consumption -Standardization -Patient, caregiver, and medical personnel Identification -Self-configuration -Scalability -Environmental impact -Exploration of new diseases -Data privacy and security
[41]	Highlighted the role of IoMT in smart medical nursing system Describes the main technologies (IoT, big data, cloud, and fog computing) and their application areas		-Intelligence in medical care -Real-time processing of data -Energy constraints, scalability, security
[43]	Proposed architecture for IoT-based smart healthcare system		
[33, 46]	Developed medical bots for educating non-medical professionals about various diseases		-Incomplete information -Encourages self-care -Complicated automated system

TABLE 14.3 (*Continued*)
Focus Areas of IoMT and Their Gaps in Healthcare

References	IoMT Applications	Focus	Gaps
			-Can increase workload and cost
			-Can reduce accessibility to human doctors
[47]	Discusses treatment for orthopedic patients, including remote care, disease detection, and monitoring		-Security -Interoperability -Limited research of IoMT systems in orthopedics
[48]	Classifies different applications of AI-based IoMT into four categories:	*i.* Diagnosis *ii.* Treatment *iii.* Data management research	-Security and privacy -Real-time feedback during remote surgery -Accessible user interface -Heterogeneity due to different users' applications and device types -Power consumption
[49]	Describes the main technologies (IoT, big data, cloud and fog computing) and their application areas		-Energy constraints -Scalability -Security

14.3.2.1 Benefits of IoMT

IoMT has several implications in the medical field and has seen increasing use in different medical domains. IoMT systems provide real-time patient data analysis to support clinicians and caregivers with recommendations to improve patient health. This can be achieved with the aid of AI-enabled technologies, clinical decision support systems tools, and electronic health records. Recent technologies assist patients with data collection, storage, and analysis in the medical field. These techniques all use AI algorithms to analyze and extract useful insights from patient information. Recently, IoT devices have been designed to use low-power and be compact, making it easy for users/patients to wear or move these devices comfortably. In addition, this IoT device reduces hospital costs and aids clinician's activity. That is, it reduces the time spent on various activities within the healthcare system. It also allows easy and efficient use of health care information by end-users. These IoT features allow patients to afford the best healthcare services, leading to improved quality of life. For example, diabetic patients can monitor their blood glucose—with the aid of IoT technologies and smartphone technologies—whereby IoT device alerts them whenever they are at risk of low or high blood glucose. Thus, IoT-based healthcare systems are affordable, easy to use, and allow users (healthcare professionals, patients, family members and other stakeholders) access to improved healthcare delivery systems.

14.3.2.2 Challenges of IoMT

Despite the successes of these IoMT technologies, several challenges are faced with these devices. Furthermore, the current limitations of IoMT are patients' privacy and data protection and security. This section will present the major issues of the IoMT system. Some of the challenges in IoT systems include but are not limited to the following: device/physical security, privacy and security concerns, network, data, server and operating system security, energy consumption, as well as others [47–50]. Table 14.4 lists the common IoMT challenges.

Energy consumption is significant to IoT-based systems. Thus, authors [33] and [51] discuss the issue of power consumption in IoMT systems. Since most IoT devices make use of batteries, it is becoming difficult to replace such batteries. Currently, researchers are looking for ways for these devices to generate power independently [51]. Thus, renewable energy sources are considered a viable solution to this problem [51]. In addition, another study proposed a new scheduling algorithm for nodes located between two or more sensing fields. This study is concerned with reducing power consumption by creating different schedules for the nodes, such as sleeping and listening schedules [52]. This reduces power consumption and extends wireless sensor networks' lifetime [52]. Thus, designing smart and effective power consumption techniques for IoMT-based systems is essential.

In addition, security is one of the most critical issues in IoMT systems. Most studies have highlighted that IoT systems are vulnerable to security issues such as cyberattacks, physical damage, unauthorized access to data, ransomware, and so on. The author of [53] presents security issues that can be physical or device security. Here, the attacker physically accesses the device and extracts important data from the device for malicious purposes [53]. Thus, it is essential for the devices not to be easily accessed. Furthermore, security issues can further be classified into four categories which are [53]:

- Network security
- Data security
- Server security
- Operating system security

Another study [33] classified data security challenges into four main categories: trust and data integrity, data privacy, vulnerability points, and data protection.

Due to the integration of different devices, such as sensors, communication networks, and processing techniques, different forms of data are generated from these techniques. Thus, to address these challenges, a study [54] highlights the DIAT scheme as a simple, scalable distributed architecture for large-scale IoT networks typically designed to overcome the interoperability issues among various IoT systems. Therefore, the IoMT issues are given in Table 14.4.

TABLE 14.4
IoMT Issues

IoMT Issues	Reference
Energy consumption	[33, 51, 52]
Transmission media, data exchange, network performance	[33, 38]
Security	[33, 38, 47, 50–52]
Human-in-the-loop	[33]
Interoperability	[35, 38, 50]
Data privacy	[33, 50]
Scalability	[33, 38]
Quality of service	[33]
Lack of standardization	[51]
Regulations	[50]
Design issues and environmental impact	[38, 47, 51]

In conclusion, some of the security issues IoT-enabled devices face can be addressed and mitigated with the help of artificial intelligence (AI) algorithms. Thus, more research needs to be done on the standard and effective ways to employ AI techniques for mitigating security risks for IoMT systems.

14.3.3 AIoMT System

The advancement of various technologies such as mobile technology, cloud computing, AIoMT systems, and blockchain has improved healthcare services. AI and IoT are becoming ubiquitous due to the increasing demand for these technologies across various medical sectors. The integration of AI and IoT in the medical field can be known as AIoMT [43]. As discussed earlier, IoT systems collect patients' Electronic Health Records (EHR) while AI uncovers a deeper understanding of patients' EHR data. The AIoMT-based system improves the decision support system for clinicians. In addition, the tool used to assist clinicians in decision-making is known as the clinical decision support system (CDSS). This CDSS tool employs IoT systems that provide efficient health records and AI models, thereby increasing the probability of generating accurate predictions (patient outcome).

Chatterjee et al. [55] defined the components of the IoT platform and decision support system as well as the application of this system to cardiovascular diseases. The authors highlighted the significance of IoT systems as well as AI models. The following technologies play an important role in CDSS: Electronic health records, IoT technologies, and AI models. The main goal for CDSS is to accurately transfer and process electronic health records efficiently to assist medical personnel in decision-making.

Shah et al. [56] highlighted the applications of IoT and AI in the healthcare field and the potential benefits of these AIoMT systems in the healthcare system. In addition, this study highlights the data security and privacy gaps of AI and IoT systems. AIoMT systems can be used to diagnose, manage, and treat patients, etc. However, data security and privacy issues need to be addressed to achieve the full potential of these systems.

Singla [57] discusses the importance of AI in the treatment of patients as well as diagnosing patients through the use of patient EHR. This study also analyses the role of AI in treating and managing different ailments such as mental health, kidney disease, diabetes, and cardiovascular diseases. This study also discusses the issues of the large volume of data collected by these IoT systems. The collection of a large volume of data can lead to the analysis of irrelevant data, which can reduce the accuracy of the results. Thus, the quality of data collected by IoT devices also determines the precision of the results.

Alshehri et al. [58] analyze various literature that encompasses the integration of IoT and IoMT, AI, edge and cloud computing, security, and medical signals technologies. This review also presents the present and future challenges of this technology. Various combinations of technologies are utilized to achieve a smart healthcare system. However, IoT and AI systems are the most predominant technologies used in the medical industry. Thus, the goal of these new technologies is to improve healthcare services.

Novel technologies implemented for healthcare systems utilize heterogeneous platforms and tools for medical systems. These heterogeneous tools cause interoperability issues within the healthcare platform. Thus, Knickerbocker et al. [59] illustrate how these technologies are employed for specific healthcare applications such as disease diagnostics. This study also highlights the significance of AI in obtaining guidance for healthcare personnel.

Thus, AIoMT technologies are mainly employed in healthcare and can be used to assist patients, caregivers and medical personnel to acheive an enhanced medical delivery system.

14.3.4 TECHNOLOGICAL CONCEPTS FOR SMART HEALTHCARE SYSTEMS

The different technologies for smart healthcare systems are given in Figure 14.3.

14.3.4.1 IoT

As discussed earlier, IoT collects vital patient information through sensors from the physical world and transfers this information to the end user (clinician, caregiver) through the internet. It uses various applications such as mobile technologies (4G/5G communication), and wireless sensor networks. This mobile technology aids the delivery of medical care by enhancing medical services and can also be used for telemedicine, emergencies, diagnosis, and treatment applications [7, 60].

14.3.4.2 AI and ML

AI is a branch of computer science that integrates logical, mathematical, and statistical knowledge and can be used to carry out complex tasks in various industries [60]. AI implements various techniques for performing such difficult tasks, including machine learning (ML) models, computer vision (CV), natural language processing (NLP), deep learning (DL), and neural networks (NN) to support clinicians by obtaining useful insights from medical data.

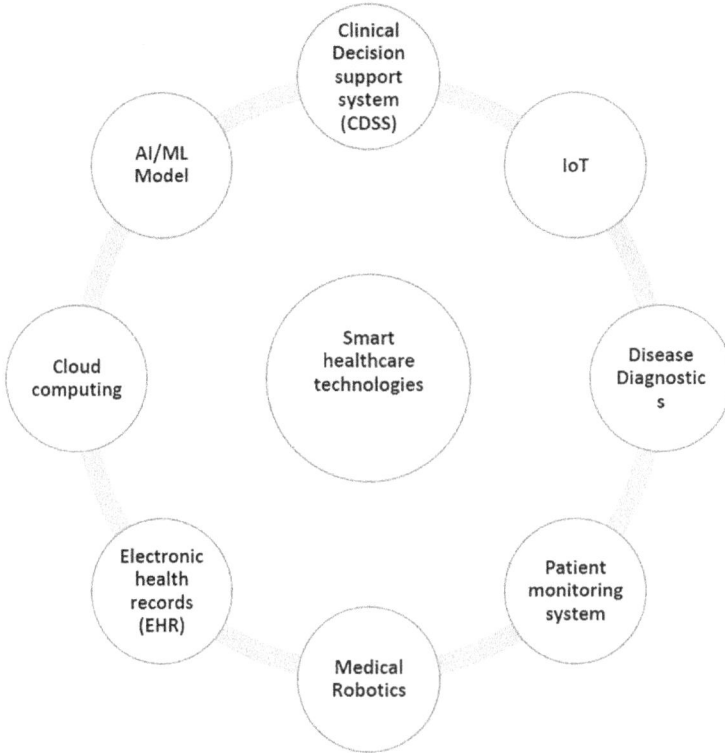

FIGURE 14.3   Different technologies for smart healthcare systems.

ML is a subclass of AI. It is used for obtaining insights from a large volume of data. It can be classified into four classes: supervised, unsupervised, semi-supervised, and reinforcement learning. Supervised learning trains labeled data, and an algorithm creates a task that matches inputs to relevant outputs [48, 61]. Thus, supervised learning is used to make predictions and can be used in medical robotics. For example, Authors of [62] have shown that supervised learning is applied to gait rehabilitation robots to teach robots how to walk physiologically. In comparison, unsupervised learning looks for patterns in a given set of data [62]. A study has highlighted the application of unsupervised learning for disease detection with the aid of endoscopic capsule robots' systems [63]. These endoscopic capsule robots are ingestible and are mainly used for body parts that are difficult to access by humans [63]. Semi-supervised learning makes use of both supervised and unsupervised learning. Semi-supervised learning enhances the performance of supervised learning by employing unsupervised learning techniques to obtain information not clearly provided in the labeled data [64]. Applications of semi-supervised in the medical field include medical imaging applications for a brain tumor and white matter hyperintensities segmentation, as discussed in ref. [64]. Reinforcement learning is employed to carry out tasks by receiving feedback to reduce or eliminate the system's drawbacks [48, 61]. Reinforcement learning has found applications in surgical robot manipulations, where surgical data is embedded into robotic simulation systems for various surgical tasks [65].

14.3.4.3   Cloud Computing and Electronic Health Record

IoT in the healthcare sector has brought about various challenges, such as data storage, transmission, management, security, and privacy concerns [66]. One solution that can address these challenges is cloud computing. Cloud computing has been the latest concept in information and computer technology [66]. Cloud computing provides computer services such as servers, databases, networking, software, and data analytics through the internet for rapid implementation, and scalability of computing resources [66].

Another useful concept for data management and analysis in the medical domain is electronic health records (EHR). Patients from developing countries and remote areas find it difficult to transport their paper medical records [67]. The development of EHR addresses the common challenges faced with keeping paper medical records. Although, these EHR systems find it difficult to integrate and transfer patient medical records from one hospital to another [67], integrating EHR and cloud computing addresses the problem of transferring EHRs over the internet, mitigating various IoT challenges.

Current studies have shown the benefits of integrating cloud computing and EHR systems. These advantages of cloud computing include access to high-quality medical resources, support for telemedicine, cost reduction, interoperability, data security and privacy, etc. [60, 66–71]. Another benefit of cloud computing is its ability to facilitate more structured and organized information sharing among medical professionals, caregivers, and patients, which reduces the likelihood of losing medical records [72].

However, integrating IoT and cloud computing with healthcare systems has limitations. These challenges include users' lack of knowledge, difficulty in integrating information from various devices and lack of administrative support, network delays for telemedicine applications, etc. [66, 69]. The summary of various issues that affect the integration of cloud computing and IoT is discussed in Table 14.5. For the integration of cloud computing to be completely adopted in the medical field, these challenges need to be addressed.

Meanwhile, another cloud computing concept has been introduced, known as fog computing (decentralized concept), while cloud computing is known as the centralized concept [66]. Fog computing performs data analytics on edge devices and addresses real-time processing issues by improving data privacy concerns and reducing costs [66]. Furthermore, it enables heterogeneous devices to connect to a network reliably and efficiently. Fog computing also has a high response time and low latency since data transmission occurs from device to device, unlike cloud, where transmission occurs from cloud to device [66]. Thus, fog computing addresses some of the limitations of cloud computing.

14.3.4.4   Clinical Decision Support System (CDSS)

As mentioned earlier, AI is used to assist clinicians in making decisions, especially in cumbersome areas for humans to make decisions. For example, A 2021 study

TABLE 14.5
Cloud Computing and IoT Challenges in Healthcare

References	Cloud computing challenges	Description
[69]	Users lack knowledge of cloud computing systems	Most healthcare administrators lack the expertise of recent cloud computing technology in the healthcare domain. Thus, training healthcare administrators on cloud computing techniques in the healthcare domain is important.
[66–68, 70]	Low response time and high latency	Cloud computing experiences communication issues that cause network delays and interruptions. This could lead to a life-threatening situation for telemedicine applications requiring real-time information processing.
[66]	Lack of standardization	Due to the different frameworks and devices (IoMT and cloud computing systems), and different regulatory bodies, there is a need for standardized policies for these systems to work effectively.
[70]	Security and privacy	Various IoMT devices and cloud computing systems have increased the possibility of cyberattacks. Thus, it is important for cybersecurity experts and developers of these IoMT systems to develop frameworks to mitigate these security and privacy challenges.

concluded that AI-based CDSS assists clinicians by identifying patients at increased risk of venous thromboembolism (VTE), applying adequate preventative measures, and ensuring compliance with the American College of Chest Physicians (ACCP) guidelines [73]. AI-based CDSS can also be known as data-driven CDSS. In addition, AI-based CDSS can be used to detect heart failure. According to [73], AI-CDSS showed high diagnostic accuracy for heart failure. The use of AI systems for decision-making can help reduce hospital costs and save time. Although AI-based CDSS has contributed significantly to the medical system, a survey on ML-based CDSS suggested that in-depth patient data can enhance the performance of this ML-based CDSS. In addition, studies indicated that missing data could lead to results biases. Thus, it is important to consider the data quality while using ML algorithms for CDSS and general medical fields. Therefore, more research needs to be carried out to determine an effective way of collecting and utilizing patient data for CDSS. In general, CDSS consists primarily of three layers, as shown in Figure 14.4.

14.3.4.5 Electronic Health Records (EHR)

Electronic health records are a system for electronically collecting patient information and past medical data history. EHR consists of patient information such as patient demographic information, and past medical conditions. It reduces costs and allows patient information to be retrieved by authorized users (medical practitioners) in real time. EHRs have advantages such as reliability, cost reduction, patient data

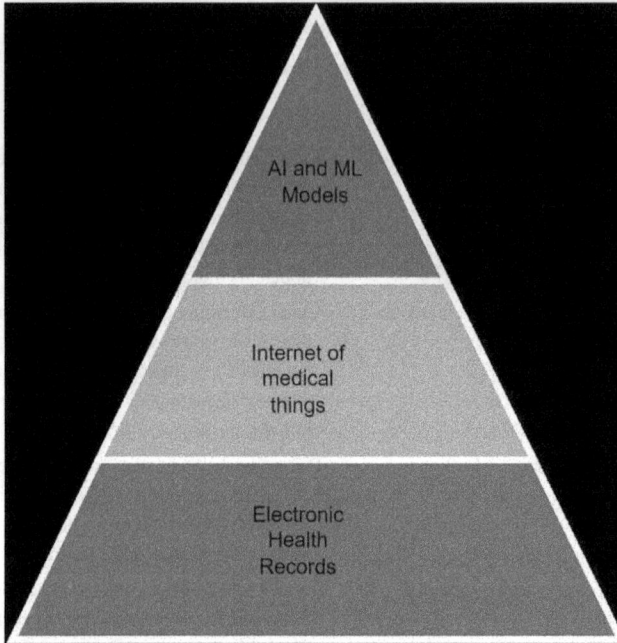

FIGURE 14.4 CDSS layers.

safety, and efficiency [74], since clinical support system employs software techniques to compare patient data with electronic medical records to extract useful recommendations for clinicians [74]. However, implementing an EHR system has its drawbacks, such as heterogeneity and complexity.

Furthermore, since EHR contains detailed patient information, obtaining useful information from this system is difficult. Thus, robust techniques such as AI can be used to interpret EHR data to predict and extract useful insights from the data [75]. For example, cardiology studies have generally employed AI systems for heart failure detection [75]. Thus, the integration of EHR, AIoMT, and CDSS tools will improve patient care and the healthcare delivery system. Thus, EHR systems can be used to enhance medical decisions, particularly when patient data is complete.

14.3.4.6 Disease Diagnostics

The application of AI in EHR can be used for disease diagnosis and real-time monitoring of patients' vitals (e.g., heart rate, blood glucose level). AI in healthcare assists clinicians by making recommendations for patients' treatment. For example, studies have highlighted the application of IBM's "Watson for Oncology," a cloud-based AI system used to keep patients' cancer records to discover the best possible treatments for individual patients based on past patient data [76, 77]. However, scholars have recently criticized Watson for inaccuracies and ineffectiveness in various applications in the medical field [76, 77].

14.3.4.7 Patient's Remote Monitoring System

Remote monitoring is essential, particularly for patients with chronic diseases and life-long ailments such as diabetes. Remote monitoring system assists clinicians and/or carers by providing real-time information of patients' vital information such as pulse rate, heart rate, blood pressure, blood oxygen volume, heart disease, and neurological disease [78]. These patient monitoring systems can be used for monitoring diabetes, dementia, migraine, etc. [79, 80]. In addition, the remote monitoring system can also be used for monitoring postoperative patients, elderly patients, fall detection systems, and mobility-related ailments with the aid of smart sensors, robotic systems, IoT, and decision-making techniques [78–81]. Researchers have highlighted the significance of remote monitoring systems, including swift detection of patients' deteriorating health and improvement of clinical outcomes [78, 80]. Thus, patient remote monitoring system integrates the following technologies: IoT systems, smart wearable devices, fog and cloud computing, AI systems, etc. This AIoT technology aims to acquire patients' information in real-time to manage patients' medical conditions effectively and accurately without being invasive to patients, unlike traditional patient monitoring systems. In addition, AI models can be applied to decision-making and for identifying various patient activities [80]. Examples of such AI techniques include ML and deep learning techniques such as neural networks (NN).

14.3.4.8 Medical Robotics

Due to recent technological advances, robots are designed to perform various tasks in the medical field [9]. With the aid of AI-enabled systems, there has been a wide increase in robot development, particularly in the healthcare system. Thus, medical robots are designed to perform tasks that are difficult to perform by humans. Medical robots have found various applications in rehabilitation systems, robotic-assisted surgeries, drug discovery, disease diagnostics, patient care, etc. Thus, medical robotics are often known for their application in surgery with robots and software to precisely handle surgical tools through minimally invasive incisions [9].

14.3.5 AIoMT IN MEDICAL ROBOTICS—OVERVIEW

AIoMT technologies have the potential to revolutionize the healthcare system. Recently, the use of AIoMT in healthcare has significantly improved the medical systems, particularly during the COVID-19 pandemic. These technologies supported medical personnel and patients through remote monitoring of patients, diagnosis of diseases, and in telemedicine applications. In addition, AI technologies were also used to classify mild, severe, and moderate cases of the COVID-19 pandemic, thereby reducing the number of patients to be admitted. Also, IoMT devices such as pulse oximeters were used to monitor and check patients' blood oxygen saturation levels [5]. Thus, AIoMT systems were beneficial for managing the COVID-19 pandemic and other diseases.

Another area of technological innovation that is impacting healthcare is the field of robotics. This technology is majorly used to carry out tasks that are challenging or time-consuming for humans to complete. Medical robotics is the application of robotics in the medical field. As mentioned earlier, they can be used for physical rehabilitation, prosthetics, therapy, and surgery, among others. They are proficient at completing physical tasks. The application of AI and IoT to the field of robotics has brought about new opportunities for the healthcare field. The next subsection discusses various applications of AIoMT in robotics.

14.3.6 APPLICATION OF AIoMT IN MEDICAL ROBOTICS—EMERGENCE OF AIoMRT

Kavidha et al. [82] classified the applications of AI, IoT, and robotics in medicine in surgical robots, exoskeletons, prosthetics, artificial organs, drug management and hospital automation robots, and social robots. The significance of this robot-assisted surgery is to improve precision and enhance surgical skills. Robot-assisted surgeries are carried out using 3D vision, robotic arms, and algorithms to control the movement of the arm. This robotic surgical system filters the surgeons' hand tremors and controls the robotic arm [82]. [32] also discusses the benefits and gaps of robotic surgeries. Some benefits include surgeons being less prone to infection, and fatigue. [32]. However, researchers have highlighted the cost, machine malfunction, and security of surgical robotics systems as the predominant issues. Surgical robotics is expensive to set up. In addition, there is also a trade-off between human control and machine control. For example, one of the main functions of this robotic system is to minimize human errors while humans also try to limit machine errors. Thus, both humans and machines work together to limit surgical errors in order to improve patient outcomes.

Another notable application of AI, IoT, and robotics is in exoskeleton, prosthetics, and rehabilitation. With the aid of wearable robotic technologies, patients with disabilities can move without human assistance. In addition, this system can also be used in prosthetics applications. Technologies such as IoT and cloud computing will be employed for future applications of these robotic systems [82]. Sivaparthipan et al. [83] defined the role of robots in Parkinson's disease. It also discussed how AI and IoT can be used to improve gait performance. Thus, AIoMRT technologies can be used to improve patients' mobility.

Other application areas include ingestible capsules and artificial organs; these robotic systems are usually embedded or swallowed. They are controlled by external algorithms (e.g., AI/ML); this technology raises regulatory concerns since these systems are controlled externally. Another application area of AIoMT in robotics is for hospital and pharmacy automation and drug management. Some robots are designed to draw blood as well as disinfect the hospital, thereby limiting human errors in healthcare facilities. These AIoMT technologies in robotics have the capability of displacing healthcare personnel in the near future.

Furthermore, social robots can aid in treatment of patients with psychological and cognitive issues. Social robots are used as a therapy for patients through human-robot interaction. Social robots can detect human moods and encourage interaction between robots and humans mainly for therapeutic purposes [84]. For example, ML-based robots can be used for children with autism [85, 86]. The framework of this system consists of the following: sensing unit, perception unit, and interaction unit. For the sensing unit, the child's mood can be detected by obtaining the child's facial expression, voice, and/or language through video, audio, and pictorial means [85, 87]. This data is collected with the use of IoT devices. For perception, ML algorithms detect the child's behavior and the robot interacts with the child based on the perception of the child's behavior [85].

In summary, AI, and IoT in medical robotics are used for monitoring, diagnosis, drug management, therapeutic, assistive, and surgical robotic systems. Recent technological advancement in surgical robotics has paved the way for autonomous surgeries. These autonomous surgeries are carried out (with the aid of AIoMT) with little to no human assistance. Research is still being carried out on this autonomous system to determine its performance and accuracy for future surgical applications [82].

14.4 CURRENT LIMITATIONS OF AIoMRT AND FUTURE DIRECTIONS

AIoMRT is a relatively new field, and only a few studies are available. In this chapter, we will classify the major challenges of AI, IoT, and robotics in Figure 14.5.

According to research, the prevalent challenges of IoT include compatibility with various devices, cyberattacks, privacy and security concerns, etc. Technologies such as fog and cloud computing address some of these issues in healthcare. For instance, addressing security and privacy issues, can reduce the cost of frequent hospital visits by improving telemedicine applications. Fog computing improves the network bandwidth and real-time data collection, transmission, and analysis [41].

The increasing number of IoMT systems has led to a large volume of data generation. Thus, managing this large data is difficult without compromising patients' privacy and safety. A study has proposed data anonymization to protect patients' privacy, leading to data loss [88]. Another way to ensure patient data privacy and

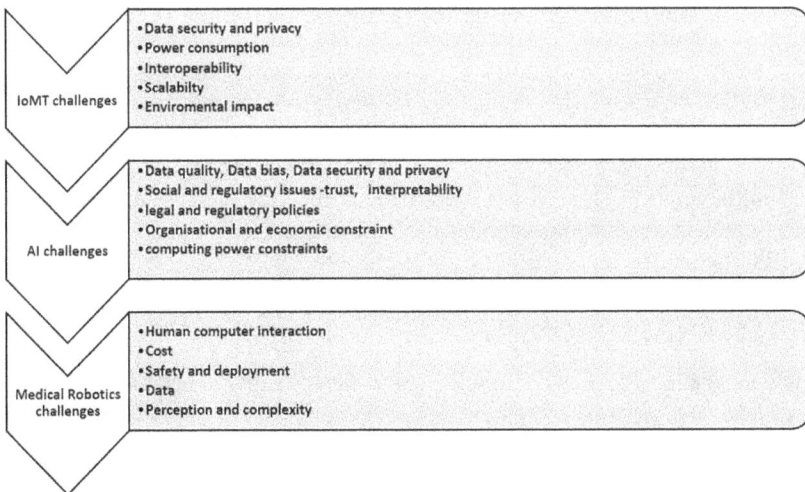

FIGURE 14.5 AIoMRT challenges.

security is to employ blockchain technology. Recent studies have highlighted the importance of blockchain for data security. [89] presented a multi-agent system as the solution to IoMT challenges where the IoMT device acts as an agent, and the blockchain ensures patient data is confidential. Furthermore, with various IoMT devices, applications, and data types, sharing data from different platforms can lead to data fragmentation. However, the development of blockchain solves this data fragmentation issue. It also ensures the safe and secure sharing of sensitive medical data. Thus, blockchain technology addresses various issues that hinder stakeholders (healthcare practitioners, patients, and caregivers) from fully utilizing the potential of IoMT systems [90–93].

Other AI challenges for healthcare systems include computing power, data bias, lack of interpretability, privacy, and security concerns since AI and ML models utilize vast computational techniques. Thus, computing power is a challenge due to the volume of data generated. AI technology has to rely on other technologies to attain the necessary computing demands, such as cloud computing, IoT. AI must be adaptable to meet the demands of these fast-growing real-world challenges. Another common problem with AI in healthcare is the lack of interpretability of the results [32]. For critical applications in the healthcare field, the reasons behind an AI decision must be known to prevent misdiagnosis or other life-threatening errors. Also, healthcare personnel rarely question the decision of AI models (which is known as automation bias), making it prone to unseen errors. Thus, there is a need for AI/ML models to be explainable to know the reasons behind AI decisions [32, 82]. In addition to technologies for patient data privacy and security concerns, there are regulatory agencies that address these issues, for example, Health Insurance Portability and Accountability Act (HIPAA) and the Health Information Technology for Economic and Clinical Health (HITECH) Act. Compliance with these acts is important to safeguard health information privacy, security, and confidentiality [80, 94]. Thus, AI models need more training to detect cyberattacks and cybersecurity concerns in the medical field.

Also, for medical robotics, human-computer interaction has to improve for better patient outcomes. Most ML-based simulations fail when transferred to robots. Thus, a study proposed the addition of noise into the training data set to make it more robust [95]. Robotics systems could also experience an equipment failure. Hence, it is important to develop robust features for future application of AIoMRT technologies

Current studies have shown that safety and privacy are one of the major challenges in the application of AIoMT for medical robotics. Thus, there is a need for more research in this field in order to determine the best techniques for solving these AIoMRT challenges.

14.5 LEARNED LESSONS

For the application of AIoMRT in the medical field, there is a need to integrate new technologies such as cloud computing, fog computing, and edge computing. For future applications of AIoMRT systems, it is important that the systems are designed to be adaptable to new technologies. Also, according to research, these systems' privacy and security concerns must be addressed to achieve the full potential of AIoMRT. Blockchain technology plays a major role in securing patients' data and privacy. For telemedicine or remote surgery applications, real-time data processing is critical. Thus, fog computing addresses the high latency and high delays of cloud computing.

14.6 CONCLUSION

The implementation of IoT, robotics, ML technologies, and cloud computing technologies in the medical field can lead to improved patient outcomes. Hence, researchers need to develop robust systems to address issues faced in AIoMRT. All these issues can be addressed by implementing technologies suitable for AIoMRT applications. For example, for robotic manipulation, researchers are beginning to focus on microbots to allow easy and swift manipulation of the robotic arm. While privacy and security concerns are the most prevalent issues, researchers need to explore a suitable system for addressing these issues. One of the limitations of this study is that the simulation studies for AI and IoT in robotics were not discussed. Thus, scholars need to do more research on integrating IoT, AI, cloud computing, and blockchain technologies in medical robotics.

ACKNOWLEDGMENT

The work of Agbotiname Lucky Imoize is supported in part by the Nigerian Petroleum Technology Development Fund (PTDF) and, in part, by the German Academic Exchange Service (DAAD) through the Nigerian-German Postgraduate Program under grant 57473408.

REFERENCES

[1] Li S, Xu LD, Zhao S. The internet of things: a survey. *Information Systems Frontiers.* 2015;17(2):243–259.
[2] Kumar S, Tiwari P, Zymbler M. Internet of things is a revolutionary approach for future technology enhancement: a review. *Journal of Big Data.* 2019;6(1):1–21.
[3] Lueth KL. IoT basics: getting started with the internet of things. *White Paper.* 2015:1–9.
[4] Mavrogiorgou A, Kiourtis A, Perakis K, Pitsios S, Kyriazis D. IoT in healthcare: achieving interoperability of high-quality data acquired by IoT medical devices. *Sensors.* 2019;19(9):1978.
[5] Chatterjee P, Tesis A, Cymberknop LJ, Armentano RL. Internet of things and artificial intelligence in healthcare during COVID-19 pandemic—a South American perspective. *Frontiers in Public Health.* 2020;8:600213.
[6] Imoize AL, Gbadega PA, Obakhena HI, Irabor DO, Kavitha KVN, Chakraborty C. Artificial intelligence-enabled internet of medical things for COVID-19 pandemic data management. In *Explainable Artificial Intelligence in Medical Decision Support Systems*, 1st ed., AL Imoize, J Hemanth, D-T Do, and SN Sur, Eds. London: The Institution of Engineering and Technology, 2022, pp. 357–380.
[7] Joyia GJ, Liaqat RM, Farooq A, Rehman S. Internet of medical things (IoMT): applications, benefits and future challenges in healthcare domain. *Journal of Communications.* 2017;12(4):240–247.
[8] Wazid M, Das AK, Rodrigues JJ, Shetty S, Park Y. IoMT malware detection approaches: analysis and research challenges. *IEEE Access.* 2019;7:182459–182476.

[9] Gyles C. Robots in medicine. *The Canadian Veterinary Journal*. 2019;60(8):819.

[10] Guo Y, Chen W, Zhao J, Yang GZ. Medical robotics: opportunities in China. *Annual Review of Control, Robotics, and Autonomous Systems*. 2022;5:361–383.

[11] Troccaz J, Dagnino G, Yang GZ. Frontiers of medical robotics: from concept to systems to clinical translation. *Annual Review of Biomedical Engineering*. 2019;21:193–218.

[12] Kim Y, Lee J, Kang J, Park S, Jang D. A study on the development of medical robotics technology commercialization model [J]. *Journal of Advances in Information Technology*. 2021;12(2).

[13] Taylor RH, Menciassi A, Fichtinger G, Fiorini P, Dario P. Medical robotics and computer-integrated surgery. In *Springer Handbook of Robotics*, Cham: Springer 2016, pp. 1657–1684.

[14] Alessandri E, Gasparetto A, Valencia Garcia R, Martinez Béjar R. An application of artificial intelligence to medical robotics. *Journal of Intelligent and Robotic Systems*. 2005;41:225–243.

[17] Beyaz S. A brief history of artificial intelligence and robotic surgery in orthopedics & traumatology and future expectations. *Joint Diseases and Related Surgery*. 2020;31(3):653.

[18] Ma R, Vanstrum EB, Lee R, Chen J, Hung AJ. Machine learning in the optimization of robotics in the operative field. *Current Opinion in Urology*. 2020;30(6):808.

[19] Moglia A, Georgiou K, Georgiou E, Satava RM, Cuschieri A. A systematic review on artificial intelligence in robot-assisted surgery. *International Journal of Surgery*. 2021;95:106151.

[20] Vallès-Peris N, Barat-Auleda O, Domènech M. Robots in healthcare? What patients say. *International Journal of Environmental Research and Public Health*. 2021;18(18):9933.

[21] Kalan S, Chauhan S, Coelho RF, Orvieto MA, Camacho IR, Palmer KJ, Patel VR. History of robotic surgery. *Journal of Robotic Surgery*. 2010;4:141–147.

[22] Kasina H, Bahubalendruni MR, Botcha R. Robots in medicine: past, present and future. *International Journal of Manufacturing, Materials, and Mechanical Engineering (IJMMME)*. 2017;7(4):44–64.

[23] Nawrat Z. MIS AI-artificial intelligence application in minimally invasive surgery. *Mini-invasive Surgery*. 2020;4:28.

[24] Yoon SN, Lee D. Artificial intelligence and robots in healthcare: what are the success factors for technology-based service encounters? *International Journal of Healthcare Management*. 2018;12(3):218–225.

[25] Zhang A, Guo L, Jarc AM. Prediction of task-based, surgeon efficiency metrics during robotic-assisted minimally invasive surgery. In *2019 International Symposium on Medical Robotics (ISMR)*. Atlanta, GA: IEEE, 2019, pp. 1–7.

[26] Di Lallo A, Murphy R, Krieger A, Zhu J, Taylor RH, Su H. Medical robots for infectious diseases: lessons and challenges from the COVID-19 pandemic. *IEEE Robotics & Automation Magazine*. 2021;28(1):18–27.

[27] Kucuk S. Introductory Chapter: Medical Robots in Surgery and Rehabilitation [Internet]. Medical Robotics - New Achievements. *IntechOpen*. 2020. Available from: http://dx.doi.org/10.5772/intechopen.85836.

[28] Dupont PE, Nelson BJ, Goldfarb M, Hannaford B, Menciassi A, O'Malley MK, Simaan N, Valdastri P, Yang GZ. A decade retrospective of medical robotics research from 2010 to 2020. *Science Robotics*. 2021;6(60):eabi8017.

[29] Boubaker O. Medical robotics. *Control Theory in Biomedical Engineering*. 2020:153–204.

[30] Hayda RA, Hsu RY, DePasse JM, Gil JA. Radiation exposure and health risks for orthopaedic surgeons. *JAAOS-Journal of the American Academy of Orthopaedic Surgeons*. 2018;26(8):268–277.

[31] Yang L, Wang T, Weidner TK, Madura JA, Morrow MM, Hallbeck MS. Intraoperative musculoskeletal discomfort and risk for surgeons during open and laparoscopic surgery. *Surgical Endoscopy.* 2021;35(11):6335–6343.

[32] Rufai AT, Dukor KF, Ageh OM, Imoize AL. XAI robot-assisted surgeries in future medical decision support systems. In *Explainable Artificial Intelligence in Medical Decision Support Systems*, 1st ed., AL Imoize, J Hemanth, D-T Do, and SN Sur, Eds. London: The Institution of Engineering and Technology, 2022, pp. 167–195.

[33] Farhan L, Kharel R, Kaiwartya O, Quiroz-Castellanos M, Alissa A, Abdulsalam M. A concise review on internet of things (IoT)-problems, challenges and opportunities. In *2018 11th International Symposium on Communication Systems, Networks & Digital Signal Processing (CSNDSP)*. Budapest: IEEE, 2018, pp. 1–6.

[34] Vishnu S, Ramson SJ, Jegan R. Internet of medical things (IoMT)-an overview. In *2020 5th International Conference on Devices, Circuits and Systems (ICDCS)*. Coimbatore: IEEE, 2020, pp. 101–104.

[35] Beardslee LA, Banis GE, Chu S, Liu S, Chapin AA, Stine JM, Pasricha PJ, Ghodssi R. Ingestible sensors and sensing systems for minimally invasive diagnosis and monitoring: the next frontier in minimally invasive screening. *ACS Sensors.* 2020;5(4):891–910.

[36] Paoli R, Fernandez-Luque FJ, Doménech G, Martinez F, Zapata J, Ruiz R. A system for ubiquitous fall monitoring at home via a wireless sensor network and a wearable mote. *Expert Systems with Applications.* 2012;39(5):5566–5575.

[37] Naranjo-Hernandez D, Roa LM, Reina-Tosina J, Estudillo-Valderrama MA. Personalization and adaptation to the medium and context in a fall detection system. *IEEE Transactions on Information Technology in Biomedicine.* 2012;16(2):264–271.

[38] Joyia GJ, Liaqat RM, Farooq A, Rehman S. Internet of medical things (IoMT): applications, benefits and future challenges in healthcare domain. *Journal of Communications.* 2017;12(4):240–247.

[39] Alam MGR. CNN based mood mining through IoT-based physiological sensors observation. 한국정보과학회 학술발표논문집. 2017:1301–1303.

[40] Ahmad E. Meezaj: an interactive system for real-time mood measurement and reflection based on internet of things. *International Journal of Advanced Computer Science and Applications.* 2020;11.

[41] Huang CH, Cheng KW. RFID technology combined with IoT application in medical nursing system. *Bulletin of Networking, Computing, Systems, and Software.* 2014;3(1):20–24.

[42] Arbat H, Choudhary S, Bala K. IOT smart health band. *Imperial Journal of Interdisciplinary Research.* 2016;2(5).

[43] Yu L, Lu Y, Zhu X. Smart hospital based on internet of things. *Journal of Netwroks.* 2012;7(10).

[44] Kumar DD, Venkateswarlu P. Secured smart healthcare monitoring system based on IOT. *Imperial Journal of Interdisciplinary Research.* 2016;2(10).

[45] W. D. de Mattos and P. R. L. Gondim, "M-Health Solutions Using 5G Networks and M2M Communications," in *IT Professional*, vol. 18, no. 3, pp. 24–29, May-June 2016, doi: 10.1109/MITP.2016.52. New Jersey, USA.

[46] Fischer M, Lam M. From books to bots: using medical literature to create a chat bot. In *Proceeding of First Workshop on IoT-enabled Healthcare and Wellness Technologies and Systems*, New York: Association for Computing Machinery, 23–28, June 30, 2016. https://doi.org/10.1145/2933566.2933573.

[47] Singh RP, Javaid M, Haleem A, Vaishya R, Ali S. Internet of medical things (IoMT) for orthopaedic in COVID-19 pandemic: roles, challenges, and applications. *Journal of Clinical Orthopaedics and Trauma.* 2020;11(4):713–717.

[48] Dhillon A, Singh A. Machine learning in healthcare data analysis: a survey. *Journal of Biology and Today's World*. 2019;8(6):1–10.

[49] Aceto G, Persico V, Pescapé A. Industry 4.0 and health: internet of things, big data, and cloud computing for healthcare 4.0. *Journal of Industrial Information Integration*. 2020;18:100129.

[50] Dash SP. The impact of IoT in healthcare: global technological change & the road-map to a networked architecture in India. *Journal of the Indian Institute of Science*. 2020;100(4):773–785.

[51] Pradhan B, Bhattacharyya S, Pal K. IoT-based applications in healthcare devices. *Journal of Healthcare Engineering*. 2021;2021:1–18.

[52] Saha D, Yousuf MR, Matin MA. Energy efficient scheduling algorithm for S-mac protocol in wireless sensor network. *International Journal of Wireless & Mobile Networks*. 2011;3(6):129–140.

[53] Shamila M, Vinuthna K, Tyagi AK. A review on several critical issues and challenges in IoT based e-healthcare system. In *2019 International Conference on Intelligent Computing and Control Systems (ICCS)*. Madurai: IEEE, 2019, pp. 1036–1043.

[54] Sarkar C, S.N. AUN, Prasad RV, Rahim A, Neisse R, Baldini G. DIAT: a scalable distributed architecture for IoT. *IEEE Internet of Things Journal*. 2015;2(3):230–239.

[55] Chatterjee P, Cymberknop LJ, Armentano RL. IoT-based decision support system for intelligent healthcare—applied to cardiovascular diseases. In *2017 7th International Conference on Communication Systems and Network Technologies (CSNT)*. Nagpur: IEEE, 2017, pp. 362–366.

[56] Shah R, Chircu A. IoT and AI in healthcare: a systematic literature review. *Issues in Information Systems*. 2018;19(3).

[58] Alshehri F, Muhammad G. A comprehensive survey of the internet of things (IoT) and AI-based smart healthcare. *IEEE Access*. 2020;9:3660–3678.

[59] Knickerbocker JU, Budd R, Dang B, Chen Q, Colgan E, Hung LW, Kumar S, Lee KW, Lu M, Nah JW, Narayanan R. Heterogeneous integration technology demonstrations for future healthcare, IoT, and AI computing solutions. In *2018 IEEE 68th Electronic Components and Technology Conference (ECTC)*. San Diego, CA: IEEE, 2018, pp. 1519–1528.

[60] Lu ZX, Qian P, Bi D, Ye ZW, He X, Zhao YH, Su L, Li SL, Zhu ZL. Application of AI and IoT in clinical medicine: summary and challenges. *Current Medical Science*. 2021;41(6):1134–1150. doi:10.1007/s11596-021-2486-z.

[61] Shailaja K, Seetharamulu B, Jabbar MA. Machine learning in healthcare: a review. In *2018 Second International Conference on Electronics, Communication and Aerospace Technology (ICECA)*. IEEE, 2018, pp. 910–914.

[62] Menner M, Neuner L, Lünenburger L, Zeilinger MN. Using human ratings for feedback control: a supervised learning approach with application to rehabilitation robotics. *IEEE Transactions on Robotics*. 2020;36(3):789–801.

[63] Turan M, Ornek EP, Ibrahimli N, Giracoglu C, Almalioglu Y, Yanik MF, Sitti M. Unsupervised odometry and depth learning for endoscopic capsule robots. In *2018 IEEE/RSJ International Conference on Intelligent Robots and Systems (IROS)*. IEEE, 2018, pp. 1801–1807.

[64] Chen S, Bortsova G, García-Uceda Juárez A, Tulder GV, Bruijne MD. Multi-task attention-based semi-supervised learning for medical image segmentation. In *International Conference on Medical Image Computing and Computer-Assisted Intervention*. Cham: Springer, 2019, pp. 457–465.

[65] Xu J, Li B, Lu B, Liu YH, Dou Q, Heng PA. SurRoL: an open-source reinforcement learning centered and dVRK compatible platform for surgical robot learning. In *2021*

IEEE/RSJ International Conference on Intelligent Robots and Systems (IROS). IEEE, 2021, pp. 1821–1828.

[66] Dang LM, Piran MJ, Han D, Min K, Moon H. A survey on internet of things and cloud computing for healthcare. *Electronics*. 2019;8(7):768.

[67] Mirza H, El-Masri S. Cloud computing system for integrated electronic health records. In *Proceedings of the International Conference on Bioinformatics & Computational Biology (BIOCOMP)*. The Steering Committee of The World Congress in Computer Science, Computer Engineering and Applied Computing (WorldComp), Athens, 2012, p. 382.

[68] Mutlag AA, Abd Ghani MK, Arunkumar NA, Mohammed MA, Mohd O. Enabling technologies for fog computing in healthcare IoT systems. *Future Generation Computer Systems*. 2019;90:62–78.

[69] Ahmadi M, Aslani N. Capabilities and advantages of cloud computing in the implementation of electronic health record. *Acta Informatica Medica*. 2018;26(1):24.

[70] García-Valls M, Calva-Urrego C, García-Fornes A. Accelerating smart eHealth services execution at the fog computing infrastructure. *Future Generation Computer Systems*. 2020;108:882–893.

[71] Zhang Z, Han Y. Detection of ovarian tumors in obstetric ultrasound imaging using logistic regression classifier with an advanced machine learning approach. *IEEE Access*. 2020;8:44999–45008.

[72] Islam SMR, Kwak D, Kabir MH, Hossain M, Kwak K. The internet of things for HealthCare: a comprehensive survey. *IEEE Access*. 2015;3:678–708.

[73] Zhou S, Ma X, Jiang S, Huang X, You Y, Shang H, Lu Y. A retrospective study on the effectiveness of Artificial Intelligence-based Clinical Decision Support System (AI-CDSS) to improve the incidence of hospital-related venous thromboembolism (VTE). *Annals of Translational Medicine*. 2021;9(6):491. doi:10.21037/atm-21-1093.

[74] Mills S. Electronic health records and use of clinical decision support. *Critical Care Nursing Clinics of North America*. 2019;31(2):125–131. doi:10.1016/j.cnc.2019.02.006.

[75] Lin WC, Chen JS, Chiang MF, Hribar MR. Applications of artificial intelligence to electronic health record data in ophthalmology. *Translational Vision Science & Technology*. 2020;9(2):13.

[76] Lee D, Yoon SN. Application of artificial intelligence-based technologies in the healthcare industry: opportunities and challenges. *International Journal of Environmental Research and Public Health*. 2021;18(1):271.

[77] Ross C, Swetlitz I. IBM's Watson supercomputer recommended 'unsafe and incorrect' cancer treatments. *Internal Documents Show*. STAT+. 25 July 2018. Available online: www.statnews.com/wp-content/uploads/2018/09/IBMs-Watsonrecommended-unsafe-and-incorrect-cancer-treatments-STAT.pdf (accessed on January 16, 2023).

[78] Kantipudi MV, Moses CJ, Aluvalu R, Kumar S. Remote patient monitoring using IoT, cloud computing and AI. In *Hybrid Artificial Intelligence and IoT in Healthcare 2021*. Singapore: Springer, 2021, pp. 51–74.

[79] Nwaneri SC, Yinka-Banjo C, Uregbulam UC, Odukoya OO, Imoize AL. Explainable neural networks in diabetes mellitus prediction. In *Explainable Artificial Intelligence in Medical Decision Support Systems*, 1st ed., AL Imoize, J Hemanth, D-T Do, and SN Sur, Eds. London: The Institution of Engineering and Technology, 2022, pp. 313–334.

[80] Jeddi Z, Bohr A. Remote patient monitoring using artificial intelligence. In *Artificial Intelligence in Healthcare*. London, UK: Academic Press, 2020, pp. 203–234.

[81] Shaik T, Tao X, Higgins N, Li L, Gururajan R, Zhou X, Acharya UR. Remote patient monitoring using artificial intelligence: current state, applications, and challenges. *Wiley Interdisciplinary Reviews: Data Mining and Knowledge Discovery*. 2023:e1485.

[82] Kavidha V, Gayathri N, Kumar SR. AI, IoT and robotics in the medical and healthcare field. In *AI and IoT-Based Intelligent Automation in Robotics*, New Jersey, USA: Wiley-Scrivener, 2021, pp. 165–187.

[83] Sivaparthipan CB, Muthu BA, Manogaran G, Maram B, Sundarasekar R, Krishnamoorthy S, Hsu CH, Chandran K. Innovative and efficient method of robotics for helping the Parkinson's disease patient using IoT in big data analytics. *Transactions on Emerging Telecommunications Technologies*. 2020;31(12):e3838.

[84] Gyrard A, Tabeau K, Fiorini L, Kung A, Senges E, De Mul M, Giuliani F, Lefebvre D, Hoshino H, Fabbricotti I, Sancarlo D. Knowledge engineering framework for IoT robotics applied to smart healthcare and emotional well-being. *International Journal of Social Robotics*. 2021:1–28.

[85] Rudovic O, Lee J, Dai M, Schuller B, Picard RW. Personalized machine learning for robot perception of affect and engagement in autism therapy. *Science Robotics*. 2018;3(19):eaao6760.

[86] Riek LD. Robotics technology in mental healthcare. In *Artificial Intelligence in Behavioral Health and Mental Health Care*, D Luxton, Ed. San Diego, CA: Elsevier, 2015, pp. 185–203. http://doi.org/10.1016/B978-0-12-420248-1.00008.

[87] Denecke K, Baudoin CR. A review of artificial intelligence and robotics in transformed health ecosystems. *Frontiers in Medicine (Lausanne)*. 2022;9:795957. doi:10.3389/fmed.2022.795957.

[88] Puiu A, Vizitiu A, Nita C, Itu L, Sharma P, Comaniciu D. Privacy-preserving and explainable AI for cardiovascular imaging. *Studies in Informatics and Control*. 2021; 30(2):21–32.

[89] Połap D, Srivastava G, Woźniak M. Multi-agent architecture for internet of medical things. In *Artificial Intelligence and Soft Computing: 19th International Conference, ICAISC 2020, Zakopane, Poland, October 12–14, 2020, Proceedings, Part II 19 2020*. Cham: Springer, 2020, pp. 49–58.

[90] Dhillon A, Singh A. Machine learning in healthcare data analysis: a survey. *Journal of Biology and Today's World*. 2019;8(6):1–10.

[91] Imoize AL, Irabor DO, Gbadega PA, Chakraborty C. Blockchain technology for secure COVID-19 pandemic data handling. In *Smart Health Technologies for the COVID-19 Pandemic: Internet of Medical Things Perspectives*, 1st ed., C Chakraborty and JJPC Rodrigues, Eds. London, UK: The Institution of Engineering and Technology, 2022, pp. 141–179.

[92] Kumar RL, Wang Y, Poongodi T, Imoize AL, Eds., *Internet of Things, Artificial Intelligence and Blockchain Technology*, 1st ed. Switzerland, AG: Springer Nature, 2021.

[93] Iguoba V, Imoize AL, The psychology of explanation in medical decision support systems. In *Explainable Artificial Intelligence in Medical Decision Support Systems*, 1st ed., AL Imoize, J Hemanth, D-T Do, and SN Sur, Eds. London: The Institution of Engineering and Technology, 2022, pp. 489–506.

[94] Moore W, Frye S. Review of HIPAA, part 1: history, protected health information, and privacy and security rules. *Journal of Nuclear Medicine Technology*. 2019;47(4):269–272.

[95] El-Shamouty M, Kleeberger K, Lämmle A, Huber M. Simulation-driven machine learning for robotics and automation. *TM-Technisches Messen*. 2019;86(11):673–684.

15 AIoMT on Intelligent Location and Clustering of Medical Units

Pablo Rodríguez de León, María Dolores Torres Soto, Aurora Torres Soto, Eunice Esther Ponce de León Sentí, and Carlos Ochoa Zezzatti

15.1 INTRODUCTION

New technologies will dramatically change the medical industry on an international level. At the same time, it happens in the field of manufacturing and computing; artificial intelligence, blockchain, the Internet of Things, etc. Those will be the tools that will enable the digital transformation of medicine and people's healthcare.

So far, Industry 4.0 technologies are not yet widely accepted in the healthcare sector, but there is some impulse to promote their use. Some specialists are enthusiastic about its uptake and implementation due to its capacity and capability for disease detection, prediction as well as medical information management.

The Health Services Institute of Aguascalientes State (ISSEA) has three jurisdictional health offices in Aguascalientes, Rincón de Romos, and Calvillo. These jurisdictional offices manage and monitor personnel, manage, and distribute supplies, equipment and medications to 89 health centers in 11 municipalities [1]. Each of the jurisdictional health offices has its own distribution centers, administrative offices, communications, warehouses, etc.

By using an automated process, communities' information was collected from MSSQL Server servers from which information was obtained from 89 health centers and 3 jurisdictions, data such as location, longitude, and latitude, as well as general information of the total number of patients from each health center also, as well as significant and contrasting information on patients classified as probable and confirmed with the pathology of diabetes mellitus.

Working with Haversine distances, the Haversine formula is used to determine the great circle distance between two points on a sphere, given their longitude and latitude [2]; a modified version of the K-means algorithm was developed with four centroids of which three are the fixed centroids representing the current jurisdictional offices and the variable represent the new health jurisdiction called fourth health Jurisdiction; these four centroids use the latitude and longitude coordinates to define their geographic position.

DOI: 10.1201/9781003370321-15

In addition, this research implemented TOPSIS technique to intelligently select one of the six candidate localities or communities close to the geographical point obtained by the modified K-means algorithm, where the new health jurisdiction 4 will be established.

It is important to propose the creation of Health Jurisdiction 4, which will help to reduce the distance to improve the distribution of supplies and medicines, and the transfer of health center maintenance staff, doctors, and administrative employees who travel daily from Jurisdiction 4 to the health centers. Other advantages are better diabetic patient care, improving and speeding up the supply of medicines and medical material, and reduction of fuel consumption of vehicles of the health jurisdiction.

In the new health jurisdiction 4, 14 health centers that belonged to health jurisdictions 1 and 2 were grouped together; with this new health jurisdiction 4, 65,568 patients will be treated, of which 30,595 patients were from health jurisdiction 1 and 34,973 from health jurisdiction 2. In relation to the pathology of diabetes mellitus, health jurisdiction 4 will attend to 3,475 confirmed diabetic patients and 3,125 patients with prediabetes.

In addition, there is currently a deficit of direct links to health jurisdictions. Through health jurisdiction 4, direct links will be installed to generate daily backups of the electronic clinical record, as well as the daily report generated for the health secretary.

This work is novel because it has the conjunction of several techniques in which a modified version of the K-means clustering technique with fixed and mobile centroids using Haversine distance is implemented, as well as the advice of an expert in urban planning to determine and weigh the values of the variables with which the TOPSIS method was fed and the best option was determined to propose the establishment of the Sanitary jurisdiction 4.

This research work has the limitation that there is not included restricted and private information on operating costs and inputs of health jurisdictions and health centers, so data published by ISSEA and INEGI (National Institute of Statistics and Geography) were used and presented, as well as data calculated by methods explained in this research.

15.1.1   KEY CONTRIBUTIONS OF THE CHAPTER

The following are the significant contributions of this chapter:

i. A novel and effective algorithm based on K-means, with which it works with fixed and mobile centroids.

ii. A new distribution of health units and the inclusion of a new health jurisdiction, to reduce times and distances between them and have a better and faster distribution of supplies and transfer of medical and administrative staff.

iii. By reducing the transportation time of patients, which will improve care and early detection of diseases such as diabetes mellitus.

15.1.2 Chapter Organization

Section 15.2 presents the related concepts on the selection of location and clustering units. Section 15.3 presents the related work of clustering medical units using K-means, other techniques, and Haversine distance techniques. Section 15.4 presents materials and methods through conceptual design, methodology, and data collection. Section 15.5 presents the processing clustering software, which is composed of modified K-means algorithm from fixed and mobile centroids and TOPSIS variables and process. Section 15.6 presents the discussions and Section 15.7 presents the conclusions.

15.2 RELATED CONCEPTS

15.2.1 Multi-Criteria Decision-Making Methods

Industry 4.0 integrated artificial intelligence, Machine Learning, Big Data, and cloud computing, among other tools, are transforming the health sector, where they are helping to make better decisions, reduce costs, optimize resources, detect, and cure diseases.

A challenge for the health system is the increase in pathologies, such as diabetes and hypertension, but due to modern medicine and the implementation of industry 4.0 tools, life expectancy has grown impressively in recent years.

There are applications of Industry 4.0 that are currently in use in the medical sector, some of them are Machine Learning and artificial intelligence, in the field of diagnosis by imaging systems, consultation systems, and disease prediction, which integrate algorithms capable of learning through experience, something that is of vital importance for the recognition of pathologies and images for their early diagnosis.

15.2.2 Multi-Criteria Decision-Making Methods

There are several options for decision-making methods, so it is essential to know and understand the differences and contributions of each of the available options. These methods use numerical techniques, which help decision-makers to select from a discrete set of alternative decisions.

These methods are based on the impact of the alternatives. Comparing these decision methods to choose the best one is often a complicated task; these models have been used extensively despite the criticisms that exist around them.

Among the most used models, we can find one of the oldest, the weighted sum model (WSM), A modification to this model is that its weak points are the weighted product model (WPM). Another model is the one proposed by Saaty, the analytical hierarchical process (AHP). Other widely used methods are the ELECTRE and TOPSIS methods.

To use a decision-making method that involves a detailed numerical analysis of the options, three steps must be followed:

1. Criteria and options are determined.
2. Numerical measures are assigned to the relative importance of the criteria and to the consequences of the options on these criteria.
3. The numerical values are processed, and a ranking of each option is determined.

15.2.3 TOPSIS

Within the diversity of techniques to support selection under multi-criteria conditions is TOPSIS, the Technique for Order Preference by Similarity to Ideal Solution [3]. The main concept of TOPSIS is that the best solution is the one with the shortest distance to the ideal solution and the one with the longest distance to the anti-ideal solution [4]. TOPSIS was developed by Hwang and Yoon in 1981 [5].

TOPSIS technique has been applied to a diverse range of decision problems, for example, in financial investment support, advanced manufacturing systems, robotic process selection applications, neural network approaches, and fuzzy set extensions; it has also been used to compare the performance of companies and the performance of financial ratios in specific industries [4]. This is an interesting tool because it requires subjective input from the decision-makers involved, and this primary subjective input is the weights.

Hwang et al. [6] propose TOPSIS based on the optimal option being as close as possible and the negative ideal option being as far away as possible. The methodology is represented by the following diagram in Figure 15.1 based on Kolios, Mytilinou, Lozano, and Salonitis [7].

Seven blocks are linked with arrows, one following the other, forming a process chain from the first block of the definition of alternative and criteria, the second block is decision matrix, the third block is normalized matrix, the fourth block is weighted and normalized matrix, the fifth block is the positive and negative ideal solutions, the sixth block is the relative closeness, and the seventh and final block is the definition to the ranking of solutions, and together are the TOPSIS process.

The TOPSIS technique can be executed through the following steps.

1. Building of the decision matrix: Starting from m alternatives Ai, i=1, 2, . . ., m that will be evaluated based on the criteria Cj, j=1, 2, . . ., n.
2. Performance data are obtained for the n alternatives on k criteria. These measures should be standardized by some method of normalization.
   a. Distributive normalization.
   b. Ideal normalization.

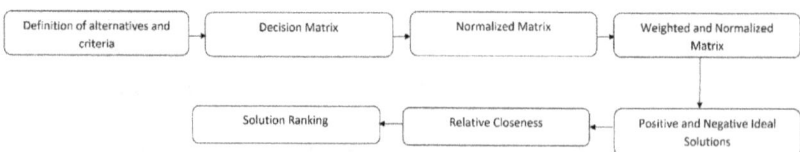

FIGURE 15.1 TOPSIS methodology [7].

$$n_{ij} = \frac{x_{ij}}{\sqrt{\sum_{j=1}^{m}\left(x_{ij}\right)^2}}, j = 1,\dots n, i = 1,\dots m \qquad (15.1)$$

3. A set of significant weights is developed for each one of the criteria. The base for these weights may be some feature but may have some relative significance.

$$v = w \, x \, nj = ni = m \qquad (15.2)$$

4. The scores of the weights are compared with each action as either an ideal action or an anti-ideal virtual action. There are three different ways to define these virtual actions.
   a. Obtaining the best and worst result in each criterion of the normalized decision matrix.

$$A^+ = \left\{v_1^+,\dots,v_n^+\right\} = \left\{\left(\max_i v_{ij}, j \in J\right)\left(\min_i v_{ij}, j \in J\right)\right\} \qquad (15.1)$$

$$A^- = \left\{v_1^-,\dots,v_n^-\right\} = \left\{\left(\min_i v_{ij}, j \in J\right)\left(\max_i v_{ij}, j \in J\right)\right\} \qquad (15.2)$$

   b. Assuming an absolute ideal and anti-ideal point, which are defined without considering the actions of the decision problem.
   c. The ideal and anti-ideal points are defined by the decision maker.

5. A distance measure is calculated for each criterion, ideal and anti-ideal alternatives.

$$d_i^+ = \left\{\sum_{j=1}^{n}\left(v_{ij} - v_j^+\right)^2\right\}^{\frac{1}{2}}, i = 1,\dots m \qquad (15.3)$$

$$d_i^- = \left\{\sum_{j=1}^{n}\left(v_{ij} - v_j^-\right)^2\right\}^{\frac{1}{2}}, i = 1,\dots m \qquad (15.4)$$

6. For each alternative, the proximity coefficient is determined as equal to the distance to the anti-ideal divided by the sum of the distance to the anti-ideal and the distance to the ideal.

$$R_i = \frac{d_i^-}{d_i^+ + d_i^-}, i = 1,\dots m \qquad (15.5)$$

7. The obtained alternatives are sorted by maximizing the proximity coefficient of step 5.

15.2.4 K-MEANS

Clustering makes it possible to recognize groups in which the elements have similarities between them and other differences with the elements of other groups [8]. MacQueen in 1967 created the K-means algorithm, which is the most famous and widely used clustering algorithm because, despite its simplicity, it is effective.

K-means classifies a group of elements into a certain number of K groups, which is defined previously. It is named K-means because it relates elements by the mean of centroids. Centroid is a recognized statistical and graphical concept. A cluster is therefore determined by its centroid, which is located right in the center of the elements that constitute the cluster [9].

The K-means technique can be separated into the following four steps [10]:

1. K elements that form the initial K groups are randomly selected. The initial value of the center for each group k is Xi, at that moment this would be the only object that belongs to the group.
2. The elements must be assigned to the group, each element is assigned to the closest group, considering a distance measurement.
3. Once all the elements are located, the centroids of the K groups are calculated. These new centroids represent the average of the total number of objects assigned to the group.
4. Repeat steps 2 and 3 until there is no difference in reassignment of elements in other groups.

This algorithm always reaches an end, but there is not a guarantee of getting the optimal solution. It is recommended to run the algorithm several times to get optimal results.

15.2.5 HAVERSINE'S FORMULA

The measurement of the distance from one point to another on the earth's surface is affected by the curvature of the earth. Haversine's formula is a fundamental equation in navigation [11].

It is a formula to know the distance between two points considering that the earth is not a plane, but it is a plane of degree of curvature and has a radius of 6,271 km. To implement Haversine's formula, four variables must be known: the longitude and latitude of geographic point 1 and the longitude and latitude of geographic point 2 [12].

The Haversine formula is a procedure for calculating the distance determined conveniently and accurately from geographic points [10]. Haversine's formula is presented next:

$$d = 2r.arcsen\sqrt{sen^2\frac{\theta_2 - \theta_1}{2} + \cos\theta_1 . \cos 2.sen^2\frac{\varphi_2 - \varphi_1}{2}} \qquad (15.6)$$

where
> $r = 6271$ km
> θ *is latitude*
> φ *is longitude*

Latitude is the line that measures the distance between the north and south of the Earth from the equator line; longitude is a line that measures the distance between the west and east of the Earth from the main meridian line.

In Figure 15.2, the relationship between the latitude and longitude can be observed.

15.2.6 FIRST LEVEL OF HEALTHCARE IN AGUASCALIENTES STATE

The Health Services Institute of Aguascalientes State ISSEA has two levels of healthcare: the first level of healthcare is divided into three health jurisdictions; they are responsible for 89 health centers distributed throughout the state. The second level of care is composed of five general hospitals, eight mental healthcare centers, and two centers of hemodialysis [14].

This research uses information from the first level of healthcare and its three health jurisdictions. Health jurisdictions manage and distribute supplies, equipment, and medicines, as well as managing and monitoring the workforce of the health centers.

We will name health jurisdiction 1, health jurisdiction 2, and health jurisdiction 3 to the current jurisdiction locations in Aguascalientes state.

Health jurisdiction 1 is in the municipality of Aguascalientes and is responsible for the health centers that belong to the municipalities of Aguascalientes, Jesús María, El Llano, and San Francisco de los Romo.

Health jurisdiction 2 is in the Rincón de Romos municipality, and it is responsible for the health centers in the municipalities of Cosío, Tepezalá, San José de Gracia, Pabellón de Arteaga, and Asientos.

Health jurisdiction 3 is in Calvillo, and it is responsible for the health centers that belong to the municipality of Calvillo; Table 15.1 shows this information.

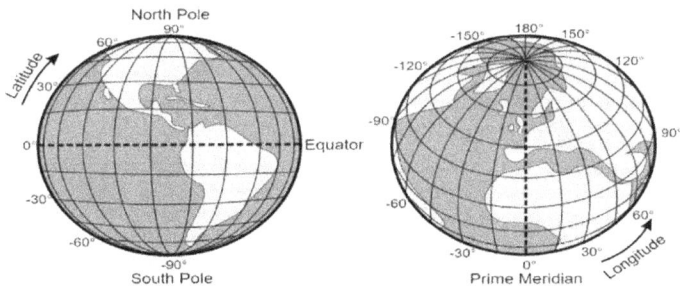

FIGURE 15.2   Hemisphere, latitude and longitude [13].

TABLE 15.1
Current Distribution of Units and Health Jurisdictions

Jurisdiction	Municipality	Units
1	Aguascalientes, Jesús María, El Llano, and San Francisco de los Romo	45
2	Cosío, Tepezalá, San José de Gracia, Pabellón de Arteaga, and Asientos	30
3	Calvillo	14
Total		**89**

In the history of Aguascalientes state, health jurisdictions have been added according to the growth of the number of health centers, but the distance from the health center to the jurisdictional office has not been considered.

15.2.7 Territorial Integration, Urban Environment, and Community Consultation System (SCITEL)

The National Institute of Statistics and Geography (INEGI) elaborates and provides the results of the 2020 Population and Housing Survey (2020 Survey), as well as the main results determined by Basic Geostatistical Areas (AGEB).

SCITEL is a dynamic consultation system that provides sociodemographic information national or by entity, based on the country's inhabited localities, AGEBs, and urban blocks [15].

The user of SCITEL can search sociodemographic indicators defined for the 2020 survey, as well as historical survey and intercensal information from 1990 to 2010.

SCITEL has a total of 221 indicators with the results of the characteristics of the population, houses for the AGEBs, and urban blocks of the country.

This system allows selecting indicators and geographic variables from a municipality or territorial demarcation level and even up to a locality level; the result of the query can be exported to Excel (XLSX) or CSV [15].

15.3 LITERATURE REVIEW

The literature review was performed by using bibliographic mining, where references of relevant articles were reviewed to extract the relevant sources in which the K-means technique, calculation of distances between geographic points with Haversine formula and studies that implemented the TOPSIS method were used and compared.

In the work of Hankir and Samar [16], the process of hierarchical analysis and TOPSIS is used to select the location of a plastics manufacturing plant in Alexandria, Egypt, in order to increase their productivity and grow their business; this work considers seven different locations of new land and facilities already prepared. These have their strengths and weaknesses, for there is a certain budget of money and features to meet, as well as a weighting for each criterion such as investment cost, availability of labor, energy, water, and transportation.

In this work, Analytic Hierarchy Process AHP method was used to evaluate the alternatives with the selected criteria, and TOPSIS was used to rank the alternatives with the intention of finding the ideal solution; these results were compared to obtain the best results.

This chapter concludes that the application of evaluating multiple decision factors with AHP and TOPSIS strategies allows a more adaptive use of existing data on possible locations in a facility siting problem.

Another interesting work was proposed by Senvar, Otay, and Bolturk [17], who present a model that included the CRITIC (Criteria Importance Through Intercriteria Correlation), TOPSIS (Technique for Order Preference by Similarity to Ideal Solution), EDAS (Evaluation based on Distance from Average Solution), and CODAS (Combinative Distance-based Assessment) methods; in this work a tool was created for effective decision-making of the alternatives for the location of a new hospital.

The CRITIC method was used to calculate the objective weights of the selection criteria to analyze the decision matrix and obtain all the information contained in the selection criteria. The TOPSIS, EDAS, and CODAS methods were implemented to rank the site alternatives for the proposed locations of the new hospital. The most fascinating and novel aspect of this study is the use of CRITIC in conjunction with the TOPSIS, EDAS, and CODAS techniques since these methods had not been used for hospital site selection problems.

The work concludes that the three methods offer advantages; the TOPSIS method has two advantages in terms of mathematical simplicity and flexibility for defining the set of options. The EDA method requires fewer calculations in comparison to other methods. Like the TOPSIS method, the EDAS method is also proficient solving complex decision-making problems.

Kuppersmith [18] developed an algorithm for drawing new neighborhood boundaries in urban areas that accurately evidence uniformity in spaces for some data sets. For simplicity, to measure reported crime cases using aggregate reported whole crime using available data such as census demographic data.

The available spatial data for the city was explored; this included data cleaning and processing, then an accurate grid representation was made, each of these small squares containing the information. A success metric was then defined using distance from the ground and standard deviation to measure the uniformity of crime within each of the 96 neighborhoods.

The first experiment of redrawing neighborhood boundaries using K-means clustering revealed several problems with this method. So, they proceeded to implement a new K-means algorithm with Haversine distances of geographic precision and vector distances of the available data.

This preliminary model leads to the proposal of the new algorithm, which uses the K-means structure with modified distance calculations to generate neighborhoods that are homogeneous and smoothly contiguous.

This research concludes that the model generates good and reproducible results, regarding the K-means algorithm, it is concluded that although the randomness of the centroid is imperfect, the result is consistent and high performance, particularly the final clustering model.

In the work of Ayah [19], a system is designed and implemented, which easily and accurately locates the nearest healthcare units in Sudan. With this system, the patient can get information about nearby healthcare units as, specifically, Sudan lacks information about healthcare units on the internet, and this lack of information has made the patient search for a long time on the location of nearby medical services. The author proposes a system that locates the nearest healthcare units by using a K-means clustering algorithm because this technique was selected for its ease, simplicity, ease of editing, and ease of improvement.

In another work where three multicriteria decision-making techniques are compared, the authors Niyazi and Tavakkoli [20] create the solution for the facility location problem; in this research the techniques of Additive Ratio Assessment (ARAS), Complex Proportional Assessment (COPRAS), and the Technique for Order of Preference by Similarity to Ideal Solution (TOPSIS) were implemented, in which the three techniques reach the same result, highlighting the TOPSIS technique over the other two techniques for the ease and simplicity of its implementation and execution.

Hartanto, Furqan, Siahaan, and Fitriani [12] developed an application to locate the nearest mosque to the user. This idea comes from the need of the Muslim community to locate the nearest mosque to their homes or workplaces, as they may have several options to locate the nearest mosque and even choose which one to attend; this problem is especially experienced by the immigrant Muslim community. For this application, they used Haversine's formula, which calculates the distance between geographical points. In this case, the application considers the distance between the user and the nearest mosques from which the user can choose which one to attend; the application provides information of the mosque, the location, and even the route to follow based on a Google Maps service.

Awotunde, Adeniyi, Ajagbe, Imoize, Oki, and Misra [21] present a work in which artificial intelligence can support medical decision-making, which is a challenging job, but through explainable artificial intelligence it is possible to achieve decision support systems to help improve patient well-being and improve the standard of care.

Among other studies employing Haversine distance calculation are two studies; the first one is by Syaripudin, Fauzi, Uriawan, Budiawan, and Rahman [22], which had the purpose to create an application to determine the nearest school based on the zoning system using the Haversine's formula as a calculation of the distance between school and home position, and the Location Based Service as a service to pinpoint the initial position using the Global Positioning System (GPS). The result of the research shows that the accuracy of this tool is 98% comparing its results with those of Google.

The second study was by Purnomo, Putra, Kusmara, Priatna, and Mukharom [23]. It was proposed to bring pet stores together with the population in the care and grooming of animals, particularly cats and dogs in the city of Bekasi. Using Haversine's formula to find the nearest pet store and, with the help of Google Maps API, a route to the pet store is determined from the app user. The result is an application called ZuPet that uses the waterfall methodology and Haversine's formula.

A summary of the literature review is presented in Table 15.2.

TABLE 15.2
Literature Review Summary

Published in	Paper Title	Authors	Techniques	Key Conclusions
2014	Solving a Facility Location Problem by Three Multi-Criteria Decision-Making Method.	• Nizary Moghaddam [20]	Additive Ratio Assessment ARAS Complex Proportional Assessment COPRAS Technique for Order of Preference by Similarity to Ideal Solution TOPSIS	Resolving a facility location selection problem while ranking the performance of three known MCDM methods: ARAS, COPRAS, and TOPSIS, which was performed in this investigation
2016	Hospital site selection with distance-based multi-criteria decision-making	• Senvar • Otay Bolturk [17]	Criteria Importance Through Intercriteria Correlation CRITIC. Technique for Order Preference by Similarity to Ideal Solution TOPSIS Evaluation based on Distance from Average Solution EDAS. Combine Distance-based Assessment CODAS	The principal target of this study is the selection of the best hospital location by taking into consideration the organization's needs. To reach this target, three distance-based MCDM methods are used
2017	Haversine Method in Looking for the Nearest Masjid	• Hartanto • Furqan • Siahaan [12]	Haversine formula	Haversine search is useful for locating nearby masjids, especially when Muslims are almost out of prayer time. The congregation can decide which masjid they will go to

(Continued)

TABLE 15.2 (Continued)
Literature Review Summary

Published in	Paper Title	Authors	Techniques	Key Conclusions
2018	Healthcare E-Guide System using K-means Clustering Algorithm.	• Saleh [24]	K-means clustering	The major goal we have achieved is to provide search for nearest healthcare center shortly and accurately. The system provides several search options to help patients to find what they need
2019	Geographic Clustering for Neighborhood. Boundaries: A Spatial Analysis of Chicago Using Public Data	Kuppersmith [18]	K-means clustering Haversine Formula	This research goes to produce a scientific process for re-drawing neighborhood boundaries in urban areas. More meaningful neighborhood design can help to facilitate more significant and insightful neighborhood-based studies and can help to differentiate a city into its key areas This can then provide a better understanding of cities and the driving factors of urban phenomena
2020	Facility Location Selection Using AHP and TOPSIS	• Hankir • Samak [16]	Analytic Hierarchy Process AHP Technique for Order of Preference by Similarity to Ideal Solution TOPSIS	The paper showed the use of AHP and TOPSIS methods to select the best area for a plastic manufacturing company to set another production line or to develop existing one among several options contemplating various criteria
2021	Haversine Formula Implementation to Determine Bandung City School Zoning Using Android Based Location Based Service	• Syaripudin • Fauzi • Uriawan • Budiawan • Rahman [22]	Haversine formula, Rational Unified Process (RUP)	Haversine Formula as the calculation of the distance between the school position and home, and the Location Based Service as the service to pinpoint the initial position using GPS

Published in	Paper Title	Authors	Techniques	Key Conclusions
2022	Explainable artificial intelligence (XAI) in medical decision support systems (MDSS)	• Awotunde • Adeniyi • Ajagbe • Imoize • Oki • Misra	Artificial Intelligence, Explainable Artificial Intelligence, Decision Support Systems	Develop decision support systems through explainable artificial intelligence and machine learning
2022	Haversine Formula to Find the Nearest Pet shop	• Purnomo • Putra • Kusmara • Priatna • Mukharom	Haversine formula	Find the nearest pet shop using Haversine's formula and, with the help of Google Maps API, a route to the pet shop

15.4 MATERIAL AND METHODS

15.4.1 CONCEPTUAL DESIGN

This research was based on a conceptual design, which is integrated by four main processes, as presented in Figure 15.3. The following steps are presented in order to research and obtain GPS points and general data of the health units.

1. K-means processing, obtaining four clusters and new centroid 4
2. Search of communities near to new centroid, selection of criteria, and data collection
3. Processing of criteria information by means of TOPSIS
4. Results and discussions

15.4.2 METHODOLOGY

These are the steps to follow in the methodology.

a. Obtaining the location of the jurisdictions, municipal capitals, and health centers that will be centroids and individuals
b. Specification of GPS coordinates (latitude and longitude) of each fixed centroid, ISSEA units, and determination of the initial positions of the mobile centroids
c. Design and development of database for storage of GPS location points and general data of ISSEA units and patient data
d. Import of GPS data information from ISSEA units and centroids into the database
e. Processing of the information through the modified K-means algorithm developed for clustering
f. Proposal of communities close to the geographic position point determined by the modified K-means algorithm
g. Obtaining and researching information of interest from the communities proposed to establish the new Health Jurisdiction 4
h. Implementation of TOPSIS for intelligent multi-criteria selection through in-formation processing of the proposed communities to establish the new Sanitary Jurisdiction 4
i. Discussion of results

This research implements a methodology presented in Figure 15.4.

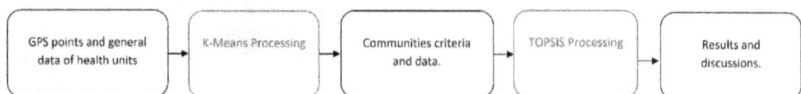

FIGURE 15.3 Conceptual design.

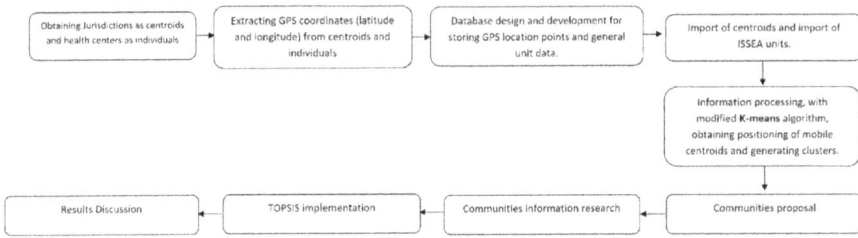

FIGURE 15.4 Methodology.

15.4.3 DATA COLLECTION

To obtain general data from the health centers and totals of patients who belong to these centers, ISSEA provided access to the information in each of the databases by performing programmed tasks to obtain the most recent and current information.

The process of obtaining, collecting, and processing data from the 89 ISSEA health centers is detailed as follows.

1. Development, design, and creation of the database Datos_recoleccion in MS SQL Server [4].
2. Development and design of tables to contain the collection of data in the database Datos_recoleccion.
3. Development and testing in a test database of queries of the required data to be collected.
4. Development of script for the insertion and update of data obtained by the queries in the file Datosrecoleccion.sql.
5. Scheduling collection tasks in MS SQL Server through the execution of scheduled tasks and data transformation services (DTS), which are executed in each restoration of the databases of the 89 health units of the ISSEA. These restores are performed automatically on weekdays, through dedicated links.
6. Review of confirmation of execution of scheduled tasks and execution data, transfer rate, percentages, statistics, etc.
7. Review of the data inserted or updated daily in the tables of Datos_recoleccion.

15.4.4 SCITEL DATA COLLECTION

Information on multiple criteria was obtained through the SCITEL, which will be used for the TOPSIS technique, the SCITEL data were obtained in the following way:

1. Access SCITEL at www.inegi.org.mx/app/scitel/Default?ev=9.
2. Select the state to query, this system includes the 32 states of the republic to select.

3. Select the desired variables, SCITEL allows the selection of 57 variables out of a total of 277, which are organized by the following groups: geographic identification, population, age and sex structure, fertility, migration, ethnicity, disability, education, economic characteristics, health services, marital status, religion, census homes, and housing.
4. Apply the filter for each desired variable. In this step, specialized filters can be selected for each of the selected variables with relational operators such as greater than, greater than and equal to, less than, less than and equal to, and equal to or different from.
5. Export filtered information, in this part, an initial accumulation of the total data to be exported is generated.
6. If information from another location is required, repeat from step 4.
7. Export the whole result of the queries to Excel (.xlsx) or Csv (.csv) format.

15.5   RESULTS

15.5.1   Processing Clustering Software Framework

As a result, an information processing clustering software framework was created, which is formed by two techniques, one of them is K-means with which the geographical position of the health jurisdiction 4 will be located, and the TOPSIS technique to intelligently select the location with the best characteristics. This framework is composed of the following steps:

1. Importing centroids and ISSEA units.
2. K-means:
   a. Creation of the distance matrix by calculating distances with the Haversine formula.
   b. Group matrix creation.
   c. Positioning of fixed centroids.
   d. Group matrix ordering by shortest distance.
   e. Calculation of new centroid position.
   f. Repeat from a–e until there are no differences in the previous group matrix.
3. Obtaining new centroids of K Groups.
4. TOPSIS:
   a. Locations are proposed, criteria are researched, information is discretized, and an expert is consulted to determine the weights of each of the criteria.
   b. The decision matrix is created.
   c. Normalized matrix is created.
   d. Weight matrix is created.
   e. Positive and negative ideal solutions are generated and analyzed.
   f. Relative closeness is calculated and analyzed.
   g. Ranking of solutions is performed.
5. Results are analyzed and discussed.

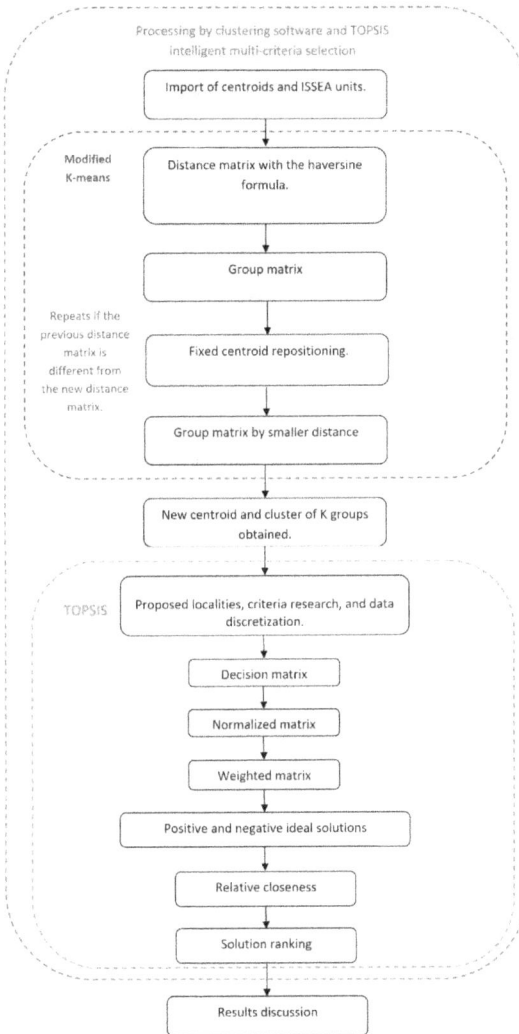

FIGURE 15.5 Information processing framework.

The design, development, and implementation of the information processing framework are presented in Figure 15.5.

15.5.2 MODIFIED K-MEANS ALGORITHM FOR FIXED AND MOBILE CENTERS

One of the results of this research is the implementation of the modified K-means algorithm for fixed and mobile centroids that are mentioned in [25] and shown next.

Modified K-means algorithm.
M = total centroids
n = variable centroids

1. GET individuals.
2. GET fixed and mobile centroids.
3. WHILE the previous group matrix differs with the new group matrix.
   a. CLEAN matrix of previous groups with zeros.
   b. CLEAN matrix of new centroids.
   c. TRAVEL all the lines of individuals and COMPARE with centroids and GENERATE a matrix of resulting distances.
   d. READ all the distance lines and COMPARE which is the smallest and GENERATE a new group matrix.
   e. SET 1-m fixed centroids.
   f. READ all the lines of groups (m + 1) -n and ADD the ones that are 1 in their respective individuals and GENERATE a new position of mobile centroids.
4. IF, the previous group matrix is different from the new group matrix.
5. YES.
   a. CLEAN new group matrix with zeros.
   b. EQUALS matrix of previous centroids to matrix of new centroids.
   c. CLEAN matrix of new centroids.
   d. REPEAT 3 and 4.
6. NO.
   a. ENDS.

15.5.3 NEW HEALTH JURISDICTION 4 HEALTH CENTERS DISTRIBUTION

Currently, 89 health centers take care of a total of 658,904 registered patients distributed as shown in Table 15.3.

Figure 15.6 shows the current distribution of health centers in each jurisdiction, in blue those belonging to jurisdiction 1; in red those belonging to jurisdiction 2; and in purple those belonging to jurisdiction 3.

TABLE 15.3
Actual Population Distribution

Jurisdiction	Units	Pre-diabetics	Diabetics	Total, Patients
I	45	25,430	26,933	461,058
II	30	8,172	8,177	126,633
III	14	6,812	6,103	71,213
All	89	40,414	41,213	658,904

The proposed distribution for registered patients for each of the jurisdictions would be redistributed as shown in Table 15.4.

Figure 15.7 shows the proposed distribution of the 89 health centers in 4 jurisdictions: in blue, those belonging to jurisdiction 1; in red, those belonging to jurisdiction 2; in purple, those belonging to jurisdiction 3; and in green, those belonging to the called health jurisdiction 4.

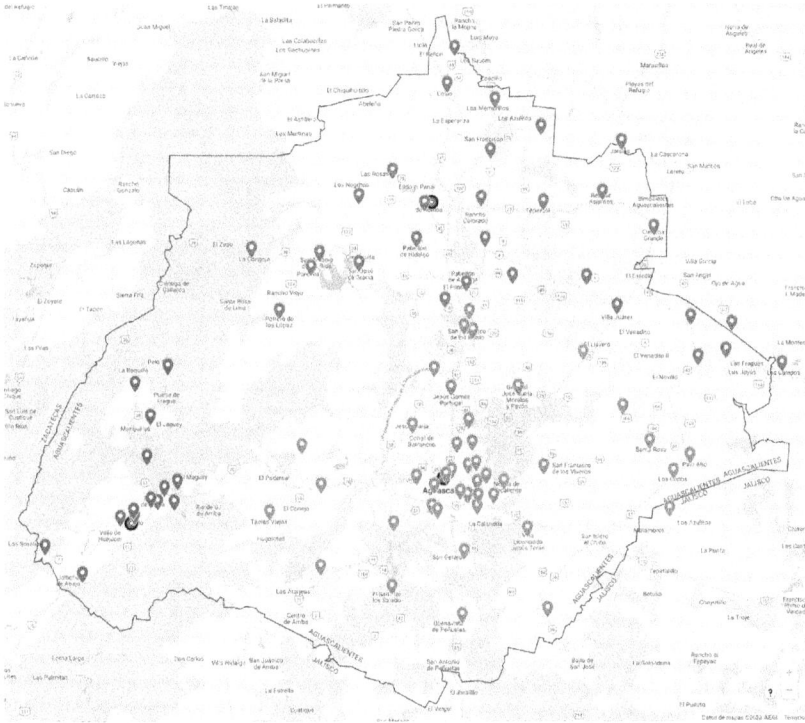

FIGURE 15.6   Current distribution and location of ISSEA health centers.

TABLE 15.4
Proposed Population Distribution

Jurisdiction	Units	Pre-diabetics	Diabetics	Total, Patients
I	35	23,868	25,105	430,463
II	26	6,609	6,530	91,660
III	14	6,812	6,103	71,213
IV	14	3,125	3,475	65,568
All	**89**	**40,414**	**41,213**	**658,904**

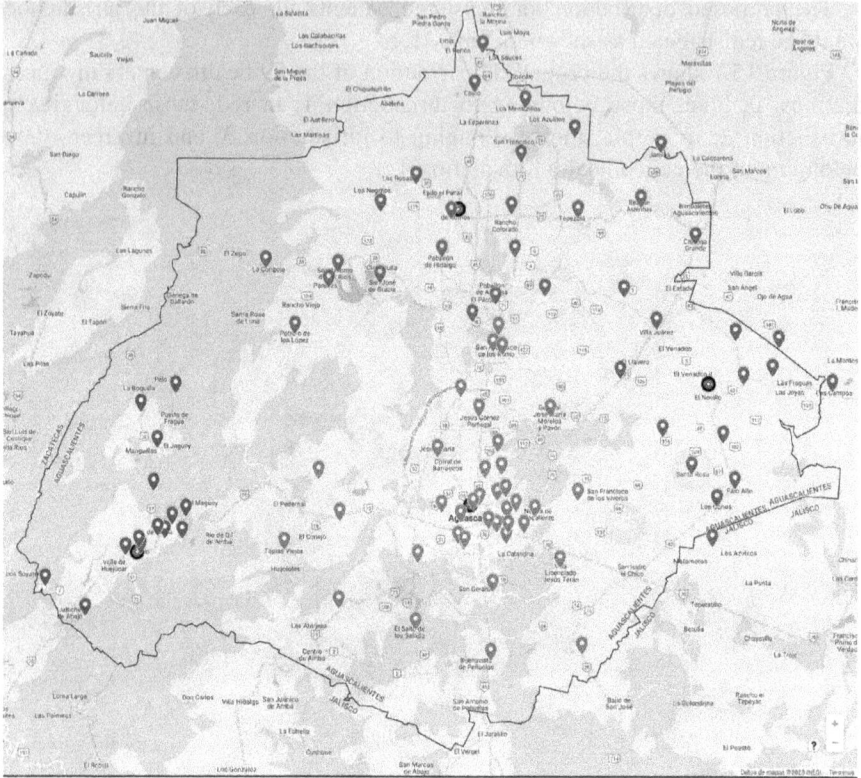

FIGURE 15.7 New clustering proposed of ISSEA health centers.

As a result of the algorithm, the inclusion of health jurisdiction four as a new centroid was proposed, thus having four clusters in total, The distance from the point of the new sanitary jurisdiction 4 that was determined by the algorithm was the position (22.037063, -102.003551) that we will call the point of attention or POA to the nearby communities with the necessary services to operate a Jurisdictional office.

This research has the support of a master's in urban planning who selected six nearby localities (10 km max distance) and the important variables to be used in the TOPSIS, the localities are listed in Table 15.5.

15.5.4 TOPSIS VARIABLES AND PROCESS

The following is the list of variables used in the multi-criteria analysis; some variables were extracted from SCITEL, and others were generated from the instructions of the expert in urban planning to support the research.

TABLE 15.5
Eligible Localities

Number	Locality	Municipality
1	El Terremoto	El Llano
2	La Luz	El Llano
3	Santa Rosa	El Llano
4	Lic. Jesús Teran	El Llano
5	Pilotos	Asientos
6	Amarillas de Esparza	Asientos

1. *Total inhabitants*: A scale of total inhabitants based on territorial information provided and determined by the INEGI.
2. *Number of houses*: A scale of the total number of houses related to the number of inhabitants and territorial information in the locality.
3. *Electricity service*: A portion determined by the number of houses with electricity service and land area information of the locality.
4. *Drainage service*: Rate of the number of housing units with drainage and sewage service.
5. *Potable water service*: Scale of the number of households that have potable water service related to land area information.
6. *Population with health services*: It is a ranking of the locality based on the number of people who have some type of health service.
7. *Size of locality*: It is a portion of the scale of localities determined by INEGI.
8. *Road distance*: It is the measurement of distance by road, the total sum of the locality to its health centers of responsibility.
9. *Linear distance*: It is the linear distance measurement, total sum of the locality to all its health centers of responsibility.
10. *Roads and highways*: It is a scale ranking based on the roads and highways inter-connected to the locality.
11. *Existence of ISSEA infrastructure*: This variable determines whether there is a health center or ISSEA building to establish the new health jurisdiction 4.

In this research, the TOPSIS analysis technique was applied, by which a classification was made according to the criteria that were proposed at the beginning together with the weight of each of them that were selected by the expert about urbanization and on these considerations a series of steps were made to achieve a rating that would give us the ideal solution to the problem.

Tables 15.6 and 15.7 present the data obtained from catalogs determined by INEGI as well as from SCITEL data qualified by the urban planning expert; this table includes the weights determined for each characteristic.

TABLE 15.6
Criteria Decision Matrix 1

Number	Locality Name	1. Total Inhabitants	2. Number of Houses	3. Electricity Service	4. Drainage Service	5. Potable Water Service	6. Population with Health Services
1	El Terremoto	6	7	6	5	7	6
2	La Luz	5	5	7	5	5	7
3	Santa Rosa	7	5	9	7	5	9
4	Licenciado Jesús Terán	6	7	5	6	7	5
5	Pilotos	8	7	9	8	7	9
6	Amarillas de Esparza	7	6	5	7	6	5
	Weight	**0.10**	**0.20**	**0.05**	**0.05**	**0.05**	**0.05**

TABLE 15.7
Criteria Decision Matrix 2

Number	Locality Name	7. Size of Locality	8. Road Distance	9. Linear Distance	10. Roads and Highways	11. Existence of ISSEA Infrastructure
1	El Terremoto	5	7	6	5	7
2	La Luz	5	5	7	5	5
3	Santa Rosa	7	5	9	7	5
4	Licenciado Jesús Terán	6	7	5	6	7
5	Pilotos	8	7	9	8	7
6	Amarillas de Esparza	7	6	5	7	6
	Weight	0.10	0.10	0.10	0.10	0.10

The first step to obtain the values given by TOPSIS is to identify the values assigned to the criteria, so the proposed values must be normalized to obtain a measure of the correct value, then we proceeded to evaluate with the weight given by the urban planning expert and obtain a matrix with the same values already normalized in all the criteria, which is presented in Tables 15.8 and 15.9.

Once we created the normalized matrix with the corresponding weights, the next step in the TOPSIS technique finds the positive ideal solution and the anti-ideal solution, this matrix is shown in Tables 15.10 and 15.11.

Then we obtained the proximity related to the absolute solution, which is shown in Table 15.12.

Finally, Table 15.13 shows the results obtained in the last step of implementing TOPSIS, which was the creation of the ranking list of solutions.

15.6   DISCUSSIONS

It is important to mention that the inclusion of a new jurisdiction is feasible since the distance between the health jurisdiction and its health centers will be reduced by at least half, and more than 65,000 patients will be assisted. More than 3,000 patients with confirmed diabetes and more than 3,000 patients with prediabetes will be cared for, which is important considering that diabetes mellitus was the ninth leading cause of mortality worldwide in 2019 according to the World Health Organization [26] and the second cause of death in Mexico from January to August 2020 (99,733 deaths), with a national rate of 7.8 and a state rate of 5.8 and a state rate of 5.5. 8 and a state rate of 5.2 deaths per 10,000 inhabitants [27], and second cause in general mortality in Aguascalientes in 2018, with 14.67% of total deaths according to the Government of the State of Aguascalientes [28].

By including health jurisdiction 4, 30,595 patients from health jurisdiction 1 and 34,973 from health jurisdiction 2 will be attended, reducing the workload of health jurisdictions 1 and 2 by 5.5% and 27%, respectively.

In the analysis of the possible localities to establish health jurisdiction 4, it is concluded that there is no restriction rule on the position of the jurisdictional office; however, it was found that the conformation of a health jurisdiction is determined by regionalization, in order to plan the provision of services, provide the optimal use of resources, and respond to the particular healthcare needs [29] so the TOPSIS technique was determinant to select the locality.

It can be concluded that the weights for each characteristic in TOPSIS were given by the urban planning expert and through the advice of the urban planning expert, a level of importance was established for the characteristics analyzed by TOPSIS:

- *Total inhabitants*: This characteristic has a dynamic and depends on two factors: natural and social, which are birth and mortality as well as migration. The size of the population has four basic parameters: birth, mortality, emigration, and immigration. Additionally, several secondary characteristics of the population can be determined, such as the sex ratio, age distribution, spatial distribution pattern, etc. The size of the locality is determined by the ratio of population and territorial size; commonly this variable is

TABLE 15.8
Normalized Matrix 1

Number	Locality Name	1. Inhabitants	2. Number of Houses	3. Electricity Service	4. Drainage Service	5. Potable Water Service	6. Health Services
1	El Terremoto	0.3728	0.4586	0.3482	0.3175	0.4586	0.3482
2	La Luz	0.3107	0.3276	0.4062	0.3175	0.3276	0.4062
3	Santa Rosa	0.4350	0.3276	0.5222	0.4445	0.3276	0.5222
4	Licenciado Jesús Terán	0.3728	0.4586	0.2901	0.3810	0.4586	0.2901
5	Pilotos	0.4971	0.4586	0.5222	0.5080	0.4586	0.5222
6	Amarillas de Esparza	0.4350	0.3931	0.2901	0.4445	0.3931	0.2901

TABLE 15.9
Normalized Matrix 2

Number	Locality Name	7. Size of Locality	8. Road Distance	9. Linear Distance	10. Roads and Highways	11. ISSEA Infrastructure
1	El Terremoto	0.3175	0.4586	0.3482	0.3175	0.4586
2	La Luz	0.3175	0.3276	0.4062	0.3175	0.3276
3	Santa Rosa	0.4445	0.3276	0.5222	0.4445	0.3276
4	Licenciado Jesús Terán	0.3810	0.4586	0.2901	0.3810	0.4586
5	Pilotos	0.5080	0.4586	0.5222	0.5080	0.4586
6	Amarillas de Esparza	0.4445	0.3931	0.2901	0.4445	0.3931

TABLE 15.10
Positive Ideal Solution and Anti-Ideal Solution Matrix 1

Concept	1. Inhabitants	2. Number of Houses	3. Electricity Service	4. Drainage Service	5. Potable Water Service	6. Health Services
V+	0.0497	0.0917	0.0261	0.0254	0.0229	0.0261
V-	0.0311	0.0655	0.0145	0.0159	0.0164	0.0145

TABLE 15.11
Positive Ideal Solution and Anti-Ideal Solution Matrix 2

Concept	7. Size of Locality	8. Road Distance	9. Linear Distance	10. Roads and Highways	11. ISSEA Infrastructure
V+	0.0508	0.0459	0.0522	0.0318	0.0459
V-	0.0318	0.0328	0.0290	0.0508	0.0328

TABLE 15.12
Related Proximity to the Absolute Solution Matrix

Number	Locality Name	+SOL	-SOL	RP
1	El Terremoto	0.0326	0.0005	0.0150
2	La Luz	0.0456	0.0008	0.0182
3	Santa Rosa	0.0364	0.0008	0.0213
4	Licenciado Jesús Terán	0.0347	0.0003	0.0079
5	Pilotos	0.0191	0.0006	0.0323
6	Amarillas de Esparza	0.0364	0.0000	0.0000

TABLE 15.13
Ranking List of Solutions

Number	Locality Name	Solution Ranking
1	El Terremoto	4
2	La Luz	3
3	Santa Rosa	2
4	Licenciado Jesús Terán	5
5	Pilotos	1
6	Amarillas de Esparza	6

linked to better job opportunities and access to services, and number of houses.

- *Roads and highways*: Sum of linear and road distances, in this case of distances based on the principle of centrality of Christaller's theory [30] in which urban spaces that provide certain services to the population of a peripheral area in a space are distributed and classified.
- *The population with electricity, drainage, drinking water, and health services*: Since only together and not separately, they determine the consolidation of the locality [31]; these characteristics are commonly linked to dependence on population size and community size and territorial dispersion, characteristics that are considered to be more important [32].

15.7 CONCLUSIONS

By integrating tools such as K-means and multi-criteria selection techniques in industry 4.0 applied in the health sector, health centers will bring together each and every one of the factors that involve challenges starting with complicated logistics in time and form, in addition to diverse processes with different demands, with different levels of complexity of protocols, to function in an organized, efficient way, with a point of view of improving care in terms of quality, early detection of pathologies, and cost reduction.

Based on the results obtained, it can be concluded that the modified K-means algorithm is a solid tool that can be conditioned to different conditions for distribution and clustering. In this research, it was adapted to work with fixed and mobile centroids due to the nature of the problem, and a very positive result was obtained.

It is concluded that given the characteristics of the locality of Pilotos, municipality of Asientos, it is the ideal locality since unlike the other possible localities, it has a population of more than 1,000 people, has the basic services (electricity, water, drainage, telephone) necessary to operate a jurisdiction, has road access through federal highway 43, and also has a health center currently operating, with the facilities to be able to establish the health jurisdiction 4.

It is important to mention that this research is a proposal based on available and freely accessible data, since it is not possible to access information on operating expenses and budgets of health centers and health jurisdictions.

For future work and to experiment with different results, we are considering to use more than one variable centroid to integrate and geographically locate other new jurisdictions in the state, in addition to the comparison of results with other exhaustive search techniques like Gaussian Mixture Model or Density-Based Spatial Clustering of Applications with Noise (DBSCAN) techniques.

REFERENCES

[1] C. Díaz de León Castañeda and J. Góngora Ortega, *eSalud en servicios de salud públicos en México: estudio de caso*, 32nd ed., vol. 32. Aguascalientes: región y sociedad, 2020.

[2]   E. Maria, E. Budiman, Haviluddin, and M. Taruk, "Measure distance locating nearest public facilities using Haversine and Euclidean Methods," *J. Phys. Conf. Ser.*, vol. 1450, no. 1, 2020, doi:10.1088/1742-6596/1450/1/012080.

[3]   E. Triantaphyllou, "Multi-criteria decision making methods," pp. 5–21, 2000, doi:10.1007/ 978-1-4757-3157-6_2.

[4]   D. L. Olson, "Comparison of weights in TOPSIS models," *Math. Comput. Model.*, vol. 40, no. 7–8, pp. 721–727, 2004, doi:10.1016/j.mcm.2004.10.003.

[5]   A. Ishizaka and P. Nemery, "Topsis," in Multi-Criteria Decision Analysis: Methods and Software, vol. 1, West Sussex: John Wiley & Sons, Ltd, 2013, pp. 213–221.

[6]   K. P. Yoon and C.-L. Hwang, "Multiple Attribute Decision Making," in Methods for Qualitative Data, Thousand Oaks, California: SAGE Publications Inc., 1995, p. 23

[7]   A. Kolios, V. Mytilinou, E. Lozano-Minguez, and K. Salonitis, "A comparative study of multiple-criteria decision-making methods under stochastic inputs," *Energies*, vol. 9, no. 7, pp. 1–21, 2016, doi:10.3390/en9070566.

[8]   F. H. Salcedo López, "Minería de Datos para segmentación de clientes en la empresa tecnológica Master PC," p. 184, 2015 [Online]. Available: http://dspace.unl.edu.ec/jspui/ bitstream/123456789/10462/1/Chamba Jiménez%2C Sairy Fernanda.pdf.

[9]   Z. Mamani, "Aplicación de la minería de datos distribuida usando algoritmo de clustering K-means para mejorar la calidad de servicios de las organizaciones modernas," Universidad Nacional Mayor de San Marcos, 2015.

[10] F. A. Cifuentes Ramos, "Clasificación automática de Tweets utilizando K-NN y K-Means como algoritmos de clasificación automática, aplicando TF-IDF y TF-RFL para las ponderaciones," Pontificia Universidad Católica de Valparaíso, 2016. *Informática*, 2016.

[11] N. Chopde and M. Nichat, "Landmark based shortest path detection by using A* and haversine formula," *GH Raisoni Coll. Eng.*, vol. 1, no. 2, pp. 298–302, 2013, [Online]. Available: www.ijircce.com/upload/2013/april/17_V1204030_Landmark_H.pdf.

[12] S. Hartanto, M. Furqan, A. Putera, U. Siahaan, and W. Fitriani, "Haversine method in looking for the nearest masjid," *Int. J. Recent Trends Eng. Res.*, vol. 3, no. 8, pp. 187–195, 2017, doi:10.23883/ijrter.2017.3402.pd61h.

[13] Wikipedia, "Coordenadas geográficas," 2016. Available: https://es.wikipedia.org/wiki/ Coordenadas_geográficas.

[14] D. Administrativo, "Primer Nivel de Atención," 2020. Available: www.aguascalientes. gob.mx/isea/prinivel.html.

[15] INEGI, "Sistema de Consulta De Integración Territorial Scitel," *INEGI*, vol. 1, no. 1, p. 26, 2020.

[16] M. Hankir and O. Samak, "Facility Location Selection Using AHP and TOPSIS." Abdullah Gul University, Kayseri, Turquía, p. 17, 2020, doi: 10.13140/RG.2.2.22879.07849.

[17] O. Senvar, I. Otay, and E. Bolturk, "Hospital site selection via hesitant fuzzy topsis," *IFAC-Papers on Line*, vol. 49, no. 12, pp. 1140–1145, 2016, doi:10.1016/j.ifacol.2016.07.656.

[18] J. B. Kuppersmith, *Geographic Clustering for Neighborhood Boundaries: A Spatial Analysis of Chicago Using Public Data*. Cambridge, MA: Harvard University Press, 2019.

[19] Y. A. Mohamed, "Healthcare E-Guide System using K-means Clustering Algorithm اكلا - محروا ُ تجمعي نظام ماظن لليلدا لإلكترونيد للرعايا زكارمل الصحيا ةياحصلا مادختساب خوارزميا ةيمزراوخ," Sudan University of Science and Technology, 2018.

[20] M. Niyazi and R. Tavakkoli-Moghaddam, "Solving a facility location problem by three multi-criteria decision making methods," *Int. J. Res. Ind. Eng.*, vol. 3, no. 4, pp. 41–56, 2014.

[21] J. Bamidele Awotunde, E. A. Adeniyi, S. A. Ajagbe, A. L. Imoize, O. A. Oki, and S. Misra, "Explainable artificial intelligence (XAI) in medical decision support systems (MDSS): applicability, prospects, legal implications, and challenges," in Explainable Artificial Intelligence in Medical Decision Support Systems, First edit., Institution of Engineering and Technology, 2023, p. 545.

[22] U. Syaripudin, N. Fauzi, W. Uriawan, W. Z, and A. Rahman, "Haversine formula implementation to determine bandung city school zoning using android based location based service," *Eur. Alliance Innov.*, vol. 11, p. 11, 2021, doi:10.4108/eai.11-7-2019.2303558.

[23] R. Purnomo, T. D. Putra, H. Kusmara, W. Priatna, and F. Mukharom, "Haversine formula to find the nearest petshop," *JATISI (Jurnal Tek. Inform. dan Sist. Informasi)*, vol. 9, no. 3, pp. 2205–2221, 2022, doi:10.35957/jatisi.v9i3.2434.

[24] B. Zhou et al., "Worldwide trends in diabetes since 1980: A pooled analysis of 751 population-based studies with 4.4 million participants," *Lancet*, vol. 387, no. 10027, pp. 1513–1530, 2016, doi:10.1016/S0140-6736(16)00618-8.

[25] P. Rodríguez de León, M. D. Torres Soto, A. Torres Soto, and E. E. Ponce de León Sentí, "Proposals for Grouping Health Centers and Health Jurisdictions in the State of Aguascalientes Using Haversine Distance and K-Means Algorithm," *Res. Comput. Sci.*, vol. 150, no. 9, p. 12, 2021, [Online]. Available: https://rcs.cic.ipn.mx/.

[26] World Health Organization, "Diabetes notas descriptivas," *Notas Descriptivas*, 2021. Available: www.who.int/es/news-room/fact-sheets/detail/diabetes.

[27] Instituto Nacional de Estadística y Geografía, "Características de las defunciones registradas en México durante enero a agosto de 2020 [Comunicado de prensa]," vol. 1, no. 2, p. 45, 2021 [Online]. Available: www.inegi.org.mx/contenidos/saladeprensa/boletines/2021/EstSociodemo/DefuncionesRegistradas2020_Pnles.pdf.

[28] Gobierno del Estado de Aguascalientes, "Informe de Gobierno del Estado de Aguascalientes 2019.," vol. 1, no. 1. Gobierno del Estado de Aguascalientes, Aguascalientes, p. 183, 2019, [Online]. Available: https://www.aguascalientes.gob.mx/cplap/Docs/datos/DATOS.pdf.

[29] P. Ejecutivo and D. E. L. Estado, "Manual de organización tipo de jurisdicción sanitaria," *Gac. del Gob.*, no. 308, p. 40, 2011.

[30] L. G. B. Valbuena, "Microeconomics approaches in the christaller's central places theory," *Ensayos Sobre Polit. Econ.*, vol. 31, no. 70, pp. 67–120, 2013.

[31] G. F. Cuesta, "Problemas teóricos sobre la definición de unidades espaciales de análisis," *Ería*, pp. 213–225, 1985 [Online]. Available: www.uniovied.net/reunido/index.php/RCG/article/download/907/837%5Cnhttps://onedrive.live.com/edit.aspx/Documentos2/Doctorado?cid=14f67daccc40b137&id=documents?&wd=target(Papers/Er?a.one%7CD72C4EE8-18E7-45CF-8314-7A4FBA3714E3/Problemas te?ricos sob.

[32] Secretaria Distrital de Desarrollo Económico, "Diagnóstico: ALTERNATIVAS DE LA POBLACIÓN RURAL EN POBREZA PARA GENERAR INGRESOS SOSTENIBLES," vol. 1. SECRETARÍA DE DESARROLLO SOCIAL 1, Aguascalientes, p. 49, 2010, [Online]. Available: https://docplayer.es/5150587-Diagnostico-alternativas-de-la-poblacion-rural-en-pobreza-para-generar-ingresos-sostenibles.html.

16 AIoMT Training, Testing, and Validation

*Vitalis Afebuame Iguoba and
Agbotiname Lucky Imoize*

16.1 INTRODUCTION

Through artificial intelligence (AI), computers are powered to carry out a task that requires human intelligence. This application cuts across science and the engineering domain. Considering scientific competitions like ImageNet's large-scale visual recognition proves that computers exhibit human-like image recognition competence. Much recent research has proven that AI can perform diagnostics on medical images at a similar level to experienced clinicians [1]. Machine learning and deep learning algorithms have provided the current development and improved workflows in radiology or offered vital assistance to the radiologists by helping with tasks automation like medical imaging qualification, and prioritizing the radiologist work list is part of the workflow improvements [2].

Inter-connected networks of medical devices enable healthcare monitoring. Machine learning is the algorithm of artificial intelligence, and interfacial sensors provide autonomous healthcare service without human intervention Via IoMT devices. The provision of remote access, process, and the transmission of medical data through a secured network is known as IoMT technology. This provides patients with a connection with clinicians in a medical device. The IoMT technology aims to reduce the non-required hospital visits and stays, which also minimizes healthcare costs by providing wireless monitoring of the essential health parameters [3].

Healthcare is being revolutionized by the recent advances in artificial intelligence (AI), 3D printing, robotics, nanotechnology, etc. The new digital healthcare system offers numerous advantages, including reducing human errors, improving clinical procedures, and large data generation and tracking. The diagnosis and treatments of various diseases, proper medical record keeping, and new optimized clinical outlooks were facilitated by AI methods from machine learning (ML) and deep learning (DL) [4]. Randomized controlled trials (RCTs) usually provide a wider evaluation of diagnosis or treatment procedures. RCTs are a new concept in AI. Despite the different training, validation, and testing steps available for AI tool development, the standard recommendations for the AI—tools used for diagnostic and predictive modeling in the biomedical setting are not available [5]. Nowadays, artificial AI and machine learning have provided a wide range of applications, such as robot control, game playing, software bugs, aid handicaps, enhanced student learning, and hacker detection [6].

DOI: 10.1201/9781003370321-16

Machine learning, or "statistical learning," involves collecting regression and classification techniques for predictive analytics. The prediction of quantitative data is called regression, while classification is when categorical data are predicted [7]. The machine learning (ML) domain is the meeting point of computer science and statistics. ML identifies patterns from a large dataset and is used to predict numerous outcomes from unseen data. Some application of machine learning [ML] in medicine is effectively predicting the diagnosis and prognosis of numerous diseases using clinical data [9]. The choice of any validation method is essential in analyzing the outcome of predictive models in machines considering comparable small data samples [10]. As the applications of AI continue to penetrate more domains in human existence, a huge challenge is also posed by it in both economic and regulatory terms [12]. The technical reproducibility method involves precisely implementing the computational steps (using the same code, dataset, etc.) to obtain the results as reported [13].

Big data is a new innovative technology aimed to modernize the traditional healthcare system and further improve the current healthcare system. Other data sources include mobile phones, body area sensors, patients, hospitals, researchers, healthcare providers, and other organizations currently responsible for generating a large volume of medical data [14]. The interpretation of medical information is a hugely challenging task. This applies to experienced medical practitioners and young doctors with little experience. Due to the limited clinicians' available time, new diseases are evolving, patient dynamics are changing with time, and the diagnostics process is becoming more complex. An accurate diagnostic process can provide timely treatment and adequate patient care [18].

These aim to improve the current benchmarks using deep convolutional networks to actualize the available computer vision tasks. In Figure 16.1, an AI model is presented, indicating the importance of data training, testing, and validation on the overall performance of an AI model. The performance difference exhibited by a model when evaluated concerning the previously seen data (training data) and testing data is called generalizability. Overfitting of the training data occurs due to poor generalizability. A plot of the training versus validation accuracy at any epoch during training provides the overfitting condition. Data augmentation, which is survey-based, is not the only technique available to checkmate overfitting [19]. Many real-world tasks are characterized by probabilistic and uncertain data that is difficult to comprehend and process by humans. Machine learning and knowledge extraction help turn abstract information into useful information to realize various applications like image recognition, scene understanding, decision-support systems, and so on [21]. The innovation in computer applications has resulted in natural language processing. A computer can now respond to human inquiry, and its ability to decipher and translate human language is termed natural language processing [25, 26].

16.1.1 Key Contribution of the Chapter

The following are the significant contributions of this chapter:

  i. Examined the key challenges of big data in AI performance improvement
  ii. Outlined the procedures for model training, testing, and validation and their emerging challenges

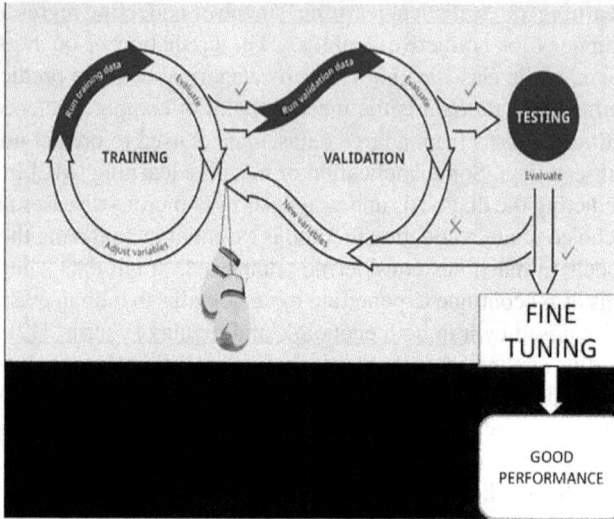

FIGURE 16.1   Model for AI data training, validation, and testing.

   iii. Highlighted some key applications of AI in the healthcare domain
   iv. Outlined some AI prediction algorithms and models.

16.1.2   CHAPTER ORGANIZATION

Section 16.2 presents the related works on the Artificial Intelligence of the Internet of Medical Things (AIoMT). Section 16.3 presents AIoMT training. Section 16.4 presents AIoMT testing. Section 16.5 presents AIoMT validation. Section 16.6 presents discussions and lessons learned, and Section 16.7 presents the conclusion and future scope.

16.2   RELATED WORK

Machine learning (ML) is not new. Algorithms like Fischer's linear discriminate analysis existed back in 1936. Later, several other models existed, such as the generalized linear models in the 1970s, and numerous non-linear algorithms like classification and regression trees emerged in the 1980s. These innovations' advantages are increased computation power, calculation power, memory storage, and available data [8]. The author evaluates the impacts of train test split variation stability of machine learning (ML) model performance in a series of validation techniques, considering only two real-world cardiovascular imaging data sets. This study focuses on the split variation methods, providing the highest range of AUC and noticeable statistical differences. Still, this approach's limitation is the high-performance instability [10]. It deals with the three central risks of AI training data: data, quality, discrimination, and innovation [11]. The author in [13] reviewed and summarized the impacts of big data and related techniques, highlighting the available standards and AI technologies for big data and the future direction for the next generation of AI.

In April 2021, European Union (EU) Commission published its proposals for an artificial intelligence act (AIA). It properly highlighted the important problems encountered in AI system applications or in relation to the EU. Article 10 of the AIA proposes a governing authority for training, validation, and test data (termed training data) used to realize AI systems with high risk [1]. The expansion of the Internet of Things (IoT) and the availability of "Big Data" have enabled the emergence of new AI tool applicants to increase its adoption [15]. The author considered the limitations of quantitative surveys as follows: first, by refusing to demand quantitative predictions of AI experts. Second, AI expertise diversification in their sample size, expanding the notion of AI experts relevant to AI, such as neuroscience, cognitive science, philosophy, and mathematics. Third, evaluation of expert disagreement considering extraction of reasons and arguments. In [16], the authors described the existing relationship between AI and neuroscience. More recently, this interaction seems less common, as both subjects have recorded much growth and disciplinary boundaries have solidified.

In [17], Chuanqi et al. suggested the Public Road Urban Drivers (PROUD) test was carried out from the University campus in Parma to the town Centre using different scenarios, such as urban, rural, and highway roads, and the challenges encountered in the intelligence test were presented in four aspects. A recent literature review also showed that most AI studies lack the recommended design characteristics for the robust validation of AI. It is, therefore, essential to develop frameworks validating the performance and safety of AI applications with respect to external datasets [20]. Waheeb [27] developed a model based on color decomposition techniques, innovative visual color, and encryption with wavelet technology to convert a color image to a grey image with important features. This chapter extensively considers the existing research trend and highlights procedures for data training, testing, and validation and the associated challenges.

In summary, Table 16.1 examines the limitations of some of the existing surveys and our contributions in this chapter to fill the knowledge gap.

16.2.1 THE ARCHITECTURAL DESIGN OF AIoMT

Machine learning applications' data are categorized into training, validation, and test sets. In machine learning, it is imperative to note that computer programmers do not create the learning algorithm's rules. Machine learning is a process of making training data into a learning algorithm. The learning algorithm usually generates a new set of rules, with the inferences drawn from the data.

Conventional statistics can be used to deal effectively with simpler datasets, whereas machine learning predictive analytics is used to handle complex datasets. Machine learning algorithms modeling concept is used to deal with model predictions. The prediction model requires the exact relationship between the observation (patients) and variables (independent variables). The prediction used some accuracy measures to evaluate the data quality and predict the outcome following

TABLE 16.1
Limitations of Some Related Work

Ref.	Focus and Coverage	Limitations	This chapter
[16]	Artificial intelligence: Learning and limitations, the learning mechanism of AI and the limitations	The scope was only limited to artificial neural networks, and the real-world application was not clearly stated	We considered the prospects and limitations of AI learning methods and primary healthcare in real-world applications
[17]	Quality validation of an image recognition system	The approach's limitations and the research's future direction were not stated	We presented the emerging challenges of AI technologies and the future direction for data training
[18]	Understanding and review of AI algorithms as a component for medical diagnostics	The scope of the study was not clearly stated, and the typical disease condition it can be used to handle	We presented a clear scope for our study and the typical real-world AI model training, testing, and validation
[19]	Used image data augmentation to deal with the problem of insufficient or inexistence data	The future research direction and applications are not stated	We highlighted the future research direction in the area of AI models
[20]	Presented the key seven steps specifying to ensure AI validation	Application is limited to breast cancer, and the performance metrics are not clearly explained	We presented numerous real-world applications of AI models
[24]	Proposed a mirror environment to tackle the problem of insufficient data	The study is only limited to the improvement of automation networks	We presented AI model testing techniques, and categorization of datasets

the observation [28]. Machine learning algorithms are categorized into three, namely:

i. *Supervised learning*: The labeled data is given to the learning algorithm and the expected outcome. For example, pictures of motor cars labeled "motor car" will enable the algorithm to identify and classify images relating to motor cars.

   Supervised learning is applicable for classification, aiming to directly map the input to the output. It is beneficial for regression; mapping inputs to consistent output is required.

   Both classification and regression are used to determine the relationship between inputs and output. However, the prediction of a trained model will be poor when noisy or incorrect labels are used. Examples of supervised learning algorithms are Support Vector Systems (SVM), Artificial neural networks (ANN), Naïve Bayes, and Random Forest [31].

TABLE 16.2
Definition of Some AI Technical Terms

1) Validation data	The available data is used for learning the selected model.
2) Test data	Data is being used to generate an unbiased estimate of the generalized error. However, it is recommended that test data should not be used for learning.
3) Validation error	This is the model error that occurred on the validation set. This differs from the data, which is an unbiased estimate of the generalized error. It is used for fine-tuning and model selection of hyperparameters.
4) Test error	The model error derived from the test data is called a test error. This error will help us to deal with the model prediction deficiencies.
5) Model validation	This is used for evaluating the validation error of a model. Validation will provide a picture of whether the model can meet the intended purpose.
6) Model evaluation	This is a way of evaluating the test error of a model. The performance measurement is necessary.
7) internal evaluation	Local test data that are used to evaluate the model.
8) External evaluation	This exist when external test data are used to evaluate the model [8].

ii. *Unsupervised learning*: The learning algorithm is given unlabeled data, and the algorithm is required to identify patterns in the input data. For example, in the recommendation system of virtual medicine, the learning algorithm can predict and recognize related diagnoses and prognoses.

iii. *Reinforcement learning*: The dynamic environment and algorithm interaction generates feedback regarding rewards and punishment. For example, a robot that performs a successful task can be rewarded. The summary and the definitions of some AI technical terms are presented in Table 16.2.

16.2.2 THE CHALLENGES OF BIG DATA IN AI APPLICATIONS

Figure 16.2 shows the steps needed for the clinical validation of AI models. With examples in Table 16.3, big data in medicine gathers information through different sections, followed by overseeing, investigating, picturing, and conveying data for dynamics. The characteristics of big data in healthcare include volume, variety, velocity, veracity, variability, and value. Big data is variable. Due to its variability, big data storage, analysis, and retrieval face huge challenges. The capacity and variability of big data made traditional databases not applicable for storing, processing, or retrieving data. However, big data analysis is faced with the following:

i. Data storage and quality
ii. High-quality data analysis
iii. Skilled analysts
iv. Security, privacy, and data sources [22]

Many challenges accompany the application of AI in healthcare. Acquiring training data is difficult due to medical data confidentiality and privacy issues. Training data

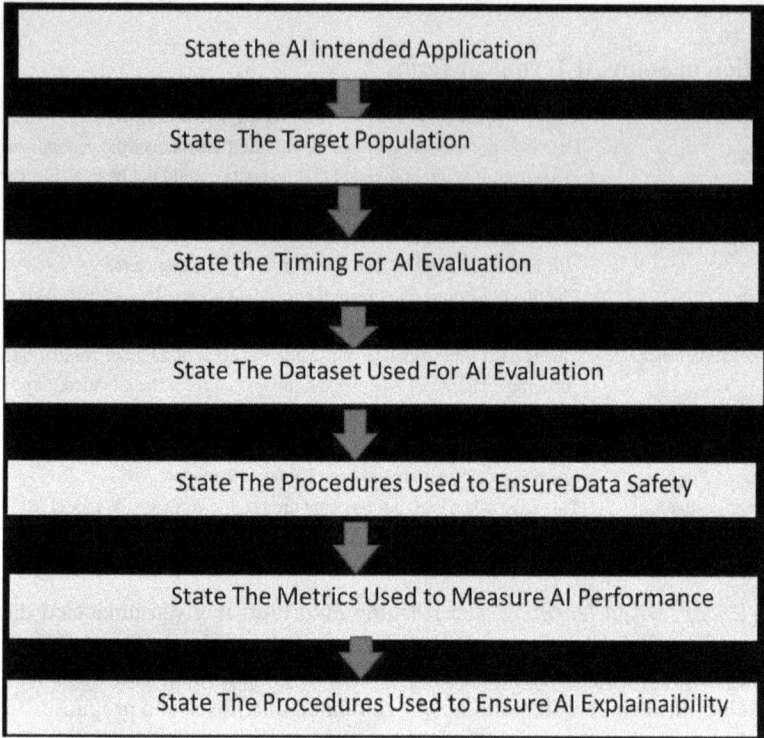

FIGURE 16.2 The steps needed for the clinical validation of AI techniques.

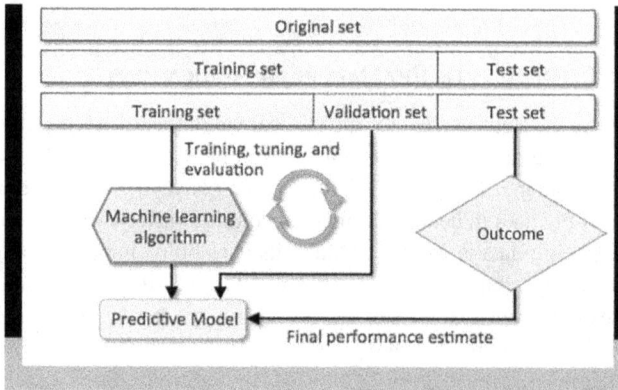

FIGURE 16.3 Machine learning algorithm.

are not readily available compared to other fields, such as natural language processing and computer vision. The computational and processing resources lead to healthcare costs. Furthermore, also highlighted the challenges of training issues, lack of explainability, interoperability, and bounding performance, and uncertainty in generality [23].

TABLE 16.3
Key Benefits of AI

S/N	Application	Description
1.	Email filtering	Artificial intelligence (AI) is being used to filter incoming emails. AI users can train their spam filters by classifying some emails as "spams."
2.	Personalization	Many online applications such as Amazon and Ali Express use artificial intelligence to personalize your demand, "learn" from your previous order the purchases made by others to recommend new stock.
3.	Fraud detection	With artificial intelligence, banks can detect if there is unusual activity in your bank account. Such unusual activities include foreign transactions and the withdrawal of large sums of money different from the usual patterns of withdrawals. AI algorithm could flag these kinds of activities.
4.	Speech recognition	Some artificial intelligence applications, such as intelligent personal assistants like Apple's "Siri," use artificial intelligence to improve their speech recognition functions [11].
5.	Medical imaging	Medical imaging is a new technology in the medical field used by a radiologist to recreate images of various parts of the body for diagnostics or prognostics purposes. This technology is quite promising for the future healthcare outlook because its non-invasive diagnostics method enables the clinician to diagnose or treat illness without an intrusive test. Some of the key applications include: a *Non-invasive diagnostics* approach for detecting diabetes using diabetic retinopathy in retinal fundus images. These techniques can also detect other ailments like eye and cardiovascular diseases. Early screening for diabetic retinopathy is essential as it will help to prevent vision loss. Hence, the importance of this screening and expert analysis cannot be overemphasized. A special optics called fundus camera is used to take several images in different orientations. b *Cancer detection:* Skin cancer is gradually becoming a threat to human existence. The most severe skin cancer with the highest fatality rate is called melanoma, which accounts for 75% of cancer-related deaths. Early detection of melanoma is a critical health issue, as this non-invasive diagnosis only requires photographic images, which can be taken by individuals' smartphones and then forwarded for analysis. Unfortunately, the traditional clinical invasive diagnostic technique has poor accuracy for melanoma diagnosis.
6.	Manufacturing robots	This category of AI is deployed to cover manufacturing requiring high precision or risk for humans to undertake them.
7.	Autonomous driving systems	The self-driven vehicles are built with the AI technology.
8.	Natural language processing	This branch of AI provides the computer's ability to interact with humans and respond to human inquiry.

TABLE 16.3 *(Continued)*
Key Benefits of AI

S/N	Application	Description
9.	Risk prediction	Certain diseases, such as cardiovascular disease, cancer, and diabetes, which seem to be silent killers, can easily be predicted by AI, even early.
10.	Virtual assistant nursing.	E-medicine or remote medical attention is now available via artificial intelligence.
11.	Smart assistant	The robots can now perform numerous functions, such as human assistants, assisting the doctor in attending to medical calls, text messages, etc.
12.	Precision medicine	Many high-risk diseases, such as cancer and diabetes, can be detected early by body scans or images.
13.	Chatbots	This is the process where AI uses computer programs to simulate human conversation by voice or text messages to solve a health-related problem.
14.	Robotic surgery	Currently, robots are used to conduct remote surgery for patients.
15.	Health monitoring and data management	Analyzing the present and past medical information is essential for medical treatment. The robot can collect, store, and trace data for faster access and medical attention [11, 37].

TABLE 16.4
AI Technologies with Example

Type	Descriptions with example
Computer vision	The ability of computers to carry out object identification and scene recognition. A good example is medical imaging and facial recognition.
Machine learning	This enhances computer task performance by data application without pre-programmed.
Natural language processing	The ability of computers to interact and respond to human inquiries. The computer can provide answers to questions asked by humans. An example is spam identification and the analysis of customer feedback.
Robotics	The branch of AI deals with the design and construction of robots, for example, unmanned aerial vehicles (UAV), selective services, and toys.
Internet of things/optimization	Physical components with inbuilt sensors are linked with other data collection and transmission devices—for example, anomaly detection and optimization.
Internet of things/optimization	This branch of AI involves developing machines that can do complex tasks such as reason, plan, and improve decision-making. This application can be used to solve mathematics theorems.
Neuromorphic computing	This can mimic biological neural networks to improve hardware efficiency and robustness of computing powers [25].

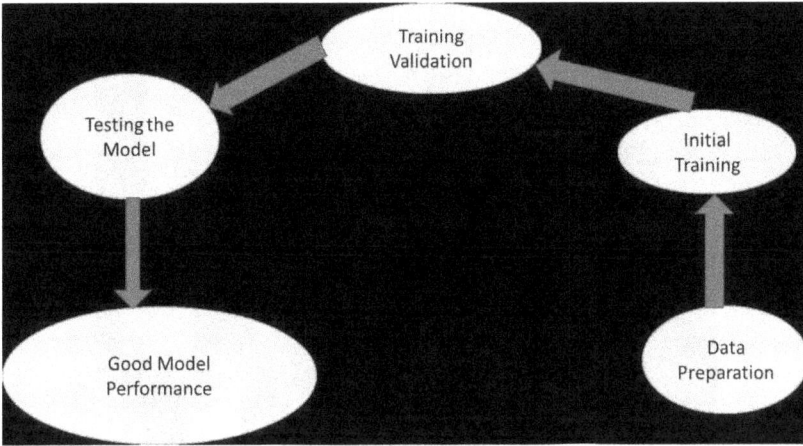

FIGURE 16.4 The basic data training procedures, for AI data training.

16.2.3 THE BASIC STEPS FOR AI DATA TRAINING

The key factors that influence the development and growth of artificial intelligence (AI) and machine learning are related to the following: data availability, computing power, and algorithm optimization. The innovation and development of new machine learning techniques, such as the layered neural networks, termed "deep learning," have provided new AI applications. The level of training acquired by an AI model determines the performance characteristics. Therefore, the outlook of an AI tool reflects the available data and the training acquired. Figure 16.4 presents the basic data training procedures for AI data training, and the procedures required to train the AI tool were properly outlined. Data preparation is the foundation of any AI model because poor and inaccurate data cannot provide an accurate predictive model. Testing and validation were also considered because these two parameters help to evaluate whether AI design can meet the intended purpose.

16.3 AIOMT TRAINING

In Figure 16.5, a machine learning prediction model is given, indicating the impact of the suitable and accurate dataset on the outcome of an AI model. A new dataset is used for training the model. The quality of training, which depends on the available data, determines the model's prediction accuracy. Training is a process of transferring knowledge to the AI model. A model cannot perform better than the level of training it acquired. Thus, the quality of training given to a model determine the overall performance efficiency. The model performance can be evaluated by measuring the errors across the data sets. The test error is a good criterion for measuring the generalization error (errors made by the model in dealing with unseen data). It is imperative to note that the test data are not

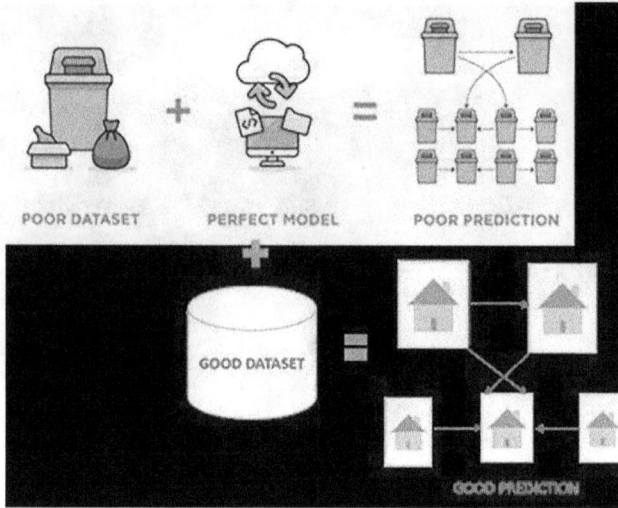

FIGURE 16.5   Machine learning prediction model.

used for training and fine-tuning the model. In the ML model, Bayes errors exist, overfitting and underfitting, soft errors, and errors due to insufficient training. The main objective is data cleaning and evaluation to provide high-quality raw data [17].

The IoT requires large or small data segments linked to its devices. The time interval between data transmission and processing of a decision needs to be relatively short; otherwise, it will be meaningless. Conventional data analysis seems inefficient in actualizing the purpose of a decision of extensive data in real-time. Hence, the scale of possible links and interactions between the various data of consideration in any research cannot be handled manually. AI techniques can adequately manage such extensive big data. Algorithms are used to categorize patients' diseases from the training dataset, and the classification rules are used to form patterns [24].

EHR data are typical real-world data (RWD), noisy, heterogeneous, structured, unstructured, and dynamic. EHRs have provided unexpected opportunities for data-based approaches to learning patterns. The first phase of data mining is business understanding. This involves setting project objectives and targets, assessing the execution plans, and risk assessment. The second phase considers the data source, acquisition, initial data collection, familiarization, and evaluation problems in the collected data [29].

16.3.1 CHALLENGES OF AI DATA TRAINING

One of the major problems of AI data training is the missing values in the datasets. However, the CLUMSTIMP method dealt with the problem of missing values in the datasets. The CLUMSTIMP method is a clustering-based imputation technique used to handle the problem of missing values, unbalanced classes, and other problems. The following schemes are used to tackle these challenges: (1) Marginalization scheme, the data sample containing the missing values is eliminated or removed from the dataset. (2) The Imputation scheme, this process estimates the missing values. The marginalization scheme is the reason for the imbalance problem, while this problem does not exist in the imputation method. The unsupervised learning algorithm estimates the missing values [30].

16.4   AIOMT TESTING

A developed AI model must undergo adequate testing to verify whether the model can meet its intended purpose. This AI model testing must meet certain criteria before it can be deployed to perform its intended task. Validation only occurs after successful training, and the training also meets the success criteria. The first stage involves passing a new data set and proceeding to the final testing stage if the results are good. The software makes additional passes through the data. The ML model or the training manager automatically modifies the parameters until no new patterns are observed. Test data quality evaluation, a targeted domain-specific application, is being examined by several researchers. In ML model applications, we are concerned with facilitating AI system quality problems [17]. Several approaches, such as pragmatic clinical trials (PCT), target trials, adoption, and the use of ML and AI techniques require further exploration.

PCT are trials developed to test the effectiveness of any clinical intervention in the real-world clinical domain. In RWD analysis, statistical models and inferential approaches are essential to make RWD meaningful, deriving a relationship, testing/validating hypotheses, and generating a regulating guide to inform policymakers and regulators in decision-making [25]. Data testing is categorized into two types: (1) in manual testing, the testers carry out their test manually without applying tools or scripts. Under this condition, the tester assumed the end user's position and tested the model to identify unusual behavior or bug. (2) Automated testing using software tools is the opposite of manual testing [31].

16.4.1   CHALLENGES OF AI DATA TESTING

The challenges of AI data testing include (1) identifying test data, (2) a lack of testable specification (3) and splitting data into training and testing sets.

1. Identifying test data in the AI domain and training and testing any model before being deployed into real-world applications is necessary. The engineer or data scientist deals with the model training and testing. Poorly sampled training data cannot represent the real-world application well.
2. Lack of testable specification, the black box technique is the most straightforward method of testing an AI model because it can be used to eliminate the inner working of an AI. The design intent of an AI model is to produce a generalized behavior. Validation of an AI application involves testing the accuracy or quality of the algorithm's prediction [39].

16.5   AIOMT VALIDATION

Validation confirms the model's accuracy using the real system. It is a process of confirming that a model achieves its intended design purpose. The model must comply with the defined predictive rules for evaluating a trained model using a testing data set. Training quality validation is the quality that could be manual or semiautomatically generated data for training sets. Data validation aims to consistently check and monitor ML data quality during the life cycle. Anomalies and errors are detected during this life cycle before the data are processed into model training. Error detection in the dataset is difficult because the data are enormous and might also contain bits of errors.

Insufficient data in ML results from insufficient data cleaning and validation tools compared with traditional software processing. The consequence of the tool is due to the errors in the data used [32, 33]. In Figure 16.6, the ML algorithm indicating the AI training stages was presented, and the AI training stages are outlined.

The following types of cross-validation are available in machine learning; K-fold cross-validation, holdout cross-validation, stratified k-fold cross-validation, leave-p-out cross-validation, leave-one-out cross-validation, and Monte Carlo cross-validation [17]. In cross-validation, data resampling is being used for ML model evaluation. The goal of cross-validation is to provide an unbiased estimate of model performance. In comparison, the holdout validation approach seems to be more accurate [8]. As AI development unfolds, it will equally have a broad social and global impact [34–36]. Several challenges were identified in data training, testing, and validation. However, the effectiveness of the AI methods used to handle these challenges is unknown. This area is still open for further research to determine the reliability of the AI methods used to handle data issues.

As the data types and algorithms, are accompanied by numerous challenges. it is difficult to sum up all the uncertainties in PHM. However, the Bayesian technique is designed to minimize uncertainties [37]. Proper attention should be given to the various AI techniques used for building the machine learning algorithm. The analytic data

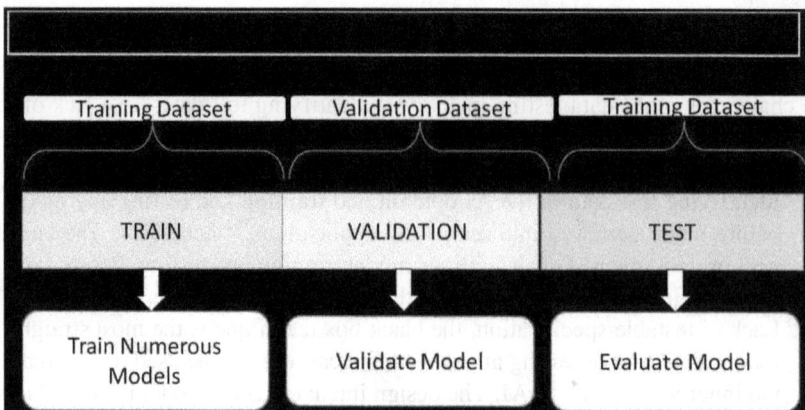

FIGURE 16.6   ML algorithm indicating the AI training stages.

tools for big data will be the turning point for AI technology [38]. Data validation is a major component of an ML system. Obtaining clean and quality data is a huge task in the pipeline process, and data validation prevents biased in ML models [39–47].

16.6 CONCLUSIONS AND FUTURE SCOPE

This chapter highlighted AIoMT training, testing, and validation using machine learning techniques. Predicting and timely diagnosis of various health issues can positively affect the patient's treatment in real-time. Several challenges have been identified in data training, testing, and validation. However, the effectiveness of AI methods in handling these challenges requires further investigations. This area is still open for further research to determine the reliability of the AI methods used to handle complex data issues. Data validation is a significant component in ML systems. Obtaining clean and quality data is a huge task in the pipeline process, and data validation prevents bias in the ML model. Future works would consider the development of cost-effective model training, testing, and validation techniques.

ACKNOWLEDGMENT

The work of Agbotiname Lucky Imoize is supported in part by the Nigerian Petroleum Technology Development Fund (PTDF) and, in part, by the German Academic Exchange Service (DAAD) through the Nigerian-German Postgraduate Program under grant 57473408.

REFERENCES

[1] Dolores Derrington, *Artificial Intelligence for Health and Health Care*, JSR-17-Task-002 JASON the MITRE Corporation, December, 2017, 1–7.
[2] Martin J. Willemink, et al. Preparing Medical Imaging Data for Machine Learning. *Radiology*, 2020, 295(4), 1–4. https://doi.org/10.1148/radiol.2020192224.
[3] Pandiaraj Manickan, et al. Artificial Intelligence (AI) and Internet of Medical Things (IoMT) Assisted Biomedical System for intelligent Healthcare. *Biosensors MDP*, 2022, 12, 1–2. https://doi.org/10.3390/bios1280562.
[4] Yogesh Kumar, Apeksha Koul, Ruchi Singla, Mahammed Faza Ijaz. Artificial Intelligence in Disease Diagnosis: A Systematic Literature Review, Synthesizing Framework and Future Research Agenda. *Journal of Ambient Intelligence and Humanized Computing*, 2021, 1–3. https://doi.org/10.007/52652-02/03612-Z.
[5] G. C. M. Siontis, R. Sweda, P. A. Noseworthy, Paul A. Friedman. Konstantinos and Chirag J Pate Development and Validation Pathways of Artificial Intelligence Tools Evaluated in Randomized Clinical Trials. *BMJ Health Care Information*, 2021, 2–8.
[6] Jeremy Straub. Machine Learning Performance Validation and Training Using a 'Perfect' Expert System. *Elsevier, B.V*, 2021, 8, 1–4. https://doi.org/10.106/j.mex.2021.101477.
[7] Christian Ruiz, *Improving Data Validation using Machine Learning, United Nations Economic Commission for Europe, Conference of European statisticians, workshop on statistical Data Editing* (Neuchatel, Switzerland, 18–20 September 2018) (Swiss Federal Statistical office, Switzerland), 2–3.

[8] Farhad Maleki, Nikesh Muthukrishan, Katie Ovens, Caroline Reinhold, Reza Forghani. Machine Learning Algorithm Validation: From Essentials to Advanced Applications and Implications for Regulatory Certification and Development. *Neuroimaging Clinics of North America*, 2020, 30, 1–6.

[9] Vikash Singh, Michael Pencina, Andrew J. Einstein, Joanna X. Liang, Daniel S. Berman, Piotr Slomka. Impact of Train/Test Sample Regimen on Performance Estimate Stability of Machine Learning in Cardiovascular/Image. *Scientific Report*, 2021, 1–5, https://doi. org/10.1038/541598-021-9365, www.Nature.com/scientific report/open-access.

[10] Philipp Hacker. A Legal Framework for AI Training Data from First Principle to the Artificial Intelligence Act. *Law, Innovation and Technology Routledge Taylor and Francis Group Publisher*, 2021, 13(2), 257–301.

[11] *Artificial Intelligence and Machine Learning: Policy Paper*, 2017, 3–5, https:// en.wikipedia.org/wiki/Artifitial_intelligence Internet society.org.

[12] Sophia Y. Wang, Suzan Pershing, Aaron Y. Lee. Big Data Requirement for Artificial Intelligence. *Current Opinion in Ophthalmology*, 2020, 31(5), 318–323, https://doi. org/10.1097/ICU.00000.00000.000676.

[13] Jenny Yang, Andrew A. S. Soltan, David A. Clifton. Machine Learning Generalizability Across Healthcare Settings: Insights from Multi-Site COVID-19 Screening. *NPJ Digital Medicine*, 2022, 5(69), 1–6. https://doi.org/10.10./1038/541746-022-006149.

[14] M. Ambigavathi, D. Sridharan. A Survey on Big Data in Healthcare Applications. *ResearchGate*, 2022, 1–5. https://doi.org/10.007/978-981-13-8618-3-77.

[15] Carla Zoe Cremer. Deep Limitations, Examining Expert Disagreement Over Deep Learning. *Progress in Artificial Intelligence*, 2021, 10, 449–464. https://doi. org/10.1007/5/3748

[16] Alisson Paulodede Oliueira, Hugo Ferreira Tadeu Braga. Artificial Intelligence: Learning and Limitations. *WSEAS Transactions Engineering Education*, 2020, 17, 10.

[17] Milad Mirbabaie, Stefan Stieglitz, Nicholas R.J Frick. Artificial Intelligence in Disease Diagnostics: A Critical Review and Classification on the Current State of Research Guiding Future Direction. *Health and Technology*, 2021, 11, 1–6.

[18] Conor Shorten, Taghi M. Khoshgoftaar. A Survey on Image Data Augmentation for Deep Learning. *Journal of Big Data*, 2019, 6(60), 1–10.

[19] Rosy Tsopra et al. A Framework for Validating AI in Precision Medicine: Consideration from the European ITFOC Consortium. *BMC Medical Informatics and Decision Making*, 2021, 21, 1–5.

[20] Lukas Fisher et al. AI Systems Engineering—Key Challenges and Lessons Learned. *Machine Learning and Knowledge Extraction*, 2021, 3.

[21] Shreyas Nopany, S. Manonmani. Applications of Big Data Analytics in Healthcare Management Systems. *International Journal of Scientific Research and Engineering Development*, 2021, 4(4), 2–6.

[22] A. L. Imoize, O. Adedeji, N. Tandiya, et al. 6G Enabled Smart Infrastructure for Sustainable Society: Opportunities, Challenges, and Research Roadmap. *Sensors*, 2021, 21.

[23] L. K. Ramasamy, F. Khan, M. Sha, B. V. V. S. Prasad, C. Iwendi, C. Bamba. Secure Smart Wearable Computing through Artificial Intelligence-Enabled Internet of Things and Cyber-Physical Systems for Health Monitoring. *Sensors*, 2022, 22, 1076. https://doi. org/10.3390/s2203176.

[24] F. Liu, Demosthenes Panagiotakos. Real-world Data: A Brief Review of the Methods, Applications, Challenges and Opportunities. *BMC Medical Research Methodology*, 2022, 22, 287. https://doi.org/10.1186/s12874-022-01768-6.

[25] Junya Tang, Kuo-Yi Lin, Li Li. Using Domain Adaptation for Incremental SVM Classification of Drift Data, *MDPI*, 2022, 10, 4–15.

[26] Rasha A. Waheeb. APP Innovation to Control Projects Risks Management During Crises. *Endorsed Transaction on Internet of Things*, 2022, 8(30). https://doi.org/10.4108/eetiotv8i30.

[27] S. K. Dhillion, M. D. Ganggayah, S. Sinnadurai, P. Lio, N. A. Taib. Theory and Practice of Integrating of Machine Learning and Conventional Statistics in Medical Data Analysis. *Diagnostics*, 2022, 12, 2526. https://doi.org/10.3390/diagnostics12102526.

[28] Darius Nahavani, Roohallah Alizadesani, Abbas Khosravi, U. Rajendra. Acharya, Application of Artificial Intelligence in Wearable Devices: Opportunities and Challenges. *Journal of Computer Methods and Programs in Biomedicine*, 2021, 9. https://doi.org/10.1016/j.cmpb.2021.106541.

[29] A. M. Rahmani, E. Yousefpoor, A. Haider, M. Hosseinzadeh, R. Ali Naqvi. Machine Learning (ML) in Medicine: Review Applications and Challenges. *Mathematics*, 2021, 9, 2970. https://doi.org/10.3390/math9222970.

[30] Zubair Khaliq, Sheik Umar Farooq, Dawood Ashraf Khan. Artificial Intelligence in Software Testing: Impact, Problems, Challenges and Prospects. *Elsevier*, 2022, 3–4.

[31] Di Li, Kazuak Akash, Haruhisa Nozue, Kenichi Tayama. A Mirror Environment to Produce Artificial Intelligence Training Data. *IEEE Access*, 2022, 10, 2–5.

[32] Ram Mohan Vadavalasa. Data Validation Process Learning Pipeline. *International Journal of Science and Research Development*, 2020, 8(4), 2321–2613.

[33] M. Supriya, A. J. Deepa. Machine Learning Approach on Healthcare Big Data: A Review, Big Data Inform. *Analytics*, 2020, 5, 16–18.

[34] Andrew C. Scot, Jose R. Solórzano, Jonathan D. Moyer et al. The Future of Artificial Intelligence. *The International Journal of Artificial Intelligence and Machine Learning*, 2022, 2(1), 18–30.

[35] Sunday Ochella, Mahmood Shafiee. Performance Metrics for Artificial Intelligence (AI), Algorithm Adopted in Prognostics and Health Management of Mechanical Systems. *Journal of Physics: Conference Series*, 2021, 1828(1), 3–4.

[36] Azra Pasic, Alija Pasic, Lejla Pasic. The Artificial Intelligence Based Assistant-AIDA. *2022 IEEE 21st Mediterranean Electrotechnical Conference (MELECON)*. Palermo, Italy. https://doi.org/10.1109/MELECON53508.2022.9843070.

[37] V. Iguoba, A. L. Imoize. The Psychology of Explanation in Medical Decision Support Systems. In *Explainable Artificial Intelligence in Medical Decision Support Systems*, 1st ed., A. L. Imoize, J. Hemanth, D.-T. Do, and S. N. Sur, Eds. London: The Institution of Engineering and Technology, 2022, pp. 489–506.

[38] Kishore Sugali, Chris Sprunger, Venkata N Inukollu. Software Testing: Issues and Challenges of Artificial Intelligence. *International Journal of Architecture, Arts and Applications*, 2021, 12, 1. https://doi.org/10.5121/ijaia.

[39] A. Zia, M. Aziz, I. Popa, S. A. Khan, A. F. Hamedani, A. R. Asif. Artificial Intelligence-Based Medical. Data Mining. *Journal of Personalized Medicine*, 2022, 12, 1359. https://doi.org/10.3390/jpm12091359.

[40] O. B. Ayoade et al. Explainable Artificial Intelligence (XAI) in Medical Decision Systems (MDSSs): Healthcare Systems Perspective. In *Explainable Artificial Intelligence in Medical Decision Support Systems*, 1st ed., A. L. Imoize, J. Hemanth, D.-T. Do, and S. N. Sur, Eds. London: The Institution of Engineering and Technology, 2022, pp. 1–43.

[41] J. B. Awotunde, E. A. Adeniyi, S. A. Ajagbe, A. L. Imoize, O. A. Oki, S. Misra. Explainable Artificial Intelligence (XAI) in Medical Decision Support Systems (MDSS): Applicability, Prospects, Legal Implications, and Challenges. In *Explainable*

Artificial Intelligence in Medical Decision Support Systems, 1st ed., A. L. Imoize, J. Hemanth, D.-T. Do, and S. N. Sur, Eds. London: The Institution of Engineering and Technology, 2022, pp. 45–90.

[42] S. C. Nwaneri, C. Yinka-Banjo, U. C. Uregbulam, O. O. Odukoya, A. L. Imoize. Explainable Neural Networks in Diabetes Mellitus Prediction. In *Explainable Artificial Intelligence in Medical Decision Support Systems*, 1st ed., A. L. Imoize, J. Hemanth, D.-T. Do, and S. N. Sur, Eds. London: The Institution of Engineering and Technology, 2022, pp. 313–334.

[43] A. T. Rufai, K. F. Dukor, O. M. Ageh, A. L. Imoize. XAI Robot-Assisted Surgeries in Future Medical Decision Support Systems. In *Explainable Artificial Intelligence in Medical Decision Support Systems*, 1st ed., A. L. Imoize, J. Hemanth, D.-T. Do, and S. N. Sur, Eds. London: The Institution of Engineering and Technology, 2022, pp. 167–195.

[44] Y. Sei, A. Ohsuga, A. L. Imoize. Statistical Test with Differential Privacy for Medical Decision Support Systems. In *Explainable Artificial Intelligence in Medical Decision Support Systems*, 1st ed., A. L. Imoize, J. Hemanth, D.-T. Do, and S. N. Sur, Eds. London: The Institution of Engineering and Technology, 2022, pp. 401–433.

[45] A. L. Imoize, D. O. Irabor, P. A. Gbadega, C. Chakraborty. Blockchain Technology for Secure COVID-19 Pandemic Data Handling. In *Smart Health Technologies for the COVID-19 Pandemic: Internet of Medical Things Perspectives*, 1st ed., C. Chakraborty and J. J. P. C. Rodrigues, Eds. London: The Institution of Engineering and Technology, 2022, pp. 141–179.

[46] A. L. Imoize, P. A. Gbadega, H. I. Obakhena, D. O. Irabor, K. V. N. Kavitha, C. Chakraborty. Artificial Intelligence-enabled Internet of Medical Things for COVID-19 Pandemic Data Management. In *Explainable Artificial Intelligence in Medical Decision Support Systems*, 1st ed., A. L. Imoize, J. Hemanth, D.-T. Do, and S. N. Sur, Eds. London: The Institution of Engineering and Technology, 2022, pp. 357–380.

[47] R. L. Kumar, Y. Wang, T. Poongodi, and A. L. Imoize, Eds. *Internet of Things, Artificial Intelligence and Blockchain Technology*, 1st ed. Switzerland, AG: Springer Nature, 2021.

17 AIoMT for Medical Image Steganalysis

Oluyemi Paul Adejumo, Aderonke Favour-Bethy Thompson, and Arome Junior Gabriel

17.1 INTRODUCTION

Communications have taken a new surge—from formerly known traditional method to a modern-day style, where the use of internet anchors the transfer of information from one place to another. As much as information transmission becomes easier and faster with the present cyberspace technology, it has similarly instigated breaches in information security. The information security issues and loss of privacy are rising concerns in global information sharing [1]. Thus, Information can easily be accessible and intruded by unauthorized individuals. This crack sinks the authentication of information that is transmitted from a sender to another receiver via internet.

To avert a possible influence of third party, data hiding techniques are used to concealed messages to be sent from a sender to the intending receivers. Data hiding techniques increase with more effective approach to provide a necessary end-to-end protection required for safe data exchange [2]. The concepts of cryptography and steganography are the two commonly used data hiding techniques to produce a secured information transmission via networks system. In cryptography, the encrypted plaintext data is changed to unreadable form called ciphertext, then transfer via internet to the receiving end, and decryption is performed on the ciphertext by the recipient.

The ciphertext generated in cryptography may not really make much sense to the view of the intruders; it naturally raises the prying level of a malicious hacker to conduct cryptanalysis attacks on the ciphertext in order to reveal the secret information and make it readable. Although, virtual cryptography scheme has been recognized capable of addressing the inadequacies that are associated with the conventional cryptography technique [3], it is still not as effective when data are concealed in another innocent object.

A well encrypted message transmission can be achieved with the use of harmless cover files to obscure the data. This has proven to be an upgraded data-hiding concept due to its ability to hide messages without raising any attention to itself, as an object of scrutiny. With such techniques, the hidden information cannot be easily suspected by unintended recipients of the cover media. This idea summarizes the concept of steganography. It simply describes the practice of obscuring information by embedding secretly within other innocent files like image, audio, or video.

DOI: 10.1201/9781003370321-17

Steganography provides a platform by which news and information can be transmitted in conserved manner that offers no clue about the embedded data, therefore eliminating all worries that may arise from the identity of the sender being revealed [4]. While protecting the security of information, these cover-up systems may also be used by criminals to transmit some malicious information, thus bringing potential risks to cyberspace security [5]. This technique is also in constant use by those who are well-known for their illegal practices in the society. Consequently, both legal and illegal communication activities are also best practice using steganography data hiding scheme due to the volume of stored data with little or no change to the properties of the cover medium.

Among all the cover files available for steganography, digital images have been recognized to be the most popular and effective in steganographic system, due to its large amount of redundant data that are beneficial to steganographic data hiding [6]. Also, the expansion of the internet has greatly increased the use of digital images and made it readily available. Images with hidden message are easy to penetrate into the world wide web or in newsgroups since most websites support free flow image dissemination, due to a reduced minimum resources consumption compared to other media sources.

Image steganalysis is the reverse process of image steganography that determines whether an image contains an embedded secret message. Its goal is to identify suspected image packages and distinguish between those ones that have payloads from ordinary ones. It begins by identifying the artifacts that exist in the suspect image stego file, which has formed as a result of embedding a message.

The interrupted data in cryptanalysis often contains a message, while steganalysis system presents a bundle of suspect data files that cannot be differentiated from each other, in terms of those files containing payload. The steganalyst is usually something of a forensic statistician and must start by reducing this set of data files (which is often quite large; in many cases, it may be the entire set of files on a computer) to the subset most likely to have been altered [7].

Image steganalysis methods usually relate to image repositories to extract images that have steganographic alterations with the aid of high-pass filters (HPF) to detect images that contain artifacts in addition to their original contents. Researches on this field carefully consider the image statistical properties that cannot be traced to stego-system paving way to find out whether an image is in its ordinary form or not. Thus, a successful steganalysis system can be identified as long as it has a higher degree of probability to predict the images that are stego as stego and the cover as cover [8].

Various algorithms such as support vector machine (SVM), Naive Bayes, and CNN are being used in image steganalysis with the idea of learning the original features of the carrier medium. Among these algorithms, convolutional neural network has recently show superiority in discerning the stego image from its cover counterpart [9]. It outperforms conventional methods due to its capability to learn the input features with deep layers of neuron structures without manual supervision [10]. While all CCN architectures are developed using key principles, several models differ in their depth and structure. CNN has equally been identified to be beneficial when working with visual data and have high potential for applications in medical fields that utilize imagery data [11]. Özdi and Yilmaz [12] reported that CNN architectures have high potential on extracting features from thermal images. Generally, the introduction of artificial intelligence (AI) to the Internet of Medical Things (IoMT) has enabled the autonomous operation of machine that provides a favorable and secure environmental landscape to healthcare personnel and patients [13].

CNN image steganalytic algorithm operates in two steps to solve various problems. The objective of the first step is to capture ample data on the input images by striding and mapping through the set of features. The second step aims at classifying the images into either stego or cover in line with the extracted values of certain features, which can be used to provide a decision-making system. The importance of decision support system (DSS) is not only valuable in information security system but also has been recognized to be beneficial in medical image segmentation to assist medical related activities [14]. A decision-making system can be clinically enabled by AI algorithms and software to produce a predictive analytical algorithm that aims at checking for patterns from complex data for conclusions characterized with a reliable degree of probability that enable the healthcare service provider to make quality decisions within a short time [15]. Medical decision support systems have played a crucial role in systems' attempts to improve patient well-being and the standard of care, particularly for non-communicable illnesses [16].

Precisely, the two steps steganalysis machine can be summarized into training and testing phases [17]. The training phase extract features from the input data to form of feature matrix of size $n \times m$ through mapping. This feature matrix is then used to train the CNN classifier. The testing phase provide the platform by which the trained CNN can be used to perform image classification into stego and cover image.

17.1.1 KEY CONTRIBUTIONS OF THE CHAPTER

The significant contributions of this chapter are represented as follows:

i. This research work proposes a JPEG color image steganalysis using adaptive momentum optimizer to explore the deep power of CNN with careful consideration of the choice of filter size and number, the CNN layers arrangement in order to both knob the requirements for sufficient feature extractions and add effective regularization effect to circumvent overfitting to produce a practical minimum number of parameters at the final feature map.

ii. It also focuses on producing a bling image steganalysis system that can work with the vast JPEG images that are commonly available on the internet with the aim of differentiating images that are ordinary from those which have messages hiding in them.

iii. The study explores the flexibility of CNN filter to extract and reserve feasible image features, as well as the suitability of concatenated rectified linear units (CReLU) to preserve the phase information of CNN in negative and positive set-ups, which make it possible to achieve both non-saturate and non-linearity. CReLU has an exceptional nature that allows a reconstruction property of the convolution layer to be characterized mathematically. This indicates the expressiveness and generalization of the corresponding CNN features

iv. The use of Adaptive Momentum (Adam) technique optimizes the model to produce adaptive learning rate for all parameters, "leading to faster computational time with fewer parameter for tunning."

The computational efficiency and simple technique of the Adaptive Momentum (Adam) characterized by first-order gradient and less memory requirement for stochastic optimization is a useful tool in implementing the proposed CNN model. High-dimensional parameter space and huge data set machine learning contest are best addressed using Adam optimization technique.

17.1.2　Chapter Organization

Section 17.2 presents a comprehensive review of the related works; Section 17.3 focuses on mathematical background of the research methodology and the system design. Section 17.4 discusses system implementation and evaluation. Finally, Session 17.5 highlights the conclusion and recommendations.

17.2　RELATED WORK

Chen *et al.* [18] explored steganalysis approach with the use of a phase split to work on how to reduce error probability and then improved the detection accuracy of image steganalysis. An augmented database was used by Yedroudj *et al.* [19] to advance the training face of CNN. Also, Zhang *et al.* [20] worked on efficient feature learning and multi-size image steganalysis based on CNN inspired by the need to amplify the noise components of images by reducing the strength of the signal-to-noise ratio of the steganalysis feature map arbitrary image size steganalysis challenge. A joint multi-domain feature learning for image steganalysis based on CNN was equally developed by Wang *et al.* [21], with the use of joint domain detection mechanism and a nonlinear detection mechanism. Kang *et al.* [22] modelled a CNN-Based ternary classification for image steganalysis. The study proposed a convolutional neural network method needed to provide a ternary classifier that could identify WOW and UNIWARD steganographic algorithm in the final output of the stego images. "The research experiment is inspired by inability of binary CNN-based classifier to separate and identify the stego image encrypted by WOW and UNIWARD steganographic algorithm, since most classifiers are designed to discriminate cover files with hidden data from their ordinary counterparts."

However, the aforementioned CNN steganalysis model are gray-scale image oriented, and not suitable for color image steganalysis. Considering gray image steganography, there are two major limitations associated with their usage: first, the image data holding capacity is small due to its eight-bit holding volume; second, most of the gray images are in BMP file format and hence are not web friendly like current RGB images. Consequently, color image steganalysis has recently attracted attention since the majority of images produced by digital cameras and those which are found on several social media are in color and JPEG format.

Zeng *et al.* [23] proposed a WISERNet color image steganalysis model using convolutional neural networks. This model focuses on constructing a wide CNN rather than making it deep for better discriminations between stego and cover image files. The proposed WISERNet model performs best in discriminating CMD-C steganographic algorithm designed recently for color images. WISERNet model is relatively shallow and does not explore the deep attribute of the convolutional neural. It is not suitable for blind steganalysis system, where no prior knowledge of the embedding algorithm is given.

Jin *et al.* [24] worked on deep learning a large number of parameters, and its weak pertinence to adaptive steganography algorithms to produce image adaptive steganalysis via convolutional neural network combined with selection channel (IAS-CNN). The objective of this work is to produce an IAS-CNN model that focuses on adaptive steganalysis. The proposed methodology contains a pre-processing layer that runs a residual calculation before the use of SRM filters to extract residual features of the image. The features are then combined with the selection channel as output.

The experimental results show that IAS-CNN accuracy increases with an increase in payload, making it efficient at high payload. IAS-CNN also presents a better model due to its fewer convolutional computation when compared to ZhuNet and YeNet with higher calculations due to its network depth. The model performance is low with low payload and is not suitable for other steganographic algorithms except HUGO and WOW.

Yan *et al.* [25] proposed an image steganalysis using different filters with squeeze-and-excitation convolutional neural networks. The study was inspired by CNN diversity of filter size and number, which has not been previously utilized completely.

The objective is to find an effective way of capturing the hidden artifacts through a new network of modules called " diverse filter modules (DFMs) and squeeze-and-excitation modules (SEMs). The methodology is made up of one pre-processing layer coupled with seven convolutional layers, six of which can be found in DFSE modules. A fully connected layer and softmax layer are used to give the final classification probability. The main function of the squeeze-and-excitation module in the architecture is to learn feature weight with respect to the loss in the training.

The superiority of the model was compared with the state-of-the-art approaches of the traditional classical method. DFSE-Net has better detection performance than other methods to detect steganographic algorithms of WOW and S-UNIWARD, at payloads of 0.2 and 0.4 bpp. Its computing power limitation placed a restriction on the size of the input image (256 × 256). The model is also limited to WOW and S-UNIWARD steganalysis with specified payloads.

The performance credibility of the model was determined using the traditional classic model, with DFSE-Net having superior performance in terms of its ability to detect WOW and S-UNIWARD steganographic algorithm with payloads for 0.2bpp and 0.4bpp. However, its computing power is limited to an input image size of 256 × 256.

The model is also limited to detecting WOW and S-UNIWARD with specified payloads.

The proposed research study is inspired by Zeng *et al.* [21] to propose a JPEG color image steganalysis with no prior knowledge of the embedding algorithm, using adaptive momentum optimizer to explore the depth strength of CNN with careful consideration of the choice of filter size and number; the CNN layers arrangement in order to both knob the requirements for sufficient feature extractions and add effective regularization effect to circumvent overfitting to produce a workable minimum number of parameters at the final feature map.

17.3 MATERIALS AND METHODS/METHODOLOGY

The proposed steganalysis system is made up of four phases: data collection, pre-processing phase, and CNN model training,

17.3.1 DATA COLLECTION PHASE

All of the training and testing image datasets are acquired from github.com image repository named IStego100K. The selected image dataset for the purpose of this research work is 4,187, which is divided into 2,631 cover images and 1,551 stego images.

17.3.2 PRE-PROCESSING PHASE

The noise content added to the image is considered to be much weaker than the image content. A high pass filter is first applied to the input datasets to make the model aware of the embedded data rather than the image contents. High-pass filter is a tool to make an image appear sharper. These filters emphasize fine details in the image; small and faint details are greatly exaggerated. Thereafter, the filtered images are normalized using min-max method as depicted in Equation 17.1.

$$x' = \frac{x - mean(x)}{\max(x) - \min(x)} \tag{17.1}$$

17.3.3 CONVOLUTIONAL NEURAL NETWORKS MODEL TRAINING PHASE

The background concept of convolutional neural networks uses convolutional layers to extract the sets of features through mapping of kernels with two-dimensional input data like image, to produce a sufficient future map that can be used by the fully connected layer to carry out the final classification, consequently giving a better representation of the original input data.

The proposed convolutional neural network architecture comprises six basic convolutional blocks and a fully connected layer. In this architecture, each of the first three convolutional blocks will be made up of four components. These are convolutional layers with filter size (5 × 5), concatenated rectifier linear unit (CReLU) activation function, pooling layer, and batch normalization. While the last three convolutional blocks will contain three components as the previous blocks except for the pooling layer. These latter three convolutional segments will affect the deep learning concept characterized by accurate classification. Filters at each convolution layer perform the convolution process of input-image transformation into the output feature maps.

In the convolutional layer, let C^{kl} represent the future map result extracted from the first layer of the convolution with the k-th kernel. From the input image, the weighting matrix, W^{kl} yields Equation 17.2.

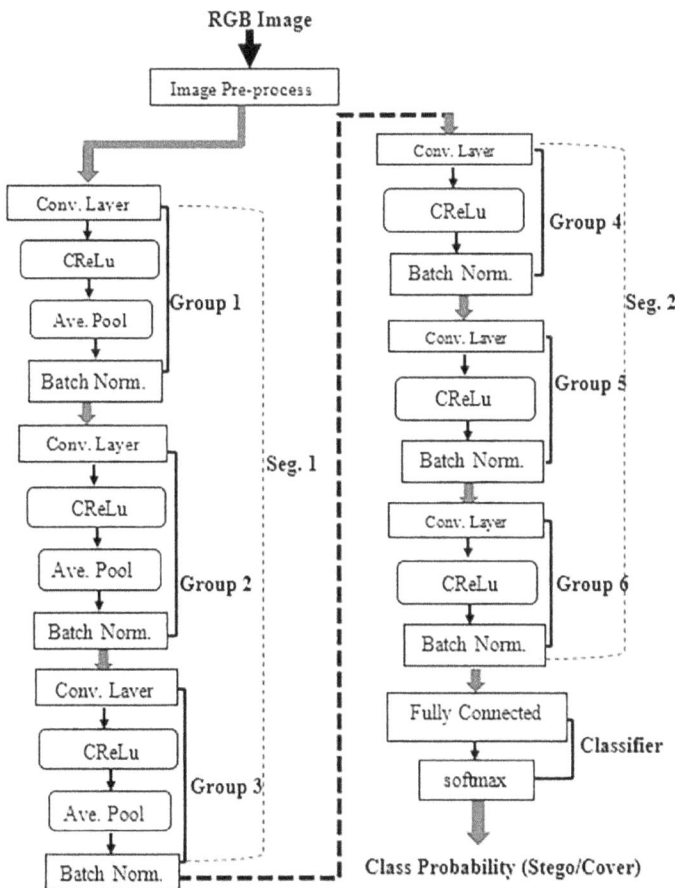

FIGURE 17.1 Proposed architecture for image steganalysis. (Adapted from [26].)

$$C^{kl} = \sum_{m=1}^{K^{l-1}} \left(W^{kl} * F^{m(l-1)} \right) \tag{17.2}$$

where $*$ denotes convolution product, K^{l-1} is the number of kernels in the previous layer, and $F^{m(l-1)}$ is the m-th final feature map produced by the layer l. For the first convolutional layer, i.e., when $l = 1$, $K^{l-1} = K^0 = 1$, and $F^{1(l-1)} = F^{1(0)} = I$, which is the input-image. W^{kl} is the size of the matrix filter, which implicitly defines the size of the region of interest.

Stride and padding are the two parameters that influence the output size of convolutional operations. While stride determines the number of steps to be taken between neighboring fields of both width and height spatial dimensions, padding allows maintaining the borders of the input feature map $F^{m(l-1)}$ or image I with the addition of zeros. S as a stride value allows the convolutional operation to be applied by shifting the weighing matrix W^{kl} from S units. Small feature maps are easily produced by a large stride. Thus, let be given a stride value S and a padding value P, we obtain for a square input image/map $F^{m(l-1)}$ an output C^{kl} such that:

$$\dim(C^{kl}) = (\dim(F^{m(l-1)}) - \dim(W^{kl}) + 2 \times P)/S + 1 \tag{17.3}$$

to keep C^{kl} at the same dimensional size as the input data $F^{m(l-1)}$, $(\dim(C^{kl}) = (\dim(F^{m(l-1)})$, the stride and padding values must be set to 1 and $\dim(W^{kl})/2$, respectively.

17.3.4 ACTIVATION FUNCTION

Activation function introduces non-linearity into the CNN so that the CNN will be configured to learn deep and effects its multi-layers strength of CNN. A variation of ReLU called "concatenated rectified linear unit" (CReLU) is used for a better performance, while reducing the number of parameters to be learned by removing redundancies

Each convolutional layer C^{kl} with an activation function f^{kl} (CReLU) to ensure its non-linearity and reduce the number of parameters by half when compared with the regularly used ReLU activation function in the model. Equation 17.4 describes the how activation function can be modeled with various possible choices.

$$f(x) = \frac{e^{-x^2}}{\sigma^2} \tag{17.4}$$

For each kernel, a bias, b^{kl} in Equation 17.5 will yield parameter optimization in layer l. Ultimately, resulting in A^{kl} with f^{kl} as the function for each kernel.

$$A^{kl} = f^{kl}(C^{kl} + b^{kl}) \qquad (17.5)$$

17.3.5 POOLING LAYER

Pooling operation in CNN basically reduces the parameters by dropping the dimension of the output feature map. To preserve enough feature information after subsampling, we applied average pooling in the first three convolutional layers resulting to a direct participation of pooling operation in all layers may lead to loss of important features, which would have effect on the classification output. Average pooling enhances the generalization ability of the network.

During the pooling step, "a 2D map will be down-sampled into $Pl \times Pl$ dimensional regions, and each region will be substituted with the mean or the maximum value." The feature mapping is achieved when pooling operation applied satisfied equations:

$$F^{kl} = pooling(A^{kl}) = pooling(f^{kl}(C^{kl} + b^{kl})) \qquad (17.6)$$

$$F^{kl} = pooling\left\{ f^{kl} \left[\sum_{m=1}^{K^{l-1}} \left(W^{kl} * F^{m(l-1)} \right) + b^{kl} \right] \right\} \qquad (17.7)$$

$$= pooling\left(f^{kl} \left(W^{kl} * I + b^{kl} \right) \right) \qquad (17.8)$$

where I is the original input-image.

17.3.6 BATCH NORMALIZATION

Batch normalization is used in all the convolution blocks to tackle the effect of overfitting. Batch normalization effect smoothens the loss function and gives some stability to the learning process by reducing the training epochs number required to train the CNN networks. This increases the training process and also plays an important role in adding generalization effect.

17.3.7 FULLY CONNECTED LAYER

Finally, the fully connected layer performs a comprehensive feature evaluation based on the convolution layers and generates an N-dimensional probability vector, where N is the number of the classification targets. The proposed architecture used one fully connected layer coupled with drop-out to suppress the effect of overfitting.

17.3.8 SOFTMAX FUNCTION

This module contains SoftMax function, which displays the classification result in accordance with the system performance. The final classification probability of the SoftMax function is used to generate results to discriminate between the cover images and their stego counterparts. This is represented by Equation 17.9.

$$\Pr\left(Y_i = K\right)\frac{e^{\beta_K.X_i}}{\sum_{k=1}^{K}e^{\beta_{k.X_i}}} \tag{17.9}$$

where Y_i represents the probability sets, β_k is the set of regression coefficients associated with outcome K, and X_i the set of explanatory variables associated with observation i.

17.3.9 ADAPTIVE MOMENTUM ESTIMATE (ADAM)

The hugeness and complexity of data involved in color image steganalysis require a suitable optimization technique for performance enhancement. In the case of RGB images of three channels, they contain 24 bits, "making them computationally complex in addition to the amount of data involve in image steganalysis training." Consequently, this research adopts Adam optimization technique to enhance the system's performance.

The computational efficiency and simple technique of the Adaptive Momentum (Adam) characterized by first-order gradient and small memory requirement for stochastic optimization is a useful tool to implement a high-dimensional parameter space and huge data set machine learning classification. Mathematically, Adam can be represented as follows:

$$x_t = \delta_1 * x_{t-1} - \left(1 - \delta_1\right) * g_t \tag{17.10}$$

$$y_t = \delta_2 * y_{t-1} - \left(1 - \delta_2\right) * g_t^2 \tag{17.11}$$

$$\Delta\omega_t = -\eta\frac{x_t}{\sqrt{y_t + \epsilon}} * g_t \tag{17.12}$$

$$\omega_{t+1} = \omega_t + \Delta\omega_t \tag{17.13}$$

η denotes initial learning rate, g_t is the gradient at time t along ω^t, x_t the exponential average of gradient along ω^t, y_t exponential average of squares of gradient along ω^t, and δ_1, δ_2 the hyperparameters.

17.4 SYSTEM IMPLEMENTATION AND EVALUATION

17.4.1 DATASET DISTRIBUTIONS

The datasets used were divided into training and test set. Seventy percent was used as the training set, while the remaining 30% was assigned to test the model. The training datasets were used to ensure that the CNN is accustomed to the vastness of features to be used in the classification process. "Consequently, a higher percentage of the datasets is required to train the model. On the other hand, the testing dataset is to validate the performance of the model." The training sample constituted 2,930 images, while the test sample constituted 1,257 images of three-dimensional shapes, respectively. Precisely, the dataset required to train the model contains 1,089 stego images and 1,841 cover images. In the test set, there are 790 cover images and 467 stego images as given in Table 17.1:

TABLE 17.1
Image Dataset Distribution

Total Images	Training Set (2,930)	Testing Set (1,257)
Cover Images	1,089	790
Stego Images	1,841	467

17.4.2 TRAINING AND VALIDATION

Data preprocessing and augmentation were performed before imputing the data into the CNN model for training. The entire image datasets were resized to 70 × 70 dimensional space, in order to make it suitable to train and test the model, since the fully connected layer of the convolutional neural networks required a fixed image size. Two thousand nine hundred and thirty images were randomly selected from github.com image repository, containing both stego and cover images, with no consideration of the embedding algorithm and rate to reflect the real-world image steganalysis when it comes to exposing images to know how they really appear to be.

To train the model, the learning was set to 1.0 with 20 training epochs, which is the configurable hyperparameter used in training the neural networks. Learning rate generally controls the adaptation of the model to the problem at hand with respect to its size. "The higher the learning rates the lesser the number of epochs required to train a neural networks. large training epochs is directly connected to smaller learning rate and vice versa." The choice of this learning value creates a hybrid of oscillation between high- and low-learning rates so as to sidestep any of the difficulties encountered by both.

17.4.3 PERFORMANCE EVALUATION

The performance of the steganalysis model is evaluated based on its predictive accuracy using three different set-ups in order to depict the effect of each of these settings on the model structural arrangement. These scenarios are the training and validation accuracy without parameter tuning, the training and validation accuracy with parameter tuning, and the training and validation accuracy graph with parameter tuning and discreet wavelength transform. These are represented in Figures 17.2, 17.3, and 17.4, respectively.

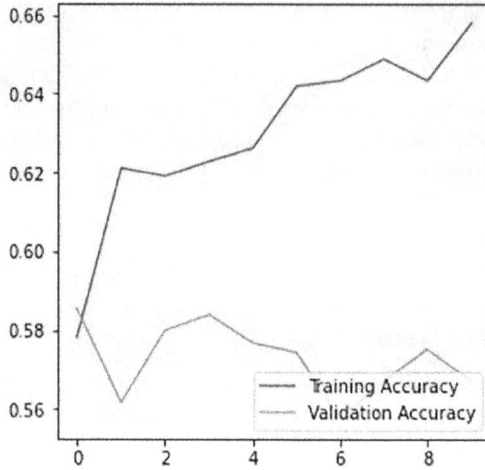

FIGURE 17.2 Training and validation accuracy without parameter tuning.

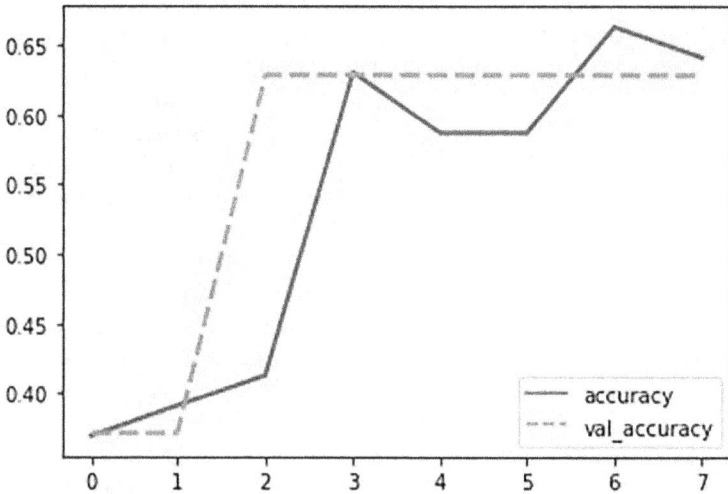

FIGURE 17.3 Training and validation accuracy graph with parameter tuning.

17.5 DISCUSSIONS

To ensure a CNN structural arrangement that the model responds well to the proposed task, we first considered how more features could be extracted from the input data at the initial fragment of the convolutional layers, and the second part to deal with the reduction of the resulting parameters in the extracted feature map from the input image. The bi-segmental method with different structural arrangements

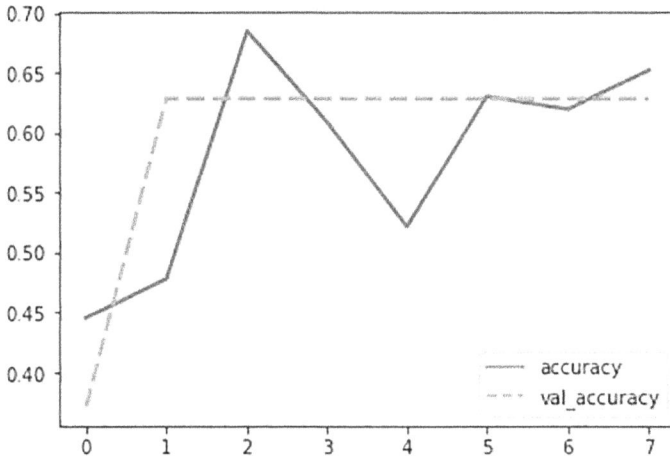

FIGURE 17.4 Training and validation accuracy graph with parameter tuning and discreet wavelength transform.

TABLE 17.2
Data Plot on Training and Validation Data

Epoch	Train-Loss	T-Accuracy	Valid-Loss	V-Accuracy	Time
1	0.8097	0.3696	0.7397	0.3715	00.88
2	0.7223	0.3913	0.7012	0.3715	00.87
3	0.6977	0.4130	0.6782	0.6385	00.86
4	0.6760	0.6304	0.6640	0.6385	00.89
5	0.6847	0.5870	0.6650	0.6385	00.87
6	0.6834	0.5870	0.6647	0.6385	00.89
7	0.6459	0.6630	0.6600	0.6385	00.87
8	0.6429	0.6413	0.6608	0.6385	00.87

allowed the proposed CNN model to have sufficient features for classification while neutralizing the effect of a possible increase in accumulated parameters. Therefore, adopting a different convolution filter size (5 × 5) in the first segment and (3 × 3) in the last segment significantly reduced the effect of large parameters size on the classification outcome of the proposed model.

The restriction of pooling operation only to the first segment of the model also prevented the possibility of data loss in the output feature map, which may affect the classification probability. The choice of average pooling over max pooling support feature maps down sampling with better abstraction with a reduction in the size of feature map and enlargement of the receptive fields. It also enhances the generalization ability of the network.

TABLE 17.3
Predicted Outcomes of Different Epochs for Each Graph Instance

Graph Chart	Epochs	Training Accuracy	Validation Accuracy
Graph results without parameter tuning	1	62.00%	56.30%
	2	61.80%	58.00%
	3	62.20%	58.20%
	4	62.40%	57.80%
	5	63.80%	57.70%
	6	64.00%	57.20%
	7	64.40%	57.00%
	8	64.00%	56.80%
Graph results with parameter tuning	1	20.00%	15.00%
	2	42.00%	63.00%
	3	63.00%	63.00%
	4	57.50%	63.00%
	5	57.50%	63.00%
	6	63.00%	63.00%
	7	65.00%	63.00%
Graph results with parameter tuning and DWT	1	48.00%	63.00%
	2	68.00%	63.00%
	3	57.00%	63.00%
	4	53.00%	63.00%
	5	63.00%	63.00%
	6	62.00%	63.00%
	7	65.00%	63.00%

TABLE 17.4
Proposed Model Performance Comparison with Existing Models

Model Name with Dataset	Proposed Model Accuracy (Github image dataset)	WiserNet Model Accuracy (BOSS-PPG, AHD-LAN)		Ye's Model Accuracy (BOSS-PPG, AHD-LAN)		Xu's Model Accuracy (BOSS-PPG, AHD-LAN)	
Data embedding rate	Not specify	0.2bpc	0.4bpc	0.2bpc	0.4bpc	0.2bpc	0.4bpc
Accuracy	0.6285	0.725	0.8411	0.6844	0.8031	0.7055	0.8118

A variation of ReLU activation function called "concatenated rectified linear unit" (CReLU) doubles the output dimension of positive x (x, 0) and negative x (0, x), "which supports the performance of the proposed model by reducing the number of parameters to be learned, removing the redundancy of learning separate filters."

17.5.1 PARAMETER TUNING

In the first segment of the proposed model, the convolutional layer contains 16 kernels of 5 × 5-dimensional size, with 26 parameters of weight and bias, resulting in 416 (16 × 24).

The second and third layers are equally configured with 32 kernels of dimensional size 5 × 5. The previous layer gives the output of 16 images in batches, which result in a combination of 16 images with 12 × 25 input and kernel size weight, respectively, plus bias. This result in each kernel having 401 parameters. The resultant total number of parameters for the layer produced is 12,832 (401 × 32), for each convolution layer.

For the second segment, the number of parameters for each convolutional is calculated as ((input size (32) × kernel size (9)) +1) × 64 = 18,4896.

The input of the dense layer is extracted from the result of the flattened layer, taking 64 × 16 images from the pooling layer, and then mapped to a flat array of 64 × 16 to give 1,024.

The output size is computed as 64, and the number of parameters is 64 × (1,024 weights + bias) = 65, 600, with the final layer having a parameter of 128 (64 × 1) × 2.

The output size is computed as 64 to produce a parameter of 65,600 resulting from 64 × (1,024 weights + bias). Likewise, the final layer yields a parameter of 128, i.e., (64 × 1) × 2.

In Figure 17.2, the training accuracy is well executed with an irregular validation accuracy. The anomalies in the validation accuracy are consequent effect of overfitting, where the mode only performs well in training data. This rationalizes the importance of fine-tuning the parameters for effective representations. The changes made to the parameters resulted in a well-ordered graph as represented in Figure 17.3. The graph indicated that the training accuracy started to gradually increase from the starting point of zero before it rapidly picked up from 0.40 down to 0.63 with no significant stability. On the other hand, there was no increase in the validation accuracy until the starting point of one, when it began to rise until it becomes constant at 0.63.

In Figure 17.4, training and validation accuracy graph with parameter tuning and discreet wavelength transform that provides the special and frequency domain information of the image presents a different performance attribute. There was no training outcome from the start of the training accuracy until 0.45 where it rose to 0.68 and fell with no further significant stability. The validation accuracy begins from zero and become constant at maximum level of 0.63. Comparing the three diagrams using the various performances of both training and validation accuracy, the training and validation accuracy with parameter tuning gives a suitable stability that is best for the proposed model.

Table 17.4 shows a comparison between the proposed model and WISERNet, Ye and Xu's model was carried out using their respective validation accuracy. The results revealed that the proposed steganalysis model gives a better abstraction of real-word image steganalysis with a good representation of what image steganalysis should characterize in information security.

The real-world steganalysis system stands on the basis that steganography detectors will not have any prior knowledge of the embedding algorithm or rate of the affected images. The blind steganalysis can best be a problem solver concept that is much effective in cyber space security. With a detection accuracy above average, we conclude that our proposed model outperforms the previous since it is based on inserting and testing. The used datasets were completely taking foreign to the model development. The CNN configuration is made to be suitable for blind steganalysis that is a better problem solver in image steganalysis. The concept of using adaptive optimizer with a thoughtful CNN structural arrangement is advantageous in actualizing a reliable level of accuracy.

17.6   CONCLUSIONS AND FUTURE SCOPE

Convolutional neural networks (CNN) conspicuous performance in computer-related tasks like object detection, image recognition, and image retrieval has made it more superior to other classifiers in the field of image steganalysis. This research work has successfully explored the profound power of convolutional neural networks to produce a suitable model for image steganalysis, with careful consideration of the choice of filter size and number, the convolutional neural network layer arrangement in order to both knob the requirements for adequate feature extraction and a prolific minimum number of parameters at the final feature map. Future image steganalysis system should be structured to further improve the detection accuracy as well as build a model to classify illicit image embedded within another image.

REFERENCES

[1]   A. J. Gabriel, A. O. Adetunmbi, Preye Obaila, A two-layer image-steganography system for covert communication over enterprise network, *Computational Science and Its Applications.* https://doi.org/10.1007/978-3-030-58817-5_34

[2]   S. Yadav, N. Tiwari, Privacy preserving data sharing method for social media platforms, *PLoS ONE.* 18(1), e0280182, 2023. https://doi.org/10.1371/journal.pone.0280182

[3]   A. Thompson, A. Abayomi, A. J. Gabriel, Multi IoT authentication system for smart homes using visual cryptography, digital memory, and blockchain technologies, in *Blockchain Applications in the Smart Eras*, S. Misra and A. Kumar Tyagi, Eds., EAI/Springer Innovations in Communication and Computing. Cham: Springer. https://doi.org/10.1007/978-3-030-89546-4_147

[4]   A. K. Jain, S. R. Sahoo, J. Kaubiyal, Online social networks security and privacy: Comprehensive review and analysis, *Springer Link.* 7, 2157–2177. https://link.springer.com/content/pdf/10.1007/s40747-021-00409-7.pdf

[5]   K. T. Smith, L. M. Smith, M. Burger, E. S. Boyle, Cyber terrorism cases and stock market valuation effects, *Information and Computer Security*, 2023. https://doi.org/10.1108/ICS-09-2022-0147

[6]   M. S. Taha, M. S. M. Rahem, M. M. Hashim, H. N. Khalid, High payload image steganography scheme with minimum distortion based on distinction grade value method, *Multimedia Tools and Applications.* 81, 25913–25946, 2022. https://doi.org/10.1007/s11042-022-12691-9

[7]   G. Li, B. Feng, M. He, J. Weng, W. Lu, High-capacity coverless image steganographic scheme based on image synthesis, Elsevier. 111, 2023. https://doi.org/10.1016/j.image.2022.116894

[8]   M. Bouzegza, A. Belatreche, A. Bouridane, M. Tounsi, A comprehensive review of video steganalysis, *IET Image Processing.* 16(13), 3407–3425, 2022. https://doi.org/10.1049/ipr2.12573

[9]   D. S. Sakkeena, S. Murugavalli, L. Jabasheela, V. Anitha, Ceaseless steganographic approaches in machine learning, *Measurement: Sensors*. 25, 100622, 2023. https://doi.org/10.1016/j.measen.2022.100622

[10] I. H. Sarker, Deep learning: A comprehensive overview on techniques, taxonomy, applications and research directions, *SN Computer Science*. 2(6), 1–20, 2021. https://doi.org/10.1007/s42979-021-00815-1

[11] M. C. Schielein, J. Christl, S. Sitaru, A. C. Pilz, R. Kaczmarczyk, T. Biedermann, T. Lasser, A. Zink, Outlier detection in dermatology: Performance of different convolutional neural networks for binary classification of inflammatory skin diseases, *Journal of the European Academy of Dermatology & Venereology*. 37(S2), 2023. https://doi.org/10.1111/jdv.18853.

[12] A. Özdil, B. Yilmaz, Medical infrared thermal image based fatty liver classification using machine and deep learning, Quantitative InfraRed Thermography Journal, 2022. https://doi.org/10.1080/17686733.2022.2158678.

[13] A. L. Imoize, P. A. Gbadega, H. I. Obakhena, D. O. Irabor, K. V. N. Kavitha, C. Chakraborty, Artificial intelligence-enabled internet of medical things for COVID-19 pandemic data management, in *Explainable Artificial Intelligence in Medical Decision Support Systems*, 1st ed., A. L. Imoize, J. Hemanth, D.-T. Do, and S. N. Sur, Eds. London: The Institution of Engineering and Technology, 2022, pp. 357–380.

[14] O. B. Ayoade *et al.*, Explainable artificial intelligence (XAI) in medical decision systems (MDSSs): Healthcare systems perspective, in *Explainable Artificial Intelligence in Medical Decision Support Systems*, 1st ed., A. L. Imoize, J. Hemanth, D.-T. Do, and S. N. Sur, Eds. London: The Institution of Engineering and Technology, 2022, pp. 1–43.

[15] V. Iguoba, A. L. Imoize, The psychology of explanation in medical decision support systems, in *Explainable Artificial Intelligence in Medical Decision Support Systems*, 1st ed., A. L. Imoize, J. Hemanth, D.-T. Do, and S. N. Sur, Eds. London: The Institution of Engineering and Technology, 2022, pp. 489–506.

[16] J. B. Awotunde, E. A. Adeniyi, S. A. Ajagbe, A. L. Imoize, O. A. Oki, S. Misra, Explainable artificial intelligence (XAI) in medical decision support systems (MDSS): Applicability, prospects, legal implications, and challenges, in *Explainable Artificial Intelligence in Medical Decision Support Systems*, 1st ed., A. L. Imoize, J. Hemanth, D.-T. Do, and S. N. Sur, Eds. London: The Institution of Engineering and Technology, 2022, pp. 45–90.

[17] D. A. Shehab, M. J. Alhaddad, Comprehensive survey of multimedia steganalysis: Techniques, evaluations, and trends in future research, *Faculty of Computing and Information Technology*. 14(1), 117, 2022. https://doi.org/10.3390/sym14010117

[18] M. Chen, V. Sedighi, M. Boroumand, J. Fridrich, JPEG-phase-aware convolutional neural network for steganalysis of JPEG images, in *Proceedings of IH&MMSec'17*, Philadelphia, PA, 2017, pp. 75–84. https://doi.org/10.1145/3082031.3083248

[19] M. Yedroudj, M. Chaumont, F. Comby, How to augment a small learning set for improving the performances of a CNN-based steganalyzer? *IS&T International Symposium on Electronic Imaging Science and Technology*, 2018. https://arxiv.org/abs/1801.04076

[20] R. Zhang, F. Zhu, J. Liu, G. Liu, Efficient feature learning and multi-size image steganalysis based on CNN. 2, 1–10, 2018. http://arxiv.org/abs/1807.11428

[21] Z. Wang, M. Chen, Y. Yang, Joint multi-domain feature learning for image steganalysis based on CNN, *EURASIP Journal on Image and Video Processing*. 7, 2020. https://doi.org/10.1186/s13640-020-00513-7

[22] X. Yan, Y. Lu, S. Wang, Image steganalysis via diverse filters and squeeze-and-excitation convolutional neural network, *Mathematics*. 9, 189, 2021. https://doi.org/10.3390/math9020189

[23] S. Kang, H. Park, J. II Park, CNN-based ternary classification for image steganalysis, *Electronics (Switzerland)*. 8(11), 1–15, 2019. https://doi.org/10.3390/electronics8111225

[24] J. Zeng, S. Tan, G. Liu, B. Li, J. Huang, WISERNet: Wider separate-then-reunion net-
      work for steganalysis of color images, *IEEE Transactions on Information Forensics
      and Security*, Images: A Review. *Journal of Artificial Intelligence*. 10, 1–21 https://
      arxiv.org/pdf/1803.04805.pdf
[25] Z. Jin, Y. Yang, Y. Chen, Y. Chen, IAS-CNN: Image adaptive steganalysis via convo-
      lutional neural network combined with selection channel, *International Journal of
      Distributed Sensor Networks*. 16(3), 3, 2020. https://doi.org/10.1177/1550147720911002
[26] M. Sharifzadeh, C. Agarwal, M. Aloraini, D. Schonfeld, Convolutional neural network
      steganalysis's application to steganography, in *2017 IEEE Visual Communications
      and Image Processing, VCIP 2017, 2018-Janua*, 2018, pp. 1–4. https://doi.org/10.1109/
      VCIP.2017.8305045

18 Case Studies in AIoMT Applications

A Secure Medical Cyber-Physical System for the Monitoring and Diagnosis of Lassa Fever

Adebowale Joseph Adelakun, Boniface Kayode Alese, Aderonke Favour-Bethy Thompson, and Olufunso Dayo Alowolodu

18.1 INTRODUCTION

The introduction of technology in the field of medicine has taken a new dimension with numerous attendant benefits. Advancement in internet technologies, artificial intelligence, and their operations in the medical field has produced what is now called Artificial intelligence of Medical Things (AIoMT). This is the operation of IoT in healthcare. AIoMT can make the remote monitoring and diagnosis of diseases possible to lower healthcare costs and offer better services [1–5].

In this study, we proposed using sensor technology for monitoring Lassa fever cases, cloud technologies and machine learning algorithms to develop a framework for the monitoring and diagnosis of Lassa fever. Cyber-physical systems (CPS) involve the combination of physical systems with computing to control or monitor operations [6]. The physical parts, such as cameras and detectors, are integrated with the cloud to continuously cover the changes in the physical terrain. CPS operations are utilized in healthcare, smart grid, automotive systems, and aerospace. MCPS is a distinct sphere of cyber-physical systems and it is made possible by the advancement of ICT and cyber/cloud technology. It has been described as a physical system consisting of control devices, network capabilities, embedded software, and complex physiological dynamics of cases in medicine [7]. MCPS operations are classified as assisted or controlled applications; the former involves monitoring the health of patients without controlling their normal living and the latter is employed for medical support in intensive care and hospitals [8].

This work intends to apply an assisted MCPS in the monitoring and diagnosis of Lassa fever (LF). Lassa fever, an acute viral hemorrhagic fever (VHF), caused

DOI: 10.1201/9781003370321-18

by a single-stranded RNA virus [9] was first encountered in Lassa village in Borno State of Nigeria. It has spread across West African nations like Serra Leone, Liberia, Guinea, Liberia, and Nigeria. Humans are infected by LF through contact with items in the household or food defiled with the urine or faeces of rodents. It is also possible for person-to-person infections and laboratory transmission to happen [10, 11].

Lassa fever has been named one of the top bio-threats in the world [12]. According to the National Centre for Disease Control (NCDC), an estimated three hundred thousand to five hundred thousand cases and five thousand related deaths happen annually in West Africa where it is recognized to be endemic but some incident has occurred in countries like the UK, USA, and Germany, considered as non-endemic [11]. Nigeria recorded the largest number of cases ever in 2018, with over 600 verified cases and over 170 deaths; case casualty rates ranged from 3% to 42% but remained between 20% and 25% from 2019 to 2022 [11]. There is presently no approved vaccine but early care with rehydration and treatment based on observed symptoms improves survival. The symptoms, according to NCDC, which are generally noticed between 2 and 21 days after contact with the virus, include fever, headache, sore throat, nausea, chest, and muscle pain, vomiting and diarrhea, and swelling of the face, and after it has become severe there could be bleeding from parts of the body like the nose, mouth, vagina, or gastrointestinal tract and a body temperature that is around 38°C [11].

An important strategy in the control of outbreaks of contagious diseases is contact tracing [13]. It is the process of locating all individuals who have had significant exposure to verified or probable cases during the time before and after the onset of symptoms [2].

Manual contact tracing is not only a time-consuming, and error-prone process but has some limitations such as confidentiality and privacy, ethics and the law, and the issues of fear of social stigmatization by society [14]. From our discussions with the experts treating Lassa Fever in the Federal Medical Centre Owo, some specific challenges of the manual contact monitoring employed were observed such as the cost of transportation for health officials to visit contacts daily for three weeks, free medicals to check their temperature and to warn the health official or if health official identify any symptoms of Lassa fever in which case they are moved to treatment centers for immediate attention, and contact may also give fake addresses so they are lost. Paramilitary officials and traditional or religious leaders are occasionally involved in furnishing health officials with the details of contacts.

Due to the foregoing, the need for the use of technology becomes desirable. Digital contact tracing is the operation of technology such as smartphones and detectors and apps to identify contacts and notify them of their exposure to infected persons. This technology has been proposed as a complement and to enhance manual contact tracing and not as an alternative [15].

18.1.1 THE CHAPTER CONTRIBUTION

The significant contribution of the chapter is as follows:

   i. The chapter discussed the importance, significant challenges, and the prospect of AIOMT in health care and research contribution with the application of AI.

ii. An algorithm for screening and diagnosis of Lassa cases is presented.

iii. The implementation of a prediction model for Lassa fever based on machine learning and the performance evaluation of the framework using a real-world medical dataset was discussed.

iv. A secured model for a real-time sensor-based monitoring system, including cloud computing technologies, was presented.

18.1.2 CHAPTER ORGANIZATION

Section 18.2 presents the works on the application of artificial Intelligence in the diagnosis and prediction of diseases, security issues of IoTs/AIoMTs, and the challenges and motivation for the research; Section 18.3 discusses the design of the prediction model for Lassa fever; Section 18.4 gives the details of results and discussions. Finally, Section 18.5 draws conclusions and makes recommendations and proposals for further research.

18.2 REVIEW OF RELATED WORK

This section focuses on reviewing related works to present what others have done, identify the limitations, and provide the motivation and need for this study.

18.2.1 REVIEW OF RELATED WORKS

Artificial intelligence (AI) has been applied in health care delivery and has been extensively reported [30–40]. The security and confidentiality of patients' records had also been a subject of a wide range of research [28, 29]. Miah et al. [16] developed a cloud-based health model for monitoring diabetes. Anonymous ID and password were used to ensure the privacy and security of data. Sailunaz *et al.* [17] worked on a cloud-based medical framework to monitor rural health and utilized Identity Based Encryption (IBE). The relevance of machine learning algorithms in diagnosis of diseases has been studied [1–5, 28–34]. Otoom *et al.* [2] proposed a model which utilized the Internet of Things (IoTs) and machine learning techniques to detect and monitor COVID-19 Cases. There has been the operation of artificial intelligence and demonstration of Explainable Artificial Intelligence (XAI) using the Explainable Neural Network (XANN) model in the prediction of diabetes mellitus. Zahid and Mona [18] employed features ranking of symptoms to detect chronic kidney disease (CKD) and carried out performance evaluation of some classification models. K-Nearest Neighbour (K-NN) had the best performance in comparison to others. The application of prediction models in enhancing the diagnosis of Lassa fever has also been extensively reported [30–35]. Oluwole and Nkonyana [19] applied Decision Tree (DT), and k-Nearest Neighbour (k-NN) models to provide prompt surveillance of outbreaks of Lassa Fever (LF) and to forecast cases. Imanov and Asengi [20] designed a ruled-based intelligent system to diagnose Lassa fever in collaboration with medical experts. Nnebe *et al.* [21] proposed an ML model to effectively diagnose suspected Lassa fever cases. The model was recommended for diagnosing other diseases.

The use of IoT detectors in health and environmental monitoring was demonstrated by Arroyo *et al.* [22], which proposes a model for uploading data via a gateway to the cloud to monitor air pollution. It also included the employment of machine learning algorithms for the classification of air content. According to Poongodi *et al.* [23] detectors can be employed in medical devices for collecting data over a wireless network for faster and cheaper healthcare services. The security of the data collected through these detectors as IoT and applied as AIoMT has been proposed [24], intelligent approaches which can be enhanced with machine learning (ML) and deep learning (DL) should be introduced beyond just securing communication among IoT components. Alowolodu *et al.* [25] recommended that cloud computing applications could be secured with Elliptic Curve Cryptography (ECC). The result was described as one of the fastest, most robust, and lower key-needed forms of cryptography for use. Alabi *et al.* [26] also proposed combining Advanced Encryption Standard (AES) and Elliptic Curve Cryptography (ECC) as a hybrid encryption algorithm for the security of information stored in the Cloud. Thompson *et al.* [27] proposed a multi-factor security technique for smart systems to overcome the difficulty that users may suffer in remembering their Personal Identification Numbers (PINs). This was based on blockchain technologies, digital memory, and visual cryptography.

18.2.2 SUMMARY OF ANALYSIS OF RELATED WORK

TABLE 18.1
Summary of Reviewed Literature and Related Work

Author/References	Problem Type	Remarks/Limitations
Akinnuwesi *et al.* [1]	SVM algorithm for early detection of prostate cancer	Only SVM and random forest were tested.
Otoom *et al.* [2]	IoT solution for early detection of COVID-19	The work did not consider the issues of security/privacy of the patient and focused mainly on COVID-19 detection and do not consider scalability to other diseases.
Kajan *et al.* [3]	Applied ANN in the diagnosis of breast cancer, cardiac arrhythmia disease, and Parkinson's disease	Only ANN was tested and it was not extended to Lassa fever.
Miah *et al.* [16]	e-health solution for diabetic patients to be accessed remotely by patients and medical officials	Machine learning techniques were not employed to enhance the diagnostic system.
Sailunaz *et al.* [17]	Cloud-based medical framework to monitor rural health	The main weakness of the system is the weak security of the system.
Oluwole and Nkonyana [19]	ML Model to provide prompt surveillance of outbreaks of Lassa fever (LF) and forecasting of future cases	The focus was on surveillance of Lassa fever (LF) outbreaks and forecasting and not on diagnosis.

TABLE 18.1 (*Continued*)
Summary of Reviewed Literature and Related Work

Author/References	Problem Type	Remarks/Limitations
Imanov and Assengi [20]	A computer-aided diagnosis system for oral squamous cell carcinoma	Machine learning was not employed to enhance the system and accuracy of the diagnosis.
Nnebe *et al.* [21]	Diagnosis of Lassa fever using ML	The proposed architectural framework was not implemented.
Thompson *et al.* [27]	A multifactor approach to security based on digital memory, visual cryptography, and blockchain technology	This can be used to enhance the authentication process of any system.

18.2.3 RESEARCH MOTIVATION AND OBJECTIVES

Lassa fever, a hemorrhagic fever, remains a prevalent threat to human health after over 50 years of its onset [10]. The prevalence of Lassa fever and Ebola virus attacks, the recent outbreak of diseases in African countries, has remained a serious challenge [41]. The dependence on manual monitoring systems, which are subject to human error or negligence for such deadly diseases, calls for a more efficient monitoring system. The proposed model would be able to handle and eliminate these errors by providing a more efficient system of monitoring. The need for a real-time alarm or alert system for timely intervention by medical personnel based on reported measurement to the central server and/or through the distributed systems. This work is hence, motivated to extend the study of [2] to cover Lassa fever such that it could be scalable to other diseases by combining digital monitoring of Lassa fever patients with machine learning algorithms for the diagnosis of the disease.

This work is aimed at designing a Secure Medical Cyber-Physical System (MCPS) from existing models for the monitoring and diagnosis of Lassa fever, and the objectives are as follows:

  i. Developing a secure Medical Cyber-Physical system for contact monitoring and diagnosis of Lassa Fever Patients (MCPS-Lassa)
 ii. Developing a machine learning predictive model for the diagnosis of Lassa fever
iii. Evaluating the developed systems

18.3 METHODOLOGY

The section discusses the methods and techniques employed in the research, the development of algorithms, the proposed architecture, and the machine learning models.

18.3.1 PROPOSED ALGORITHMS FOR THE DIGITAL MONITORING OF LASSA FEVER CONTACTS

The monitoring of Lassa fever contacts (infected or exposed individuals) in Ondo State, Nigeria, in this study will include the following steps: digital monitoring, data collection, and data analytic procedures/techniques. This work also proposes a Lassa fever monitoring and diagnosis system. Real-time data from a wearable sensor would be collected and uploaded to the cloud through a secured gateway to identify potential Lassa fever cases from the collected data. Five classifiers, namely Naïve Bayes, artificial neural network, support vector machine, decision table, and k-nearest neighbor were applied for classifying the dataset to propose a suitable model. The performance evaluation was done using standard metrics with the view to determine the most suitable for implementing the diagnostic model.

As a result of interaction with the medical experts on the procedure for screening, monitoring and alerting health officials for further action on suspected contacts of Lassa fever, an algorithm was developed. A high-level language of the algorithm is outlined in Figure 18.1.

18.3.2 The Proposed AIoMT Framework

Our proposed AIoMT-based framework would be used to monitor potential and suspected Lassa fever patients. Figure 18.2 shows the AIoMT conceptual diagram. It has

Step 1: Initialize patient data and wearable sensor

Step 2: Read the patient's temperature using a wearable sensor

Step 3: If the temperature is >= 38°C:

    Step 3.1: Label the patient as a "Suspect"

    Step 3.2: Temperature Last for 3 days

    Step 3.3: Trigger Alarm to Health Authority

Step 4: If the patient is labeled as "Suspect":

    Step 4.1: Check for symptoms (a1, a2, a3, ... , an)

    Step 4.2: If symptoms are present:

        Step 4.2.1: Administer Rivabirin

    Step 4.2.2: Admit for PCR test

        Step 4.2.3: If the PCR test is positive:

        Step 4.2.3.1: Label the patient as "Confirmed"

        Step 4.2.3.2: Continue treatment

    Step 4.3: Else:

        Step 4.3.1: Screen the patient as a contact

    Step 4.3.2: Monitor for 21 days

FIGURE 18.1   The algorithm of the proposed contact monitoring system

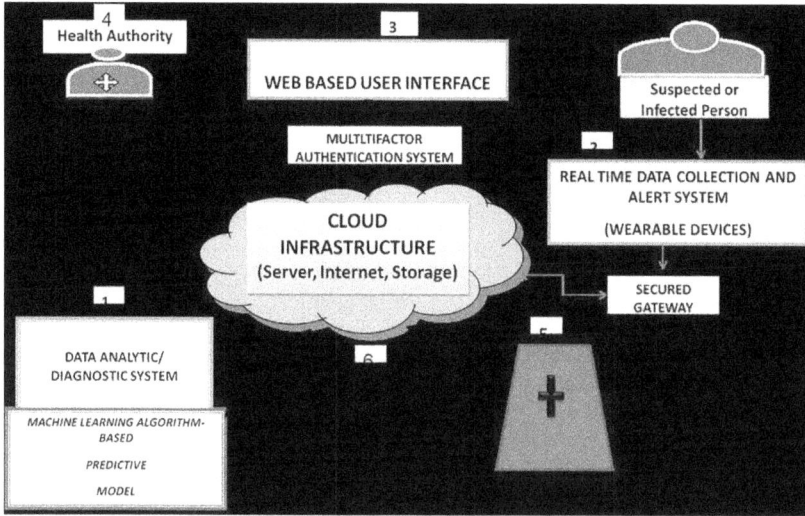

FIGURE 18.2 Proposed AIoMT architecture for Lassa fever.

six major elements: Real-Time Data Collection and Alert System, Diagnostic System, Isolation Centre, a Web-based interface App for Users and the Health Authority, the Security System (authentication, secured gateway), and the cloud infrastructure.

18.3.2.1 Real-Time Data collection and Alert System

A wearable device that can measure vital signs is attached to the body of the suspected/infected person to collect and transfer this data for storage in the cloud [23]. This is analyzed through a diagnostic feature in the MCPS—Lassa App, which is a web-based app for users' registration and virtualization of the log data/result of analysis to guide health authority/caregivers. In addition, an integrated alerts system is designed to trigger caregivers and patients when the machine learning model confirms a patient is infected or the condition becomes serious to be declared an emergency based on the analysis of vital signs uploaded through the wearable device(s).

The alarm is set out to the health authority and/or the patient for immediate action when the measurement goes above agreed thresholds.

18.3.2.2 Data Analytic/Diagnostic System

The data analytic/diagnostic system is a machine learning-based model that would be used to classify Lassa fever cases based on collected real-time data. These would aid accurate and timely identification of infected users and recommend appropriate action to users or the health authority. It would make the health authorities or assistants to be more efficient in helping the Lassa patients.

18.3.2.3 The Isolation Centre

The patients diagnosed as suspected cases are either self-quarantined or moved to the isolation center and connected to the real-time data collection system. The patients

confirmed infected are held in the isolation center and monitored through the real-
time data collection system.

18.3.2.4   The Cloud Infrastructure

The cloud hosts the storage and the needed communication resources to which the
system is connected via the internet. In addition, the real-time data from wearable
sensors on the suspected cases are uploaded and personal health records, predictions
results, and physician recommendations are stored.

18.3.2.5   The Web-Based Interface

The patients and health authority access the analyzed data or prediction result
through the web-based interface from the cloud. The physician or caregiver could act
fast on suspected cases.

18.3.2.6   The Secure Gateway

The users and health officials use their faces and fingerprints to access the system
through a multifactor authentication process. The data collected are secured through
a hybrid encryption scheme.

18.3.3   The Machine Learning Predictive Model

The machine learning predictive model was based on the raw data collected. This
was pre-processed and used to train five machine learning algorithms. Finally, their
performances were evaluated using standard metrics.

18.3.3.1   Dataset

The model proposed in this work was implemented using a dataset collected from
Federal Medical Centre Owo, in Ondo State, Nigeria. The collected data was in a raw
format not suitable for machine learning processes and had to be pre-processed. The
data contains various information, but our focus was on the symptoms and outcome
of the initial result of the Polymerase Chain Reaction (PCR) tests to confirm whether
the patients are infected or not. We also observed the record of the outcome of treatment with RIVABIRIN after ten days and the outcome whether they were discharged
after recovery, referred to other medical facilities or death. The data acquired had
70 features/symptoms and 439 instances (corresponding to 439 patients). This was
reduced to 47 features/symptoms manually in consultation with the experts and consultants; by employing the information gain feature ranking to remove redundant and
irrelevant data, which included features like age, sex, profession, date of admission,
and so on, the attributes were finally reduced to 27, including the class.

18.3.3.2   Pre-Processing Data

The dataset has cases from which we got 47 symptoms and 3 other features (Treatment
with Rivabirin, PCR result after 10 days, and Final Outcome). The total case or
instances was 440 giving 27,897 data records. It should be noted that the cases were
based on suspected cases due to a baseline temperature of 38°C and above. Feature

ranking and selection were carried out on the data to determine the most relevant symptoms for the diagnosis of Lassa fever by applying an information gain ranking filter on all training datasets. Based on the feature ranking the first 26 symptoms were extracted as shown in Table 18.2.

18.3.3.3 Predictive Model

The predictive diagnostic model for Lassa fever was built by using the preprocessed dataset. The model estimates whether Lassa Fever infects a suspected case or individual based on Five ML classifiers namely Naïve Bayes (NB), Artificial Neural Networks (ANN)), Support Vector Machine (SVM), k-nearest neighbors (kNN), and Decision Tables (DT) [1–5, 34]. Cross-fold validation method for measuring the performance of classification models was used in this work to measure their

TABLE 18.2
The Symptoms of Lassa after Feature Selection

S/N	SYMPTOMS/FEATURES
1.	Headache
2.	General weakness
3.	Body pain
4.	Chills and rigor
5.	Fever
6.	Sore throat
7.	Bitter taste
8.	Vomiting blood
9.	Vomiting
10.	Oedema on face/neck
11.	Abdominal pain
12.	Baseline systolic BP
13.	Chest pain
14.	Cough
15.	Difficulty in breathing
16.	Restlessness
17.	Hematuria/coke-colored urine
18.	Renal complications
19.	Contact with confirmed +
20.	Loss of consciousness
21.	Dizziness
22.	Loss of appetite
23.	Diarrhea, watery Stool
24.	Bleeding from any part of the body
25.	Convulsion
26.	Temperature
27.	Class: PCR Test

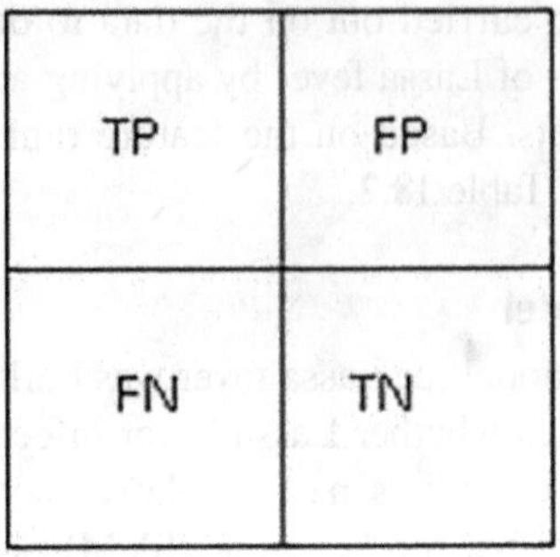

FIGURE 18.3 Confusion matrix notation.

performances. The labelled dataset was split into K-folds such that one of the folds is used for testing and the remaining for training. In this work, the tenfold cross-validation technique was used. The data instances were divided into tenfold; ninefold were used for training and the remaining one was used for testing [2].

18.3.3.4 The Confusion Matrix

This is a result of the evaluation of the trained dataset with the test dataset using any of the splitting techniques. The four notations are represented in Figure 18.4. Here, TP (True Positive) predicts a condition as positive which is actually positive; TN (True negative) predicts a negative condition as negative; FP (False Positive) is when a condition is negative and it is predicted as positive; FN (False Negative) is when a condition is positive it is predicted to be negative by the classifier.

18.3.3.5 The Metrics for Performance Evaluation

The performance evaluation of the models or classifier is carried out based on the confusion matrix notations in Figure 18.4. Equations 18.1, 18.2, 18.3, 18.4, 18.5, and 18.6 were used to calculate the Accuracy, Precision, Recall, F1 Score, and Specificity, True/False Positive respectively. The ROC curve was plotted using Equations 18.6 and 18.7. The results for the five classifiers in this study are shown in Table 18.3.

$$\text{Accuracy} = \frac{\text{TP} + \text{TN}}{\text{TP} + \text{FP} + \text{TN} + \text{FN}} \times 100\% \tag{18.1}$$

$$\text{Precision} = \frac{\text{TP}}{\text{TP} + \text{FP}} \times 100\% \tag{18.2}$$

$$\text{Recall} = \frac{\text{TP}}{\text{TP} + \text{FN}} \times 100\% \tag{18.3}$$

$$\text{F1 Score} = 2 \times \frac{\text{Precison} \times \text{Recall}}{\text{Precision} + \text{Recall}} \tag{18.4}$$

$$\text{Specificity} = \frac{TN}{TN + FP} \times 100\% \qquad (18.5)$$

$$\text{True Positive} = \frac{TP}{TP + FN} \qquad (18.6)$$

$$\text{False Positive} = \frac{FP}{FP + TN} \qquad (18.7)$$

18.4   THE RESULTS AND DISCUSSIONS

The results from the study are presented in this section, and it also discusses the proposed model evaluation results and makes recommendations for its application and future research work.

18.4.1   CONFUSION MATRICES

The confusion matrices for the five selected classifiers are shown in Figure 18.5. A high-top left corner (TP) with a high lower right corner is good (TN), while a higher top right corner (FP) and higher lower left corner (FN) are not good.

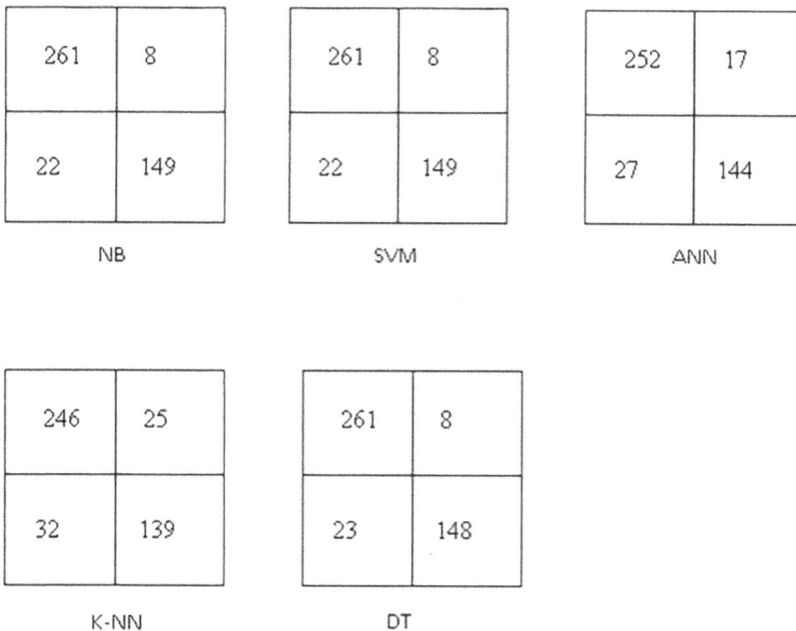

FIGURE 18.4   Showing the confusion matrixes of the models: Naïve Baiyes (NB), Support Vector Machine (SVM), Artificial Neural Networks (ANN), K-Nearest Neighbour (K-NN) and Decision Table (DT).

TABLE 18.3
The Summary of Performance of the Models

Base Classifiers	Accuracies	Recall	Specificity	Precision	F1 score	AUC
NB	**93.2**	92.2	94.9	**97.0**	94.6	**92.9**
SVM	**93.2**	92.2	**94.9**	**97.0**	94.6	**92.9**
DT	**93.0**	91.9	**94.9**	**97.0**	94.4	90.0
ANN	90.0	90.3	89.4	93.3	92.0	91.4
K-NN	87.5	88.5	85.8	91.4	89.9	87.7

The first column has the Base classifier as NB, SVM, DT, ANN, and KNN, respectively. And calculated figures are listed for each of them, respectively.

18.4.2 ROC CURVES

The result is shown in Figure 18.6. ROC, which means Receiver Operating Characteristics (ROC), is a measure of the performance of the model at all given thresholds. This is the graph where the True Positive Rate (Equation 18.6) as Y-axis, is plotted against the False Positive Rate (Equation 18.7) as X-axis. The areas under the ROC curve AUC is a measure of how good the model is.

18.4.3 THE PERFORMANCE RESULT

The performance result of the evaluation of the five models is good. The accuracy, precision, recall, and specificity of the models are from 90% and above except for the k-NN model with an Accuracy of 87.5% and an AUC measure of 87.7%. Naïve Bayes and SVM have the same performance with an Accuracy of 93.2 %, Precision of 93.2, and AUC of 92.9%.

The clinical diagnosis record from our dataset shows that out of the 440 Cases screened 269 were confirmed to be positive after the PCR test. Using simple mathematical methods, the performance was 61%. Evaluating the NB or SVM model with the calculated performance shows that the proposed model performs better, and its adoption would reduce the cost and time of testing, which has the potential of saving many patients infected by Lassa fever and also control this deadly epidemic in West Africa. The implementation of real-time data acquisition and modification for the digital monitoring of contacts is ongoing.

18.5 CONCLUSIONS

The proposed model is suitable as a secure medical cyber-physical for monitoring Lassa fever, and both the NB and SVM machine learning model is recommended to improve the accuracy of diagnosis of Lassa fever, which can be very useful in this era of the pandemic. The potential of using feature ranking on the dataset can be implemented to predict whether a confirmed case would recover or not. It is recommended that an ensemble approach to combine the four (NB, SVM, DT, and ANN) could

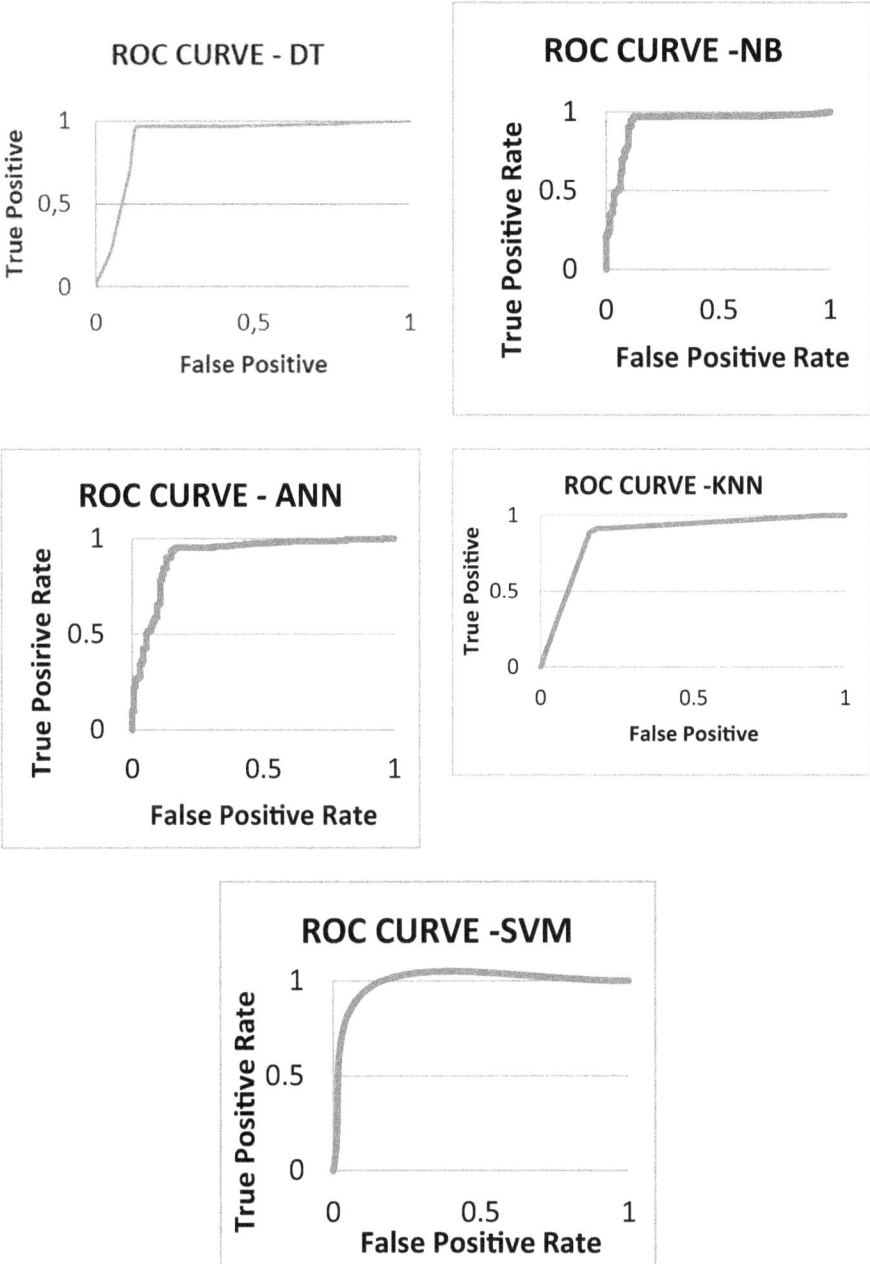

FIGURE 18.5 ROC curves for the models.

be investigated for a better-performing model. Future work should also involve the performance evaluation of the security system in our model against known attacks. There is also the need for the production of a standard dataset for Lassa fever which can be a subject of further study.

REFERENCES

[1]   Akinnuwesi, B. A., Olayanju, K. A., Aribisala, B. S., Fashoto, S. G., Mbunge, E., Okpeku, M., and Owate, P. (2022). Application of support vector machine algorithm for early differential diagnosis of prostate cancer. *Data Science and Management*. https://doi.org/10.1016/j.dsm.2022.10.001.

[2]   Otoom, M., Otoum, N., Alzubaidi, M. A., Etoom, Y., and Banihani, R. (2020). An IoT-based framework for early identification and monitoring of COVID-19 cases. *Biomedical Signal Processing and Control, 62*, 102149. https://doi.org/10.1016/j.bspc.2020.102149

[3]   Kajan, S., Pernecký, D., and Goga, J. (2015). *Application of Neural Network in Medical Diagnostics.* www2.humusoft.cz/www/papers/tcp2015/030_kajan.pdf. Last visited February 2023.

[4]   Verma, A. K., Chakraborty, M., and Biswas, S. K. (2021). Breast cancer management system using decision tree and neural network. *SN Computer Science, 2*(234). https://doi.org/10.1007/s42979-021-00644-2.

[5]   Kakhi, K., Alizadehsani, R., Kabir, H. D., Khosravi, A., Nahavandi, S., and Acharya, U. R. (2022). The internet of medical things and artificial intelligence: Trends, challenges, and opportunities. *Biocybernetics and Biomedical Engineering, 42*(3), 749–771. https://doi.org/10.1016/j.bbe.2022.05.008.

[6]   Rajkumar, R., Lee, I., Sha, L., and Stankovic, J. (2010). Cyber-physical systems: The next computing revolution. In *Proceedings—Design Automation Conference*, 731–736. https://doi.org/10.1145/1837274.1837461.

[7]   Chen, F., Tang, Y., Wang, C., Huang, J., Huang, C., Xie, D., Wang, T., and Zhao, C. (2022). Medical cyber-physical systems: A solution to smart health and state of the art. *IEEE Transactions on Computational Social Systems, 9*(5), 1359–1386.

[8]   Dey, N., Ashour, A. S., Shi, F., Fong, S. J., and Tavares, J. M. R. S. (2018). Medical cyber-physical systems: A survey. *Journal of Medical Systems, 42*(4), 74. https://doi.org/10.1007/s10916-018-0921-x

[9]   WHO (2023). www.who.int/emergencies/disease-outbreak-news/item/lassa-fever-united-kingdom-of-great-britain-and-northern-ireland. Last visited February, 2023.

[10] CDC (2023). www.cdc.gov/vhf/lassa/pdf/factsheet.pdf. Last visited on 31st January, 2023

[11] NCDC (2023). www.ncdc.gov.ng/diseases/info/L

[12] Pal, M., Gutama, K. P., Gowda, L., and Dave, P. (2022). Lassa fever: An emerging and re-emerging fatal viral disease of public health concern. *American Journal of Public Health Research, 10*(4), 143–146.

[13] Ejembi, J., Emma-Ukaegbu, U., Garba, I., Omale, A., Dogo, B., and Taiwo, L. (2019). Contact tracing in Lassa fever outbreak response, an effective strategy for control?. *Online Journal of Public Health Informatics, 11*(1), e378. https://doi.org/10.5210/ojphi.v11i1.9854

[14] Chakraborty, P., Maitra, S., Nandi, M., and Talnikar, S. (2020). *Contact Tracing in Post-Covid World, A Cryptologic Approach*, 1st ed., Springer Singapore, 2020, ISBN 981159726X, 9789811597268

[15] Kahn, P. J. (2020). *Digital Contact Tracing for Pandemic Response; Ethics and Governance Guidance*, Johns Hopkins University Press, Baltimore, MD, 21218–4363.

[16] Miah, S. J., Hasan, J., and Gammack, J. G. (2016). On-cloud healthcare clinic: An e-health consultancy approach for remote communities in a developing country. *Telematics and Informatics, 34*(1), 311–322. https://doi.org/10.1016/j.tele.2016.05.008

[17] Sailunaz, K., Alhussein, M., Shahiduzzaman, M., Anowar, F., and Mamun, K. A. A. (2016). CMED: Cloud-based medical system framework for rural health monitoring in developing countries. *Computers & Electrical Engineering, 53*, 469–481. https://doi.org/10.1016/j.compeleceng.2016.02.005

[18] Ullah, Z., and Jamjoom, M. (2023). Early detection and diagnosis of chronic kidney disease based on selected predominant features. *Journal of Healthcare Engineering, 2023.* Article ID 3553216. https://doi.org/10.1155/2023/3553216

[19] Oluwole, A. S., and Nkonyana, T. (2022). Forecasting Lassa fever outbreak progression with machine learning. In *Int. l Conference on Electrical, Computer, Communications and Mechatronics Engineering. (ICECCME)*, Maldives, pp. 1–5. https://doi.org/10.1109/ICECCME55909.2022.9987787

[20] Imanov, E., and Asengi, F. J. (2021). Artificial intelligence for Lassa fever diagnosis system. In Aliev, R. A., Kacprxyk, J., Pedrycz, W., Jamshidi, M., Babanli, M., and Sadikoglu, F. M. (eds.), *14th International Conference on Theory and Application of Fuzzy Systems and Soft Computing—ICAFS-2020—ICAFS 2020. Advances in Intelligent Systems and Computing*, vol. 1306. Springer, Cham. https://doi.org/10.1007/978-3-030-64058-3_67.

[21] Nnebe, S. E., Okoh, N. A. O., Otumu, J. A. M., and Oshoiribhor, E. O. (2019). A neuro-fuzzy based reasoning framework for detecting Lassa fever based on observed symptoms. *American Journal of Artificial Intelligence, 3*(1), 9–16. https://doi.org/10.11648/j.ajai.20190301.12

[22] Arroyo, P., Herrero, J., Suárez, J., and Lozano, J. (2019). Wireless sensor network combined with cloud computing for air quality monitoring. *Sensors, 19*(3), 691. MDPI AG. https://doi.org/10.3390/s19030691

[23] Poongodi, T., Gupal, R., and Saini, A. (2021). IOT architecture, communication technologies, and its application. In Lakshmana Kumar, R., Wang, Yichuan, Poongodi, T., and Imoize, Agbotiname Lucky (eds.), *The Internet of Things, Artificial Intelligence and Blockchain Technology*, Springer Nature, Switzerland.

[24] Al-Garadi, M. A., Mohamed, A., Al-Ali, A. K., Du, X., Ali I., and Guizani, M. (2020). A survey of machine and deep learning methods for internet of things (IoT) security. *IEEE Communications Surveys & Tutorials, 22*(3), 1646–1685. https://doi.org/10.1109/COMST.2020.2988293.

[25] Alowolodu, D. O., Alese, B. K., and Adetunmbi, A. (2016). Secured cloud application platform using elliptic curve cryptography. In *Proceeding of the World Congress of Engineering and Computer Science 2016. Vol I WCECS 2016, October 19–21*, San Francisco. https://www.iaeng.org/publication/WCECS2016/WCECS2016_pp208-213.pdf

[26] Alabi, O., Thompson, A., Alese, B., and Gabriel, A. (2020). Cloud application security using hybrid encryption. *Communications on Applied Electronics, 7*, 25–31. https://doi.org/10.5120/cae2020652866.

[27] Thompson, A., Abayomi, A., and Gabriel, A. J. (2016). Multifactor IoT authentication systems for smart homes using visual cryptography, digital memory and blockchain technologies. in *Blockchain Applications in the Smart Eras*, S. Misra and A. Kumar Tyagi, Eds., EAI/Springer Innovations in Communication and Computing. Cham: Springer. https://doi.org/10.1007/978-3-030-89546-4_147

[28] Imoize, A. L., Irabor, D. O., Gbadega, P. A., and Chakraborty, C. (2022). Blockchain technology for secure COVID-19 pandemic data handling. In Chakraborty, C., and Rodrigues, J. J. P. C. (eds.), *Smart Health Technologies for the COVID-19 Pandemic: Internet of Medical Things Perspectives*, 1st ed., London: The Institution of Engineering and Technology, pp. 141–179.

[29] Imoize, A. L., Gbadega, P. A., Obakhena, H. I., Irabor, D. O., Kavitha, K. V. N., and Chakraborty, C., Artificial intelligence-enabled internet of medical things for COVID-19 pandemic data management. In Imoize, A. L., Hemanth, J., Do, D.-T., and Sur, S. N. (eds.), *Explainable Artificial Intelligence in Medical Decision Support Systems*, 1st ed., London: The Institution of Engineering and Technology, pp. 357–380.

[30] Osaseri, R. O., and Osaseri, E. I. (2016). Soft computing approach for diagnosis of Lassa fever. *World Academy of Science, Engineering and Technology International Journal of Computer and Information Engineering, 10*(11). https://publications.waset. org/abstracts/51743/soft-computing-approach-for-diagnosis-of-lassa-fever.

[31] Cong, J., Wei, B., He, Y., Yin, Y., and Zheng, Y. (2017). A selective ensemble classification method combining mammography images with ultrasound images for breast cancer diagnosis. *Computational and Mathematical Methods in Medicine, 2017*, 4896386. https://doi.org/10.1155/2017/4896386.

[32] Ajenaghughrure, I. B., Sujatha, P., and Akazue, M. I. (2017). Fuzzy-based multi-fever symptom classifier diagnosis model. *European Journal of Comput. Science in Information Technology, 9*(10), 13–28.

[33] Aminu, E. F., Ajani, A. A., Rabiu, I. O., Anda, I., Isah, A. O., and Zubairu, H. A. (2018). A diagnosis system for Lassa fever and related ailments using fuzzy logic. *Journal of Science Technology, Mathematics and Education (JOSTMED), 14*(2), 18–30.

[34] Steur, N. A. K., and Mueller, C. (2019). Classification of viral hemorrhagic fever focusing Ebola and Lassa fever using neural networks. *International Journal of Machine Learning and Computing, 9*(3), 334–343.

[35] Osarumwense, A. S., and Eromosele, B. M. (2020). A machine learning-based approach for detecting dengue Hemorrhagic fever. *International Journal of Academic and Applied Research, 4*(5), 13–25.

[36] Sourab, S. Y., Shuvo, H. R., Hasan, R., and Masruf, T. (2021). Diagnosis of COVID-19 from chest X-ray images using convolutional neural networking with K-fold cross validation. In *IEEE International Power and Renewable Energy Conference (IPRECON)*, Kollam, India, pp. 1–5. https://doi.org/10.1109/IPRECON52453.2021.9640744.

[37] Casiraghi, E., Malchiodi, D., Trucco, G., Frasca, M., Cappelletti, L., Fontana, T., Esposito, A. A., Avola, E., Jachetti, A., Reese, J., Rizzi, A., Robinson, P. N., and Valentini, G. (2020). Explainable machine learning for early assessment of COVID-19 risk prediction in emergency departments. *IEEE Access, 26*(8), 196299–196325. https://doi. org/10.1109/ACCESS.2020.3034032.

[38] Ireye, F., Aigbiremolen, A. O., Famiyesin, O. E., Ireotoi, G., Ogbaini-Emovon, E., Irowa, O., Imafidon, O., and William, W. (2021). Contact tracing and profile of Lassa fever contacts in Edo state, Nigeria: Implications for the control of Lassa fever outbreaks. *Journal of Health Sciences & Surveillance System, 9*(1), 20–25. https://doi.org/10.30476/ jhsss.2020.87640.1124

[39] Nwaneri, S. C., Yinka-Banko, C., Uregbulum, U. C., Odukoya, O. O., and Imoize, A. L. (2022). Explainable neural networks in diabetes mellitus prediction. In Imoize, A. L., Hemanth, J., Do, D. T., and Sur, S. N. (eds.), *Explainable Artificial Intelligence in Medical Decision Support Systems*, 1st ed., London: The Institution of Engineering and Technology, pp. 313–334.

[40] Deif, M., Attar, H., Amer, A., Elhaty, I., Khosravi, M., and Solyman, A. (2022). "Diagnosis of oral squamous cell carcinoma using deep neural networks and binary particle swarm optimization on histopathological images: An AIoMT approach. *Computational Intelligence and Neuroscience, 2022*. http://doi.org/10.1155/2022/6364102.

[41] National Library of Medicine. www.ncbi.nlm.nih.gov/pmc/articles/PMC7866331/. Last visited February 2023

19 AIoMT-Assisted Telemedicine

A Case Study of eSanjeevani Telemedicine Service in India

Ambili Parathra Sreedharan Pillai

19.1 INTRODUCTION

Globalization and uncontrolled population growth are forcing humankind to face complex challenges. The diseases such as infectious, chronic diseases, trauma, and mental health issues are becoming dynamic with large-scale variants and posing challenges to researchers, scientists, medical practitioners, and decision-makers in addressing them [1, 2]. As per the available statistics of the data taken from Global Health Workforce Statistics database of World Health Organization (WHO), approximately 40 million new jobs to be created in health and social care fields globally to address United Nations 2030 agenda of healthcare-related Sustainable Development Goals (SDGs) [3]. There is an additional need for 18 million health workers, in rural areas with low-resource settings, to ensure necessary healthcare services to ensure medication for all [4]. The most alarming situation as per data is that the healthcare infrastructure and availability of healthcare workforce is concentrated in urban areas, whereas rural coverage is only nominal. Figure 19.1 is a representation of the statistics of region-wise count of medical workforce taken per 10,000 population.

Quality healthcare treatment is not reaching rural areas, compared to the technologies such as the internet or mobile and other service sectors. Epidemic such as COVID-19 has given a severe warning to humankind and highlighted the necessity of preparedness to face challenges in the health sector. Due to the higher expenses, traditional healthcare facility creation and management is a great challenge with respect to rural areas. Technological innovations in the health sector can address the lack of trained and skilled resources. Internet of Things (IoT)-based health sensing technologies have become more demandable in healthcare systems as they can reach remote areas and aid in smart monitoring of patients. The number of connected devices in IoT networks is growing quickly and points to the need for healthcare applications [5]. It can process enormous medical data and handles efficiently and intelligently.

Artificial intelligence (AI) methods can further aid to achieve early warning and auxiliary diagnosis as well as automatically transfer vital data collected during

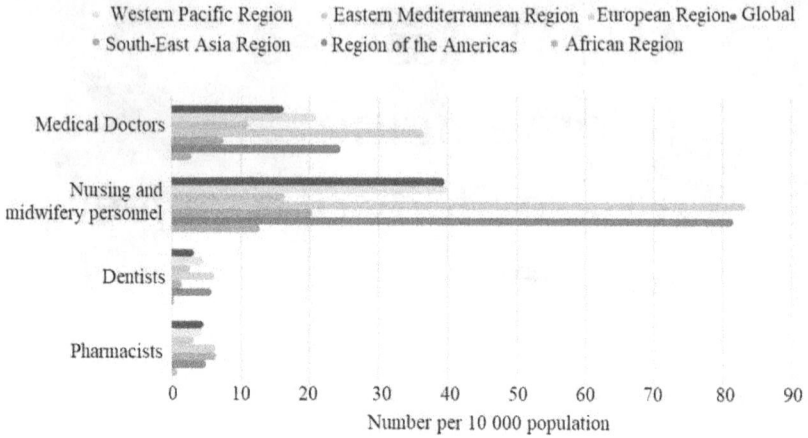

FIGURE 19.1 Region-wise count of medical workforce per 10,000 population.

Source: WHO National Health Workforce Accounts Database, 2022 [3]

health investigation, which helps in timely and effective diagnosis [6]. The integration of medical sensors and AIoT is named Artificial Intelligence of Medical Things (AIoMT) and will be a future development toward the Internet of Medical Things (IoMT). AIoMT is also helpful for providing remote diagnosis, real-time decision-making, and a reliable and affordable healthcare system. AIoMT technologies can obtain a great ability to predict the future conditions of patients, prescribe potential medicines, and prevent further damage through remote monitoring by physicians and provide self-control options to the monitored persons [7]. The remote medical image analysis and pervasive medical systems through medical sensors are key features in an internet of medical things (IoMT)-based intelligent healthcare platform. This points to AIoMT filling the gap of lack of availability of medical professionals and the scope of these technologies in telediagnosis and telemedicine. Adopting advanced devices and technologies such as the internet of medical things (IoMT) can boost sustainable healthcare 5.0 [8]. This chapter focuses on the technological interventions in the medical field, healthcare applications, different innovative AIoMT architectures and offers insights for potential research directions in this field. This chapter precisely presents a study of eSanjeevani, a successful national telemedicine service provided by the government of India.

19.1.1   KEY CONTRIBUTIONS OF THE CHAPTER

The significant contributions presented in this chapter:
    The key objectives of this study are as follows:

i. A comparative analysis of the earlier telemedicine systems with the telemedicine technology powered with AI and IoT. This includes the limitations of the earlier telemedicine systems and the effective use of AI-powered chatbots, kiosks, or robotic assistance with IoT-enabled assistive devices.

ii. How potential machine learning/deep learning algorithms can be effectively integrated for affordable and reliable healthcare in AIoMT?

- The ML/DL algorithms can help analyze clinical data, find relevant patterns in the data for better diagnosis, and can effectively give recommendations.
- A detailed study on the working of such algorithms, distributed architecture of such systems, and how to integrate it with IoT for Intelligent diagnosis.

iii. The challenges of next-generation IoT networks that effectively contribute to healthcare towards Sustainable Healthcare 5.0.Cloud/Edge integrated, and AR/VR enabled IoT network with AI for effective remote health support.

A comparative study on the limitations of contemporary telemedicine and future of AIoMT is also presented in the study. Architecture, operations, and features of eSanjeevani, a successful national telemedicine service provided by the government of India, is presented as a case study.

19.1.2 CHAPTER ORGANIZATION

Section 19.2 is a presentation of the related work on the role of AIoMT in telemedicine. Further, the related literature of study is presented in the corresponding sections itself for better understanding. Section 19.3 gives architectural design of AI-powered telemedicine system with specific concentration on brain tumor analysis. It discusses in detail the role of deep learning in intelligent remote diagnosis and precision medication. Section 19.4 discusses how AI-powered conversational chatbots help telemedicine. Section 19.5 presents a detailed study of the architecture and process flow of eSanjeevani, a telemedicine portal of Government of India. Section 19.6 gives the conclusion and future directions of AIoMT enabling telemedicine.

19.2 RELATED WORK

The rapid development of digital innovations in medical field integrating artificial intelligence techniques, IoT, and cloud computing on top of high-speed wireless 5G communications, during the pandemic period and beyond, opened the door of opportunities in the field of AI-powered telediagnosis and telemedicine [9]. People opted for a moving away from the traditional time-consuming hospital visits to a system of getting their health-related problems being solved at home itself. Early and accurate prediction of critical diseases can be made possible with machine learning techniques over the internet in a remote manner [10]. The related literature of study is presented in the corresponding sections.

19.3 ARCHITECTURAL DESIGN OF AI-POWERED TELEMEDICINE SYSTEM

AI-powered telemedicine systems can intelligently interact with patients and can provide results fast and accurately. The key areas of telemedicine where AI is applied are diagnosis, medicine prescription, patient monitoring, and extended continued support in treatment. New models such as AI-powered voice chatbots and AI-powered robotic instruments can be adopted for achieving this: Oneremission—an Oncology support system, Babylon—an integrated AI-powered medical support system, Florence—Health tracker and Medication reminder system are a few of the examples of AI-powered Chatbots.

AI-powered telemedicine systems mostly make use of machine learning, deep learning algorithms, or the capability of natural language processing to find undiscovered patterns and relationships in data and to arrive at intelligent decisions [11, 56]. The scope of efficient integration of AI and Medical imaging in neurodegenerative diseases and possible tele advice is a current focus of research [12]. Detection of neurodegenerative diseases at the initial stage forms a key aspect of medication and recovery. Figure 19.2 depicts the general representation of the proposed system architecture where the test results or clinical reports form the input, and using deep learning methodologies it can be processed to get the medication prescribed, which can be stored and made available to users on request.

By thoroughly surveying current developments, the authors attempt to present a most suitable deep learning model to be adopted for precision neural disorders medication, which can extend help in tele-diagnosis and tele-medicine. In most of the neural disorder cases, the input will be images like X-rays/EEG or MRI, and according to reliable data there can be 2.4 million features associated with a color image that measures 800×1000 pixels [13]. Deep learning algorithms are very effective in detecting edges and colors for image representation, the convolutional layers can efficiently translate the representations into numerical values and thus interpret and find relevant patterns for accurate results. Figure 19.3 depicts the general representation of the process flow in the proposed system architecture, where the test results or clinical reports form the input and using deep learning methodologies it can be

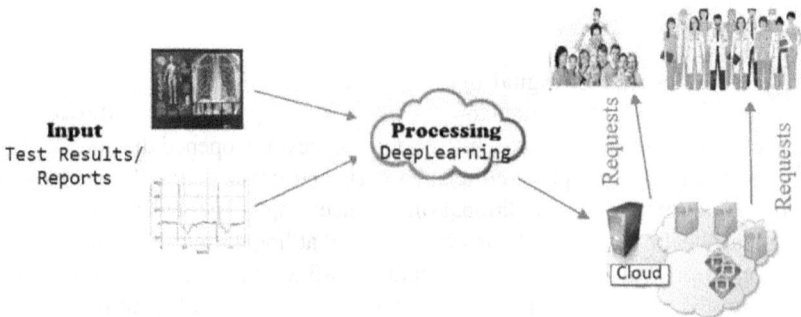

Input
Test Results/
Reports

Processing
DeepLearning

Requests

Requests

Cloud

FIGURE 19.2   A general system architecture.

processed to get the medication prescribed, which can be stored and made available to users on request.

19.3.1 AIoMT in Brain Tumor Diagnosis

Brain tumor is a critical brain disorder where abnormal growth is identified in parts of brain. This can be malignant growth, resulting in brain damage, to be fatal or non-cancerous tumors. The key challenges associated with the diagnosis process are to identify the location of the growth in the central organ of the nervous system,

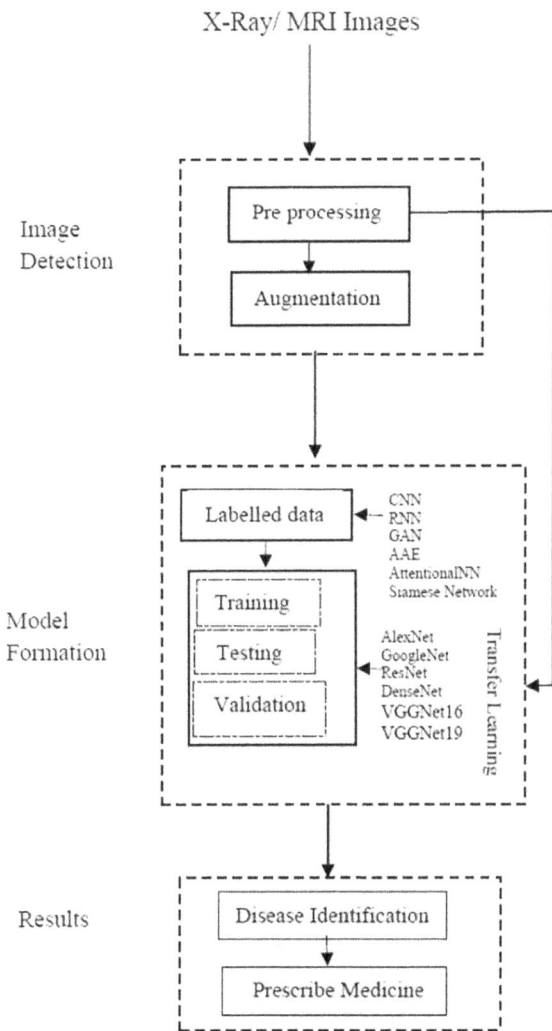

FIGURE 19.3 The precision medication system process flow.

Input Image Acquisition/ PreProcessing	→	Skull Stripping	→	Region of Interest Segmentation	→	Deep Feature Extraction	→	Deep Model

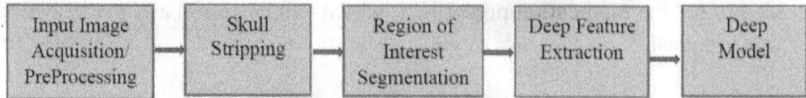

FIGURE 19.4   Steps in brain tumor diagnosis.

classification of tumor based on grading, malignancy, types, and subtypes as of the World Health Organization (WHO) specifications [14, 15].

Figure 19.4 represents the different steps involved in the deep learning approach for brain tumor diagnosis.

19.3.1.1   Image Acquisition and Pre-Processing

In the telediagnosis process employing deep learning, image acquisition and preprocessing the image without noise is an important primary step. The X-Ray/PET Scan/ MRI images intensity variations adjustment can adopt smoothing as preprocessing operation [16]. In order to avoid misclassification and wrong image acquisition effective filtering, many filtering techniques can be applied, for example, Weiner Filter [17, 18], an efficient adaptive edge noise-filtering techniques, and Iterative Gaussian filter [19], which have proven precision with MRI images.

19.3.1.2   Skull Stripping

In the scanned MRI and other brain imaging-generated pictures, other regions such as skin, neck, and eyeballs are mostly present. In automatic detection and getting precision results using learning algorithms, it is essential to have clear images of brain parts only. Skull stripping is a robust technique by which the extra tissues in the MRI images, such as skull, skin, neck, and eyeballs, can be intensely removed.

The main challenges involved in the skull stripping process include absence of Voxel to identify each edge accurately; the gray and white histograms, which result in central and right-side peaks, respectively; and scan noises and fluid presence. The key deep learning approaches employed are central pixel segmentation, which is done in voxel-by-voxel manner through the CNN layers and entire image segmentation, where the entire image gets segmented by the FCN (Fully Convolutional Networks). Apart from False Positive and False Negative, Performance analysis of the stripped skull images is done with various other techniques including Containment Index, Volume Error Rate, Surface Distance Deviation, Boundary Voxel Error, etc. A literature survey of a few deep-learning algorithms for skull stripping is presented in Table 19.1.

19.3.1.3   Region of Interest Segmentation

For diagnosing the presence of abnormalities from the stripped and processed brain images, deep learning algorithms work by segmenting the region of interest (ROI). This learning is done to extract features of the affected part. Many methods could be employed for segmentation and hybrid models, which give more probability of

2D Skull Stripping   3D Skull Stripping

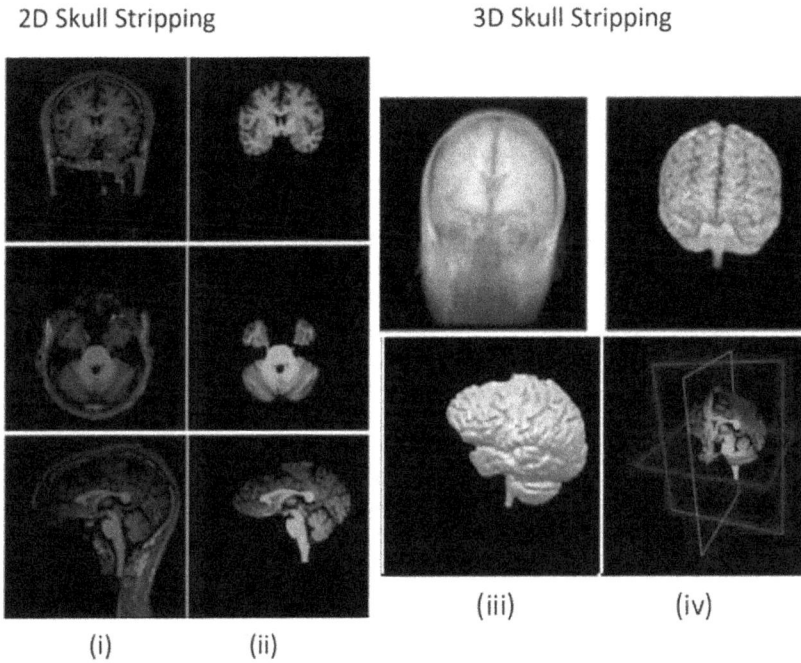

(iii)   (iv)

(i)   (ii)

FIGURE 19.5   Images of 2D and 3D skull stripping.

(i) 2D MRI image

(ii) Skull-stripped image slice

Similarly (iii) and (iv) MRI brain volume and the corresponding skull-stripped representation.

[NFBS dataset (20)]

TABLE 19.1
Few Deep Learning-Based Algorithms in Skull Stripping

Algorithm	Year	Authors	Performance Measures
SegNet	2017	Roberto Cipolla et al. [21]	Very useful deep convolutional encoder decoder learning algorithm for joint feature learning. Works in a semantic pixel-wise and feed-forward manner.
Yolo	2016	Joseph Redmon et al. [22]	Computer vision and pattern recognition, real-time object detection algorithm.
SMOTE	2003 & 2018	Nitesh V. Chawla et al. [23, 24]	Works excellently on unbalanced data sets. Very fast and as it can be trained on the entire image.
ASM-CNN	2018	N H M Duy et al. [25]	Active Shape Model (ASM) integrated with CNN for effective skull stripping of MRI images. Works by processing image sequences in 2D plane.

(Conitnued)

TABLE 19.1 *(Continued)*
Few Deep Learning-Based Algorithms in Skull Stripping

Algorithm	Year	Authors	Performance Measures
NeuroNet	2018	Rajchl et al. [26]	Intelligent multi-output segmentation tool that automatically segments brain tissue and cortical and other structures with the help of standard neuroimaging pipelines.
MeshNet	2017	A Fedorov et al. [27]	A deep learning technique using volumetric dilated convolutions for reducing processing time and possibility of errors in MRI segmentations.
SLANT	2019	Yuankai Huo et al. [28]	SLANT is very effective and fast method for high-resolution segmentation of whole images of brain. High-speed multiple 3D deep neural networks, which work independently. All contents available for research in https://github.com/MASILab/SLANTbrainSeg
FRnet	2019	Qian Zhang et al. [29]	Flattened Residual Network (FRNet), an efficient technique for infant brain image segmentation for skull stripping. Boundary loss function for separating brain tissues and nonbrain regions.
Improved BET	2019	L Wang et al. [30]	To overcome error possibilities vertex displacement is done after each iteration and to ensure surface reconstruction process independently new search path is added and embedded.
MONSTR	2017	Snehashis Roy et al. [31]	Multi-cONtrast brain STRipping or MONSTR can be a tool for skull-stripping of metacontrast MR brain images. A target brain mask is created, and the process gives highly accurate stripped images.
VoxResNet	2018	Hao Chen et al. [32]	Voxelwise Residual NETwork effectively does 3D segmentation. Since it has 25 layers, produces representative features of variations in brain tissues. Multimodal and multilevel combining of information done in this learning system.
U-Net	2020	Yen-Yu Ian Shih et al. [33]	Intelligent algorithm that automatically identifies brain boundaries found in the MRI of animals like rat. Effectively does skull stripping by resolution identified from scalp distance and variation in tissues around the skull. Can be applied efficiently in human brain images. Link to the U-Net skull stripping tool:https://github.com/CAMRIatUNC/RodentMRISkullStripping.

accurate results are also used. Table 19.2 presents a survey of few ROI segmentation techniques.

19.3.1.4 Deep Feature Extraction and Deep Models

This step in the process of diagnosis ensures the automatic detection of key features. Ensemble learning, transfer learning isolated CNNs, and deep block fine tuning strategies are found to be very effective in brain tumor deep feature extraction

TABLE 19.2
Few ROI Segmentation Techniques for Brain Tumor Diagnosis

Method	Authors	Feature extraction
Edge-based segmentation techniques	Asra Aslam et al. (2015)	Closed contour-based techniques for improved edge detection. Effectively detects shapeless tumor growth by working with boundaries of connected regions [34].
	Min Jiang et al. (2021)	Automatic accurate edge-based segmentation called DDU-net. The issue of class imbalance is solved with CE loss and novel edge extraction. Even small abnormalities can be extracted [35].
Region-based segmentation	Shidong Li et al. (2022)	Initially 2D U-Net architecture employed to segment regions for brain tumor diagnosis. Better visualization of the ROI done with 3D U-Net afterwards. Hausdorff distance measurement for error reduction [36].
	P Dhage et al. (2015)	Watershed Segmentation techniques use Multiparameter calculations and multicolor mapped segmentation to ensure diagnosis accuracy [37].
ARHE	Saravanan S et al. (2021)	Adaptive Region-based Histogram Enhancement (ARHE) uses independent component analysis for extraction and enhancement of features. To deal with the abnormal findings morphological based segmentation is done [38].
Semantic Segmentation	Gokay Karayegen et al. (2021)	Automatic segmentation technique giving high accuracy rate. 3D imaging and Augmented segmentation for exactly diagnosing the affected part [39].
Brain Extraction Tool Algorithm	Zeynettin Akkus et al. (2020)	Employs two filters, first a sequential convolutional filter that can represent classes by considering the lower dimensional region and in the second convolutional filters decodes and reconstruct the image. The tool is very fast and represented accurate results [40].

(Continued)

TABLE 19.2 (Continued)
Few ROI Segmentation Techniques for Brain Tumor Diagnosis

Method	Authors	Feature extraction
Brain metastases automatic segmentation	Charron O et al. (2018)	3D CNNs do the learning and separation of metastases are done from necrotic parts of multimodal MRI images [41, 42].
	Endre Grøvik et al. (2019) Hsu DG et al. (2021)	3D V-Net CNN learns and segments brain metastases and automatically performs extraction. 3D deep learning segmentation produces precise output [43].
Fast Fuzzy C-means algorithm	Srikanth Busa et al. (2019)	Automatic detection of affected area based on many parameters. Very efficient in multiple growth diagnosis [44].
Voxel clustering algorithm	Schreibmann E et al. (2013) Ali Hamzenejad et al. (2021)	Heterogeneous responses are analyzed from tumor images for effective diagnosis and precision medication. Very effective segmentation technique for PET images by arranging classified voxels to identifiable patterns [45]. Robust PCA algorithm for clustering and automatic accurate finding of exact growth location with sensitivity factor high [46].

[47–50]. These detailing helps build deep models, which can automatically diagnose and suggest medication effectively without the support of medical practitioners. 3D deep feature learning techniques can extract various high level features from multimodal MRIs and can assist the telemedicine system by even predicting the accurate survival time of patients in critical conditions [51].

To validate the deep models, Receiver Characteristic Operator (ROC) curve is a good option and Area Under the Curve (AUC) of ROC can show how your model performs based on parameters like, Specificity, Sensitivity, Jaccard Index, Dice-Coefficient etc. [52]. Derived from True Positive (TrP), True Negative (TrN), False Positive (FsP), and False Negative (FsN) cases.

Sensitivity (Sv)

$$Sv = \left(\frac{TrP}{FsN + TrN} \right) \qquad (19.1)$$

Specificity (S_{ct})

$$S_{ct} = \left(\frac{TrN}{TrN + FsN} \right) \qquad (19.2)$$

Jaccard Index (J_{Indx})

$$J_{Indx} = \left(\frac{TrP}{FsN + FsP + TrP} \right) \qquad (19.3)$$

Dice Coefficient (Dc_{Coef})

$$Dc_{Coef} = \left(\frac{2 * TrP}{2 * TrP + FsP + FsN} \right) \qquad (19.4)$$

19.4 AI-POWERED CONVERSATIONAL CHATBOTS

AI-powered conversational chatbots, the virtual assistants, can help the healthcare sector to a great extent. Most of these chatbots provides multilingual support to present the health queries. They have a working procedure spanning mainly in three levels. The first stage is the input stage, where the voice inputs are converted to text. In the second level using artificial intelligence and natural language processing techniques, further processing is done to understand the query. In the final level, the text can be translated to voice again for output where the patient gets answers in the form of medical advice or prescription.

Google cloud platform can be used for patient access to artificial health care support. Conversational chatbots like CARO assist people with depression kind of health situation, who normally are reluctant to directly share the problems with healthcare professionals [53]. The key merits of these virtual assistants are that they support 24/7 assistance and provide user friendly interactions. Figure 19.6 represents a general architecture of AI-powered conversational chatbots in health care.

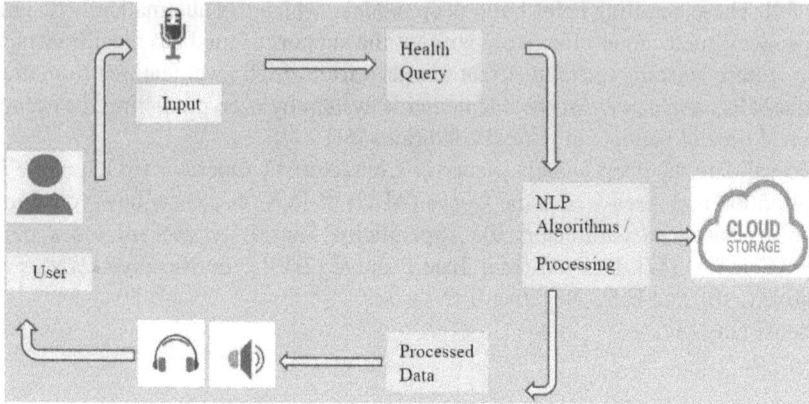

FIGURE 19.6   General architecture of AI-powered conversational chatbots in health care

19.4.1   SELF-SERVICE KIOSKS SUPPORT FOR TELEMEDICINE

Self-service kiosks can aid the growth of telemedicine and IoMT as it can provide support to patients without the help of healthcare professionals. These self-service stations at accessible public locations assists people in diagnostics, medical tests, and book appointments if required. This type of service helps in reducing the healthcare costs of hospital visits.

In this AI-powered era, the future of medical kiosks lies in incorporating deep learning algorithms for finding patterns in data, and to showcase the found anomalies to make the kiosks intelligent [54]. P. H. Leong et al. [55] proposed an AI-powered conversational agent (CA) integrated with the medical kiosks. These human computer interactions can produce very effective, accurate, and user friendly for providing fast healthcare assistance.

19.4.2   ROBOTS TO AID AIoMT

Robots as essential components of IoMT can assist doctors or autonomously work to enhance telemedicine systems. The elderly who are alone are taken care of by medical robots, where vital body conditions transfer to care givers or hospitals in emergencies, regular routine care assistance, and medicine reminder functions are taken care of [57].

Table 19.3 presents a few of the functionalities of medical robots.

19.4.3   FUTURE OF ROBOTICS IN TELEMEDICINE

Heterogeneous robotic structures help conventional inaccessible surgical methodologies accessible and possible through technology. The recent developments in edge computing and AI-powered Medical IoT can even forecast the organ functioning after surgery using scientific tools [61]. Future robotic healthcare systems

TABLE 19.3
Medical Robots Functionalities

Purpose	Function	Challenges
Medical examination	Sensor-based monitoring and reporting of examination results	Need human intervention for obstacle removal/avoiding
Heart rate monitoring	Monitoring and onscreen display of reports regularly. Blood pressure measuring functionalities	Transmission of fast and accurate results
Voice-based interactions	Assist doctors or work autonomously based on detected voice inputs and suggest medication	In medical examination of body parts, ensuring exact camera movements [58]
Surgery	Assists doctor or independently does surgeries (telesurgery). Few applications include: • Obstetrics • Gynecology • Cancer care • Liver surgery • Knee Surgery • Neurological disorders • Cardiac assistance	In gynecology surgical cases the immediate physical assistance/ feedback and clarity of visuals [59] Positional movements of robotic arm in surgery [60]

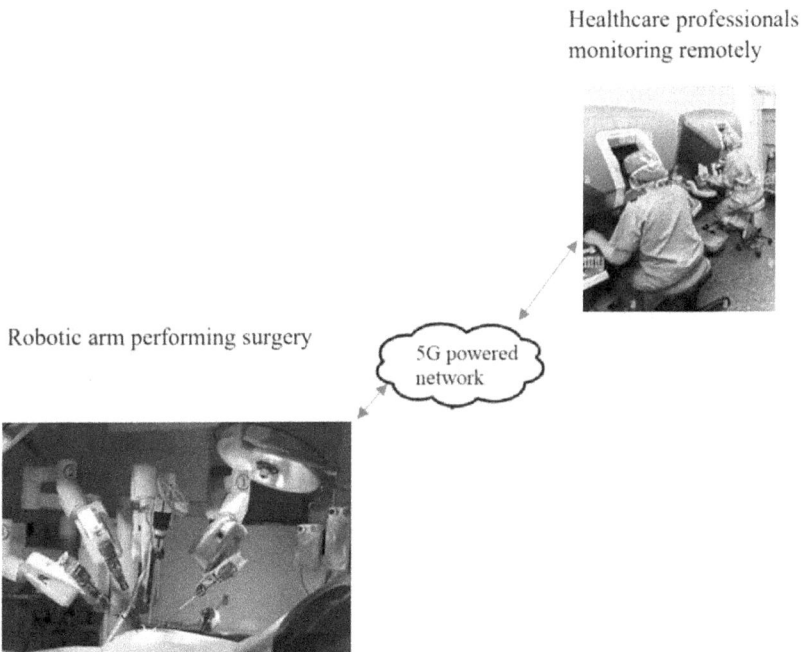

FIGURE 19.7 General architecture of robotic arm based telesurgery in a 5G network.

may include programmable settings from surgeon part over high speed 5G wireless networks [62, 63]. AR/VR integrated with AI ensures live like interactions in the virtual paradigm. The resource scheduling tasks of the network are treated as NP-hard problem and is solved with a heuristic scheme [64]. Explainable artificial intelligence methods that give better interpretations of decisions can be a future trend in robotic surgeries [65].

19.5   ESANJEEVANI—A CASE STUDY

eSanjeevani, a cloud-based telemedicine service, is a successful national e-healthcare provided by the Government of India. The system that enables audio-video consultations is developed using the open-source stack.

19.5.1   OBJECTIVES

Objectives of the system include ensuring healthcare reach in rural areas of the country, less expensive healthcare availability to the citizens, reducing long awaited queues in hospitals and primary healthcare centers, and narrowing down the divide between urban and digital healthcare services.

The potential impact of this system is the E-prescriptions made via this system are very effective and error free. eSanjeevani system is made operational through the hub and spoke type of architecture and has successfully served more than 83 million patients since its inception in November 2019 [66].

19.5.2   SYSTEM ARCHITECTURE

eSanjeevani has two functional modules:

- Provider to doctor or doctor to doctor teleconsultation
- Patient to doctor remote communication

eSanjeevani, the digital telemedicine system, reduces operational errors by the tech team conducting remote trainings to familiarize users to the platform. The process flow in eSanjeevani comprises four phases as shown in Figure 19.8. The first phase is the token-generation phase. Here, the user requests for token by registering and on confirmation through OTP; token is generated by the system with patientID and sent via SMS. The user can login to the system using this patientID and will be admitted to the waiting room. On the availability of the practitioner, the call now button in the waiting room gets enabled and the patient can start video call. The process gets completed by the consultation process where the consultation and e-prescription happen.

Further support services are provided over telephone calls and WhatsApp communications in this integrated telemedicine system. Virtual Private Server (VPS) is used to relay messages from the application to core server, data movement is guaranteed, and data security is also addressed. AI integration in this telemedicine system

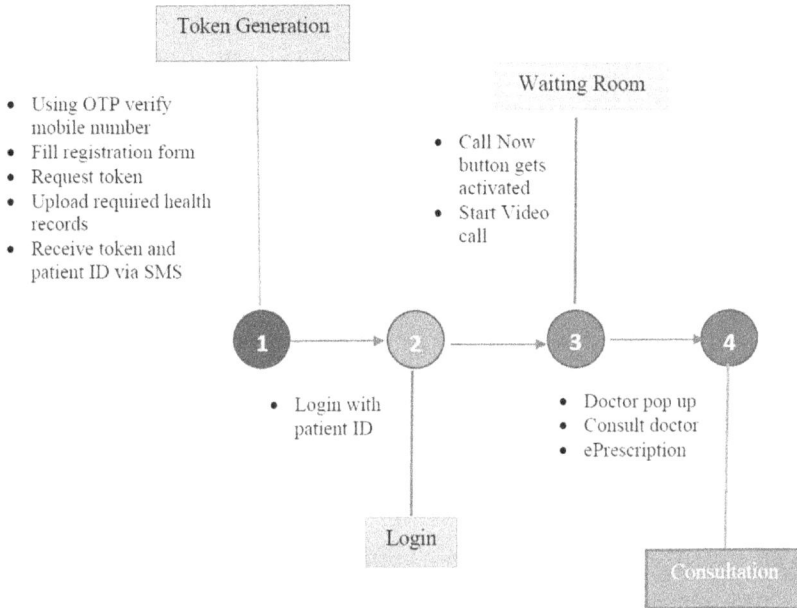

FIGURE 19.8   Process flow of eSanjeevani.

with the recently introduced 5G networks is under consideration and that can revolutionize telemedicine support in the country.

19.6   CONCLUSION AND FUTURE DIRECTIONS

The fast pace of artificial intelligence techniques enabled online platforms during the pandemic time and increased awareness about how to use these platforms with the internet capable gadgets gave the AIoMT-enabled Telemedicine a sound growth. The introduction of 5G wireless networks further boosted IoMT for telediagnosis and telemedicine. The deep learning algorithms easily preprocess, segments clinical images, and intelligently does the remote diagnosis and precision medication effectively, reducing the healthcare costs and ensuring reachability of medical system to the rural population. This study surveyed, eSanjeevani, an AWS cloud-based telemedicine service, proved as a successful national telemedicine service provided by the government of India.

Future design of tele healthcare systems may include AI-embedded programmable wearable devices, intelligent robotics in medical diagnosis, and medication and edge devices supported over high-speed 5G/6G wireless networks. Future robotic based surgery may use programmable robotic devices and does not need any assistance of remote healthcare professionals. Virtual reality-based healthcare applications with multiple sensors and virtual community for various childhood and adult psychological disorders and surgical simulation applications may contribute to the future AIoMT-based telemedicine framework.

ACKNOWLEDGMENT

The author acknowledges the support extended by Dr. Marco Cavallo, Associate Professor in Clinical Psychology (Clinical Neuropsychology), eCampus University, Novedrate (Como), Italy, for supporting the neurological disorder related queries during the preparation of this chapter.

REFERENCES

[1]   P. Lee, D. Paxman, Reinventing Public Health, *Annual Review of Public Health*, 18, 1997, pp. 1–35. https://doi.org/10.1146/annurev.publhealth.18.1.1

[2]   Jack B. Homer, Gary B. Hirsch, System Dynamics Modeling for Public Health: Background and Opportunities, *American Journal of Public Health*, 96(3), 2006, pp. 452–458. https://doi.org/10.2105/AJPH.2005.062059

[3]   World Health Statistics 2022: Monitoring Health for the SDGs, Sustainable Development Goals, *WHO's Annual World Health Statistics Report 2021*, ISBN 978-92-4-005114-0, www.who.int/data/gho/publications/world-health-statistics (First Accessed 5th September 2022).

[4]   Global Strategy on Human Resources for Health: Workforce 2030, *WHO Library Cataloguing-in-Publication Data*, ISBN 978 92 4 151113 1, www.who.int/publications/i/item/9789241511131 (First Accessed 5th September 2022).

[5]   Marc Mitchell, Lena Kan, Digital Technology and the Future of Health Systems, *Health Systems & Reform*, 5(2), 2019, pp. 113–120. https://doi.org/10.1080/23288604.2019.1583040.

[6]   Mohammed Yousef Shaheen, Applications of Artificial Intelligence (AI) in Healthcare: A Review, *ScienceOpen*, 2021. https://doi.org/10.14293/S2199-1006.1.SOR-.PPVRY8K.vl

[7]   Youcef Djenouri, Asma Belhadi, Anis Yazidi, Gautam Srivastava, Jerry Chun-Wei Lin, Artificial Intelligence of Medical Things for Disease Detection Using Ensemble Deep Learning and Attention Mechanism, *Expert Systems*, 2022, p. e13093. https://doi.org/10.1111/exsy.13093.

[8]   Elliot Mbunge, Benhildah Muchemwa, Sipho'esihle Jiyanea, John Batani, Sensors and Healthcare 5.0: Transformative Shift in Virtual Care through Emerging Digital Health Technologies, *Global Health Journal*, 5(4), 2021, pp. 169–177. https://doi.org/10.1016/j.glohj.2021.11.008

[9]   Daniel S.W. Ting, et al., Artificial Intelligence, the Internet of Things, and Virtual Clinics: Ophthalmology at the Digital Translation Forefront, *Lancet Digital Health*, 2(1), 2020, pp. e8–e9. https://doi.org/10.1016/S2589-7500(19)30217-1

[10] G. Shaheamlung, H. Kaur, M. Kaur, A Survey on Machine Learning Techniques for the Diagnosis of Liver Disease, *International Conference on Intelligent Engineering and Management (ICIEM)*, 2020, pp. 337–341, http://doi.org/10.1109/ICIEM48762.2020.9160097.

[11] J. Lotsch, F. Lerch, R. Djaldetti, I. Tegder, A. Ultsch, Identification of Disease-Distinct Complex Biomarker Patterns by Means of Unsupervised Machine-Learning Using an Interactive R Toolbox (Umatrix), *Big Data Analytics*, 3, 2018, pp. 1–17.

[12] M.A. Myszczynska, P.N. Ojamies, A.M.B. Lacoste, et al., Applications of Machine Learning to Diagnosis and Treatment of Neurodegenerative Diseases, *Nature Reviews Neurology*, 16, 2020, pp. 440–456. https://doi.org/10.1038/s41582-020-0377-8.

[13] Lawrence J. Fennelly, *Effective Physical Security*, Book • Fifth Edition • 2017, Science Direct, ISBN:978-0-12-804462-9.

[14] *WHO Classification of Tumours Editorial Board: World Health Organization Classi-fication of Tumours of the Central Nervous System.* 5th ed. Lyon: International Agency for Research on Cancer; 2021.

[15] K.J. Zulch, *Histological Typing of Tumours of the Central Nervous System*, Vol. 21. Geneva: World Health Organization; 1979.

[16] R. Vimal Kurup, V. Sowmya, K.P. Soman, *Effect of Data Pre-processing on Brain Tumor Classification Using Capsulenet*, ICICCT 2019-Springer Nature, ISBN: 978-981-13-8460-8.

[17] Jorge Samper-González, et al., Reproducible Evaluation of Classification Methods in Alzheimer's Disease: Framework and Application to MRI and PET Data, *NeuroImage*, 183, 2018, pp. 504–521.

[18] Ramesh Babu Vallabhaneni, V. Rajesh. Brain Tumour Detection Using Mean Shift Clustering and GLCM Features with Edge Adaptive Total Variation Denoising Technique, *Alexandria Engineering Journal*, 57(4), 2018, pp. 2387–2392.

[19] Mohammed Nasor and Walid Obaid, Segmentation of Osteosarcoma in MRI Images by K-means Clustering, Chan-Vese Segmentation, and Iterative Gaussian Filtering, *IET Image Processing*, 2021, https://doi.org/10.1049/ipr2.12106.

[20] B. Puccio, J.P. Pooley, J.S. Pellman, et al., The Preprocessed Connectomes Project Repository of Manually Corrected Skull-stripped T1-weighted Anatomical MRI DATA, *GigaSci*, 5(45), 2016. https://doi.org/10.1186/s13742-016-0150-5.

[21] Roberto Cipolla et al., A Deep Convolutional Encoder-Decoder Architecture for Robust Semantic Pixel-Wise Labelling, *IEEE Transactions on Pattern Analysis and Machine Intelligence*, 2017. https://doi.org/10.1109/TPAMI.2016.2644615.

[22] J. Redmon, S. Divvala, R. Girshick, A. Farhadi, You Only Look Once: Unified, Real-Time Object Detection, *2016 IEEE Conference on Computer Vision and Pattern Recognition (CVPR)*; 2016, pp. 779–788. http://doi.org/10.1109/CVPR.2016.91.

[23] N. V. Chawla, A. Lazarevic, L. O. Hall, K. W. Bowyer, SMOTEBoost: Improving Prediction of the Minority Class in Boosting, *Proceedings of 7th European Conference on Principles and Practice of Knowledge Discovery in Databases*; *Lecture Notes in Computer Science*; 2003, pp. 107–119. http://doi.org/10.1007/978-3-540-39804-2_12

[24] Nitesh V. Chawla, Alberto Fernández, Salvador García, Francisco Herrera, SMOTE for Learning from Imbalanced Data: Progress and Challenges, Marking the 15-year Anniversary, *Journal of Artificial Intelligence Research*, 61, 2018, pp. 863–905.

[25] Nguyen Ho Minh Duy, Nguyen Manh Duy, Mai Thanh Nhat Truong, Pham The Bao, Nguyen Thanh Binh, Accurate Brain Extraction Using Active Shape Model and Convolutional Neural Networks, *arXiv*, 2018, arXiv:1802.01268.

[26] Martin Rajchl, Nick Pawlowski, Daniel Rueckert, Paul M. Matthews, Ben Glocker, Neuronet: Fast and Robust Reproduction of Multiple Brain Image Segmentation Pipelines, *arXiv*, 2018, arXiv:1806.04224.

[27] A. Fedorov, J. Johnson, E. Damaraju, A. Ozerin, V. Calhoun, S. Plis, End-to-end Learning of Brain Tissue Segmentation from Imperfect Labeling, *2017 IEEE International Joint Conference on Neural Networks*, USA; 2017, http://doi.org/10.1109/IJCNN.2017.7966333

[28] Yuankai Huo, Zhoubing Xu, Yunxi Xiong, Katherine Aboud, Parasanna Parvathaneni, Shunxing Bao, Camilo Bermudez, Susan M. Resnick, Laurie E. Cutting, Bennett A. Landman, 3D Whole Brain Segmentation Using Spatially Localized Atlas Network Tiles, *NeuroImage*, 194(1), 2019, pp. 105–119. https://doi.org/10.1016/j.neuroimage.2019.03.041

[29] Qian Zhang, Li Wang, Xiaopeng Zong, Weili Lin, Gang Li, Dinggang Shen, FRNET: Flattened Residual Network for Infant MRI Skull Stripping, *arXiv*, 2019, arXiv:1904.05578.

[30] L. Wang, Z. Zeng, R. Zwiggelaar, An Improved BET Method for Brain Segmentation, *22nd International Conference on Pattern Recognition*; 2019, pp. 3221–3226. http://doi. org/10.1109/ICPR.2014.555.

[31] Snehashis Roy, John A. Butman, Dzung L. Pham, Robust Skull Stripping Using Multiple MR Image Contrasts Insensitive to Pathology, *NeuroImage*, 2017, pp. 132–147. https:// doi.org/10.1016/j.neuroimage.2016.11.017

[32] Hao Chen, Qi Dou, Lequan Yu, Jing Qin, Pheng-Ann Heng, VoxResNet: Deep Voxelwise Residual Networks for Brain Segmentation from 3D MR Images, *NeuroImage*, 170(15), 2018, pp. 446–455. https://doi.org/10.1016/j.neuroimage.2017.04.041

[33] Yen-Yu Ian Shih, L.-M. Hsu, S. Wang, P. Ranadive, W. Ban, T.-H.H. Chao, S. Song, D.H. Cerri, L.R. Walton, M.A. Broadwater, S.-H. Lee, D. Shen, Automatic Skull Stripping of Rat and Mouse Brain MRI Data Using U-Net, Frontiers in Neuroscience, *Science Brain Imaging Methods*, 2020. https://doi.org/10.3389/fnins.2020.568614.

[34] Asra Aslam, Ekram Khan, M.M. Sufyan Beg, Improved Edge Detection Algorithm for Brain Tumor Segmentation, *Procedia Computer Science*, 58, 2015, pp. 430–437. ISSN 1877-0509. https://doi.org/10.1016/j.procs.2015.08.057.

[35] Min Jiang, Fuhao Zhai, Jun Kong, A Novel Deep Learning Model DDU-net Using Edge Features to Enhance Brain Tumor Segmentation on MR Images, *Artificial Intelligence in Medicine*, 121, 2021. https://doi.org/10.1016/j.artmed.2021.102180.

[36] S. Li, J. Liu, Z. Song, Brain Tumor Segmentation Based on Region of Interest-Aided Localization and Segmentation U-Net, *International Journal Mach Learn Cybern*, 13(9), 2022, pp. 2435–2445. https://doi.org/10.1007/s13042-022-01536-4.

[37] Padmakant Dhage, M.R. Phegade, S.K. Shah, Watershed Segmentation Brain Tumor Detection, *International Conference on Pervasive Computing (ICPC)*, 2015, pp. 1–5 http://doi.org/10.1109/PERVASIVE.2015.7086967

[38] S. Saravanan, R. Karthigaivel, V. Magudeeswaran, A Brain Tumor Image Segmentation Technique in Image Processing Using ICA-LDA Algorithm with ARHE Model, *Journal of Ambient Intelligence and Humanized Computing*, 12, 2021, pp. 4727–4735. https:// doi.org/10.1007/s12652-020-01875-6.

[39] Gökay Karayegen, Mehmet Feyzi Aksahin, Brain Tumor Prediction on MR Images with Semantic Segmentation by Using Deep Learning Network and 3D Imaging of Tumor Region, *Biomedical Signal Processing and Control*, 66, 2021. https://doi.org/10.1016/j. bspc.2021.102458.

[40] Zeynettin Akkus, Petro Kostandy, Kenneth A. Philbrick, Bradley J. Erickson, Robust Brain Extraction Tool for CT Head Images, *Neurocomputing*, 392, 2020, pp. 189–195. https://doi.org/10.1016/j.neucom.2018.12.085.

[41] O. Charron, A. Lallement, D. Jarnet, V. Noblet, J.B. Clavier, P. Meyer, Automatic Detection and Segmentation of Brain Metastases on Multimodal MR Images with a Deep Convolutional Neural Network, *Computers in Biology and Medicine*, 1(95), 2018, pp. 43–54. https://doi.org/10.1016/j.compbiomed.2018.02.004.

[42] Endre Grøvik, Darvin Yi, Michael Iv, Elizabeth Tong, Daniel Rubin, Greg Zaharchuk, Deep Learning Enables Automatic Detection and Segmentation of Brain Metastases on Multisequence, *Journal of Magnetic Resonance Imaging, Wiley,* 2019. https://doi. org/10.1002/jmri.26766

[43] D.G. Hsu, Å. Ballangrud, A. Shamseddine, J.O. Deasy, H. Veeraraghavan, L. Cervino, K. Beal, M. Aristophanous, Automatic Segmentation of Brain Metastases Using T1 Magnetic Resonance and Computed Tomography Images, *Physics in Medicine and Biology*, 66(17), 2021. https://doi.org/10.1088/1361-6560/ac1835.

[44] S. Busa, N.S. Vangala, P. Grandhe, V. Balaji, *Automatic Brain Tumor Detection Using Fast Fuzzy C-Means Algorithm*, Lecture Notes in Networks and Systems, vol. 32. Singapore: Springer; 2019, https://doi.org/10.1007/978-981-10-8201-6_28

[45] E. Schreibmann, A.F. Waller, I. Crocker, W. Curran, T. Fox, Voxel Clustering for Quantifying PET-based Treatment Response Assessment, *Medical Physics*, 40(1), 2013, p. 012401. https://doi.org/10.1118/1.4764900.

[46] Ali Hamzenejad, Saeid Jafarzadeh Ghoushchi, Vahid Baradaran, Clustering of Brain Tumor Based on Analysis of MRI Images Using Robust Principal Component Analysis (ROBPCA) Algorithm, *BioMed Research International*, 2021. https://doi.org/10.1155/2021/5516819

[47] Y.E. Almalki, M.U. Ali, K.D. Kallu, M. Masud, A. Zafar, S.K. Alduraibi, M. Irfan, M.A.A. Basha, H.A. Alshamrani, A.K. Alduraibi, M. Aboualkheir, Isolated Convolutional-Neural-Network-Based Deep-Feature Extraction for Brain Tumor Classification Using Shallow Classifier, *Diagnostics*, 12(8), 2022, p. 1793. https://doi.org/10.3390/diagnostics12081793

[48] Zar Nawab Khan Swati, Qinghua Zhao, Muhammad Kabir, Farman Ali, Zakir Ali, Saeed Ahmed, Jianfeng Lu, Brain Tumor Classification for MR Images Using Transfer Learning and Fine-Tuning, *Computerized Medical Imaging and Graphics*, 75, 2019, pp. 34–46. https://doi.org/10.1016/j.compmedimag.2019.05.001.

[49] J. Kang, Z. Ullah, J. Gwak, MRI-Based Brain Tumor Classification Using Ensemble of Deep Features and Machine Learning Classifiers, *Sensors*, 21(6), 2021, p. 2222. https://doi.org/10.3390/s21062222

[50] Mesut Toğaçar, Zafer Cömert, Burhan Ergen, Classification of Brain MRI Using Hyper Column Technique with Convolutional Neural Network and Feature Selection Method, *Expert Systems with Applications*, 149, 2020. https://doi.org/10.1016/j.eswa.2020.113274.

[51] D. Nie, J. Lu, H. Zhang, et al., Multi-Channel 3D Deep Feature Learning for Survival Time Prediction of Brain Tumor Patients Using Multi-Modal Neuroimages, *Scientific Reports*, 9(1103), 2019. https://doi.org/10.1038/s41598-018-37387-9

[52] Khushboo Munir, Hassan Elahi, Afsheen Ayub, Fabrizio Frezza, Antonello Rizzi, Cancer Diagnosis Using Deep Learning: A Bibliographic Review, *Cancers Journal*, 11(9), 2019, p. 1235. https://doi.org/10.3390/cancers11091235

[53] N. Harilal, R. Shah, S. Sharma, V. Bhutani, CARO: An Empathetic Health Conversational Chatbot for People with Major Depression, *Proceedings of the 7th ACM IKDD CoDS and 25th COMAD; ACM*; 2020, pp. 349–350. https://doi.org/10.1145/3371158.3371220

[54] M.N. Kamel Boulos, G. Haywood, Opportunistic Atrial Fibrillation Screening and Detection in "Self-Service Health Check-Up Stations": A Brief Overview of Current Technology Potential and Possibilities, *Mhealth*, 7(12), 2021. https://doi.org/10.21037/mhealth-19-204.

[55] P.H. Leong, O.S. Goh, Y.J. Kumar, MedKiosk: An Embodied Conversational Intelligence Via Deep Learning, *2017 13th International Conference on Natural Computation, Fuzzy Systems and Knowledge Discovery (ICNC-FSKD)*; 2017, pp. 394–399, http://doi.org/10.1109/FSKD.2017.8393301.

[56] P.S. Ambili, Biku Abraham, A Predictive Model for Student Employability Using Deep Learning Techniques, *ECS Transactions*, 107(1), 2022, p. 10149. https://doi.org/10.1149/10701.10149ecst.

[57] N. Koceska, S. Koceski, P. Beomonte Zobel, V. Trajkovik, N. Garcia, A Telemedicine Robot System for Assisted and Independent Living, *Sensors*, 19, 2019, p. 834. https://doi.org/10.3390/s19040834

[58] Seon Mi Jang, Yeong-Joo Hong, Kyounga Lee, Sukwha Kim, Bùi Văn Chiến, Jeongeun Kim, Assessment of User Needs for Telemedicine Robots in a Developing Nation Hospital Setting, *Telemedicine and e-Health*, 2021, pp. 670–678. http://doi.org/10.1089/tmj.2020.0215

[59] S. Senapati, A.P. Advincula, Telemedicine and Robotics: Paving the Way to the Globalization of Surgery, *International Journal of Gynecology & Obstetrics*, 91(3), 2005, pp. 210–216. https://doi.org/10.1016/j.ijgo.2005.08.016.

[60] B. Eldridge, K. Gruben, D. LaRose, J. Funda, S. Gomory, J. Karidis, J. Anderson, A Remote Center of Motion Robotic Arm for Computer Assisted Surgery, *Robotica*, 14(1), 1996, pp. 103–109. https://doi.org/10.1017/S0263574700018981

[61] S. Pandya, H. Ghayvat, P.K. Reddy, T.R. Gadekallu, M.A. Khan, N. Kumar, Countersavior: AIoMT and IIoT Enabled Adaptive Virus Outbreak Discovery Framework for Healthcare Informatics, *IEEE Internet of Things Journal*, 2022. https://doi.org/10.1109/JIOT.2022.3216108.

[62] J.E.G. Villarruel, B.T. Corona, Proposal for a Remote Surgery System Based on Wireless Communications, Electromyography and Robotics, *2008 Electronics, Robotics and Automotive Mechanics Conference (CERMA '08)*; 2008, pp. 93–98. http://doi.org/10.1109/CERMA.2008.19.

[63] Brodie Andrew, Vasdev Nikhil, The Future of Robotic Surgery, *The Annals of the Royal College of Surgeons of England*, 100(7), 2018. https://doi.org/10.1308/rcsann.supp2.4

[64] Yangzhe Liao, Liqing Shou, Quan Yu, Qingsong Ai, Quan Liu, Joint Offloading Decision and Resource Allocation for Mobile Edge Computing Enabled Networks, *Computer Communications*, 154, 2020, pp. 361–369. https://doi.org/10.1016/j.comcom.2020.02.071.

[65] Imoize Agbotiname Lucky, Jude Hemanth, Dinh-Thuan Do, Samarendra Nath Sur, eds., *Explainable Artificial Intelligence in Medical Decision Support Systems: applicability, prospects, legal implications, and challenges*, Institution of Engineering and Technology (IET) Digital Library; 2022. https://doi.org/10.1049/PBHE050E_ch2.

[66] www.indiastack.global/esanjeevani (First accessed 2nd August 2022).

Index

3D convolutional neural network (3DCNN), 10
3D virtual environment, 16
3G, 4G, 5G, and GSM, 5, 226
6G wireless communication, 139, 216

A

abridged costs, xxiii
accelerometer, 6, 9
Access Control, and Ownership (LACO), 67, 130
accreditation, 31, 50
acquisition, 278, 279, 296, 310, 311
Active Shape Model (ASM), 451
adaptability, 34, 54, 101
Adaptive Momentum (Adam) Optimization, xvii, 303, 414, 420
adoption scale, 28, 32, 36, 49, 51, 55, 72, 77, 105, 107, 139
advanced AI techniques, 22, 42, 120
advanced analytics, vi, vii, 33, 51
advantages of AIoMT, ix, 140, 161, 236
advantages and disadvantages, xx, 176, 178
adversarial attacks, xxii, 157, 158, 229, 230
Adverse Drug Reaction (ADR), 180, 182
African-American race, 35, 54
Agbotiname, xvi, xxvii, xxviii, xxix, xxxv, 63, 89, 97, 121, 168, 189, 214, 241
AI Applications for Threats Response and Recovery, xi, xvi, 199, 224, 273, 274, 276, 397, 399, 403
AI in Healthcare Ecosystem, ix, 136
AIIoMT, 183, 186
ailments, 148, 176, 183, 218, 330, 350, 355, 401
AIoMT applications, 1, 64, 107, 429
AIoMT architectures, 153, 217
AIoMT concerns, 134, 153
AIoMT devices, xix, xxi, 63, 65, 68, 99, 101, 107, 110
AIoMT, i–xxvii
AIoMT security trepidation, 231
AIoMT testing, 405
AIoMT training, 392, 396, 401, 403
AIoMT training, testing, and validation, 392, 396, 401, 403, 406, 505
AIoMT validation, xvi, 396, 406
AI subsets, xxi
Akoka, xxix, xxxv
Ambient assisted Living (AAL), 180
ambient technologies, ii
Ambrose Alli University, Nigeria, xxix
anatomy, 27, 28, 47, 128
An IoMT-based healthcare application, 1
anxiety monitoring, 8

anxious, 8
applications of AIoMT in Remote Healthcare, 171, 180
applications of DT in IoMT, 296
applications, xxxiii, 1, 2, 3, 4
architectural design of AIoMT, 397
architecture of IoMT framework, 179
artificial intelligence, 68, 100, 106, 107, 109, 113, 201
artificial organs, 274
assistive robots, xxv
attack prevention techniques, xix
attacks based on adversary location, 76
attacks based on information damage level, 77
attestation-based architecture, 114, 116
audio-video consultations, xxvii, 458
Aurel Vlaicu University of Arad, Arad, Romania, xxix
auscultation, 15, 27, 28, 47
authentication protocols in AIoMTs, 160
autonomous identification of diseases, 275
AWS cloud-based telemedicine service, xxvii, 459

B

B5G, xix
Babylon, 448
batch normalization, 417, 419
battery power, 3, 5, 54, 282
behavior prediction, 6, 9
bells, xxix
benefits of the AIoMT, 33, 52
bias, 54, 101
Big Data, 8, 21, 399
bio-cryptographic key generation, 114, 116
biological specimens, 21, 41
biological traits, 35, 54
biomedical applications, ii
biometric security, 333
biomorph, 48
BLE, 5
Blockchain-assisted Secure Data Management Framework (BSDMF), 65
Blockchain Enabled Authenticated Key Management Protocol for IoMT (BAKMP-IoMT), 67
blood glucose monitoring, 3, 48
blood pressure monitoring, xxii
bluetooth low energy, 5, 69
body sensor networks (BSN), 1
body temperature, 3, 106, 181, 226, 303, 430
Boundary Voxel Error, 450
BP monitoring, 171, 185

brain tumor diagnosis, 449, 450, 453, 454
brainwave, 7
breathing rate, 3, 226
bridged, xxi, xxiii

C

cardiac electrophysiology, 174
cardiac imageries, 174
cardiovascular system, 27, 47
caregivers, 185, 347, 352, 358, 435
care-services tier (tier 4), 4
carrying capacity, i, xix
case study: deep learning-based falling detection
    for seniors living alone, 9
categories of security and privacy of data
    algorithms, 69
cellular network, 4
challenges, 14
challenges of AIoMTs, 34
challenges and future directions, 14
challenges in remote healthcare delivery, 171, 184
channel blockage, 5
chatbots, 285, 402, 447, 448, 455, 456
Cheng-Chi Lee, iii, iv, xxix
Children's Health Information (CHI), 180
chips and nano sensors, 6
chronic disease monitoring, 7
chronic kidney disease (CKD), xxii
chronic obstructive pulmonary disease, 27, 47
circular economy (CE), 173
classifying and detecting Lassa fever patients,
    xxvi
clinical decision support system (CDSS), 137,
    349, 352
clinical diagnostics, 24, 44
clinical information, 23, 145, 151, 158, 231
clinical revolution, xxiii
cloud computing, 4, 21, 31, 41, 50, 105, 197, 352,
    356, 432, 447
Cloud IoT-Health, 172
Cloudnet, 213
cognitive computing, 171, 173
communication, xix, xxviii, xxix, xxxi, xxxii,
    xxxv, 4, 5, 6, 15, 16, 23, 26, 43, 45, 68,
    69, 75, 77, 81, 84, 85, 86, 97, 98, 99,
    101, 343, 447, 458
community healthcare (CH), 180
computational capacity, xxiii, 72
computed tomography (CT), 173, 311, 325
Computer Emergency Response Team (CERT), 220
concatenated rectified linear units (CReLU), 413,
    417, 418, 424
conceptual framework for AIoMT security, 205
conclusions, 36, 56, 213, 407, 426
conclusions and future scope, 36, 56, 213, 407, 426
confusion matrix, 438, 439
congestion, xxiii, 1, 112, 157, 232

connected health sensors, 23, 43, 44, 97
Containment Index, 450
contemporary, xxiii, 447
continuous health monitoring, 7
conventional methods, xix
convergence, xxiii, xxvi, 21, 23, 34, 36, 39
convolution neural networks (CNN), xxvi
copula sample generation, 257
coronavirus, 149, 150, 151, 172, 173
Council for the Regulation of Engineering in
    Nigeria (COREN), xxix
countermeasures for smart healthcare, 280
COVID-19 pandemic, 8, 9
CRCAIEAP, ii
CRC Press, iii
cross-fertilization, 31
cross-site scripting (XSS) attack, 228
cryptographic and noncryptographic solutions,
    i, xix
cyber attacks, 64, 70, 226, 228, 229, 233
cyberattacks, 64, 70, 226, 228, 229, 233
cyberattacks on PACS, 219, 233
Cyber Incident Response Team (CIRT), 220
Cyber MDX, 78
cyber-physical systems (CPS), 429
Cybersecurity Bill of Materials (CBOM), 79
cybersecurity concerns, xxiv, 285
Cybersecurity for Smart Healthcare, 271
cyber security strategy, 220
cybersecurity, xxiv, xxxiii, 31, 50, 78, 79, 192, 195
cyberspace, 219
Cycle-Generative Adversarial Network
    (Cycle-GAN), 66

D

data collection phase, 416
data interoperability, 30, 49
data management and power issues, 35, 54
data security, 29, 33, 49
data security threats, 23, 29, 43, 49, 56
dataset distributions, 420
data storage layer, 180
Decision Tree, 248
Decision Tree with LDP Data, 248
deep feature extraction, 452
deep learning (DL) technology, 8, 450
Deloitte, 183
denial-of-service attacks (DoS), 67
Department of Electrical Engineering and
    Information Technology, xxviii
derisory management, xxi
detection mechanisms for AIoMTs networks,
    136, 160
device mobility, 31, 49, 51
devices amalgamation, 171
devices vulnerabilities and requirements, 71
diabetes, 6, 8, 48, 106

diagnosing Lassa fever, xxvi
digital integrated circuits, xxx
digitalization, 32, 51, 293
digital prescriptive maintenance (DPM), 175
digital twins, 293, 295
digital twins in AIoMT, 295
disease causes, 171
disease prediction, 367
diseases, 42, 55, 101, 119, 138, 139, 150, 152, 169,
        170, 173, 183, 185, 272, 275, 309
disposable, 23, 24, 44
disposable health sensors, 23, 24, 44
Distributed Data Storage System (DDSS), 66
distributed denial of service (DDoS) attacks,
        112, 200
DT-AIoMT enabled senior safety monitoring, 301

E

early-stage chronic disease prediction, 21
eavesdropping, 144, 145, 153, 154, 202, 219, 228,
        231, 280, 281
ECG, 3, 4, 6, 7, 8, 26, 27, 44, 46, 83, 106
echocardiography, 314, 315
edge layer, 2, 3, 4
education, xxiv, xxxi, xxxii, xxxv, xxxvi
educators, i
Efficient Privacy-preserving outsourced Support
        Vector Machine (EPoSVM), 66
elastography, 314
electrocardiogram (ECG), 116, 134
electrocardiogram monitoring (ECG), xxii
electrochemical reaction, 24, 44
electroencephalogram (EEG), 3, 26, 44
electromyography (EMG), 27, 46
electronic devices in the AIoMT, xx, xxi, 23, 28,
        43, 45, 47, 49, 51, 53, 55, 56
electronic devices, xx, xxi, 23, 28, 43, 45, 47, 49,
        51, 53, 55, 56
electronic health record (EHR), 134, 182, 192
electronic sensors in the IoMT, 43
electronic sensor traits, 23, 24, 43
electronic signals in sensors, 23, 26, 43
elliptic curve cryptography (ECC), 64, 79, 115, 432
elliptic curve integrated cryptographic algorithm,
        65
embedded internet, 335
embedded technology, 24, 44
e-medical healthcare, 9
emergencies, 1, 6, 9, 36, 55, 278, 280, 284, 300,
        350, 456
enabling technologies, 14, 16, 140
encryption, 64–67, 69, 79–88, 104, 109, 114–116,
        119, 139, 151, 155, 156, 193, 195, 197,
        199, 200–203, 207, 227, 231, 245, 281,
        283, 397, 431, 432, 436
Enhanced On-Demand Vector (EAODV)-enabled
        routing, 66

entertainment, xxiv, 5
environmental data, 3, 298
environmental impact, 29, 346, 349
environments, xx, 15, 16, 26, 46, 77, 170, 193,
        195, 280, 282, 295, 296, 337
epilepsy detection, 8
eSanjeevani telemedicine service, xxvi, 445
exoskeletons, xiii, 274, 285
experimental study, 13, 294, 302
experimental, xxvi, 13, 66, 178, 209, 222, 264,
        265, 294, 301, 302, 310, 337, 415
expert systems, ii
explainable artificial intelligence (XAI), 160, 170,
        377, 431
explainable neural network (XANN), 431
exploitation, xii, xix, xxii, xxiii, 139, 158, 229,
        230, 233, 235

F

face-to-face, 1
falling detections, 7
Fitbit watches, 27, 46
Flattened Residual Network (FRNet), 452
florence, 448
Food and Drug Administration (FDA), 78
fourth industrial revolution, xxii
frequency range, 14, 15, 26, 45
functional near-infrared spectroscopy, 315
future directions, 447, 459
future research direction, 337, 398
fuzzy logic, 106, 150

G

gait, 15, 26, 45
gait analysis, 15, 26, 45
GANs, 224
gastric juice, 24
gateway, 3, 5, 69, 82, 83, 103
Gelsenkirchen, xxvii
German Academic Exchange Service (DAAD),
        xxviii, xxix, 89, 214, 265, 331, 359
Germany, xxviii, xxix, 89, 214, 265, 331, 359
Global Health Workforce, 445
Glucose Level Detection, xxii, 171
glycemic, 3
Google's DeepMind AI system, 33, 52
guaranteeing authentication, xxiii

H

Hadamard, 12
handbook, i, ii
handling high-dimensional data, 264
hardware requirement, 4
hardware technology, 4
HAR processing, 10

Haversine distance, xxv, 365, 366, 367, 373, 374, 393
healthcare automation robots, 274
healthcare business, xxi, 78
healthcare ecosystem, i, ix, xix, 134, 135, 136, 141, 161, 174, 236
healthcare monitoring, 1, 2, 6, 7, 176, 222, 276, 394
healthcare organizations, xx, 32, 51, 97, 184, 202
healthcare-related prediction, 8
healthcare service, xx–xxiii, 30, 36, 55, 86, 432, 445, 452
healthcare systems, i–iii, 68, 139, 229, 350
health factors, 23, 42
Health Information Technology for Economic and Clinical Health (HITECH) Act, 203
Health Insurance Portability and Accountability Act (HIPAA), 203, 278, 358
health jurisdiction, xxv, 25, 365, 366, 371, 382, 388
health practitioners, 22, 42, 100, 134
heart pulse, 3, 6
higher bandwidth, 5
high infrastructure costs, 31, 50
hijacking of session, 229
hip prosthesis, 48
HRV analytics, 27, 46
human-computer interaction, 10, 138, 358
human intelligence, xxi, xxv, 394
human skin, 25, 44
Hybrid SSA-LSTM Detection and Prediction Model, xiv
Hybrid Teaching and Learning Based Optimization (HTLBO), 67

I

Identity Based Encryption (IBE), 431
IEEE 802.11x series of standards, 5
IEEE communication society, xxix
IEEE Xplore, 175
IEEE, xxix, 5
image data visualization, xiv, 320
image enhancement, 310, 317, 324, 325
image feature extraction, 10
image feature selection, 318
image segmentation, 15
images, xxiv, 10, 13, 14, 235, 310, 318
implantable device, 3, 134
implantable medical devices (IMDs), 173, 191
implantable sensors, 23, 26, 43, 45
implants, 1, 170, 274, 319
implementable, 24, 44
incorporation, 21, 41, 107, 153, 172, 197, 206, 207, 221, 222, 225, 253
independent RNN (IndRNN), 12

indoor and outdoor environments, xx
industrial automation, xx
industrial manufacturing, xxiv, 293, 295, 297
Industry 4.0, ii, 365, 367, 391
inertial measurement unit (IMU) sensors, 48
infections, xx, 23, 42, 76, 100, 275, 324, 430
ingestible, 23, 24, 43, 44, 182, 344, 346, 361
ingestible sensors, 23, 24, 43, 44, 182, 344, 346, 361
Institute of Digital Communication, Ruhr University Bochum, xxviii
Institute of Health Services of the State of Aguascalientes (ISSEA), xxv
integrated circuits (IC), 73
Intel i7 NVIDIA GeForce GTX 1080 graphics card under Windows 10, 13
intelligent, 78, 223, 365, 381, 385, 445, 456
interconnection of billions, xix
International Journal of Advanced Intelligence Paradigms (IJAIP), xxx
internet-based technologies, 22, 42
internet infrastructure, 1
internet, i–xxxiii, 1–464
Internet of Medical Things (IoMT), i–iii, 1, 41, 191, 201, 271, 309
Internet of Things, ii, vii, 41, 72, 73, 78, 139
Inter Planetary File Systems (IPFS), 65
intrusion detection algorithms, i, xix
intrusive sensors, 24, 44
IoMT environment, 15, 21, 22, 30, 41, 42, 49, 64, 65, 67, 77, 88
IoMT regulations on cybersecurity, 78
Isolation Centre, 435

J

JPEG color image steganalysis, xxvi

K

Kaggle database, xxiv
key contributions of the chapter, 2, 23, 43, 171, 294, 336, 365, 413, 446
Kinect V2 camera, 10
K-means algorithm, 365, 366, 367, 370, 373, 378, 381, 391
k-nearest neighbors, xxiii
K Nearest Neighbour (K-NN), xxvi
knee arthroplasty monitoring, 48

L

Lagos, xxviii, xxix, xxxiv
language processing, ii, 147, 171, 174, 223, 224, 350
Lassa cases, xxvi
Lassa fever (LF), 429, 431, 432

licensing challenge, 33, 52
lightweight ML models, 15
limitation of AIoMT, 23, 35
limitation of memory, xxiii
local differential privacy (LDP), xxiii, 245
logical object (LO), xxiv
long-term tracking, 1
lower frequency, 5
Lucas, xxviii
Lucius, xxviii
Lucky, xxviii
Luke, xxviii

M

MAC based, 83
machine-learning-based action detection
        methods, 9
magnetic particle imaging, 316
magnetic resonance imaging (MRI), 311
major function blocks, 300
malicious attacks in AIoMT, 157, 158
malicious intruders, xix
management system, 4, 33, 48, 52, 116, 184
man-in-the-middle attacks, 77, 119
MARS system—methodology, 10
measures of AI trustworthy in healthcare, 137
medical, 4, 8, 14, 15, 30, 33, 52, 150, 177, 277,
        288, 309, 310, 324, 459
medical data, 4, 8, 14, 15, 30, 36, 49, 64, 65
medical diagnosis, 33, 52, 150, 177, 277, 288,
        309, 310, 324, 459
medical electronics, 21, 23, 25, 27, 28, 29, 31, 33,
        35, 37
medical image processing, 309, 310, 316, 323, 330
medical image restoration, 318
medical image segmentation and lack of
        database, 15
medical image steganalysis, 411, 413, 415, 417,
        419, 421, 423, 425
medical industry, 23, 30, 37, 43, 98, 111, 115, 273,
        324, 350, 365
medical information, 63–65
medical information systems Privacy and
        Security, 63
medical information systems, xxi, 63
medical science, ii
medical specialists, xxii
medical stakeholders, xx, xxi, 37, 56
medical things, i–iii, v–viii, 100, 109, 113, 169,
        191
medical treatment, 33, 53, 97, 137, 293, 294, 402
Medicare organizations, 32, 51
Medium Access Control (MAC), 66
mental well-being, xxii
Metaverse, 16, 20
microelectronics, xx, xxi, 21, 41, 71, 100

microfabricated integrated circuit, 24, 44
missteps and errors, 35, 54
mobile internet, xx, xxi, 21, 41
mobility, 4, 9, 25, 31, 44, 49, 51, 75, 83, 217, 218,
        267, 341, 342, 355, 356
modern life, xix
modus operandi, 35, 54, 281
monitor long-term health status, 1
multi-criteria decision-making methods, 367
multilayer perceptron neural network
        (MLP—ANN), xxvi
multi-sensor action recognition-based Senior
        falling detection (MARS) system, xx,
        2, 9, 10, 14
Mutual Authentication and Key Agreement
        (MAAKA), 66

N

Naive Bayes (NB), xxvi
natural language processing (NLP), ii, 147, 171,
        174, 223, 224, 350
nature of cyberattacks, 219, 226
Near-Field Communication (NFC), 69
network segmentation, 203, 204, 281
neurodegenerative diseases, 448
next generation wireless communications, 102,
        166, 202
Nigerian Society of Engineers (NSE), xxix
NLP, ii, 147, 171, 174, 223, 224, 350
noise interference, 5
noise reduction/removal, 318
North Rhine-Westphalia, xxvii, xxviii
novel applications in the Metaverse era, 16
nuclear medicine imaging, 313

O

one-pixel attacks, 222, 229
Oneremission, 448
orchestrate, xix
ovarian cancer distinction, 7
overstretched, i, xix
overview, 1, 294, 355
oxygen level monitoring, xxii, 181
oxygen saturation monitoring, xxii, 181
oxygen, xxii, 181

P

packet transfer, 26, 45
parameter tuning, 425
patch sensors, 23, 24, 43, 44
patient empowerment, 34, 53
patient information, 22, 41, 42, 87, 174, 233, 234,
        272, 278, 344, 347, 350, 353, 354
patient retreatment, 24, 44

penetration testing, 202–205
perception layer devices, 226
performance in resource-constrained
    environments, 16
periodic management, 21
personal health monitoring, 16, 64
personalized, 33, 53, 275
personalized medicine, 33, 53, 275
Petroleum Technology Development Fund
    (PTDF), xxviii, xxix, 89, 120, 214
phonocardiography, 48
photoacoustic imaging, 314
photodiode, 27, 46
photoplethysmographic (PPG), 26, 46
photoplethysmography, 26, 46
physical object (PO), xxiv, 293
physical, xxix, 4, 26, 28, 29, 293
piezoelectric, 48
point-of-care (POC), 64, 198
Polytechnic University of Timisoara, xxix
Ponemon Institute, 30, 49
pooling operations, xxvi
potential benefits and impacts of AIoMT, 182
powered conversational chatbots, 447, 455, 456
PPG signal, 4, 116, 303, 424
precautions, 37, 57, 109
prediction accuracy, xxv, 8, 331
pre-processed data, 3
pre-processing phase, 416
privacy concerns, i, xix, 8, 34, 54, 106
Privacy Engineering Program (PEP3), 79
privacy, i, xix, 8, 34, 54, 106
prosthetics, 274, 285, 356
Proteus Digital Medicine model, 24, 44
Provably Secure and Lightweight (PSL), 66
public key infrastructure (KPI), 79
Public Road Urban Drivers (PROUD) test, 397
PubMed, 175
PUF based, 85
Python3.8, 13
PyTorch, 13

Q

qualitative, xxii, 196

R

radio frequency identification (RFID), 69, 143,
    144, 173, 179, 181, 200, 226, 335, 345
radiography (X-ray), xiv, 311
randomized controlled trials (RCTs), 394
ransomware attacks, 78, 228
rapid diagnosis, xix
real-time monitoring, 97, 106, 107
real-world scenarios, i
recurrent neural networks (RNN), 12

reduction in human error, 34, 53
reduction in medical costs, 34, 53
references, 37, 56, 69, 121, 161, 185, 214, 236, 266,
    285, 305, 331, 359, 391, 407, 426, 442, 460
regulatory challenges, 30, 50
rehabilitative, xxv, 337
remedy, 32, 51, 106, 204, 322
remote diagnosis, 4, 285, 446, 447, 459
remote healthcare delivery, 169, 184
remote health monitoring, 5, 100, 272, 320
remote sensors, 3, 161, 236
researchers, ii, 2, 36, 37, 55, 56, 88, 102, 113–116,
    120, 139, 180, 192, 229, 245–248, 253,
    272, 285, 303, 310
respiration sensor, 3
revamp, i, xix
robotic surgery, 174, 192, 273, 336, 338, 339, 340,
    342, 343, 402
robots to aid AIoMT, 456
ROC curves, xviii, 440, 441
rogue access, 229
Romania and Hungary, xxx

S

SafeTwins, xxiii, 294, 299, 300, 301, 302
safety and privacy (SNP), 77, 79, 80
scalable, 35, 348, 433
ScienceDirect, 175
SCITEL, 379, 380, 384, 385
SCITEL data collection, 379
security, 145, 149, 153, 154
security concern in application layer, 145
security intimidations to availability, 112
security risks to integrity, 110
security vulnerability, 15, 64, 78
seizure detections, 8
Semantic Medical Access (SMA), 180
senior member, xxix, xxx
senior population, 25, 44
sensor layer, 3, 10, 191, 202
server layer, 2, 4, 10
settings, 339, 421
skeleton features extraction, 10
skeleton image, 3, 10, 11, 14
skeleton image feature extraction, 10
skull stripping, 450, 451, 452
skytron, 23, 42
sleep apnea, 28, 48, 104
sleep monitoring, 7
smart\wireless technology interface tier (tier 2), 4
smart city, ii, xxii, 1, 30, 271, 273, 276, 278, 293
smart clothes, 26, 45
smart clothing, 23, 24, 26, 43, 44, 45
smart e-healthcare, 141
smartphone application, 24, 44, 102, 244
smart surveillance, 64, 98, 102, 105, 271

Soft Computing and Applications (SOFA), xxx
software-defined networking (SDN), 103, 147, 148, 166, 193, 195, 199, 207, 213, 214, 236, 287
solutions, 230, 278, 282, 285, 322
SQL injection attack, 228
standardisation, 31, 50
standardization challenges, 31, 50
standard performance metrics, 209
steganalysis, xxvi, 411, 412, 413, 414, 415, 417, 420–426
stomach, 24, 44, 182
strip-type, 24, 44
supercomputing, 28, 48
support vector machine (SVM), xxvi, 176, 277, 412, 437, 439
surface distance deviation, 450
sustainability, 4
Sustainable Development Goals (SDGs), 445
synthetic datasets, 242, 258, 265
system architecture, 299, 448
System-on-Chip (SoC), 73
systems, 350

T

tag cloning, 229
target ML model, 244
target scenario, 243
TCP/IP stacks, 78
Technique for Order of Preference by Similarity to Ideal Solution (TOPSIS), xxv, 336, 367, 368
technological processes, 1
technologies, 4, 5, 14, 16, 22, 23, 26, 30, 32, 36
technologists, 36, 55
telediagnosis, xxvii, 446, 447, 450, 459
telemedicinal services, xxvii
telemedicine frameworks, xxii, 185
telemedicine operations, 15
temperature monitoring, 3, 171, 181
temperature sensor, 3, 6, 76, 151
temporarily, 7, 103, 313
testbed dataset, 213
three-layer iomt architecture, 2
TOPSIS variables and process, 367, 384
traditional security architecture, i, xix
training database, 13
transportation, 179, 267
trust maintenance, 32, 52

U

UAVs, 172
ubiquity, xxii, xxiii, 111, 192, 201
ultrasound, 309, 311, 313, 314, 315
University of Lagos, Nigeria, xxviii, xxix
unlawful exploitation, xix
U.S. Census Bureau report, 9
utilitarian, 33, 52

V

Valentina, ii, iii
ventricular contraction, 27, 47
Verizon, 30, 49
Very Large Scale Integration (VLSI) chips, 73
VGG-16 CNN model, xxiv
viral haemorrhagic fever (VHF), 429
viral infections, 23, 42
visual image recognition, xxv
voice assistants, 36, 55, 284
volume error rate, 450

W

WAMSE, 250, 251
Wearable Device Access (WDA), 180
wearable devices, 3, 7, 9, 27, 28, 35, 47, 54, 98, 100
wearable medical electronics, 21, 23, 28
wearable sensor, xxvi, 151, 169, 183, 303, 434, 436
wearable, xx, 21, 23, 276, 459
web-based interface, 435, 436
wheelchair management, xxii, 171, 346
Wi-Fi, 5, 344, 345
wiretapping, 219, 281
World Health Organization (WHO), 445, 450
worldwide acceptance, 1
WUSTL-EHMS-2020 dataset, xxiii

X

Xerafy, 23, 42
X-rays and CT scans, 173

Z

Zigbee, 5, 180, 226

For Product Safety Concerns and Information please contact our EU
representative GPSR@taylorandfrancis.com
Taylor & Francis Verlag GmbH, Kaufingerstraße 24, 80331 München, Germany